# Percutaneous Intervention for Coronary Chronic Total Occlusion

Stéphane Rinfret
Editor

# Percutaneous Intervention for Coronary Chronic Total Occlusion

## The Hybrid Approach

Springer

*Editor*
Stéphane Rinfret
Multidisciplinary Cardiology Department
Quebec Heart and Lung Institute
Quebec
Canada

ISBN 978-3-319-21562-4 ISBN 978-3-319-21563-1 (eBook)
DOI 10.1007/978-3-319-21563-1

Library of Congress Control Number: 2015952644

Springer Cham Heidelberg New York Dordrecht London


Printed on acid-free paper

Springer International Publishing AG Switzerland is part of Springer Science+Business Media (www.springer.com)

*To Marie and Justine, for all their love and support*

# Foreword

Complete revascularization, i.e., revascularization of all ischemic myocardial regions, is the accepted goal to optimize long-term outcomes including survival and freedom from myocardial infarction. Even the most ardent interventionalist must concede that coronary bypass surgery (CABG) is currently more effective in achieving complete revascularization. This superiority is due to greater efficacy in revascularizing territories supplied by chronic total occlusions (CTOs). Thus, the ability to predictably recanalize the CTO is central for percutaneous intervention (PCI) to achieve the same degree – or greater revascularization relative to CABG. When this equality occurs (and it will), a comparison of PCI vs CABG in multivessel disease may show improved outcomes with PCI relative to the best current comparison (SYNTAX) of these two modalities.

Technical advances, including antegrade wiring approaches and dedicated CTO wires, antegrade dissection and re-entry with a dedicated system, and retrograde approaches have been key to the improved recanalization rates reported in the last decade. We can expect with current techniques a success rate of 90 % or more for lesions that are appropriate to treat for clinical indications. This success rate is particularly impressive by operators whose primary decision point is clinical need, regardless of the technical challenges.

A recent procedural advance is related more to a strategic "state-of-mind" than to a technical advance. The "hybrid approach" provides a plan to succeed. It teaches that one should nimbly move from one approach to another if progress is not being made. A pre-procedure plan is the mandatory first step, utilizing in part the "hybrid algorithm" to prioritize various technical approaches. If Plan A is not going well, then the operator moves to Plan B or based on observations during Plan A modify Plan A accordingly. The hybrid approach implies a level of mastery with each of the known techniques so the operator can move easily from one technique to the other. It also implies that the operator knows when "enough is enough" and this conclusion, in the final analysis, is an intuitive feel conditioned by experience and supported by the operator's commitment to succeed.

This book has admirably addressed the techniques required for mastering CTO recanalization, each chapter written by acknowledged experts. It is an outstanding educational resource for those interventionalists committed to full revascularization in the cath lab.

Barry F. Uretsky, MD

# Preface

Chronic total occlusions (CTOs), from a technical point of view, are used to be considered the last frontier of percutaneous coronary intervention (PCI). Because they were difficult to open, many physicians preferred to consider CTOs as a different subset of lesions that for obscure reason would not derive the same benefit if reopened compared to non-occlusive lesions, even considering the same amount of ischemia and symptoms. Ironically, CTOs have been the only lesion subset in interventional cardiology for which interventional cardiologists tried to find good reasons not to open them. On the other hand, bifurcations, multivessel disease, left main PCI found many advocates, despite the same level of evidence, likely because they were much simpler to treat technically.

Fortunately, those pioneer operators, who were considered dangerous "cowboys" by colleagues, have courageously moved the field forward. It was obviously an unjustified accusation. "Cowboys" are operators doing things beyond their skill level, without any respect to the risk to benefit ratio. CTO PCI operators cannot be cowboys; otherwise, they quickly are put out of business. This entire field has moved forward thanks to operators who have pursued their quest for excellence despite criticism, despite superficial judgment from peers, despite the lack of financial incentive, and despite the lack of recognition by the community. They were few at the beginning. With the tremendous input of very innovative and skillful Japanese operators, few American operators made a substantial effort to adapt to the western world practice, with the few and limited available devices early on. It is needless to say how pioneers such as Barry Rutherford and Barry Uretsky have paved the way, followed by the tremendous energy input from William Lombardi, Craig Thompson, Mike Wyman, and Aaron Grantham. They were among this first generation of believers who clearly wanted to share their knowledge they acquired hardly in adversity.

I consider myself one of the fortunate who have benefited from their teaching on a personal basis. I adapted some of their teaching to the Canadian environment, much more prone to work from a transradial approach. But first and foremost, we all became friends, noticing that we were all on the same page, witnessing the birth of "school of thoughts" as a result of free and enthusiastic knowledge dissemination across country borders. We all came to a conclusion that our objective was noble: to open arteries, obviously not the ones supplying non-viable myocardium, but the ones that were causing ischemia and angina, resulting in poor quality of life. We all realized that, with the time restraints that the North-American practice impose to interventional cardiologist, we had to maximize the testing of many potential successful strategies such as antegrade wiring, retrograde approach, and dissection re-entry techniques while reducing the amount of contrast and radiation in the same procedure. We were convinced this novel approach would attract many operators who were skeptical to CTO PCI. And from this seminal work led by Manos Brilakis, we came to this hybrid perspective, which we all refer to in our teaching endeavors. This approach resulted from the rejection of dogmas through a practical perspective. The hybrid approach, a new school of teaching in CTO PCI, has produced more followers than any other approaches of knowledge translation. From a dozen of centers performing high-volume CTO PCI before 2010, we can now count on hundreds of operators who clearly joined the battle.

I consider myself privileged to have learned from all those out-of-the-box thinkers I met over the last few years. This book was the opportunity to give them another platform to reach the community with this infective passion that has moved us forward. With this set of chapters, I am convinced that you will find the most up-to-date knowledge on the hybrid approach to CTO PCI.

Quebec City, QC, Canada Stéphane Rinfret, MD, SM

# Contents

1 **How to Justify CTO Revascularization** ... 1
Dominique Joyal and Samer Mansour

2 **How to Set Up a Chronic Total Occlusion Angioplasty Program** ... 13
John J. Graham and Christopher E. Buller

3 **What Equipment Should Be Available?** ... 19
Emmanouil S. Brilakis

4 **Specific Basic Techniques to Master in CTO PCI** ... 33
William J. Nicholson

5 **When and How to Perform an Antegrade Approach Using a Wire Escalation Technique** ... 43
James C. Spratt

6 **When and How to Perform an Antegrade Dissection/Re-entry Approach using the CrossBoss and Stingray Catheters** ... 53
Simon Walsh

7 **How to Deal with Difficult Antegrade Issues** ... 65
R. Michael Wyman

8 **Intra-occlusion Microinjection of Contrast: When, Why and How** ... 81
Mauro Carlino

9 **How and When to Perform the Retrograde Approach** ... 87
Stéphane Rinfret and Dimitri Karmpaliotis

10 **How to Recanalize In-Stent Chronic Total Occlusions** ... 133
Benjamin Faurie and Stéphane Rinfret

11 **How to Fix Common Problems Encountered in CTO PCI: The Expanded Hybrid Approach** ... 141
James Sapontis, Steven P. Marso, William L. Lombardi, and J. Aaron Grantham

12 **How to Improve Catheter Support During CTO PCI** ... 161
Mohamad Lazkani and Ashish Pershad

13 **When and How to Perform a Transradial Approach for CTO PCI** ... 167
Khaldoon Alaswad and Stéphane Rinfret

14 **How to Manage Radiation and Contrast During Chronic Total Occlusion Percutaneous Coronary Intervention** ... 179
Antonis N. Pavlidis and Elliot J. Smith

**15 Complications of Chronic Total Occlusion Percutaneous Coronary Intervention** . . . . . . . . . . 193
Rolf Graning and Tony DeMartini

**16 How to Prevent Perforation During CTO PCI** . . . . . . . . . . 207
Parag Doshi

**17 How to Prevent and Manage Ischemic Complications During CTO PCI** . . . . . . . . . . 211
Minh N. Vo

**18 Managing Entrapped Gear During Chronic Total Occlusion Interventions** . . . . . . . . . . 217
Creighton W. Don and William L. Lombardi

**19 How to Start and Build Your CTO Practice and Maintain Referrals in a Competitive Environment** . . . . . . . . . . 223
M. Nicholas Burke and Stéphane Rinfret

**Index** . . . . . . . . . . 227

# Contributors

**Khaldoon Alaswad, MD** Section of Cardiology, Department of Medicine, Henry Ford Hospital, Detroit, MI, USA

**Emmanouil S. Brilakis, MD, PhD** Department of Cardiology, VA North Texas Health Care System, Dallas, TX, USA

**Christopher E. Buller, MD, FRCPC** Division of Cardiology, St. Michael's Hospital, University of Toronto, Toronto, ON, Canada

**M. Nicholas Burke, MD** Department of Medicine, Minneapolis Heart Institute, Minneapolis, MN, USA

**Mauro Carlino, MD** Department of Interventional Cardiology, San Raffaele Hospital Milano, Milan, Italy

**Tony DeMartini, MD** Department of Cardiology, Advocate Heart Institute, Downers Grove, IL, USA

**Creighton W. Don, MD** Division of Cardiology, University of Washington Medical Center, Seattle, WA, USA

**Parag Doshi, MD, FACC, FSCAI** Department of Medicine, Chicago Cardiology Institute, Schaumburg, IL, USA

**Benjamin Faurie, MD** Institut Cardiovasculaire, Groupe Hospitalier Mutualiste de Grenoble, Grenoble, France

**John J. Graham, BSc(hons), MB, ChB, MRCP (UK)** Division of Cardiology, St. Michael's Hospital, Toronto, ON, Canada

**Rolf Graning, MD** Department of Cardiology, William Beaumont Hospital, Royal Oak, MI, USA

**J. Aaron Grantham, MD, FACC** Department of Cardiology, University of Missouri Kansas City, Kansas City, MO, USA

Department of Cardiology, Saint Luke's Health System's Mid America Heart Institute, Kansas City, MO, USA

**Dominique Joyal, MD** Department of Medicine, Jewish General Hospital/McGill University, Montreal, QC, Canada

**Dimitri Karmpaliotis, MD, PhD, FACC** Department of Cardiology, NYPH/Columbia University Medical Center, New York, NY, USA

**Mohamad Lazkani, MD** Department of Interventional Cardiology, Banner University Medical Center - Phoenix, AZ, USA

**William L. Lombardi, MD** Department of Cardiology, University of Washington Medical Center, Seattle, WA, USA

**Samer Mansour, MD** Department of Medicine, Centre Hospitalier de l'Université de Montréal, Montreal, QC, Canada

**Steven P. Marso, MD** Department of Internal Medicine, University of Texas Southwestern Medical Center, Dallas, TX, USA

**William J. Nicholson, MD** Division of Interventional Cardiology, WellSpan York Hospital, York, PA, USA

**Antonis N. Pavlidis, MD, PhD, FACC** Department of Cardiology, Barts Health NHS Trust, London, UK

**Ashish Pershad, MD, FACC, FSCAI** Division of Interventional Cardiology, Banner University Medical Center - Phoenix, AZ, USA

**Michael E. Rich, MD** Department of Cardiology, Banner Good Samaritan Hospital, Phoenix, AZ, USA

**Stéphane Rinfret, MD, SM** Multidisciplinary Department of Cardiology, Quebec Heart and Lung Institute, Quebec City, QC, Canada

Laval University, Quebec City, QC, Canada

**James Sapontis, BSc, MBBCh, FRACP** Department of Medicine, Monash Heart, Cardiology, Monash Medical Center, Melbourne, VIC, Australia

**Elliot J. Smith, MD, MRCP** Department of Cardiology, London Chest Hospital, Barts Health NHS Trust, London, UK

**James C. Spratt, BSc, MD, FRCP, FESC, FACC** Department of Cardiology, Forth Valley Royal Hospital, Larbert, UK

**Minh N. Vo, MD** Department of Cardiology, St. Boniface Hospital, Winnipeg, MB, Canada

**Simon Walsh, MD, FRCP, FSCAI** Cardiology Department, Belfast Health and Social Care Trust, Belfast City Hospital, Belfast, UK

**R. Michael Wyman, MD** Department of Medicine, Torrance Memorial Medical Center, Torrance, CA, USA

# How to Justify CTO Revascularization

# 1

Dominique Joyal and Samer Mansour

**Abstract**

Chronic total occlusions (CTO) are frequently found on coronary angiography but the rate of CTO percutaneous coronary intervention (PCI) has remained low in most countries. In recent years, there has been a renewed interest in CTO PCI. With the advent of novel techniques and equipment, CTO PCI has evolved into a safer and more efficient procedure. The main benefits of CTO PCI are relief of angina, improvement in quality of life and achievement of complete revascularization. Other parameters such as improvement in survival and left ventricular function, although suggested by the current literature, remain hypothesis generating. The present chapter will review the current evidence on the benefits of CTO PCI and offer an algorithm to guide the management of patients with CTO.

**Keywords**

Chronic total occlusion • Percutaneous coronary intervention • CTO PCI • CTO revascularization • LV Function • Myocardial electrical stability

Chronic total occlusions (CTO) are frequently found on coronary angiography and are considered the most challenging coronary lesions to treat. Although the general prevalence is unknown, in the selected population of patients undergoing diagnostic coronary angiography the prevalence of CTO ranges between 18 and 52 % [1–6]. In North American centres [3], the rate of CTO percutaneous coronary intervention (PCI) ranges between 6 and 9 % while in Japanese centres the rate is near 60 % [4]. Clearly, the benefits of CTO PCI are still debated by a large proportion of operators. CTOs are often found in patients with multi-vessel disease, and its presence represents an important factor in the decision toward surgical revascularization [7]. In contrast, in patients with isolated CTO, medical management is often chosen [7]. Historically, the main reasons to refrain in CTO PCI were the lack of data on hard outcomes, the increased risks of the procedure, the low success rate, the lack of specific and advanced CTO techniques and the lack of dedicated equipment. In recent years, there has been a renewed interest in CTO PCI, mainly driven from the introduction of novel devices, techniques and consequently, centers of excellence with success rate approaching regular PCI. In experienced hands, CTO PCI can now be performed in a safe and efficient manner [8].

The main benefits of CTO PCI are relief of angina, improvement in quality of life and achievement of complete revascularization. Other parameters such as improvement in survival and left ventricular function, although suggested by the current literature, remain hypothesis generating because of the quality of the current evidence (Fig. 1.1). To date, only retrospective studies are available to support hard outcome data, and most of them offer short and long term comparison of successful vs. unsuccessful CTO PCI. Thus the data is

D. Joyal, MD (✉)
Department of Medicine,
Jewish General Hospital/McGill University,
Montreal, QC, Canada
e-mail: Djoyal@jgh.mcgill.ca

S. Mansour, MD
Department of Medicine,
Centre Hospitalier de l'Université de Montréal,
Montreal, QC, Canada





S. Rinfret (ed.), *Percutaneous Intervention for Coronary Chronic Total Occlusion: The Hybrid Approach*,
DOI 10.1007/978-3-319-21563-1_1

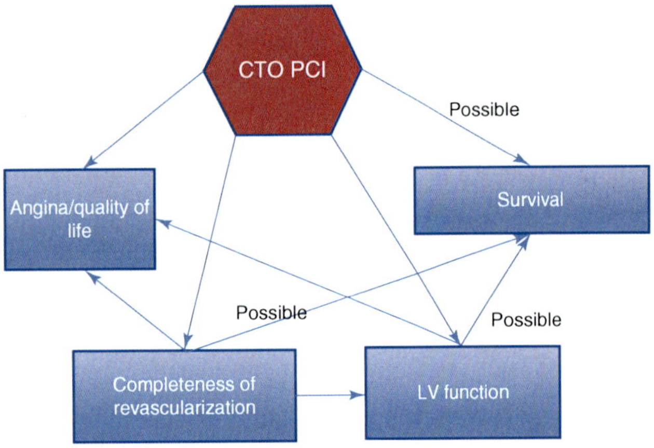


**Fig. 1.1** Interrelated benefits of CTO PCI

mostly composed of registries of patients who had a clinical indication for revascularization; this represents however the best evidence to date short of any randomized control trial (RCT). The present chapter will review the current benefit of CTO PCI and offer an algorithm to guide the management of patients with CTO.

## Symptoms and Quality of Life

Patients with obstructive coronary artery disease (CAD) and ischemic symptoms are helped from coronary revascularization. Most would not argue that in the non-CTO population, angina status is improved post PCI. This reality forms the basis for the majority of elective ad-hoc PCI. Although challenged by some for not being hard outcomes, angina relief and improvement in quality of life remain valuable and safely achievable goals. This reasoning is rarely put into question for patients with severely narrowed vessels, but yet is often challenged for occluded vessels. A sense of security is present when collaterals are well formed, ignoring the fact that myocardium remains frequently and severely ischemic. Physiologic interrogation of the distal bed of a collateralized CTO with a pressure wire reveals significant pressure gradients before and after vasodilator stimuli [9]. Such occluded vessels derive the same benefits in term of normalization of the fractional flow reserve after PCI than severely narrowed but non-occluded vessels [10]. Thus patients often remain chronically ischemic and symptomatic despite collateralization of the occluded vessel(s), and must be maintained on an intensive medical regimen.

The majority of the observational studies where angina status was assessed reported improvement in Canadian Cardiovascular Society (CCS) classification. In an analysis of six studies that reported residual/recurrent angina, successful recanalization was associated with a significant reduction in residual/recurrent angina (OR 0.45, 95 % CI 0.30–0.67) when measured in a dichotomous fashion i.e. presence or absence of angina at follow-up [11]. In one of the observational studies, patients with successful recanalization were more likely to have a negative exercise test result at follow up (73.0 % vs. 46.7 %, P=0.0001) [12]. In the prospective, randomized PRISON II trial comparing DES and BMS in CTO, the overall proportion of patients with CCS angina class ≥3 was reduced from 62 % at baseline to 25 % at 6 months after successful CTO PCI [13]. Quality of life was assessed in the FACTOR trial [14], which examined the health status benefits of successful vs. unsuccessful CTO PCI on symptoms, function, and quality of life. By using the Seattle Angina Questionnaire (SAQ), procedural success was independently associated with angina relief, improved physical function and enhanced quality of life 1 month after successful PCI. These findings were found mainly in the symptomatic patients, who derived large and clinically important improvement in reported health status. The magnitude of benefits was found to be similar to improvement of SAQ scores after surgical revascularization and PCI of non-CTO lesions. In a long-term registry of attempted CTO recanalizations, successful procedures were also associated with significant improvement in angina-related quality of life at a median follow up of 4 years [15]. Recently, a 10-center prospective registry confirmed the observation that symptoms and quality of life improve to the same degree in CTO PCI compared to non-CTO PCI [16].

The evidence thus far suggests angina reduction or disappearance with successful CTO PCI, as is frequently observed with non-CTO PCI. Quality of life, functional status, exercise capacity and medication reduction are all noble goals to consider in the care of patients with CTO (Fig. 1.1).

## Completeness of Revascularization

Historically, the presence of a CTO was a strong predictor of referral to coronary artery bypass grafting (CABG) compared to CTO PCI [5]; the purpose being a more probable achievement of complete revascularization (CR) with CABG [17]. This concept is not new as CR has been a long-standing objective in coronary revascularization. CR has been associated with better long-term outcomes with both PCI [18, 19] and CABG [20]. Most of the data however comes from the surgical literature, as surgical techniques have allowed for CR since almost their inception. Whether achieved by CABG or PCI, the goal of CR is rarely challenged unless significant co-morbidities are present to accept incomplete revascularization (IR).

The outcomes of CR have been studied in the different eras of coronary revascularization with mostly observational studies or subgroup analysis of RCT. A recent meta-analysis by Garcia et al. [21] included 35 studies and near 90,000 patients. CR was more often achieved with CABG than with PCI (75 % vs. 44 %), due to the historical difficulty in achieving CR with PCI. Overall, CR was associated with hard outcomes reductions, namely a 30 % reduction in long-term mortality and a 22 % reduction in MI. Importantly, similar mortality reductions were observed in both PCI and CABG-treated patients and were independent of the study design and definition of CR.

Designed a decade ago, the SYNTAX trial [17] compared the long-term outcomes of the two accepted and favored approaches for patients with complex multi-vessel disease i.e. CR with PCI or CR with CABG. A criterion for randomization was that equivalent anatomical revascularization could be achieved with either treatment, avoiding goal-oriented IR. CR was achieved more frequently in the CABG group (63 % vs. 57 % in PCI group) [22]. Also, the presence of a CTO was a strong predictor of IR in the PCI group (OR=2.46, 95 % CI 1.66–3.64, P<0.001) [22] reflecting the era before specialized technique and dedicated material for CTO recanalization. The residual SYNTAX score (rSS) defined as the delta between the baseline and post-revascularization SYNTAX score (SS) correlates with adversed long-term outcomes [23]. A rSS>8 was associated with 35.3 % all-cause mortality at 5-years in the SYNTAX PCI cohort [24]. Not surprisingly, the presence of at least 1 CTO was observed in half (50.7 %) of patients with a rSS>8 [24], suggesting a strong impact of failed CTO recanalization on the rSS. In a registry of patients with multi-vessel PCI, the rSS was an independent predictor of mortality, whereas the SS was not [25]. In a large all-comers DES registry, the rSS was associated with adverse cardiac events and larger rSS values were found in patients with multiple comorbidities such as diabetes, hypertension, previous PCI, and MI histories [26]; characteristics frequently found in patients with CTO. These findings suggest that the rSS is a reflection of residual ischemia burden. Significant ischemia is linked to adverse outcomes, and revascularization of patients with moderate-severe ischemia is linked to better prognosis [27, 28].

When assessing patients with multi-vessel disease and the presence of a CTO, one must assess the probability of achieving CR, which is most often derived from the probability of revascularization of the CTO. CR, as a pre-determined goal, is then a key determinant as to which revascularization approach is chosen. When multi-vessel PCI is decided, for example in low to intermediate SS, careful anatomical evaluation is done to decide the sequence of PCI procedures. Several factors come into play, such as the jeopardy score, complexity of lesions, collateral circulation etc. On many occasions the non-CTO vessels may be intervened upon first as to facilitate and improve the safety of CTO recanalization. The retrograde technique, for example, requires a reasonably healthy donor vessel which is often treated before the index contralateral CTO PCI. Hence, the subsequent CTO recanalization is then performed to achieve the pre-determined goal of CR, for the benefits described above. Failing to do so prevents the achievement of CR in patients with multi-vessel disease, in whom CABG might otherwise have been a more reasonable option.

As said, CABG is often selected over PCI for multivessel disease, especially when some arteries have total occlusions. However, the effectiveness of CABG for the revascularisation of CTOs is questioned. Although it is common for surgeons to perform CABG on totally occluded vessels, those arteries present some additional challenges compared to non-occluded vessels. As the surgeon needs to perform an anastomosis on the vessel distal to the occlusion, a CTO, which is usually associated with limited contra-lateral flow to the distal bed and significant negative remodeling (or vessel shrinkage) [29] will present additional difficulties to the surgical manoeuvres. In the large PRAGUE-4 trial, which compared off-pump vs. on-pump CABG on long-term graft patency, although all bypass grafts placed distal to a collateralized LAD CTO remained patent at 1-year, only 23 % of those grafts remained patent when placed on the LCX or the RCA system [30]. More recently, in the SYNTAX trial, 543 patients were randomized despite the presence of a totally occluded vessel. Of the 266 patients randomized to surgery, 32 % of the totally occluded vessels finally never received a graft, leading to an incomplete revascularisation. Reasons for not bypassing the totally occluded vessel were not specified in close to half of patients. Otherwise, reasons quoted by surgeons for not grafting the vessels were multiple, including a too small vessel, a too diseased vessel, having no intention to graft, etc. In the end, an incomplete revascularisation procedure, either with PCI or CABG, in the presence of a totally occluded vessel, was associated with increased mortality [31]. In summary, many CTOs will not receive a graft when referred for surgery. And in the cases where a graft was placed, there is evidence that long-term patency is poor. Therefore, effectiveness of CABG specifically for CTOs is questioned, and should be better studied.

## Survival

Thus far, the data of CTO PCI on hard outcomes is unfortunately only supported by observational studies comparing successful and unsuccessful CTO PCI. The majority of these studies have found improved survival at long-term follow-up after successful CTO PCI. Four meta-analyses, designed alike, have all yielded similar findings in terms of reduction of mortality [11, 32–34]. A summary of their major findings is depicted in Table 1.1. Additional studies have since been reported, adding to the pool of studies, but not to the quality of the data. The latest study includes data from the U.K. Central Cardiac Audit Database [35], which analyzed outcomes in over 14,000 CTO PCI procedures. Successful

**Table 1.1** Summary of outcomes data from four meta-analyses comparing successful vs. unsuccessful CTO PCI

| | # studies | Mortality | MACE | MI | CABG | Angina |
|---|---|---|---|---|---|---|
| Joyal et al. [11] | 13 | OR 0.56, 95 % CI 0.43–0.72 | OR 0.81, 95 % CI 0.55–1.21 | OR 0.74, 95 % CI 0.44–1.25 | OR 0.22, 95 % CI 0.17–0.27 | OR 0.45, 95 % CI 0.30–0.67 |
| Khan et al. [33] | 23 | RR 0.54, 95 % CI 0.45–0.65 | RR 0.70, 95 % CI 0.60–0.83 | RR 0.79, 95 % CI 0.57–1.08 | RR 0.25, 95 % CI 0.21–0.30 | NR |
| Pancholy et al. [34] | 13 | OR 0.39, 95 % CI 0.31–0.49 | NR | NR | NR | NR |
| Li et al. [32] | 16 | OR 0.50, 95 % CI, 0.38–0.65 | OR 0.69, 95 % CI 0.49–0.97 | OR 0.58 95 % CI, 0.39–0.86 | OR 0.21, 95 % CI, 0.18–0.26 | OR 0.48, 95 % CI, 0.34–0.67 |

*OR* odds ratio, *RR* relative risk, *NR* not reported

CTO PCI was again associated with improved survival (hazard ratio [HR]: 0.72; 95 % CI: 0.62–0.83; $p<0.001$), with the biggest survival advantage found in patients with complete, compared to those with partial or failed revascularization.

The major limitations of these observational studies are the presence of unmeasured confounders, with the unsuccessful CTO PCI patients likely representing a higher risk group. There will always remain a certain degree of bias that cannot be fully negated even by the statistical adjustment for the most common confounders. Patients with complex CTOs often have complex non-CTO lesions, with high atherosclerotic burden, inferring worse prognosis irrespective of the CTO itself.

However, the current body of evidence does suggest a survival benefit with CTO PCI. Some have found the survival benefit to be confined to LAD CTO PCI [36], while others have found it to be related to both LAD and CX CTO PCI [37]. The LAD supplies the largest area of myocardium and its patency has the largest effect on ventricular function and electrical stability. Proximal LAD occlusion are frequently associated with greater than 10 % of ischemic myocardium, and this threshold has been demonstrated to confer worsen prognosis [27]. It is likely and intuitive that the greatest survival benefit be associated with successful LAD (ideally proximal) CTO PCI. Until conclusive data is available, a recanalized proximal LAD supplying a large area of ischemic myocardium must be perceived as providing a better prognosis.

The presence of a CTO in a non-infarct related artery is associated with increased mortality in both patients with STEMI [38] and NSTEMI [39]. In patients with MVD and myocardial infarction, the presence of a CTO in a non-infarct related artery (IRA) is the main driver of increased mortality, while MVD without a CTO is a weaker predictor [40]. In patients undergoing primary PCI, markers of reperfusion such as ST segment resolution, TIMI −3 flow and myocardial blush are affected by the presence of a CTO [41]. The presence of a CTO in a non-infarct related artery is also predictor of hemodynamic instability and cardiogenic shock. In patients with cardiogenic shock, both MVD and the presence of a CTO affect short-term mortality, but long-term mortality is mostly affected by the presence of a CTO [38]. These findings underscore the relative fragility of the safety net provided by chronic collateral supply to a major occluded epicardial vessel, leading to coronary inter-dependence. Acute loss of a donor artery often leads to myocardial infarction in multiple interdependent territories.

Several trials are underway to determine the long-term outcomes of CTO PCI compared to optimal medical management. The EXPLORE trial [42] is evaluating the value of recanalization of a non-IRA CTO after primary PCI. The primary endpoints are left ventricular function and left ventricular end diastolic volumes at 4 months, with clinical follow up at 5 years, which should provide insight on clinical outcomes. Two trials, in different geographical regions, are assessing hard outcomes on CTO PCI vs. optimal medical therapy (OMT). The EuroCTO trial is randomly assigning 1200 European patients, with a primary endpoint of QOL at 1 year and a cumulative composite end point of all-cause death, non-fatal MI at 3 years. The estimated completion date is in 2017 but may be delayed based on slow recuitment. The DECISION-CTO is randomly assigning 1284 Asian patients, with a primary endpoint of composite outcomes of all cause death, myocardial infarction, stroke, and any revascularization at 3 years. The estimated completion date is in 2018.

Until RCT data are available to settle the controversy on survival from CTO PCI, sound clinical decision-making must be made in each patient with a CTO when considering the potential impact on survival. The extent of ischemia, the location of the CTO and the plaque burden and risk of plaque rupture in the donor vessel must be taken into account.

## LV Function

Chronic ischemia related to a CTO can cause LV dysfunction, and may lead to exercise intolerance and finally heart failure. It therefore seems logical that the opening of an occluded artery, which irrigates dysfunctional myocardium, could reverse this dysfunction. Several studies have assessed the effects of CTO PCI on LV function and remodelling. In these studies, statistically significant improvement in regional wall motion, global LV ejection fraction (LVEF) and/or decrease in LV volumes have been demonstrated at 5–6 months after the procedure [43–51]. However, the degree of LVEF improvement was generally small, typically <5 % [44–49]. The greatest LVEF gains have been limited to patients with a patent target vessel at follow-up, those without prior MI in the distribution territory of the CTO, and those with baseline regional or global LV dysfunction [44–46]. The improvement does not appear to depend on the presence of pre-existing collaterals, but probably on preserved microvascular integrity [46]. Improvement in regional and global LV function after CTO PCI has also been related to the extent of baseline transmural necrosis, as shown in studies using contrast-enhanced magnetic resonance imaging (MRI) [48–52].

The combination of multiple MRI derived viability parameters including dobutamine contractile reserve assessment, transmural extent of infarction (TEI), and segmental wall thickening (SWT) of normal residual myocardium was shown to reduce the proportion of false-positive patients, that is, patients with viable myocardium but without improvement in LV function after successful CTO PCI [49]. Indeed, this combination of parameters was a better predictor of improvement of dysfunctional segments than the single widely used parameter of TEI [48]. The expected beneficial prognostic effect of CTO PCI is thought to be associated with the amount of ischaemic myocardium, as has been observed in patients with CAD in general [27, 53, 54]. However, CTO–PCI might be beneficial in some cases despite the absence of ischemia. In one study, patients with successful CTO–PCI of the LAD coronary artery ($n=99$) were stratified according to the presence of perfusion defects on nuclear imaging before the procedure [55]. Both those with reversible ($n=40$) and those with fixed ($n=50$) perfusion defects had significant improvement at 1 year in perfusion abnormalities (−20 %, $P=0.001$ and −15 %, $P=0.041$, respectively), LVEF (6 %, $P=0.002$ and 4.1 %, $P=0.006$), quality of life measured as improved 6 min walking distance (~50 m, $P<0.05$ and ~25 m, $P<0.05$), and frequency of angina measured with the SAQ (mean score 18, $P<0.05$ and mean score 15, $P<0.05$). No benefit of CTO–PCI was observed in patients who had no perfusion defects ($n=9$) [55].

## Myocardial Electrical Stability

Currently, limited evidence is available to show that myocardial electrical stability is improved after successful CTO–PCI. However, in patients with an implantable cardioverter–defibrillator (ICD) for ischaemic cardiomyopathy ($n=162$), a CTO was significantly associated with ventricular arrhythmias requiring ICD therapy (HR 3.5, 95 % CI 1.5–8.3, $P=0.003$) [56]. Two previously established arrhythmogenic factors might be responsible for the ventricular tachycardia: ischemia owing to inadequate perfusion of the myocardium can lead to abnormal automaticity of the ventricular myocardial cells, and re-entry circuits in patients with a previous myocardial infarction and fibrous tissue interspersed with islands of viable tissue [57]. Restoring antegrade flow after successful CTO–PCI could resolve the ischemia and might, therefore, enhance electrical stability in patients with ventricular arrhythmia, regardless of the presence of an ICD, which only treats the arrhythmic defect and not the cause of ischemia.

## Procedural Success and Complications

Despite procedural complexity, increased operator volumes have led to an improved success rate of CTO-PCI from approximately 68 to 85 % [58–62], and even higher success rates with highly trained operators [59, 63–67]. This improvement is accompanied by a low risk of procedural complications, regardless of procedural success [68]. These figures are similar to non-CTO procedures, with the exception of a significantly increased use of contrast agent and fluoroscopy time [60].

Most of the potential procedural complications are clinically uneventful; the in-hospital major adverse cardiac events (MACEs) after elective CTO PCI range from 0.9 to 6.5 % [43, 60, 68]. However, recent reports from registries performed by experienced operators showed a similar in-hospital MACE rate for CTO PCI as compared to non-CTO interventions. Of note, a higher reported in-hospital mortality rate among patients in whom the PCI of the CTO failed, ranging from 1.0 to 2.6 %. The 30-day procedure-related outcomes of CTO PCI are shown (Table 1.2) and are thus far reported in only two studies [60, 69]. Thirty-day mortality in the overall CTO cohort regardless of procedure success was 1.1 %.

Hence, under experienced hands, CTO PCI have high success rate nowadays with an acceptable rate of meaningful complications. Dedicated material, improved techniques and dissemination of knowledge within the CTO community have led to safer and more efficient procedures.

**Table 1.2** Adverse event rate after CTO PCI

| 30-d event | Hoye et al. [69] | ERCTO [60] |
|---|---|---|
| Death (%) | | |
| Overall patients | 1.1 | – |
| CTO success | 0.7 | 0 |
| CTO failure | 2.0 | 1.9 |
| MI (%) | | |
| Overall patients | 0.5 | – |
| CTO success | 0.5 | 0.8 |
| CTO failure | 0.3 | 3.6 |
| MACE (%) | | |
| Overall patients | 8.7 | – |
| CTO success | 5.5 | – |
| CTO failure | 14.8 | – |

Thirty-day adverse events after CTO-PCI in the overall patient cohort and stratified according to technical success

**Table 1.3** Summary of practice guidelines on CTO

**2011 ACCF/AHA/SCAI Guideline for Percutaneous Coronary Intervention:**

Section 5.8.1. CTOs recommendations :

Class IIa:PCI of a CTO in patients with appropriate clinical indications and suitable anatomy is reasonable when performed by operators with appropriate expertise (level of Evidence : B).

*"The decision to try PCI for a CTO (vs. continued medical therapy or surgical revascularization) requires an individualized risk-benefit analysis encompassing clinical, angiographic, and technical considerations.Consultation with a cardiothoracic surgeon and use of the Heart Team approach in cases of CTO in which a large territory is subtended and/or multivessel CAD is present are frequently done."*

**2012 ACCF/AHA/ACP/AATS/PCNA/SCAI/STS Guideline for the Diagnosis and Management of Patients With Stable Ischemic Heart Disease:**

Section 4.2. General approach to therapy:

*"In general, complete revascularization leads to better outcomes than incomplete revascularization (413–418). In patients with chronic total occlusion, CABG could be preferable to PCI (419), but this is still controversial. Although the technology and techniques for PCI of chronic total occlusions are improving, there remains no current evidence that survival is improved after successful PCI of a chronic total occlusion."*

**2014 ESC Guidelines in myocardial revascularization:**

Section 14.2 Disease progression and late graft failure:

*"Percutaneous coronary intervention for a chronic total occlusion (CTO) may be indicated when ischaemic symptoms are present with evidence of significant ischaemia and viable myocardium in the territory supplied."*

Section 17.3.2. Chronic total coronary occlusions :

*Class IIa, level B:* Percutaneous recanalization of CTOs should be considered in patients with expected ischaemia reduction in a corresponding myocardial territory and/or angina relief.

*Class IIb, level C:* Retrograde recanalization of CTOs may be considered after a failed anterograde approach or as the primary approach in selected patients.

*"Treatment of CTOs should be considered in the presence of symptoms or objective evidence of viability/ischaemia in the territory of the occluded artery. (...) Ad hoc PCI is not recommended for CTOs. Observational studies suggest that successfully revascularized CTOs confer a long-term survival advantage over failed revascularization. In addition, better relief of angina and functional status was observed after successful CTO recanalization."*

**2013 ESC guidelines on the management of stable coronary artery disease:**

Section 9.7. Chronic total occlusions:

*"Revascularization needs to be discussed in patients with symptoms of occlusion or large ischaemic areas. Percutaneous coronary intervention (PCI) of CTOs is technically challenging and requires familiarity with advanced techniques and specialized equipment. Surgical treatment, with the implantation of a distal bypass graft, is also a valid option for discussion."*

## Current Guidelines

Contrary to popular belief, current American and European guidelines generally support CTO PCI for ischemic patients. Although worded differently, both the ACCF/ACC/SCAI and ESC guidelines give a Class IIa indication for CTO PCI [70, 71]. The ACCF/ACC/SCAI guidelines require "appropriate clinical indication", "suitable anatomy" and "appropriate expertise". The ESC guidelines are more liberal by mainly mentioning an "expected ischemia reduction". The ACCF/SCAI/STS/AATS/AHA/ASNC appropriateness criteria provide several scenarios to help guide in the decision making to recanalyse a CTO [70]. The 18 scenarios are based on degree of symptoms, ischemia quantification and intensity of medical regimen. However, the criteria mainly pertain to isolated CTOs, as they fail to address the issue of completeness of revascularization in patients with MVD and a CTO. Regardless, in more than 2/3 of the clinical scenarios CTO PCI is rated as either "appropriate" or "uncertain", leaving a large role to clinical judgement and discussion with patients regarding the expected benefits. A summary of the clinical guidelines and appropriateness criteria are provided in Tables 1.3 and 1.4 respectively.

**Table 1.4** ACCF/SCAI/STS/AATS/AHA/ASNC appropriateness criteria

| | | | |
|---|---|---|---|
| **Class 3-4 angina Max tx** | A | A | U |
| **Class 1-2 angina Max tx** | A | U | U |
| **Asymptomatic Max tx** | U | U | I |
| **Class 3-4 angina No or min tx** | A | U | I |
| **Class 1-2 angina No ore min tx** | U | U | I |
| **Asymptomatic No or min tx** | U | I | I |
| | High risk non-invasive test | Intermediate risk non-invasive test | Low risk non-invasive test |

A: Appropriate, U: Uncertain, I: Inappropriate, Tx: Treatment

## Proposed Algorithm

Once a diagnosis of symptomatic ischemic heart disease with the presence of a CTO is made and revascularization is desired, the decision making on whether CTO PCI is undertaken starts with the evaluation of the extent of coronary disease i.e. isolated CTO or MVD. Since LAD (ideally proximal) CTO is more likely to affect mortality, isolated CTO must be divided into either LAD or RCA and Cx CTOs. If the likelihood of success of RCA and Cx CTO is high, CTO PCI may be undertaken, unless minimal ischemia or symptoms are present. In low chance of success, medical management should be continued. Assessing LAD CTO PCI requires attention to other factors such has diabetes mellitus, left ventricular function or local expertise in minimally invasive surgical revascularization. Both PCI and CABG are currently acceptable options in isolated LAD CTO.

Patients with MVD plus the presence of a CTO must be approached differently (Fig. 1.2). One needs to address *a priori* whether the overall goal for the patient is CR or IR. If IR is acceptable based on age, comorbidities or overall frailty, PCI to non-CTO vessels is usually undertaken first. Subsequently, reassessment of ischemia and symptoms will determine whether CTO PCI is performed afterwards. If the goal is to offer CR, evaluation of complexity of disease by the SYNTAX score (SS) is important. In intermediate to high SS, strong consideration must be made for CABG, as suggested by current literature, with the current caveats of uncertainty about the effectiveness of CABG specifically for the CTO vessel, as mentioned. In low SS, the decision on CTO PCI vs. CABG will depend on several factors including diabetes and LV function, as well as the likelihood of CTO PCI success. In those patients, CTO PCI is often attempted first as to bail out to CABG if the procedure is unsuccessful. However, in many instances where the likelihood of success is high and the donor vessel is diseased, treating the non-CTO vessel first confers increased safety for the CTO PCI. Both the choices and the sequences of revascularization are dependent on the initial objective in regards to completeness of revascularization, as well as on clinical, technical and anatomical considerations.

**Fig. 1.2** Ischemic symptoms and presence of CTO

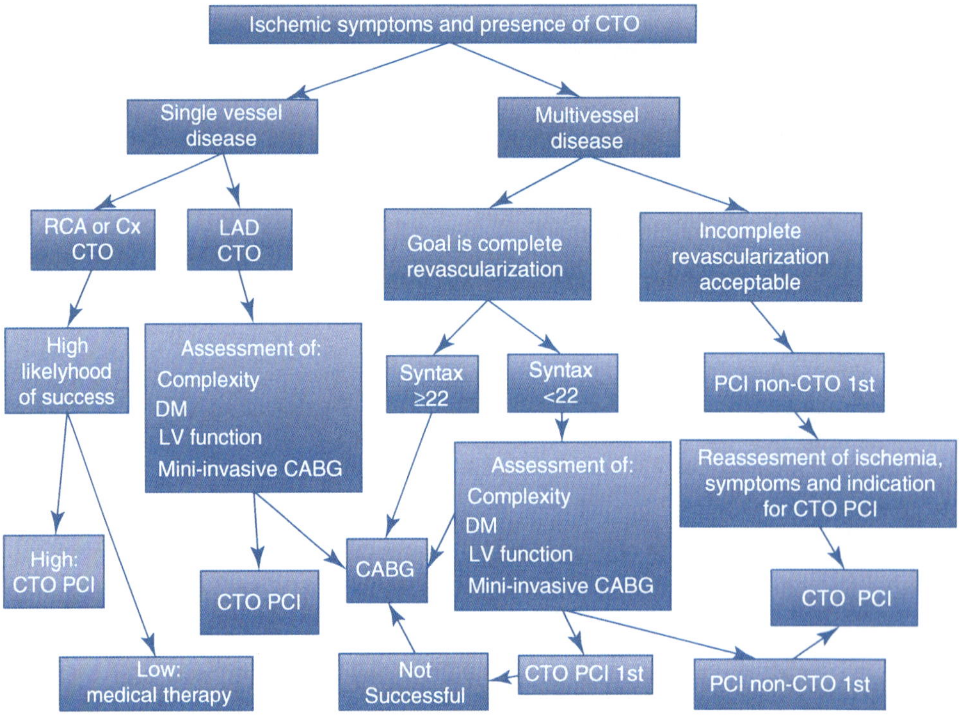


**Conclusion**

CTO PCI has evolved into a safe and efficient procedure, with observed benefits on mortality, angina and LV function. Until RCT data is available, sound clinical decision-making is needed to offer the best revascularization strategy, which may include CTO PCI in a substantial proportion of patients.

## References


1. Kahn JK. Angiographic suitability for catheter revascularization of total coronary occlusions in patients from a community hospital setting. Am Heart J. 1993;126:561–4.
2. Christofferson RD, Lehmann KG, Martin GV, Every N, Caldwell JH, Kapadia SR. Effect of chronic total coronary occlusion on treatment strategy. Am J Cardiol. 2005;95:1088–91.
3. Srinivas VS, Brooks MM, Detre KM, King SB, Jacobs AK, Johnston J, Williams DO. Contemporary percutaneous coronary intervention versus balloon angioplasty for multivessel coronary artery disease: a comparison of the National Heart, Lung and Blood Institute Dynamic Registry and the Bypass Angioplasty Revascularization Investigation (BARI) study. Circulation. 2002;106:1627–33.
4. Yamamoto E, Natsuaki M, Morimoto T, Furukawa Y, Nakagawa Y, Ono K, Mitsudo K, Nobuyoshi M, Doi O, Tamura T, Tanaka M, Kimura T. Long-term outcomes after percutaneous coronary intervention for chronic total occlusion (from the CREDO-Kyoto registry cohort-2). Am J Cardiol. 2013;112:767–74.
5. Fefer P, Knudtson ML, Cheema AN, Galbraith PD, Osherov AB, Yalonetsky S, Gannot S, Samuel M, Weisbrod M, Bierstone D, Sparkes JD, Wright GA, Strauss BH. Current perspectives on coronary chronic total occlusions: the Canadian Multicenter Chronic Total Occlusions Registry. J Am Coll Cardiol. 2012;59:991–7.
6. Jeroudi OM, Alomar ME, Michael TT, Sabbagh AE, Patel VG, Mogabgab O, Fuh E, Sherbet D, Lo N, Roesle M, Rangan BV, Abdullah SM, Hastings JL, Grodin J, Banerjee S, Brilakis ES. Prevalence and management of coronary chronic total occlusions in a tertiary veterans affairs hospital. Catheter Cardiovasc Interv. 2014;84(4):637–43.
7. Råmunddal T, Hoebers L, Henriques JP, Dworeck C, Angerås O, Odenstedt J, Ioanes D, Olivecrona G, Harnek J, Jensen U, Aasa M, Jussila R, James S, Lagerqvist B, Matejka G, Albertsson P, Omerovic E. Chronic Total Occlusions in Sweden – a report from the Swedish Coronary Angiography and Angioplasty Registry (SCAAR). PLoS One. 2014;9(8):e103850.
8. Christopoulos G, Menon RV, Karmpaliotis D, Alaswad K, Lombardi W, Grantham A, Patel VG, Rangan BV, Kotsia AP, Lembo N, Kandzari D, Carlson H, Garcia S, Banerjee S, Thompson CA, Brilakis ES. The efficacy and safety of the "hybrid" approach to coronary chronic total occlusions: insights from a contemporary multicenter US registry and comparison with prior studies. J Invasive Cardiol. 2014;26(9):427–32.
9. Werner GS, Surber R, Ferrari M, Fritzenwanger M, Figulla HR. The functional reserve of collaterals supplying long-term chronic total coronary occlusions in patients without prior myocardial infarction. Eur Heart J. 2006;27(20):2406–12.
10. Sachdeva R, Agrawal M, Flynn SE, Werner GS, Uretsky BF. Reversal of ischemia of donor artery myocardium after recanalization of a chronic total occlusion. Catheter Cardiovasc Interv. 2013;82(4):E453–8.
11. Joyal D, Afilalo J, Rinfret S. Effectiveness of recanalization of chronic total occlusions: a systematic review and meta-analysis. Am Heart J. 2010;160(1):179–87.
12. Olivari Z, Rubartelli P, Piscione F, Ettori F, Fontanelli A, Salemme L, Giachero C, Di Mario C, Gabrielli G, Spedicato L. Immediate results and one-year clinical outcome after percutaneous coronary interventions in chronic total occlusions data from a multicenter, prospective, observational study (TOAST-GISE). J Am Coll Cardiol. 2003;41:1672–8.

13. Suttorp MJ, Laarman GJ, Rahel BM, et al. Primary Stenting of Totally Occluded Native Coronary Arteries II (PRISON II): a randomized comparison of bare metal stent implantation with sirolimus-eluting stent implantation for the treatment of total coronary occlusions. Circulation. 2006;114:921–8.
14. Grantham JA, Jones PG, Cannon L, et al. Quantifying the early health status benefits of successful chronic total occlusion recanalization: results from the FlowCardia's Approach to Chronic Total Occlusion Recanalization (FACTOR) Trial. Circ Cardiovasc Qual Outcomes. 2010;3:284–90.
15. Borgia F, Viceconte N, Ali O, et al. Improved cardiac survival, freedom from MACE and angina-related quality of life after successful percutaneous recanalization of coronary artery chronic total occlusions. Int J Cardiol. 2012;161(1):31–8.
16. Safley DM, Grantham JA, Hatch J, et al. Quality of life benefits of percutaneous coronary intervention for chronic occlusions. Catheter Cardiovasc Interv. 2014;84(4):629–34.
17. Serruys PW, Morice MC, Kappetein AP, Colombo A, Holmes DR, Mack MJ, Ståhle E, Feldman TE, van den Brand M, Bass EJ, Van Dyck N, Leadley K, Dawkins KD, Mohr FW, SYNTAX Investigators. Percutaneous coronary intervention versus coronary-artery bypass grafting for severe coronary artery disease. N Engl J Med. 2009;360(10):961–72.
18. Bourassa MG, Yeh W, Holubkov R, Sopko G, Detre KM. Long-term outcome of patients with incomplete Vs. complete revascularization after multivessel PTCA: a report from the NHLBI PTCA Registry. Eur Heart J. 1998;19:103–11.
19. McLellan CS, Ghali WA, Labinaz M, et al., for the APPROACH Investigators. Association between completeness of percutaneous coronary revascularization and postprocedure outcomes. Am Heart J. 2005;150:800–6.
20. Bell MR, Gersh BJ, Schaff HV, et al. Effect of completeness of revascularization on long-term outcome of patients with three-vessel disease undergoing coronary artery bypass surgery: a report from the Coronary Artery Surgery Study (CASS) Registry. Circulation. 1992;86:446–57.
21. Garcia S, Sandoval Y, Roukoz H, Adabag S, Canoniero M, Yannopoulos D, Brilakis ES. Outcomes after complete versus incomplete revascularization of patients with multivessel coronary artery disease: a meta-analysis of 89,883 patients enrolled in randomized clinical trials and observational studies. J Am Coll Cardiol. 2013;62(16):1421–31.
22. Head SJ, Mack MJ, Holmes Jr DR, Mohr FW, Morice MC, Serruys PW, Kappetein AP. Incidence, predictors and outcomes of incomplete revascularization after percutaneous coronary intervention and coronary artery bypass grafting: a subgroup analysis of 3-year SYNTAX data. Eur J Cardiothorac Surg. 2012;41(3):535–41.
23. Généreux P, Palmerini T, Caixeta A, Rosner G, Green P, Dressler O, Xu K, Parise H, Mehran R, Serruys PW, Stone GW. Quantification and impact of untreated coronary artery disease after percutaneous coronary intervention: the residual SYNTAX (Synergy Between PCI with Taxus and Cardiac Surgery) score. J Am Coll Cardiol. 2012;59(24):2165–74.
24. Farooq V, Serruys PW, Bourantas CV, Zhang Y, Muramatsu T, Feldman T, Holmes DR, Mack M, Morice MC, Ståhle E, Colombo A, de Vries T, Morel MA, Dawkins KD, Kappetein AP, Mohr FW. Quantification of incomplete revascularization and its association with five-year mortality in the synergy between percutaneous coronary intervention with taxus and cardiac surgery (SYNTAX) trial validation of the residual SYNTAX score. Circulation. 2013; 128(2):141–51.
25. Malkin CJ, George V, Ghobrial MS, Krishnan A, Siotia A, Raina T, Morton AC, Gunn J. Residual SYNTAX score after PCI for triple vessel coronary artery disease: quantifying the adverse effect of incomplete revascularisation. EuroIntervention. 2013;8(11):1286–95.
26. Park KW, Kang J, Kang SH, Ahn HS, Kang HJ, Koo BK, Chae IH, Youn TJ, Oh BH, Park YB, Kandzari D, Kim HS. The impact of residual coronary lesions on clinical outcomes after percutaneous coronary intervention: Residual SYNTAX score after percutaneous coronary intervention in patients from the Efficacy of Xience/Promus versus Cypher in rEducing Late Loss after stENTing (EXCELLENT) registry. Am Heart J. 2014;167(3):384–92.
27. Shaw LJ, Berman DS, Maron DJ, Mancini GB, Hayes SW, Hartigan PM, Weintraub WS, O'Rourke RA, Dada M, Spertus JA, Chaitman BR, Friedman J, Slomka P, Heller GV, Germano G, Gosselin G, Berger P, Kostuk WJ, Schwartz RG, Knudtson M, Veledar E, Bates ER, McCallister B, Teo KK, Boden WE, COURAGE Investigators. Optimal medical therapy with or without percutaneous coronary intervention to reduce ischemic burden: results from the Clinical Outcomes Utilizing Revascularization and Aggressive Drug Evaluation (COURAGE) trial nuclear substudy. Circulation. 2008;117:1283–91.
28. Davies RF, Goldberg AD, Forman S, Pepine CJ, Knatterud GL, Geller N, Sopko G, Pratt C, Deanfield J, Conti CR. Asymptomatic Cardiac Ischemia Pilot (ACIP) study two-year follow-up: outcomes of patients randomized to initial strategies of medical therapy versus revascularization. Circulation. 1997;95:2037–43.
29. Galassi AR, Tomasello SD, Crea F, Costanzo L, Campisano MB, Marza F, Tamburino C. Transient impairment of vasomotion function after successful chronic total occlusion recanalization. J Am Coll Cardiol. 2012;59:711–8.
30. Widimsky P, Straka Z, Stros P, Jirasek K, Dvorak J, Votava J, Lisa L, Budesinsky T, Kolesar M, Vanek T, Brucek P. One-year coronary bypass graft patency: a randomized comparison between off-pump and on-pump surgery angiographic results of the prague-4 trial. Circulation. 2004;110:3418–23.
31. Farooq V, Serruys PW, Garcia-Garcia HM, Zhang Y, Bourantas CV, Holmes DR, Mack M, Feldman T, Morice MC, Stahle E, James S, Colombo A, Diletti R, Papafaklis MI, de Vries T, Morel MA, van Es GA, Mohr FW, Dawkins KD, Kappetein AP, Sianos G, Boersma E. The negative impact of incomplete angiographic revascularization on clinical outcomes and its association with total occlusions: the syntax (synergy between percutaneous coronary intervention with taxus and cardiac surgery) trial. J Am Coll Cardiol. 2013;61: 282–94.
32. Li R, Yang S, Tang L, Yang Y, Chen H, Guan S, Han W, Liu H, Dai J, Gan Q, Fang W, Qu X. Meta-analysis of the effect of percutaneous coronary intervention on chronic total coronary occlusions. J Cardiothorac Surg. 2014;9:41.
33. Khan MF, Wendel CS, Thai HM, Movahed MR. Effects of percutaneous revascularization of chronic total occlusions on clinical outcomes: a meta-analysis comparing successful versus failed percutaneous intervention for chronic total occlusion. Catheter Cardiovasc Interv. 2013;82(1):95–107.
34. Pancholy SB, Boruah P, Ahmed I, Kwan T, Patel TM, Saito S. Meta-analysis of effect on mortality of percutaneous recanalization of coronary chronic total occlusions using a stent-based strategy. Am J Cardiol. 2013;111(4):521–5.
35. George S, Cockburn J, Clayton TC, Ludman P, Cotton J, Spratt J, Redwood S, de Belder M, de Belder A, Hill J, Hoye A, Palmer N, Rathore S, Gershlick A, Di Mario C, Hildick-Smith D. Long-term follow-up of elective chronic total coronary occlusion angioplasty: analysis from the U.K. Central Cardiac Audit Database. J Am Coll Cardiol. 2014;64(3):235–43.
36. Safley DM, House JA, Marso SP, Grantham JA, Rutherford BD. Improvement in survival following successful percutaneous coronary intervention of coronary chronic total occlusions: variability by target vessel. JACC Cardiovasc Interv. 2008;1(3):295–302.
37. Claessen BE, Dangas GD, Godino C, Henriques JP, Leon MB, Park SJ, Stone GW, Moses JW, Colombo A, Mehran R, Multinational CTO Registry. Impact of target vessel on long-term survival after

percutaneous coronary intervention for chronic total occlusions. Catheter Cardiovasc Interv. 2013;82(1):76–82.
38. Hoebers LP, Vis MM, Claessen BE, van der Schaaf RJ, Kikkert WJ, Baan Jr J, de Winter RJ, Piek JJ, Tijssen JG, Dangas GD, Henriques JP. The impact of multivessel disease with and without a co-existing chronic total occlusion on short- and long-term mortality in ST-elevation myocardial infarction patients with and without cardiogenic shock. Eur J Heart Fail. 2013;15(4):425–32.
39. Gierlotka M, Tajstra M, Gąsior M, Hawranek M, Osadnik T, Wilczek K, Olszowski D, Dyrbuś K, Poloński L. Impact of chronic total occlusion artery on 12-month mortality in patients with non-ST-segment elevation myocardial infarction treated by percutaneous coronary intervention (from the PL-ACS Registry). Int J Cardiol. 2013;168(1):250–4.
40. Claessen BE, van der Schaaf RJ, Verouden NJ, Stegenga NK, Engstrom AE, Sjauw KD, Kikkert WJ, Vis MM, Baan Jr J, Koch KT, de Winter RJ, Tijssen JG, Piek JJ, Henriques JP. Evaluation of the effect of a concurrent chronic total occlusion on long-term mortality and left ventricular function in patients after primary percutaneous coronary intervention. JACC Cardiovasc Interv. 2009; 2(11):1128–34.
41. Claessen BE, Dangas GD, Weisz G, Witzenbichler B, Guagliumi G, Möckel M, Brener SJ, Xu K, Henriques JP, Mehran R, Stone GW. Prognostic impact of a chronic total occlusion in a non-infarct-related artery in patients with ST-segment elevation myocardial infarction: 3-year results from the HORIZONS-AMI trial. Eur Heart J. 2012;33(6):768–75.
42. Van der Schaaf RJ, Claessen BE, Hoebers LP, Verouden NJ, Koolen JJ, Suttorp MJ, Barbato E, Bax M, Strauss BH, Olivecrona GK, Tuseth V, Glogar D, Råmunddal T, Tijssen JG, Piek JJ, Henriques JP, EXPLORE investigators. Rationale and design of EXPLORE: a randomized, prospective, multicenter trial investigating the impact of recanalization of a chronic total occlusion on left ventricular function in patients after primary percutaneous coronary intervention for acute ST-elevation myocardial infarction. Trials. 2010;11:89.
43. Valenti R, Migliorini A, Signorini U, et al. Impact of complete revascularization with percutaneous coronary intervention on survival in patients with at least one chronic total occlusion. Eur Heart J. 2008;29:2336–42.
44. Dzavik V, Carere RG, Mancini GB, et al. Predictors of improvement in left ventricular function after percutaneous revascularization of occluded coronary arteries: a report from the Total Occlusion Study of Canada (TOSCA). Total Occlusion Study of Canada Investigators. Am Heart J. 2001;142:301–8.
45. Chung CM, Nakamura S, Tanaka K, et al. Effect of recanalization of chronic total occlusions on global and regional left ventricular function in patients with or without previous myocardial infarction. Catheter Cardiovasc Interv. 2003;60:368–74.
46. Werner GS, Surber R, Kuethe F, et al. Collaterals and the recovery of left ventricular function after recanalization of a chronic total coronary occlusion. Am Heart J. 2005;149:129–37.
47. Nakamura S, Muthusamy TS, Bae JH, et al. Impact of sirolimus eluting stent on the outcome of patients with chronic total occlusions. Am J Cardiol. 2005;95:161–6.
48. Kirschbaum SW, Rossi A, Boersma E, et al. Combining magnetic resonance viability variables better predicts improvement of myocardial function prior to percutaneous coronary intervention. Int J Cardiol. 2012;159:192–7.
49. Baks T, van Geuns RJ, Duncker DJ, et al. Prediction of left ventricular function after drug-eluting stent implantation for chronic total coronary occlusions. J Am Coll Cardiol. 2006;47:721–5.
50. Kirschbaum SW, Baks T, van den Ent M, et al. Evaluation of left ventricular function three years after percutaneous recanalization of chronic total coronary occlusions. Am J Cardiol. 2008;101:179–85.
51. Cheng AS, Selvanayagam JB, Jerosch-Herold M, et al. Percutaneous treatment of chronic total coronary occlusions improves regional hyperemic myocardial blood flow and contractility: insights from quantitative cardiovascular magnetic resonance imaging. JACC Cardiovasc Interv. 2008;1:44–53.
52. Kirschbaum SW, Rossi A, van Domburg RT, et al. Contractile reserve in segments with nontransmural infarction in chronic dysfunctional myocardium using low-dose dobutamine CMR. JACC Cardiovasc Imaging. 2010;3:614–22.
53. Hachamovitch R, Rozanski A, Shaw LJ, Stone GW, Thomson LE, Friedman JD, Hayes SW, Cohen I, Germano G, Berman DS. Impact of ischaemia and scar on the therapeutic benefit derived from myocardial revascularization vs. medical therapy among patients undergoing stress-rest myocardial perfusion scintigraphy. Eur Heart J. 2011;32:1012–24.
54. Piccini JP, Starr AZ, Horton JR, Shaw LK, Lee KL, Al-Khatib SM, Iskandrian AE, O'Connor CM, Borges-Neto S. Single-photon emission computed tomography myocardial perfusion imaging and the risk of sudden cardiac death in patients with coronary disease and left ventricular ejection fraction >35%. J Am Coll Cardiol. 2010;56:206–14.
55. Sun D, Wang J, Tian Y, Narsinh K, Wang H, Li C, Ma X, Wang Y, Wang D, Li C, Wu JC, Tian J, Cao F. Multimodality imaging evaluation of functional and clinical benefits of percutaneous coronary intervention in patients with chronic total occlusion lesion. Theranostics. 2012;2(8):788–800.
56. Nombela-Franco L, Mitroi CD, Fernández-Lozano I, García-Touchard A, Toquero J, Castro-Urda V, Fernández-Diaz JA, Perez-Pereira E, Beltrán-Correas P, Segovia J, Werner GS, Javier G, Luis AP. Ventricular arrhythmias among implantable cardioverter- defibrillator recipients for primary prevention: impact of chronic total coronary occlusion (VACTO Primary Study). Circ Arrhythm Electrophysiol. 2012;1:147–54.
57. Meissner MD, Akhtar M, Lehmann MH. Nonischemic sudden tachycardia death in atherosclerotic heart disease. Circulation. 1991;84:905–12.
58. Michael TT, Karmpaliotis D, Brilakis ES, Alomar M, Abdullah SM, Kirkland BL, Mishoe KL, Lembo N, Kalynych A, Carlson H, Banerjee S, Luna M, Lombardi W, Kandzari DE. Temporal trends of fluoroscopy time and contrast utilization in coronary chronic total occlusion revascularisation: insights from a multicenter United States registry. Catheter Cardiovasc Interv. 2015;85(3):393–9.
59. Patel VG, Brayton KM, Tamayo A, Mogabgab O, Michael TT, Lo N, Alomar M, Shorrock D, Cipher D, Abdullah S, Banerjee S, Brilakis ES. Angiographic success and procedural complications in patients undergoing percutaneous coronary chronic total occlusion intervention: a weighted meta-analysis of 18,061 patients from 65 studies. JACC Cardiovasc Interv. 2013;6:128–36.
60. Galassi AR, Tomasello SD, Reifart N, Werner GS, Sianos G, Bonnier H, Sievert H, Ehladad S, Bufe A, Shofer J, Gershlick A, Hildick-Smith D, Escaned J, Erglis A, Sheiban I, Thuesen L, Serra A, Christiansen E, Buettner A, Costanzo L, Barrano G, Di Mario C. In-hospital outcomes of percutaneous coronary intervention in patients with chronic total occlusion: insights from the ERCTO (European Registry of Chronic Total Occlusion) registry. EuroIntervention. 2011;7(4):472–9.
61. Morino Y, Kimura T, Hayashi Y, J-CTO RegistryInvestigators, et al. In hospital outcomes of contemporary percutaneous coronary intervention in patients with chronic total occlusion insights from the J-CTO Registry (Multicenter CTO Registry in Japan). JACC Cardiovasc Interv. 2010;3:143–51.
62. Rathore S, Matsuo H, Terashima M, et al. Procedural and in-hospital outcomes after percutaneous coronary intervention for chronic total occlusions of coronary arteries 2002 to 2008: impact of novel guidewire techniques. JACC Cardiovasc Interv. 2009;2: 489–97.
63. Rathore S, Katoh O, Matsuo H, Terashima M, Tanaka N, Kinoshita Y, Kimura M, Tsuchikane E, Nasu K, Ehara M, Asakura K, Asakura Y,

Suzuki T. Retrograde percutaneous recanalization of chronic total occlusion of the coronary arteries: Procedural outcomes and predictors of success in contemporary practice. Circ Cardiovasc Interv. 2009;2:124–32.
64. Thompson CA, Jayne JE, Robb JF, Friedman BJ, Kaplan AV, Hettleman BD, Niles NW, Lombardi WL. Retrograde techniques and the impact of operator volume on percutaneous intervention for coronary chronic total occlusions an early US. Experience. JACC Cardiovasc Interv. 2009;2:834–42.
65. Rinfret S, Joyal D, Nguyen CM, Bagur R, Hui W, Leung R, Larose E, Love MP, Mansour S. Retrograde recanalization of chronic total occlusions from the transradial approach; early Canadian experience. Catheter Cardiovasc Interv. 2011;78:366–74.
66. Karmpaliotis D, Michael TT, Brilakis ES, Papayannis AC, Tran DL, Kirkland BL, Lembo N, Kalynych A, Carlson H, Banerjee S, Lombardi W, Kandzari DE. Retrograde coronary chronic total occlusion revascularization: procedural and in-hospital outcomes from a multicenter registry in the United States. JACC Cardiovasc Interv. 2012;5:1273–9.
67. Nombela-Franco L, Urena M, Jerez-Valero M, Nguyen CM, Ribeiro HB, Bataille Y, Rodes-Cabau J, Rinfret S. Validation of the j-chronic total occlusion score for chronic total occlusion percutaneous coronary intervention in an independent contemporary cohort. Circ Cardiovasc Interv. 2013;6:635–43.
68. Werner GS, Hochadel M, Zeymer U, Kerber S, Schumacher B, Grube E, Hauptmann KE, Brueck M, Zahn R, Senges J. Contemporary success and complication rates of percutaneous coronary intervention for chronic total coronary occlusion: results from the ALKK quality control registry of 2006. EuroIntervention. 2010;6:361–6.
69. Hoye A, van Domburg RT, Sonnenschein K, et al. Percutaneous coronary intervention for chronic total occlusions: the thorax center experience 1992–2002. Eur Heart J. 2005;26:2630–6.
70. Patel MR, Dehmer GJ, Hirshfeld JW, Smith PK, Spertus JA. ACCF/SCAI/STS/AATS/AHA/ASNC/HFSA/SCCT 2012 appropriate use criteria for coronary revascularization focused update: a report of the American College of Cardiology Foundation Appropriate Use Criteria Task Force, Society for Cardiovascular Angiography and Interventions, Society of Thoracic Surgeons, American Association for Thoracic Surgery, American Heart Association, American Society of Nuclear Cardiology, and the Society of Cardiovascular Computed Tomography. J Am Coll Cardiol. 2012;59:857–81.
71. Windecker S, Kolh P, Alfonso F, Collet JP, Cremer J, Falk V, Filippatos G, Hamm C, Head SJ, Jüni P, Kappetein AP, Kastrati A, Knuuti J, Landmesser U, Laufer G, Neumann FJ, Richter DJ, Schauerte P, Sousa Uva M, Stefanini GG, Taggart DP, Torracca L, Valgimigli M, Wijns W, Witkowski A. 2014 ESC/EACTS Guidelines on myocardial revascularization: the Task Force on Myocardial Revascularization of the European Society of Cardiology (ESC) and the European Association for Cardio-Thoracic Surgery (EACTS)Developed with the special contribution of the European Association of Percutaneous Cardiovascular Interventions (EAPCI). Eur Heart J. 2014;35(37):2541–619. Authors/Task Force members.

# How to Set Up a Chronic Total Occlusion Angioplasty Program

**2**

John J. Graham and Christopher E. Buller

**Abstract**

With recent focus on chronic total occlusion angioplasty (CTO-PCI), there has been interest in the logistics of establishing a CTO PCI program. However, certain features of CTO PCI distinguish it from non-CTO angioplasty and should be considered prior to introducing a CTO PCI program. These features include vascular access (usually dual), procedure length (longer), contrast volume (higher), fluoroscopy time and radiation dose (greater), number of stents implanted (more) and complication rate (increased). These – and other – aspects result in higher cost utilization for CTO PCI procedures. With these associated increased complexities, a certain level of pre-existing PCI skill is a pre-requisite. However, as this chapter will demonstrate, with appropriate forethought, planning and with support and "buy-in" from relevant institutional programs, these potential obstacles can be overcome allowing establishment of a successful CTO PCI program.

**Keywords**

CTO • PCI • CTO PCI program • CTO PCI toolbox • CTO PCI systems

## Introduction

As the preceding chapter has highlighted, in select patients, there is compelling evidence for CTO PCI. However, historically poor CTO PCI success rates had tempered enthusiasm for this and it was recognized that presence of a CTO was a major predictor for the patient being referred for CABG or to remain unrevascularized and to persevere with medical therapy (with ongoing symptoms). Recent technical advances and increasing familiarity with these advances and with new equipment, and improved awareness of the potential benefits of revascularizing a CTO has led to increased interest in this field of interventional cardiology (which has been unhelpfully termed the "final frontier"). This chapter aims to highlight certain issues peculiar to CTO PCI that will hopefully allow the establishment of a successful CTO PCI program in your center.

Before establishing a CTO PCI program, certain considerations should be taken into account. These include personal and system factors and include operator expertise, infrastructure, support and personnel.

## Developing CTO Skills

### Operator Selection

More than ever, there are many directions to expand one's interventional horizons, and CTO PCI is but one. Whether, and in which direction to expand, depends upon local need and opportunity, experience during formal training, and personal interest. Determining whether CTO PCI is a

J.J. Graham, BSc(hons), MB, ChB, MRCP (UK) (✉)
Division of Cardiology, St. Michael's Hospital, Toronto, ON, Canada
e-mail: grahamjj@smh.ca

C.E. Buller, MD, FRCPC
Division of Cardiology, St. Michael's Hospital, University of Toronto, Toronto, ON, Canada





S. Rinfret (ed.), *Percutaneous Intervention for Coronary Chronic Total Occlusion: The Hybrid Approach*, DOI 10.1007/978-3-319-21563-1_2

good fit must start with an analysis of these practical considerations. Beyond this, however, must come reflection regarding one's strengths in lights of the unique demands of CTO PCI.

CTO PCI stretches operator technique and coronary equipment to their limits; individuals who are likely to succeed are those that have established a track record for offering PCI to patients with other forms of complex anatomy, including those deemed too complex for bypass surgery. Two-stent techniques for bifurcations, unprotected left main PCI, rotational atherectomy for severe calcification, management of long and diffuse disease, as well as management of coronary perforations and other intra-procedural complications are skills operators should feel entirely comfortable with before considering hybrid CTO training. Experientially, this level of comfort is rarely achieved before a thousand independent coronary cases, and often much later.

CTO PCI typically demands thoughtful responses to changing conditions. Adaptability, lateral thinking and creative intra-procedural problem solving are key operator attributes. CTOs are associated with greater atherosclerotic burden and its consequences including multivessel CAD, prior MI, prior CABG, peripheral vascular disease, cerebrovascular disease, ventricular dysfunction, congestive heart failure and kidney disease/renal dysfunction. CTO-PCI operators must be experienced and comfortable working with these inherently complex patients. Finally, interventionalists who succeed in building CTO programs are capable of bringing disciplined focus to long procedures without succumbing to external time pressure or distractions.

Initiating a formal CTO PCI program presents an opportunity for open discussion with colleagues regarding their own aspirations for sub-specialization. Given the requirements for competency, it is uncommon that a high-volume institution can support more than two CTO experts. We suggest that opportunities for sub-specialization within the interventional field should be distributed within a group or laboratory, and agreement to support one another's subspecialty interests is a constructive approach that fosters individual and collective excellence.

Most interventional cardiologists in practice today received only cursory exposure to CTO PCI during training. This likely consisted of observing more experienced operators employ antegrade wire techniques in highly selected patients. As such, the acquisition of advanced hybrid CTO skills often occurs years or even decades after fellowship, and so requires an experienced interventionalist to be willing to return to a training mindset that includes temporary relinquishing of the role of expert. One must willingly check one's ego at the door, at least for a period.

## One Operator or Two?

The physician model developed at our institution, and many others, involves 2 CTO operators for complex cases (employing retrograde or dissection re-entry as likely strategies), those with unusual and potentially instructive features, or with ambiguous anatomy in referral films. We believe this approach accelerates learning, identifies more technical options, and thus may improve primary success. By alternating as primary operator on longer procedures, fatigue can be managed, errors avoided, and safety improved. Importantly, a second operator is invaluable when complications occur that require more than one prompt action. Although a "buddy" system may not be possible in all centers, we recommend this model if feasible.

## Training

CTO training has become well organized in recent years, and generally includes attendance at a practical CTO course that includes live cases, in-lab proctoring, and familiarization with the relevant technical and evidentiary literature. The technical and decision-making skills required for CTO PCI have been organized into *skill sets* and algorithms that have made translation more consistently 'teachable' through didactic courses, dedicated websites (CTOfundamentals.org), in simulators or during live procedures.

There now exists a community of expert CTO operators who are willing to proctor interested and qualified interventionalists. These individuals are typically faculty members at practical courses and are readily identified. An experienced and available proctor who will commit the necessary time is an absolute requirement for any new program. It can be helpful to find a proctor who is eligible for visiting privileges in order to have the proctor participate directly in the first procedures; this can improve teaching efficiency and helps assure successful procedures during start-up. A variant of the traditional proctor model is emerging in which the visiting proctor takes primary responsibility for procedures during program start-up then gradually transfers this responsibility as the trainees' skills develop, typically over a few months.

Since consequential complications early in a nascent program could stall or halt program development, a key role of the proctor is to assist in prospective identification of general and case-specific hazards, as well as the active prevention of complications during the procedures themselves. We also recommend selecting straightforward cases during the proctor phase and especially in the immediate *post*-proctor phase of 20–25 independent cases. This textbook discusses CTO PCI risks and complications elsewhere in greater detail. Briefly, however, we recommend avoiding early on cases requiring instrumentation of epicardial or dominant collaterals, patients with low EF who will not tolerate intra-procedural ischemia, or marked renal impairment who will not tolerate considerable contrast burden.

## Infrastructure

### Cardiac Catheterization Laboratory Volume

To ensure adequate exposure to candidate patients, sufficient catheterization laboratory case volume and mix is necessary. In practice, this translates to a cardiac catheterization laboratory undertaking a minimum of roughly 2000 diagnostic angiograms and 1000 non-CTO PCIs per annum. The European CTO Club white paper suggests that at least 50 CTO PCIs per annum are necessary to maintain skill sets [1], and cardiac catheterization programs unable to provide this substrate internally will make program initiation difficult. Although 18 % of patients undergoing diagnostic angiography will harbor one or more non-acute occlusions, only a small fraction of this group is likely to be referred by colleagues, particularly during start-up [2].

### Cardiac Catheterization Laboratory

CTO procedures place unique demands upon the laboratory schedule. While hybrid techniques and training do emphasize procedural efficiency, complex CTO PCI procedures remain on average considerably longer than conventional PCIs. This is particularly true during the learning curve when procedures lasting 3–4 h are typical. Even established programs find that turnover and case preparation mean that 2–3 CTO cases usually fill an 8-h cardiac catheterization slate.

Though many successful programs eventually integrate CTO procedures into a general PCI list, we recommend assigning dedicated laboratory time to these procedures, particularly during program initiation. This arrangement removes time pressure, allows focus, and enables predictable scheduling for proctors, industry clinical specialists, selected catheterization laboratory staff, and a "CTO buddy" (see below). Doing several CTO procedures in succession enhances learning through re-enforcement.

Initiating a program in facilities that operate with a single laboratory is not recommended. The absolute need to accommodate emergency procedures, particularly primary PCI, makes prolonged CTO procedures impractical and hazardous.

CTO procedures place considerable demands on x-ray equipment. The need to visualize fine details including collaterals and microchannels requires modern flat-panel digital systems that have periodic calibration of image quality. Digital systems offer image processing and low frame rate settings (usually 7.5 frames/s) that reduce x-ray flux and dose. Aging systems prone to overheating or poor reliability are unsuitable for long complex procedures, particularly retrograde procedures where equipment cannot be safely removed blindly if X-ray imaging is lost.

### Cardiac Surgery Program

An on-site cardiac surgery program is preferred, but is not a requirement. There are now a growing number of centers with successful CTO programs in stand-alone PCI facilities. In the absence of on-site surgery, we recommend case selection that avoids undertaking procedures in those at highest risk for coronary rupture/perforation and tamponade. This complication accounts almost entirely for the excess acute risk of CTO PCI over conventional PCI. For this reasons, we believe stand-alone programs should generally avoid instrumentation of epicardial collaterals as well as patients at high risk of intra-procedural ischemic complications by virtue of coronary anatomy or LV dysfunction. CTO operators in stand-alone PCI programs should consider a liaison to a CTO program that offers on-site surgery so that such cases can be thoughtfully accommodated rather than declined.

### Non-medical Staff

The complex nature of CTO interventions places greater demands on laboratory staff, both scrubbed and circulating, thus it is important to identify, promote and mentor motivated staff that you believe will be assets to your program. For the scrubbed assistant, the active inventory of wires and catheters is typically triple that in conventional PCI and must remain organized for quick access. Two manifolds and guide catheters are typical. Over-the-wire exchanges, now unfamiliar to many cath lab assistants, are routine. For the circulating staff, a thorough knowledge of new inventory must be developed. The circulating staff in most labs is also charged with patient comfort and sedation; the duration of CTO procedures will require experienced staff that can assess these components and respond appropriately.

Once team members are identified, it is important to educate them in all aspects of CTO PCI, including terminology, equipment and potential complications. Attendance at training courses or dedicated CTO PCI conferences is strongly encouraged to fully immerse them in the field of CTO PCI. Ideally they should be actively involved in all aspects of preparing for your first case, both to help with actual case preparation and also to reinforce the idea of working as a

CTO PCI team. Regular (ideally after every case or series of CTO PCI cases) debriefs are encouraged to explain treatment choices made during a particular case, and especially following complications. Moreover, they should be encouraged to speak up when noticing something unfamiliar on screen or at the table; this way, they may help the team avoid dreaded complications. There is no place for the so-called authority gradient in a CTO team. Everybody should be allowed to speak and highlight potential problems during the procedure.

## Administrative Support

It is imperative to have the support of your institution's catheterization laboratory management executive. Given the complex nature of these interventions, when compared to conventional non-CTO PCI, they often require increased numbers of increasingly specialized (and expensive) equipment. Multiple drug eluting stents are the norm rather than the exception. Karmpaliotis et al quantified the significant additional cost of CTO PCI ($10,870 versus $7436 for non-CTO PCI), which was almost completely attributable to excess procedure costs (e.g. doubling of costs of balloon catheters and over four times the cost of guide wires) [3]. When contemplating introducing a CTO PCI program, your institution's management may reasonably express concern at this increased expenditure. However, with recent increases in the numbers of cardiac catheterization laboratories, most centers' catheterization laboratory volumes are flat (or declining). Data from established CTO PCI programs suggests that, in addition to the CTO PCI procedure itself, approximately 20 % of patients will require further procedure (s) – either following an initial set-up (or 'investment') procedure, or as follow up after the CTO PCI. Thus, leaving aside the compelling clinical argument for a CTO PCI program, a business argument can be made purely in terms of increasing laboratory volume (volume which is likely currently under-utilized). The support of your institution cannot be over-emphasized and may be pivotal in ensuring the success of your program.

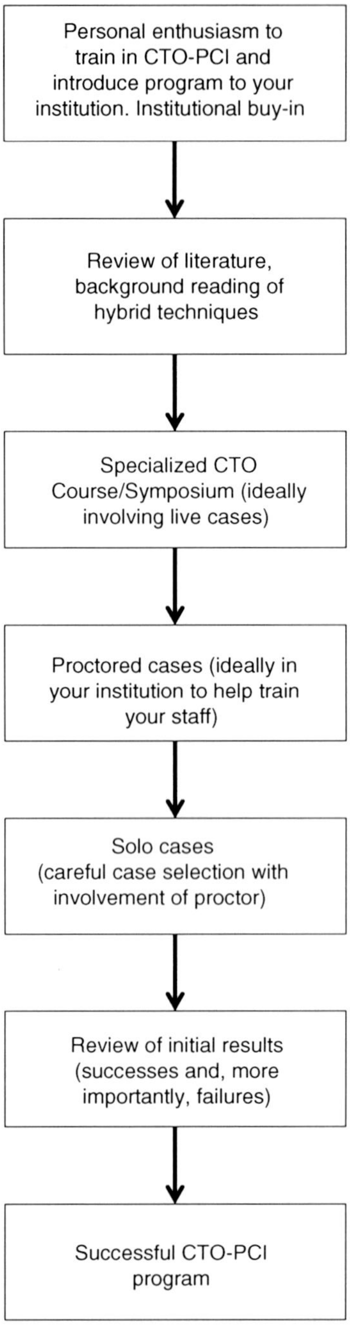


**Fig. 2.1** Suggested schema to introduce CTO-PCI program

## Practicalities

### Next Steps (Fig. 2.1)

Having expressed an interest in learning these skills and introducing a CTO PCI program (and having the support of your institution), there are a few more steps prior to undertaking your first case. We would recommend background reading around the field of CTO PCI (potentially with a book such as this!), essentially immersing you in the subject and becoming familiar with terminology and techniques. Co-incident with this reading, various online resources exist to reinforce your learning. One such resource (ctofundamentals.org) offers step-wise lectures and tutorials on various aspects of CTO PCI and allows continuous feedback via regular self-assessment tests. Also, once your program is established, this is a worthwhile resource for advice and suggestions to help overcome difficult cases and, importantly, for support and help following failure or complications. Attendance at a dedicated CTO course or symposium

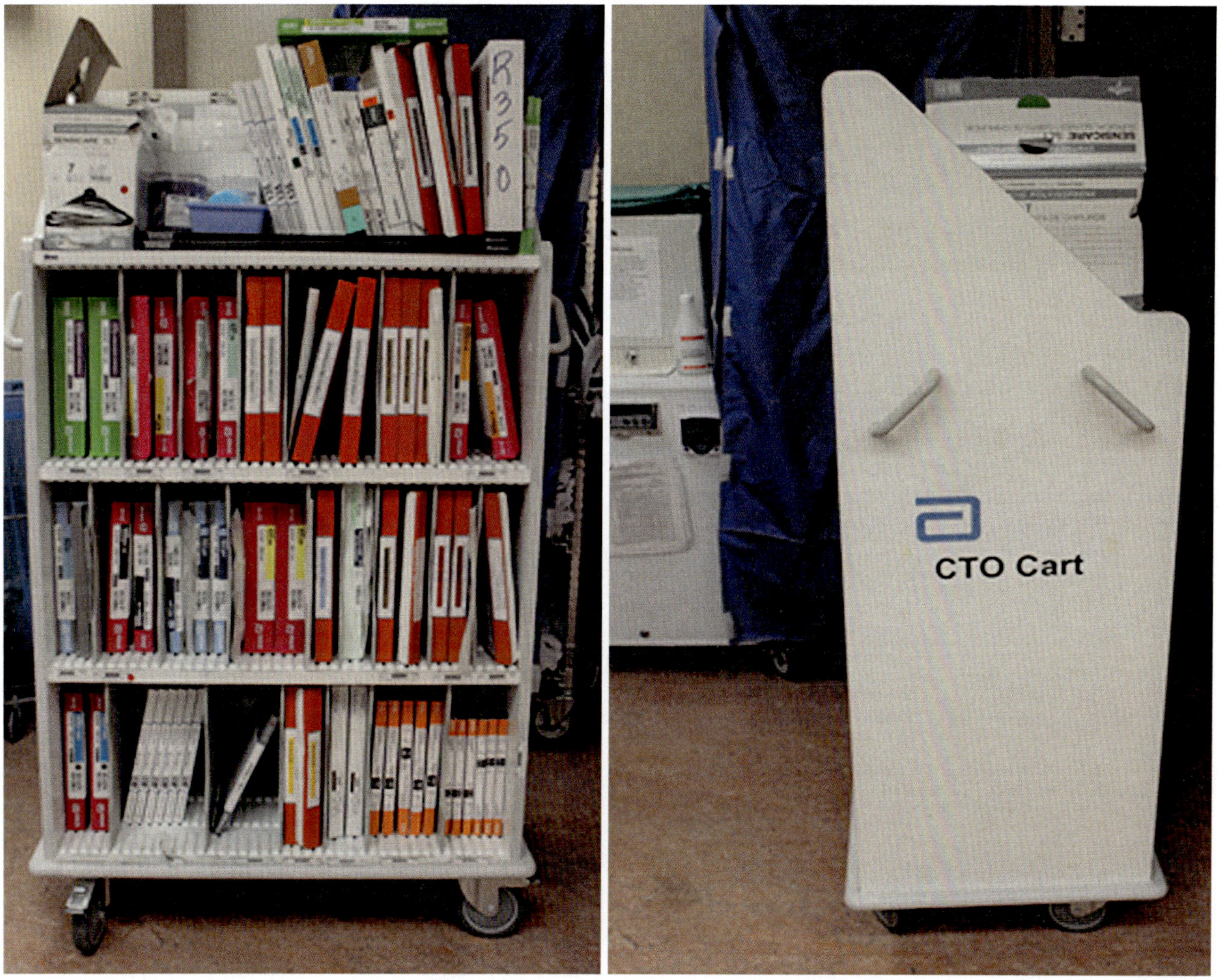


**Fig. 2.2** CTO cart containing equipment suited to CTO-PCI (short guide catheters, guidewires, microcatheters, micro-beads/embolization coils)

(ideally involving live cases) will go some way to increasing your awareness of what is possible in this field. In anticipation of your program starting (and as an early team building exercise), it is a good idea to fund your desired CTO PCI team (nurses, technicians, etc) to also attend.

Initial contact with your proctor will involve review of cases and also they will provide a "shopping list" of necessary equipment. Although equipment is covered in the next chapter, the only recommendation we would make is organizing CTO-specific equipment in an easily accessed space. At our institution we use a mobile cart that can be wheeled into whichever laboratory is being used for CTO PCI (Fig. 2.2).

During the initial proctored cases at your institution, this is an ideal opportunity to review further cases for their suitability as your first solo cases. With regard to case planning, we have found the use of CTO Planning Forms to be invaluable (see Fig. 2.3). These follow the hybrid algorithm [4] and mean that, whoever is performing the CTO PCI, a clear plan of action is delineated. Although there are no hard and fast rules, it is advisable to start slow with one or, at most, two CTO cases scheduled on your first few dedicated CTO PCI days. On each day, ensure the staff is aware of the planned procedure (antegrade, retrograde, etc). After each dedicated CTO PCI day, review the cases undertaken that day. Evaluating each step in a case is important, particularly in unsuccessful cases where understanding the mode of failure may predict future success. If unsure how to overcome difficulties, discussion with your proctor or use of one of the online resources may obtain strategies and solutions to surmount these obstacles. Once your program is established, it can be useful to connect with other CTO PCI practitioners in your area. Informal dinner meetings are an ideal forum to show planned cases and obtain opinions as to potential strategies. Also, after failures or complications, these meetings are a great way of educating your colleagues of potential pitfalls. Finally, by collating your resources, they are also an excellent mechanism for undertaking research and evaluating outcomes in this field.

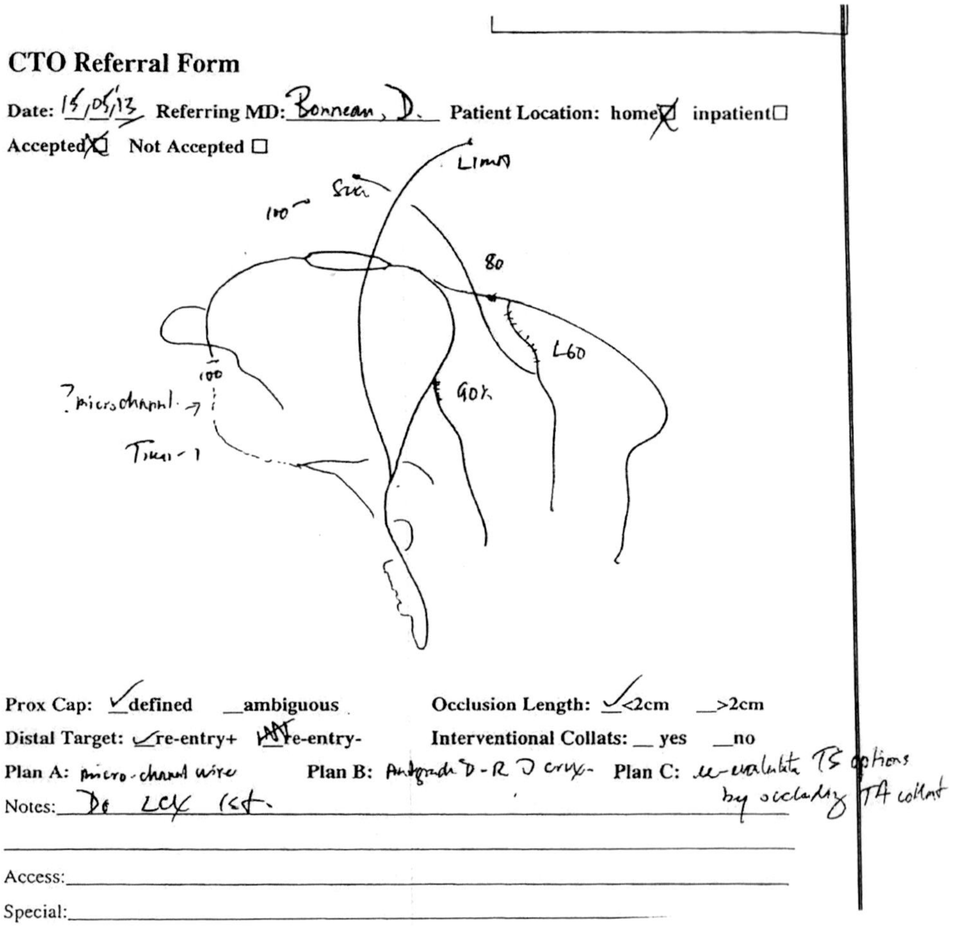
CTO Referral Form

Date: 15/05/13 Referring MD: Bonneau, D. Patient Location: home☒ inpatient☐

Accepted☒ Not Accepted ☐

Prox Cap: ✓defined __ambiguous Occlusion Length: ✓<2cm __>2cm

Distal Target: ✓re-entry+ __re-entry- Interventional Collats: __ yes __no

Plan A: micro-channel wire Plan B: Plan C:

Notes:

Access:

Special:

**Fig. 2.3** CTO-PCI procedure planning form

We firmly believe in the clinical rationale for revascularizing coronary CTOs. The skill sets necessary can be readily adopted and, as this chapter has hopefully illustrated, will allow establishment of a successful CTO PCI program in your institution.

## References


1. Di Mario C, Werner GS, Sianos G, et al. European perspective in the recanalisation of Chronic Total Occlusions (CTO): consensus document from the EuroCTO Club. EuroIntervention. 2007;3:30–43.
2. Fefer P, Knudtson ML, Cheema AN, et al. Current perspectives on coronary chronic total occlusions: the Canadian Multicenter Chronic Total Occlusions Registry. J Am Coll Cardiol. 2012;59:991–7.
3. Karmpaliotis D, Lembo N, Kalynych A, et al. Development of a high-volume, multiple-operator program for percutaneous chronic total coronary occlusion revascularization: procedural, clinical, and cost-utilization outcomes. Catheter Cardiovasc Interv. 2013;82:1–8.
4. Brilakis ES, Grantham JA, Rinfret S, et al. A percutaneous treatment algorithm for crossing coronary chronic total occlusions. JACC Cardiovasc Interv. 2012;5:367–79.

# What Equipment Should Be Available?

# 3

Emmanouil S. Brilakis

**Abstract**

The equipment necessary for performing chronic total occlusion (CTO) percutaneous coronary interventions (PCI) can be grouped into 12 categories: sheaths, guide catheters, microcatheters, guidewires, dissection/re-entry equipment, guide catheter extensions, snares, equipment for "balloon uncrossable" and "balloon undilatable" lesions, intravascular imaging, equipment for managing complications, equipment for minimizing operator radiation exposure, and stents. Use of an over-the-wire system is important for CTO PCI along with carefully selected guidewires based on the characteristics of occlusion. Antegrade dissection/re-entry is optimally performed using the CrossBoss catheter and Stingray balloon and wire. Guide catheter support can be significantly improved by using guide catheter extensions and other dedicated devices. Snares may be needed for externalization of the retrograde guidewire. Familiarity with the algorithm and equipment needed to treat balloon "uncrossable" and undilatable lesions is also important. Intravascular ultrasound can facilitate CTO crossing. Covered stents and coils are important to have available in case of perforation. Use of radiation shields can reduce operator radiation exposure and use of drug-eluting stents (especially second generation) is preferred.

**Keywords**

Equipment • Guidewire • Microcatheter • Balloon • Complications • Sheaths • Guide catheters • Snares • Laser • Rotational atherectomy • Guide catheter extensions • Covered stents • Coils • Radiation • Stents

Having the right equipment readily available for use is critical for achieving high success (and high efficiency) during CTO PCI, but also requires familiarity of each operator with each piece of equipment to enable appropriate and safe use. CTO PCI equipment is shown in Table 3.1, divided into "must have" and "good to have" categories [1–4].

E.S. Brilakis, MD, PhD
Department of Cardiology, VA North Texas Health Care System, Dallas, TX, USA
e-mail: esbrilakis@gmail.com

## Sheaths

Bilateral femoral 45-cm long sheaths are preferred by most CTO operators as they provide excellent guide catheter support and torquability by straightening the iliac artery tortuosity. Radial operators can either use 6 Fr (or rarely 7 Fr) sheaths or use a sheathless guide system (Eaucath, Asahi Intecc, Japan, available in 6.5, 7.5, and 8.5 Fr diameters, that create a puncture area equivalent to a 2 size smaller sheath). Alternatively, regular 8 Fr guides can be delivered using a 110 cm dilator that comes with a long 6 F Cook Shuttle sheath (See Chap. 13).



S. Rinfret (ed.), *Percutaneous Intervention for Coronary Chronic Total Occlusion: The Hybrid Approach*,
DOI 10.1007/978-3-319-21563-1_3

**Table 3.1** Checklist of equipment needed for CTO interventions

| Category no. | Equipment | Must have | Good to have |
|---|---|---|---|
| 1. | Sheaths | | 45-cm long sheaths (if using femoral access) |
| 2. | Guides | XB/EBU 3.0, 3.5, 3.75, 4.0<br>AL1, AL0.75<br>JR4<br>Y-connector with hemostatic valve (such as Co-pilot or Guardian) | 90-cm long<br>Side hole guides, especially AL1<br>Sheathless guides (if using radial access)<br>110 cm 6 F Cook Shuttle Sheath (for the dilator, to be inserted into an 8 F guide for sheathless transradial access) |
| 3. | Microcatheters | Finecross (150 cm for retrograde – 135 cm for antegrade)<br>Corsair (150 cm for retrograde – 135 cm for antegrade)<br>Small (1.20, 1.25, or 1.5 mm diameter) 20 mm long over-the-wire balloons of 145 cm or longer total length | Venture<br>Valet<br>MultiCross<br>Prodigy |
| 4. | Guidewires[a] | Fielder XT<br>Confianza Pro 12<br>Pilot 200<br>Sion<br>Fielder FC<br>RG3 wire (for externalization) | Miracle 3 or 12<br>Gaia wires and R350 |
| 5. | Dissection/re-entry equipment | CrossBoss catheter<br>Stingray balloon and wire | |
| 6. | Support devices | Guideliner or Guidezilla | |
| 7. | Snares | Ensnare or Atrieve 18–30 mm or 27–45 mm | Amplatz Gooseneck snares |
| 8. | Balloon "uncrossable-undilatable" lesion equipment | Small 20 mm long over-the-wire and rapid-exchange balloons<br>Tornus 2.1 and 2.6 | Rotablator<br>Laser<br>Angiosculpt |
| 9. | Intravascular imaging | IVUS (any) | IVUS (solid state) |
| 10. | Complication management | Covered stents<br>Coils + delivery microcatheters (such as Renegade or Progreat)<br>Pericardiocentesis tray | |
| 11. | Radiation protection | | Radiation scatter shields |
| 12. | Stents | Drug-eluting stents | |

[a]For radial operators, 300-cm wires or guidewire extension are needed since trapping cannot be used through a 6 Fr guide catheter for over-the-wire balloons, the CrossBoss catheter, and the Stingray balloon
Trapping through a 6 Fr guide catheter is feasible for the Finecross and the Tornus 2.1 microcatheter. Guidewire extensions (for the Asahi and Abbott guidewires) could be used instead, but long guidewires are preferred

## Guide Catheters

Dual 8 Fr guides are most commonly used for transfemoral CTO PCI, although some operators use femoral access for the antegrade and radial for the retrograde guide catheter. Using 90 cm long guides is useful if the retrograde approach is used, as it facilitates guidewire externalization. Use of supportive guide shapes is critical for success: usually XB and EBU are used for the left coronary artery and AL for the right coronary artery. Side holes can be used to minimize pressure dampening in the right coronary artery, but should not be used in an unprotected left main artery so that under perfusion of the large territory supplied by the left main is promptly recognized.

Using a Y-connector with a hemostatic valve (such as the Co-Pilot, Abbott Vascular, US or Guardian, Vascular Solutions, US) is important to minimize blood loss from back bleeding and is also easier to use.

## Microcatheters

An over-the-wire system should always be used for antegrade CTO crossing to increase wire support, and allow reshaping of the tip and easy guidewire exchanges. Although either a microcatheter or an over-the-wire balloon can be used, microcatheters are preferred because they have a marker at the tip *vs* in the middle of the shaft in 1.5 or 1.25 mm balloons and are more

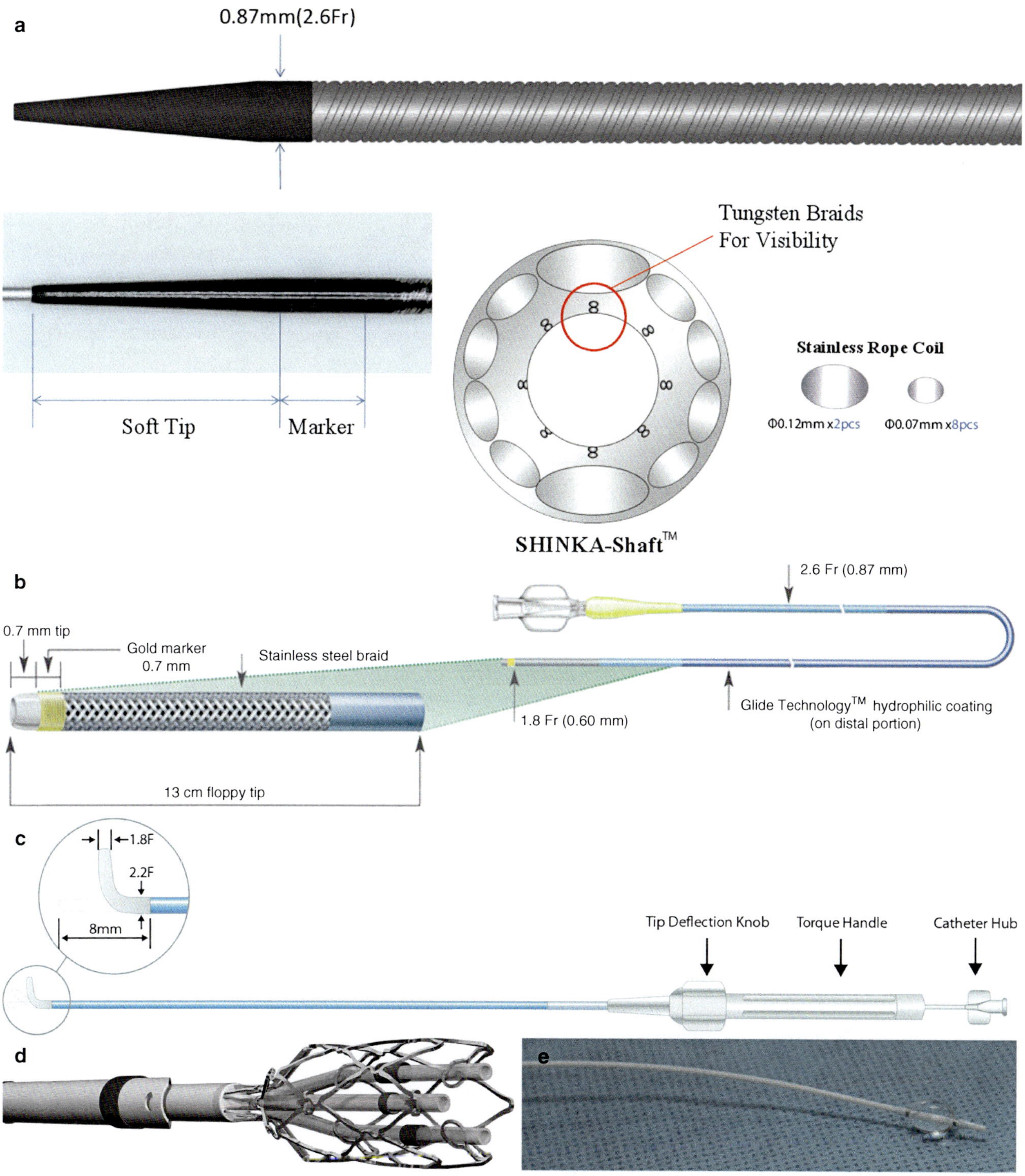


**Fig. 3.1** Illustrations of various microcatheters used for CTO PCI. (**a**) Corsair; (**b**) Finecross; (**c**) Venture; (**d**) MultiCross; (**e**) Prodigy (**a**: Reproduced with permission from Asahi Intecc.; **b**: Reproduced with permission from Terumo; **c**: Reproduced with permission from Vascular Solutions; **d**: Reproduced with permission from Roxwood Medical; **e**: Reproduced with permission from Radius Medical)

resistant to kinking. The three most commonly used microcatheters are the Corsair (Asahi Intecc, Japan), Finecross (Terumo, Japan), and Venture (Vascular Solutions, US). Two new microcatheters can facilitate antegrade crossing, the Multicross (Roxwood Medical, US) and the Prodigy (Radius Medical, US).

## Corsair

The Corsair microcatheter (Asahi Intecc, Japan) [5] has a "Shinka" shaft constructed with 8 thin wires wound with two larger wires, facilitating torque transmission (Fig. 3.1a). Its inner lumen is lined with a polymer that enables contrast injection and facilitates wire advancement. Moreover, the distal 60 cm of the catheter are coated with a hydrophilic polymer to enhance crossability. The tip is tapered and soft, contains tungsten powder to enhance visibility, and has a platinum marker coil 5 mm from the tip. The Corsair catheter is advanced by rotating in either direction, however it is braided to have better power when rotated counterclockwise. The catheter should not be over-rotated (>10 consecutive turns without release) to avoid deformation, entrapment or tip separation with the body of the catheter. The Corsair may have to be replaced if resistance to wire advancement is felt, especially after prolonged use (currently known as "Corsair fatigue").

### Turnpike

The Turnpike catheter (Vascular Solutions, US) is considered by many operators as an improved version of the Corsair catheter, with better coverage of the coils by the polymer tapered tip, reducing the risk of tip separation with the shaft of the catheter. Clinical experience is however limited. To date, most operators found the catheter to be stiffer than the Corsair. It is therefore best suited for septal than in epicardial collaterals, or for antegrade work.

### Finecross

The Finecross microcatheter (Terumo, Japan) has the lowest crossing profile available (1.8 Fr distal tip), stainless steel braid to enhance torquability and a marker located 0.7 mm from the tip (Fig. 3.1b). It is particularly useful for navigating tortuous epicardial collaterals, and is still the preferred antegrade microcatheter for many operators.

### Venture

The Venture catheter (Vascular Solutions, US, Fig. 3.1c) has an 8 mm radiopaque torquable distal tip with a bend radius of 2.5 mm [6–11]. By clockwise rotation of a thumb wheel on the external handle the tip can be deflected up to 90°. Rotating the entire catheter, enables steering in all planes. The Venture catheter is especially useful for CTOs after a severe bend, for example ostial circumflex CTOs [12]. The Venture catheter is compatible with 6 Fr guiding catheters and with 0.014″ guidewires. However, because of high shaft profile it cannot be removed using a "trapping balloon technique" unless an 8 Fr guide catheter is used [11].

### Multicross

The MultiCross catheter (Fig. 3.1d) is a tri-lumen support catheter with a nitinol scaffold to facilitate 0.014″ guidewire access across complex lesions. The scaffold anchors and centers the catheter to provide the operator with three separate 0.014″ lumen options. The clinical experience with this catheter is limited.

### Prodigy

The Prodigy catheter (Fig. 3.1e) has an elastomeric anchoring balloon mounted at the distal end that can expand up to 6 mm diameter [13]. The inflation lumen has a pressure relief valve that limits the inflation pressure to 1 mm Hg, anchoring the catheter in place while minimizing the risk for proximal vessel injury. The clinical experience with this catheter is also limited.

## Guidewires

Several guidewires are currently available for CTO PCI (Table 3.2), yet the following wires are most commonly utilized at present:

1. Fielder XT (Asahi Intecc, Fig. 3.2a): soft, polymer-jacketed, tapered wire often used as the first wire for initial antegrade crossing and for creating tight knuckles.
2. Confianza Pro 12 (Asahi Intecc, Fig. 3.2b): stiff, tapered-tip, penetrating wire, for antegrade crossing in cases with clearly identified anatomy.
3. Miracle 12 wire (Asahi Intecc, Fig. 3.2c): stiff, non-tapered tip wire, often used for equipment delivery after sub-intimal guidewire crossing, as it provides excellent support.
4. Miracle 3 wire (Asahi Intecc, Fig. 3.2c): stiff, non-tapered tip wire, which can be shaped to a smooth curve to deliver a microcatheter to a CTO cap located at a bifurcation, either retrograde or antegrade, as it prevents wire prolapse into the side branch.
5. Pilot 200 (Abbott Vascular, Fig. 3.2d): polymer jacketed and moderately stiff, non-tapered tip wire, for tortuous vessels or when the course of the target lesion and vessel is unclear. The Pilot wire can also be knuckled for sub-intimal crossing but forms wider and more powerful knuckles compared with the Fielder XT wire.
6. Sion (Asahi Intecc, Fig. 3.2d): hydrophilic, highly torquable soft guidewire with excellent shape retention for retrograde wiring through collaterals.
7. Gaia 1st, 2nd and 3rd: Gaia (Asahi Intecc) wires are the latest generation CTO that have an uncoated, distal, flexible coil, a variable (decreasing from Gaia first to third) tapered tip which is highly flexible and a tip to core design, which provides close to 1:1 torque. This wire is engineered to deflect if it encounters severe resistance and theoretically can be steered through a (relatively non-calcific) occlusion by gentle retraction and rotation when wire tip deflection is encountered.
8. Fielder FC (Asahi Intecc, Fig. 3.2a): polymer-jacketed soft wire for retrograde wiring through collaterals.

**Table 3.2** Description of coronary guidewires commonly utilized in CTO PCI

| Wire category | Tip style | Commercial name | Tip stiffness | Manufacturer | Properties |
|---|---|---|---|---|---|
| **Polymer covered** | | | | | |
| | Tapered | **Fielder XT**[a] | **1.2 g** | **Asahi Intecc** | Front-line wire for antegrade crossing. Can also be used for knuckle wire formation and for retrograde crossing |
| | Straight (non-tapered), low tip stiffness | **Fielder FC**[a]<br>Whisper LS, MS, ES<br>Pilot 50<br>Choice PT Floppy | **1.6 g**<br>0.8, 1.0, 1.2 g<br>1.5 g<br>2.1 g | **Asahi Intecc**<br>Abbott Vascular<br>Abbott Vascular<br>Boston Scientific | Used to cross through collateral vessels during the retrograde approach |
| | Straight (non-tapered), high tip stiffness | **Pilot 150 \| 200**[a]<br>Crosswire NT<br>PT Graphix Intermediate<br>PT2 Moderate Support<br>Shinobi<br>Shinobi Plus | **2.7 \| 4.1 g**<br>7.7 g<br>1.7 g<br>**2.9 g**<br>7.0 g<br>6.8 g | **Abbott Vascular**<br>Terumo<br>Boston Scientific<br>Boston Scientific<br>Cordis<br>Cordis | Antegrade crossing, especially when the course of the occluded vessel is unclear. Also useful for knuckle wire formation and for re-entry into true lumen during antegrade wire-based dissection and reentry technique |
| **Open coil (no Polymer jacket)** | | | | | |
| | Straight, low tip stiffness | **SION (hydrophilic)**[a] | **0.8** | **Asahi Intecc** | First choice guidewire for retrograde collateral navigation and crossing |
| | Tapered, low tip stiffness | Cross-it 100XT (0.010″)<br>Runthrough NS Tapered (0.008″) | 1.7 g<br>1.0 g | Abbott Vascular<br>Terumo | |
| | Tapered, high tip stiffness, hydrophilic coating | **Confianza Pro 9, 12**[a] **(0.009″ tip)**<br>PROGRESS 140 T, 200 T (0.0105″, 0.009″)<br>Persuader 9 (0.011″)<br>ProVia 9, 12 (0.009″) | 9.3 g,12.4 g<br>12.5 g, 13.3 g<br>9.1 g<br>11.8 g, 13.5 g | **Asahi Intecc**<br>Abbott Vascular<br>Medtronic<br>Medtronic | Antegrade crossing when vessel course is known |
| | Tapered, moderate tip, stiffiness, highly steerable, hydrophilic coating | Gaia First (0.010″)<br>**Gaia Second (0.011″)**[a]<br>**Gaia Third (0.012″)**[a] | 1.7 g<br>**3.5 g**<br>**4.5 g** | **Asahi Intecc** | Antegrade crossing when vessel course is known, especially when facing bends |
| | Straight tip, high tip stiffness, hydrophobic tip | **MiracleBros 3**[a], 4.5, 6<br>**MiracleBros 12**[a]<br>PROGRESS 40, 80, 120<br>Persuader 3, 6 (-philic and –phobic)<br>Provia 3, 6 (-philic and –phobic) | 3.9, 4.4, 8.8 g<br>13.0 g<br>5.5, 9.7, 13.9 g<br>5.1, 8.0 g<br>8.3, 9.1 g | Asahi Intecc<br>Asahi Intecc<br>Abbott Vascular<br>Medtronic<br>Medtronic | Antegrade crossing when vessel course is known<br>To deliver a microcatheter to a CTO cap located at a bifurcation, either retrograde or antegrade, preventing wire prolapse into the side branch<br>For device exchange when performing antegrade dissection and reentry |
| | Tapered, high tip stiffness, hydrophobic coating | Confianza 9 (hydrophobic)<br>Persuader 9 (hydrophobic)<br>ProVia 9, 12 (hydrophobic) | 8.6 g<br>9.1 g<br>11.8 g, 13.5 g | Asahi Intecc<br>Medtronic<br>Medtronic | Antegrade crossing when vessel course is known |
| Externalization wires | | Viper (0.014 tip)[a]<br>**RG3**<br>R350 | 3.6 g | CSI<br>**Asahi Intecc**<br>Vascular Solutions | 335 cm in length, 0.014" shaft<br>**330 cm in length, 0.012" shaft**<br>350 cm in length, 0.013" shaft |

Adapted from Brilakis et al. [4] with permission
[a]Most commonly utilized guidewires

9. RG3 (Asahi Intecc, Japan) wire for externalization after retrograde crossing.

Short guidewires (180–190 cm) are used in most cases and are exchanged using the trapping technique, however if 6 Fr guide catheters are used, long wires are preferred, as trapping is not always feasible. Alternatively, Abbott or Asahi guidewire extension can be used.

## Dissection/Re-entry Equipment

The CrossBoss catheter and Stingray balloon and guidewire (Boston Scientific, Fig. 3.3) are designed for sub-intimal CTO crossing and re-entry (antegrade dissection reentry or DR). The CrossBoss catheter (Fig. 3.3a) is a metallic over-the-wire catheter with a 1 mm blunt, rounded, hydrophilic-coated distal tip. It is rotated rapidly using a proximal torque device ("fast spin" technique). In approximately 1 in 3 cases the CrossBoss catheter can cross from true to true lumen [14], but if enters the sub-intimal space the Stingray catheter (Fig. 3.3b) can be used for re-entry [12, 15, 16]. The CrossBoss catheter has also emerged as the preferred catheter for true-to-true crossing of in-stent CTOs.

When inflated the Stingray balloon is 2.5 mm wide and 10 mm in length and has a flat shape with two side exit ports. The balloon is inflated at low-pressure (4 atm) resulting in self-orientation towards the true lumen [17]. The Stingray guidewire is stiff with a 20 cm distal radi-

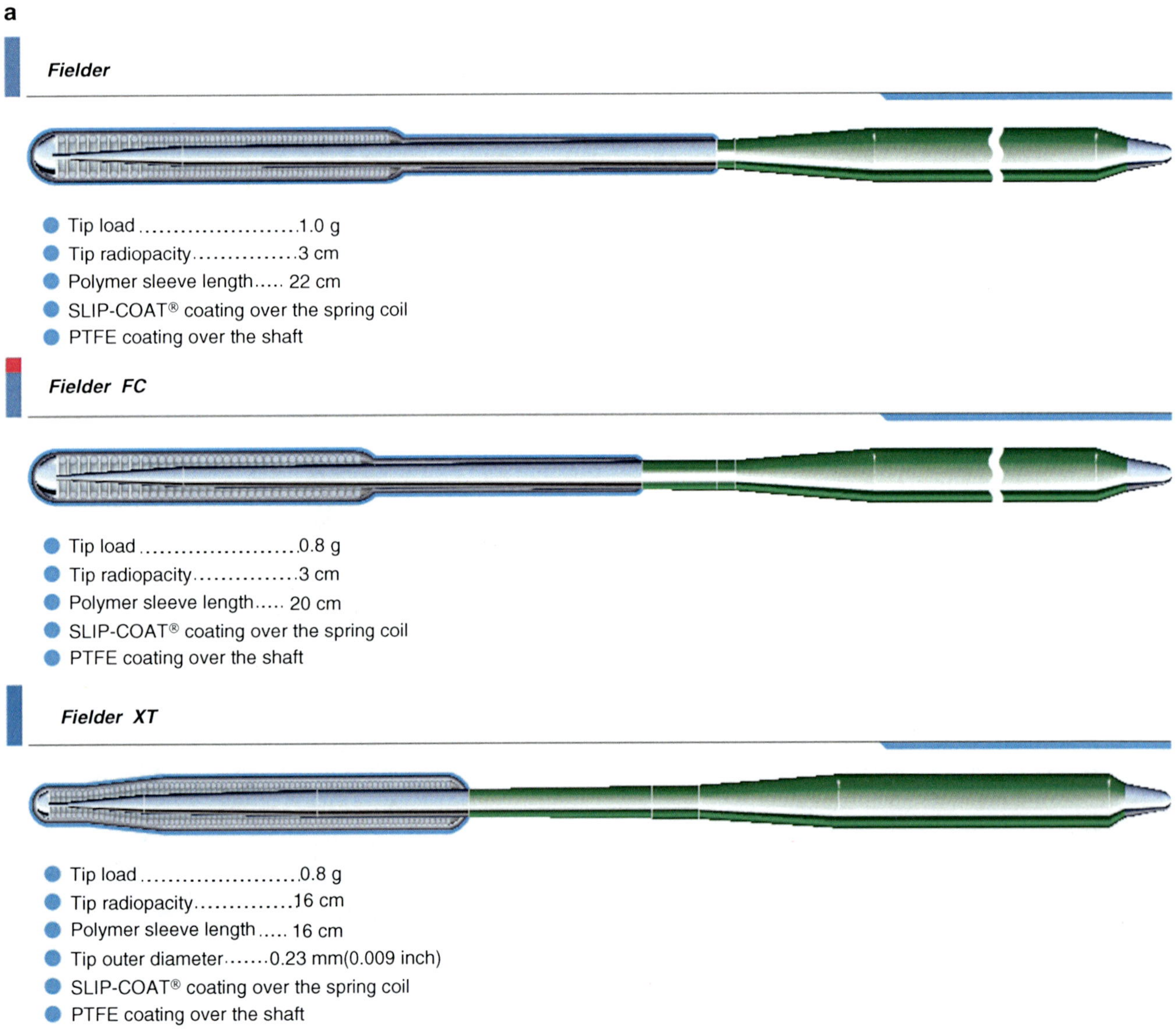


**Fig. 3.2** Illustrations of various guidewire families used for CTO PCI. (**a**) Fielder; (**b**) Confianza; (**c**) Miraclebros; (**d**) Pilot; (**e**) Sion (**a**–**c**, **e**: Reproduced with permission from Asahi Intecc.; **d**: Courtesy of Abbott Vascular. ©2014 Abbott. All Rights Reserved)

**b**

***CONFIANZA***

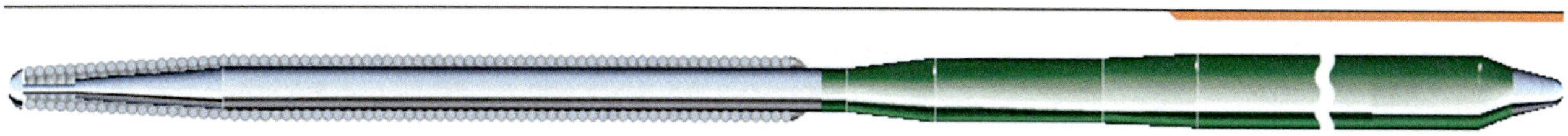

- Tip load .......................9.0 g
- Tip radiopacity............. 20 cm
- Tip outer diameter....... 0.23 mm(0.009 inch)
- PTFE coating over the shaft

***CONFIANZA PRO***

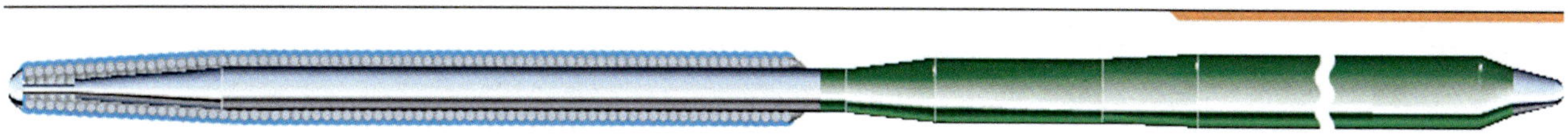

- Tip load .......................9.0 g
- Tip radiopacity...............20 cm
- Tip outer diameter....... 0.23 mm(0.009 inch)
- SLIP-COAT® coating over the spring coil
- PTFE coating over the shaft

***CONFIANZA PRO 12***

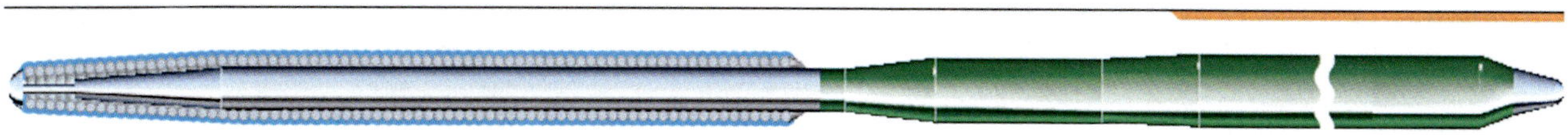

- Tip load .......................12.0 g
- Tip radiopacity...............20 cm
- Tip outer diameter..... 0.23 mm(0.009 inch)
- SLIP-COAT® coating over the spring coil
- PTFE coating over the shaft

**Fig. 3.2** (continued)

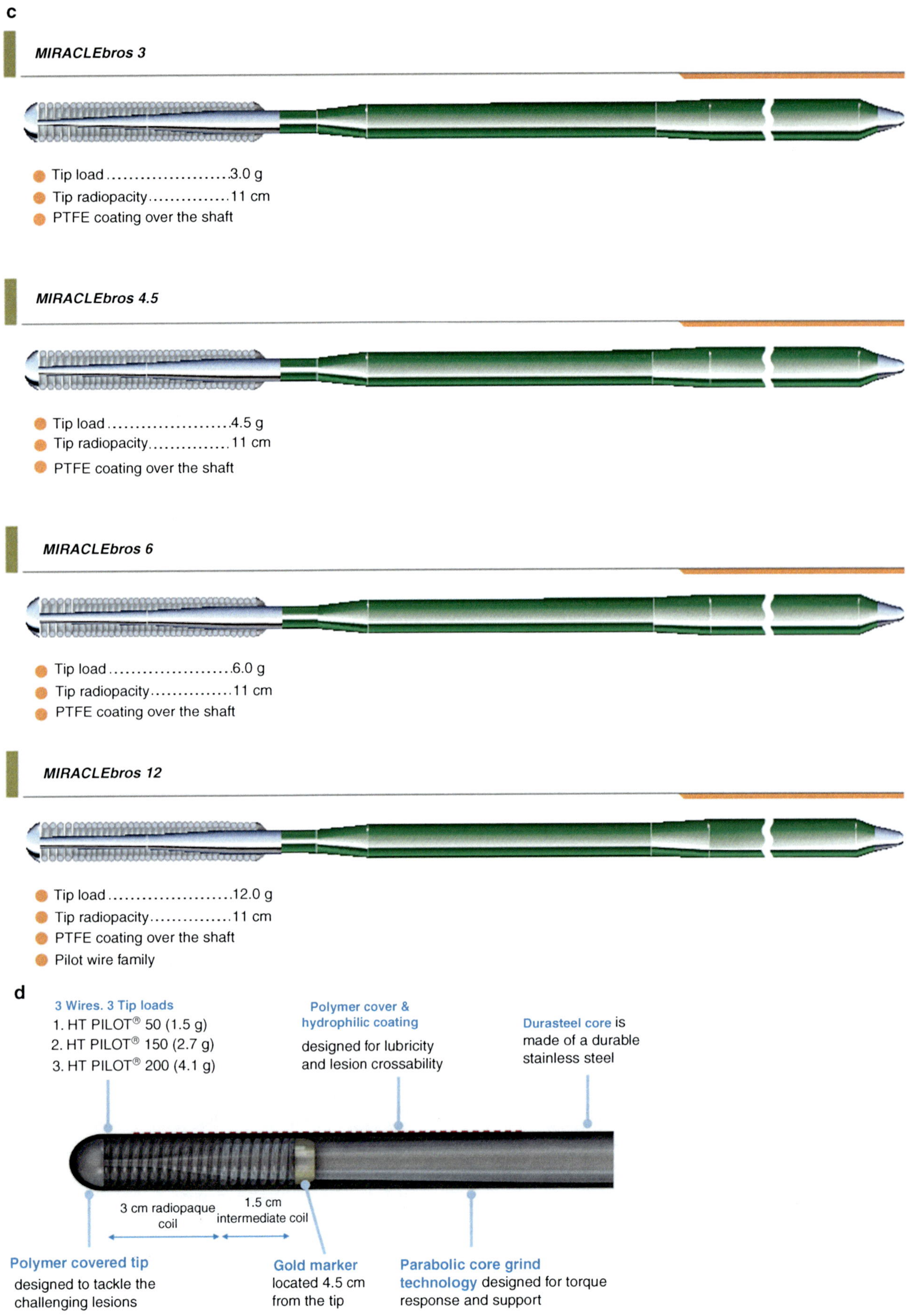


**Fig. 3.2** (continued)

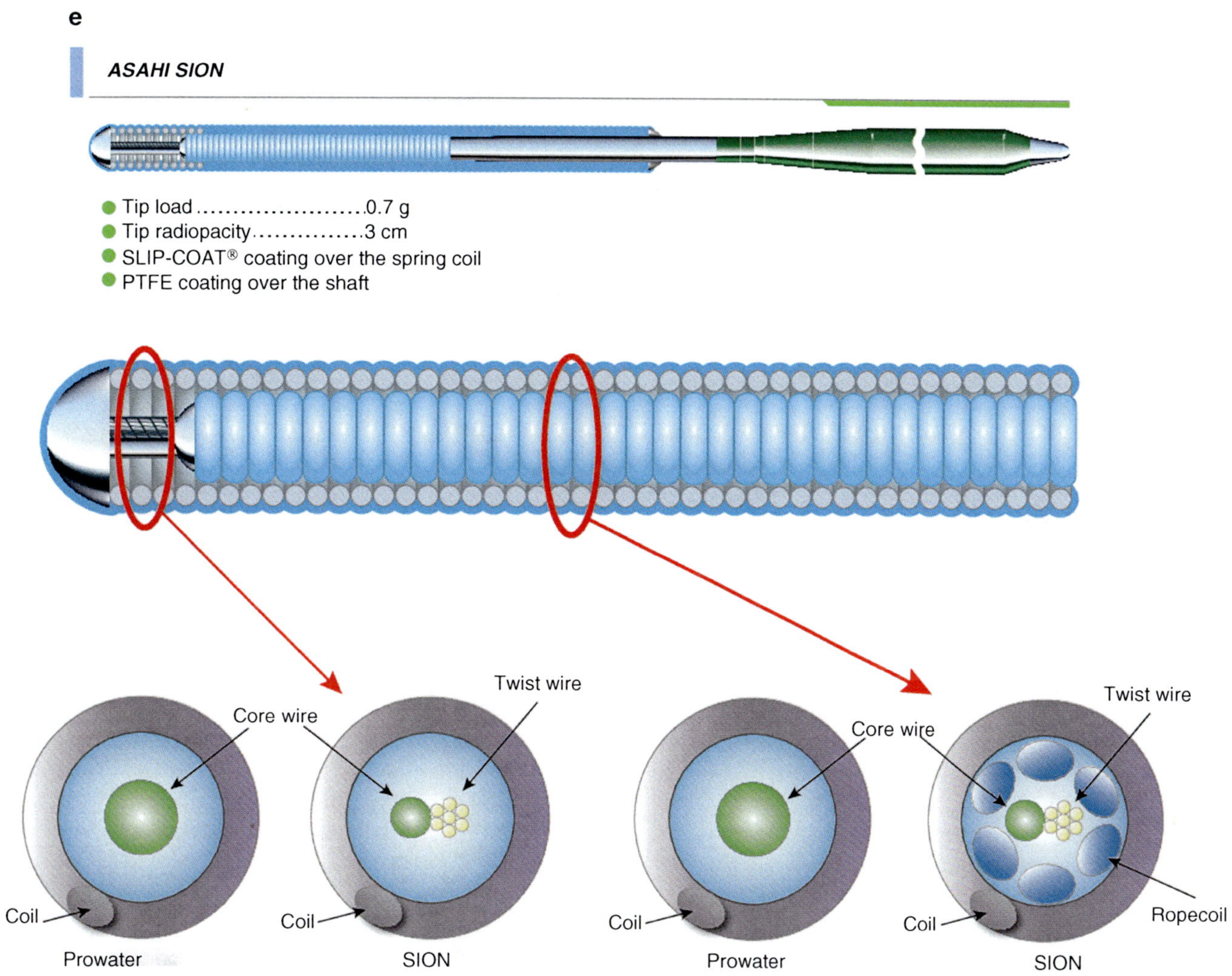


**Fig. 3.2** (continued)

opaque segment and a 0.009″ tapered tip with a 0.0035″ distal prong. The Stingray wire can be advanced towards one of the two side ports of the Stingray balloon using fluoroscopic guidance to re-enter the distal true lumen [12, 15, 16].

## Guide Catheter Extensions

There are two guide catheter extensions currently available in North America: the Guideliner V3 catheter (Vascular Solutions, US, Fig. 3.4a) and the Guidezilla (Boston Scientific, US, Fig. 3.4b). Both are rapid exchange, "mother and child" guide catheter extensions. The Guideliner V3 is manufactured in 4 sizes (5.5 Fr, 6 Fr, 7 Fr, and 8 Fr) that fit through a 6 Fr, ≥6 Fr, ≥7 Fr, and 8 Fr guide catheter, respectively, whereas the Guidezilla is only manufactured in 6 Fr size. Use of a guide catheter extension reduces the effective inner diameter of the guide catheter by approximately 1 Fr. Advancing equipment through guide catheter extensions can cause equipment loss or deformation [18], whereas deep intubation of a coronary artery carries a risk for dissection [19]. Use of a guide catheter extension can significantly facilitate completion of the balloon-assisted retrograde dissection and re-entry [20].

## Snares

Snares may be needed if the retrograde guidewire cannot be advanced into the antegrade guide catheter. Three-loop (tulip) snares, such as the Ensnare (Merit Medical, US) and the Atrieve (Angiotech), especially large ones (27–45 mm or 18–30 mm) are preferred, as they facilitate capturing the guidewire compared with the single-loop snares, such as the Amplatz Gooseneck snare (Covidien). However, smaller Gooseneck snares are useful to retrieve entrapped equipment in coronaries, like embolized stents.

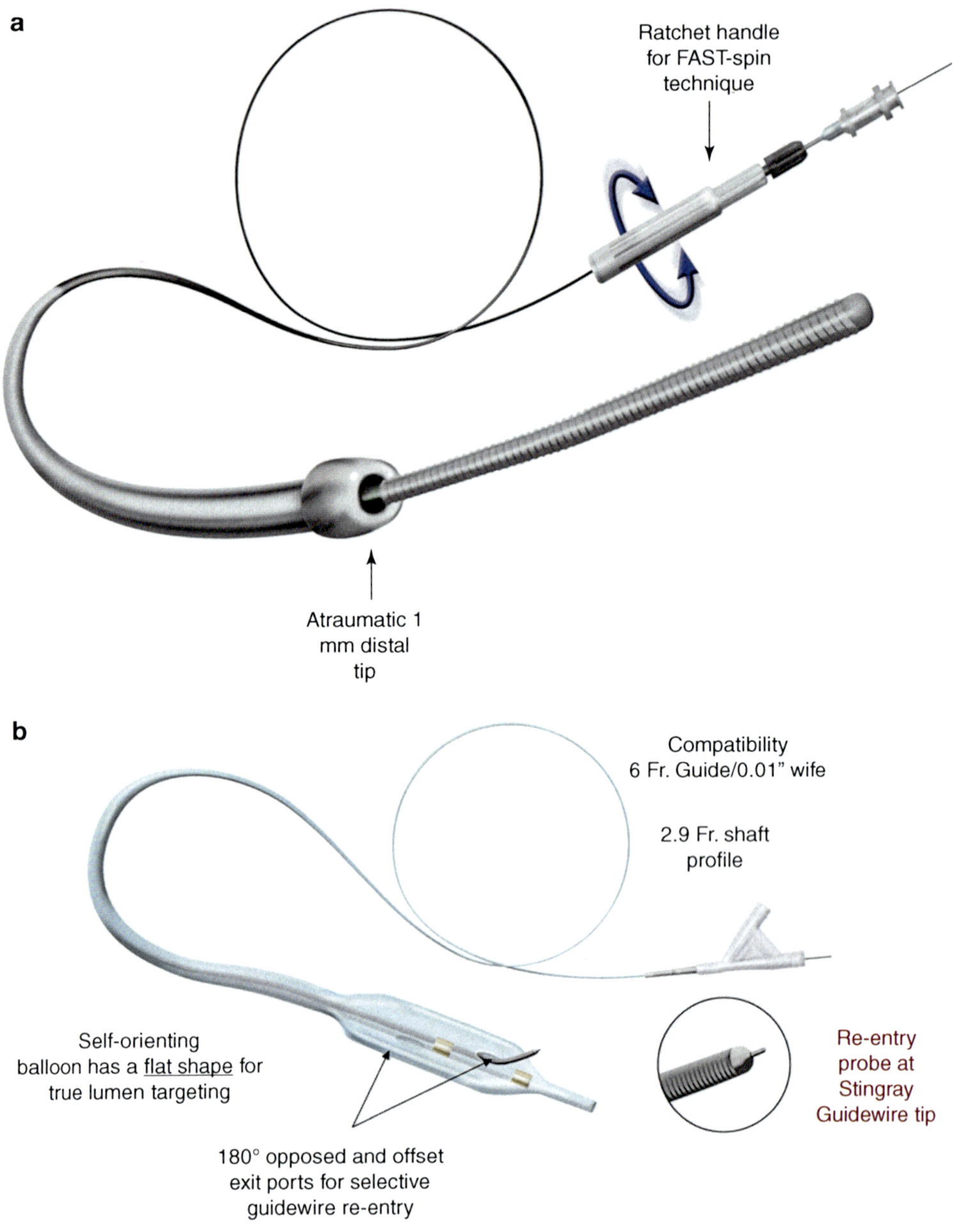


**Fig. 3.3** Illustration of the CrossBoss catheter (panel **a**) and the Stingray balloon and guidewire (panel **b**) (Image provided courtesy of Boston Scientific. © 2014 Boston Scientific Corporation or its affiliates. All rights reserved)

## Equipment for "Uncrossable – Undilatable" Lesions

Balloon uncrossable lesions can be approached with techniques that either modify the lesion (such as the Tornus catheter, laser, and rotational atherectomy), or that increase guide catheter support (such as guide catheter extensions and anchoring techniques).

The Tornus catheter (Asahi Intecc, Fig. 3.5) is manufactured with 8 stainless steel wires stranded in a coil [21]. It is available in two sizes (2.1 Fr and 2.6 Fr) and has a platinum marker 1 mm from the tip. The Tornus can be advanced by counter-clockwise rotation and withdrawn by clockwise rotation, converting rotational forces into forward advancement of the catheter. No more than 20 rotations should be done in any direction to prevent catheter kinking or unraveling. In contrast to the Corsair, contrast cannot be injected through a Tornus catheter, as it leaks through the stranded wire coils.

## Intravascular Ultrasound (IVUS)

Intravascular ultrasound can assist in several scenarios during CTO PCI, for example by identifying the proximal cap of the occlusion and confirming appropriate guidewire course, confirming true lumen entry of the retrograde guidewire, and assisting with appropriate balloon sizing during the CART and reverse CART techniques. Solid state IVUS systems are preferred to rotational systems, as imaging occurs closer to the catheter tip.

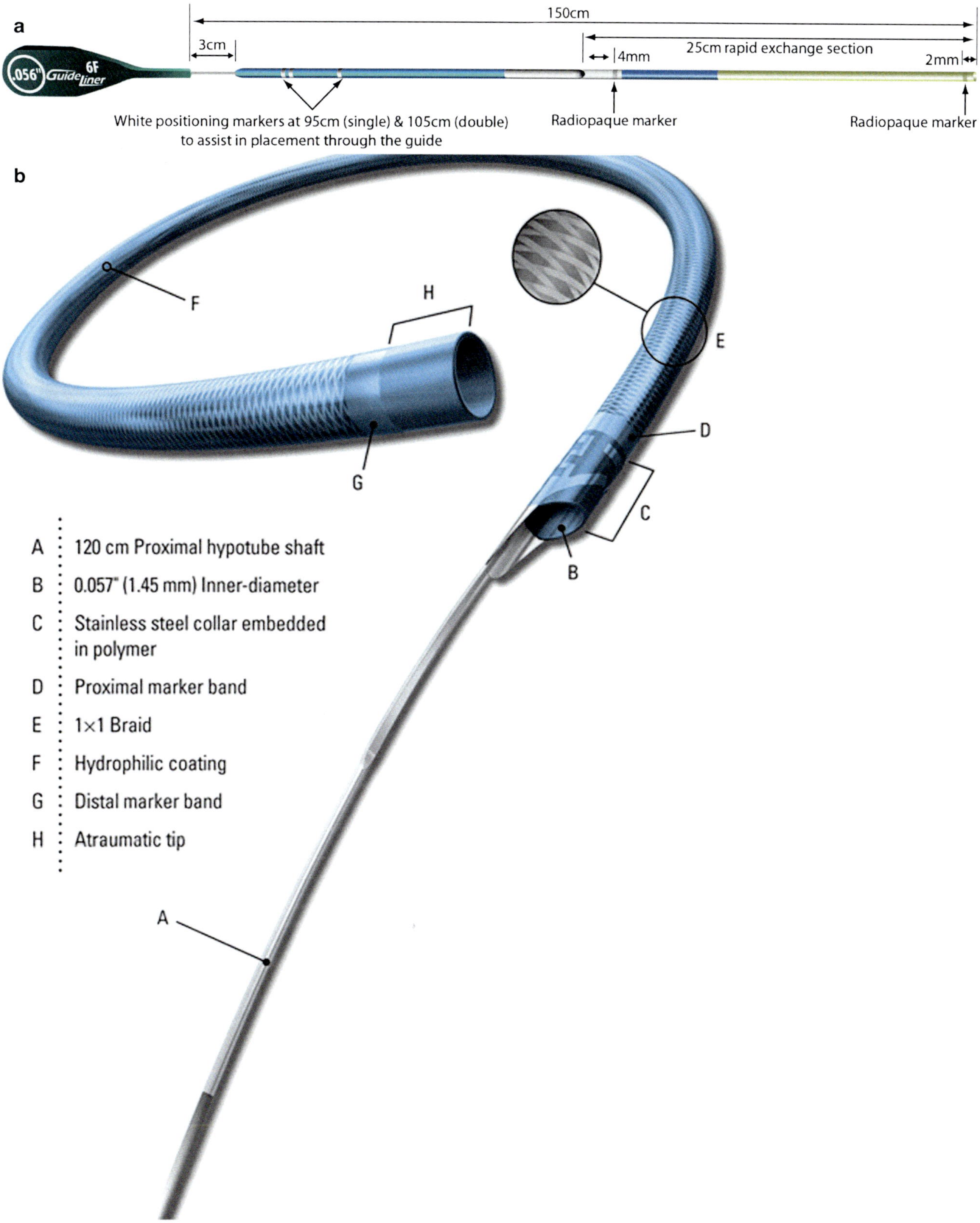


**Fig. 3.4** Illustration of the Guideliner V3 catheter (**a**) and the Guidezilla (**b**) (**a**: Reproduced with permission from Vascular Solutions; **b**: Image provided courtesy of Boston Scientific. © 2014 Boston Scientific Corporation or its affiliates. All rights reserved)

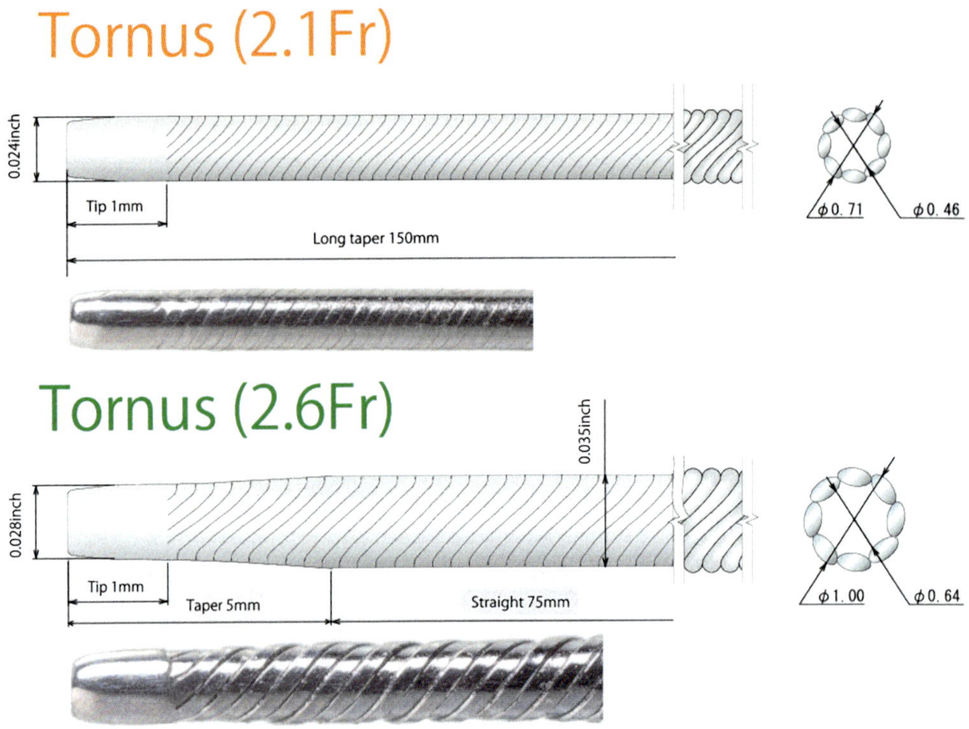


**Fig. 3.5** Illustration of the Tornus catheter (Reproduced with permission from Asahi Intecc)

## Complication Management Equipment

Covered stents and coils are important both for the CTO and non-CTO PCI to cover large vessel perforations [22]. There is only one covered stent available in the US and Canada (Jostent Graftmaster and Graftmaster Rx, Abbott Vascular), approved through a humanitarian device exemption [22, 23]. Covered stents can be challenging to deliver and require high pressure inflations (at least 15 atm but ideally higher) for adequate expansion. A 6 Fr guide catheter is required for 2.8–4.0 mm stents and a 7 Fr guide catheter for the 4.5 and 4.8 mm stents.

Coils should be available for use in case of distal branch or collateral vessel perforation [22]. Coils come into 0.014′ and 0.018′ size. Although 0.014′ coils will fit through a Finecross or Corsair microcatheter, 0.018′ ones require large microcatheters for delivery (such as the Renegade, Transit or Progreat) [24]. A coil pusher is also an asset. If coils are not available, thrombin [25] or microparticles (150–250 μm in diameter mixed with contrast to allow visualization under X-ray) can be injected instead.

## Radiation Protection Equipment

Fixed and disposable radiation shields, such as the RadPad® (Worldwide Innovations & Technologies, Inc) and radiation monitors that provide real time feedback on radiation exposure can be very useful for minimizing operator (and patient) exposure during CTO PCI.

## Stents

Drug-eluting stents should be used in all CTO PCI (unless the patient has a contra-indication to prolonged antiplatelet therapy), as they significantly reduce the risk for restenosis and reocclusion [26]. Second generation appear to be more efficacious compared with first generation drug-eluting stents [27].

Storing all CTO-related equipment on a dedicated CTO cart can facilitate their retrieval and increase the flow of the procedure See chap. 2, Fig. 2.2). Although every operator has his or her own preferences regarding equipment selection, consistent use of selected equipment is important for optimizing its use and ensuring optimal success and low complication rates.

## References

1. Brilakis ES. The essential equipment for CTO interventions. Cardiology Today's Intervention. May, June 2013.
2. Joyal D, Thompson CA, Grantham JA, Buller CEH, Rinfret S. The retrograde technique for recanalization of chronic total occlusions: a step-by-step approach. JACC Cardiovasc Interv. 2012;5:1–11.
3. Brilakis ES, Grantham JA, Thompson CA, et al. The retrograde approach to coronary artery chronic total occlusions: a practical approach. Catheter Cardiovasc Interv. 2012;79:3–19.
4. Brilakis ES, Grantham JA, Rinfret S, et al. A percutaneous treatment algorithm for crossing coronary chronic total occlusions. JACC Cardiovasc Interv. 2012;5:367–79.
5. Tsuchikane E, Katoh O, Kimura M, Nasu K, Kinoshita Y, Suzuki T. The first clinical experience with a novel catheter for

collateral channel tracking in retrograde approach for chronic coronary total occlusions. JACC Cardiovasc Interv. 2010;3:165–71.
6. McClure SJ, Wahr DW, Webb JG. Venture wire control catheter. Catheter Cardiovasc Interv. 2005;66:346–50.
7. Naidu SS, Wong SC. Novel intracoronary steerable support catheter for complex coronary intervention. J Invasive Cardiol. 2006;18:80–1.
8. McNulty E, Cohen J, Chou T, Shunk K. A "grapple hook" technique using a deflectable tip catheter to facilitate complex proximal circumflex interventions. Catheter Cardiovasc Interv. 2006;67:46–8.
9. Aranzulla TC, Colombo A, Sangiorgi GM. Successful endovascular renal artery aneurysm exclusion using the venture catheter and covered stent implantation: a case report and review of the literature. J Invasive Cardiol. 2007;19:E246–53.
10. Aranzulla TC, Sangiorgi GM, Bartorelli A, et al. Use of the venture wire control catheter to access complex coronary lesions: how to turn procedural failure into success. EuroIntervention. 2008;4:277–84.
11. Iturbe JM, Abdel-Karim AR, Raja VN, Rangan BV, Banerjee S, Brilakis ES. Use of the venture wire control catheter for the treatment of coronary artery chronic total occlusions. Catheter Cardiovasc Interv. 2010;76:936–41.
12. Brilakis ES, Lombardi WB, Banerjee S. Use of the stingray guidewire and the venture catheter for crossing flush coronary chronic total occlusions due to in-stent restenosis. Catheter Cardiovasc Interv. 2010;76:391–4.
13. Moualla SK, Khan S, Heuser RR. Anchoring improved: introduction of a new over-the-wire support balloon. J Invasive Cardiol. 2014;26:E130–2.
14. Whitlow PL, Burke MN, Lombardi WL, et al. Use of a novel crossing and re-entry system in coronary chronic total occlusions that have failed standard crossing techniques: results of the FAST-CTOs (Facilitated Antegrade Steering Technique in Chronic Total Occlusions) trial. JACC Cardiovasc Interv. 2012;5:393–401.
15. Werner GS. The BridgePoint devices to facilitate recanalization of chronic total coronary occlusions through controlled subintimal reentry. Expert Rev Med Devices. 2011;8:23–9.
16. Brilakis ES, Badhey N, Banerjee S. "Bilateral knuckle" technique and stingray re-entry system for retrograde chronic total occlusion intervention. J Invasive Cardiol. 2011;23:E37–9.
17. Michael TT, Papayannis AC, Banerjee S, Brilakis ES. Subintimal dissection/reentry strategies in coronary chronic total occlusion interventions. Circ Cardiovasc Interv. 2012;5:729–38.
18. Papayannis AC, Michael TT, Brilakis ES. Challenges associated with use of the GuideLiner catheter in percutaneous coronary interventions. J Invasive Cardiol. 2012;24:370–1.
19. Luna M, Papayannis A, Holper EM, Banerjee S, Brilakis ES. Transfemoral use of the GuideLiner catheter in complex coronary and bypass graft interventions. Catheter Cardiovasc Interv. 2012;80:437–46.
20. Vo M, Brilakis ES. Faster, easier, safer: "guideliner reverse CART" for retrograde chronic total occlusion interventions. Catheter Cardiovasc Interv. 2014;83:933–5.
21. Fang HY, Lee CH, Fang CY, et al. Application of penetration device (Tornus) for percutaneous coronary intervention in balloon uncrossable chronic total occlusion-procedure outcomes, complications, and predictors of device success. Catheter Cardiovasc Interv. 2011;78(3):356–62.
22. Brilakis ES, Karmpaliotis D, Patel V, Banerjee S. Complications of chronic total occlusion angioplasty. Interv Cardiol Clin. 2012;1:373–89.
23. Romaguera R, Waksman R. Covered stents for coronary perforations: is there enough evidence? Catheter Cardiovasc Interv. 2011;78:246–53.
24. Pershad A, Yarkoni A, Biglari D. Management of distal coronary perforations. J Invasive Cardiol. 2008;20:E187–91.
25. Kotsia AP, Brilakis ES, Karmpaliotis D. Thrombin injection for sealing epicardial collateral perforation during chronic total occlusion percutaneous coronary interventions. J Invasive Cardiol. 2014;26:E124–6.
26. Brilakis ES, Kotsia A, Luna M, Garcia S, Abdullah SM, Banerjee S. The role of drug-eluting stents for the treatment of coronary chronic total occlusions. Expert Rev Cardiovasc Ther. 2013;11:1349–58.
27. Lanka V, Patel VG, Saeed B, et al. Outcomes with first- versus second-generation drug-eluting stents in coronary chronic total occlusions (CTOs): a systematic review and meta-analysis. J Invasive Cardiol. 2014;26:304–10

# Specific Basic Techniques to Master in CTO PCI

4

William J. Nicholson

**Abstract**

CTO cap engagement and entry requires specialized guidewires and handling techniques. The four guidewire manipulation strategies of sliding, drilling and penetration are essential for successful initial progress. Leveraging the subintimal space when true lumen recanalization cannot be achieved is an essential skill employed by hybrid operators. Formation and utilization of a knuckled guidewire is one of the most common methods of entering and traveling safely in the subintimal space. When removing microcatheters and over-the-wire equipment, ensuring that distal wire position is secure is required to maintain positioning and safety. This is best accomplished by guidewire trapping during catheter exchanges.

**Keywords**

Sliding • Drilling • Penetration • Knuckle Wire • Wire Trapping • Trapping Balloon

Guidewire 'escalation' is the cornerstone of CTO crossing and recanalization. It is somewhat of a misnomer as sometimes sequential wires will go from soft to harder, but also from harder to softer. The wires utilized for crossing the CTO have unique qualities and require specialized techniques to, in some cases, safely and effectively traverse the fibrous proximal cap, and in other scenarios, facilitate leveraging the subintimal space to travel around the occlusion. The length of the lesion occlusion should guide the operator in selecting the appropriate initial crossing strategy. In general, lesions less than 20 cm are typically initially approached with true-to-true (TTT) lumen sequential wire strategy [1], while longer lesions will often require entry into the subintimal space followed by controlled re-entry strategies [2], often called dissection re-entry (DR) techniques.

**Electronic supplementary material** The online version of this chapter (doi:10.1007/978-3-319-21563-1_4) contains supplementary material, which is available to authorized users.

W.J. Nicholson, MD
Division of Interventional Cardiology, WellSpan York Hospital, York, PA, USA
e-mail: wjnichmd2@aol.com

## Approaching the CTO Segment

When approaching the CTO segment of the vessel, a workhorse non-CTO specific guidewire should be used to advance a microcatheter to the cap of the occlusion. Placing a microcatheter at the base of operation is advantageous and confers safety for several reasons. First, traversing the non-occluded, often heavily diseased, proximal vessel with CTO specific wires exposes the non-occluded segment to potential trauma due to the inherent penetrating qualities of CTO wires. Additionally, while a typical workhorse wire bend of 3 mm with a 45–75° angle is employed to navigate the patent vessel segment and advance a microcatheter to the cap of the occlusion, a CTO bend on the tip of the wire of 1 mm at a 30–50° angle will maximize the operator's ability to penetrate and navigate the occluded segment. By having the microcatheter delivered to the proximal cap when approaching the occlusion antegrade or distal cap when approaching the lesion retrograde, wire tip reshaping and exchanging for different niche specific guidewires can be done efficiently and safely. In general, most operators prefer to utilize microcatheters instead of over-the-wire balloons. Over-the-wire balloons have inherent shortcomings not intrinsic to microcatheters. As opposed to


S. Rinfret (ed.), *Percutaneous Intervention for Coronary Chronic Total Occlusion: The Hybrid Approach*, DOI 10.1007/978-3-319-21563-1_4

**Table 4.1** Guidewire handling techniques for approaching the CTO cap

| Guidewire technique | Guidewire choice (tip load) | Guidewire tip shape | Degree of torqueing | Tip force applied |
|---|---|---|---|---|
| Sliding and drilling | Fielder XT (0.8 g) | 1 mm 30–45° | Rapid spinning when facing resistance | Minimal – gentle probing and exploring the cap surface for microchannel presence |
| Controlled drilling | Pilot 200 (4.1 g)<br>Confianza Pro 12 (12 g) | 1 mm 30–45° | Controlled quick 90° clockwise and counterclockwise rotation | Intermediate – steady cap engaging force while burrowing the tip into a weak zone of the cap |
| Penetration | Confianza Pro 12 (12 g) | 1 mm 30–45° *Alternatively* 3 mm 30–45° if necessary to centralize wire tip engagement to the cap | None | Heavy – needle like approach to puncture the resistant cap |
| Push and torque | Gaia 1st, 2nd and 3rd | Pre-shaped | 90° wire redirection when the tip deflects | Intermediate – The tip will deflect when too much force applied |

microcatheters, the distal tip of over-the-wire balloons are not radiopaque and the marker on 1.5 mm and smaller balloons is a center marker, making it difficult to visualize the catheter tip's position in relation to the CTO cap. Over-the-wire balloons are also predisposed to kinking in angulated vessel segments when the wire is removed for reshaping or during exchanges, requiring removal of the balloon catheter and surrendering achieved progress.

## Wire Manipulation Techniques in CTO

Selection of the initial wire for attempted CTO crossing depends upon the morphologic characteristics of the cap. The CTO cap's appearance and response to being engaged with different tip strength guidewires will direct the operator as to which of three wire manipulation techniques will be most effective in entering and the traversing the CTO. These four common guidewire handling techniques are referred to as **sliding and drilling, controlled drilling, penetrating,** and **push and torque**. Table 4.1 outlines the wire choices and features of these three strategies. While wire selection and manipulation is different for each of these techniques, the guidewire tip shape is common to all three. The commonly referred to "CTO bend" of the guidewire tip consists of a 1 mm distal tip bent at a 30–45° angle (Fig. 4.1). Achieving this tip is accomplished by inserting the guidewire through the introducer tool exposing the distal 1 mm of the wire. The exposed wire tip is then firmly bent with the operator's finger or a syringe to avoid glove puncture. The only exception to this bending technique is with the Sion wire, when shaped for collateral crossing. This specific wire is sensitive to break if too firmly bended, so progressive and repetitive forces applied at the tip of the needle will result in a nice Sion bending without the risk of traumatizing the internal guidewire structure. This short tip with a hard angle of 30–45° cannot be

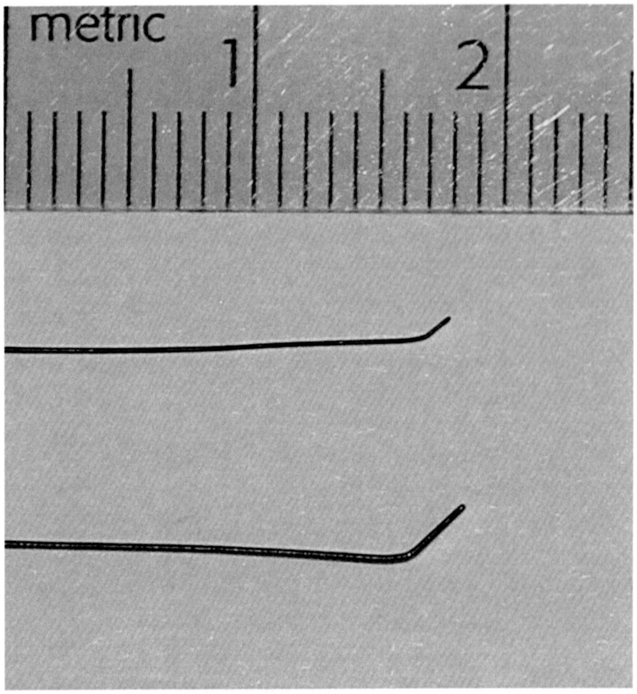


**Fig. 4.1** Typical "CTO bend" of a guidewire tip as compared to a typical "workhorse" guidewire tip used in non-CTO interventions

accomplished by shaping the wire against the side of the introducer tool with one's finger, as many operators prefer to do when shaping normal workhorse wires for non-CTO intervention. The Gaia wire comes pre-shaped with this typical CTO bend.

**Sliding and drilling** is usually the initial CTO crossing strategy attempted. Pathologic examination of CTO's reveal that there are often 160–230 μm vessel channels permeating through the proximal cap that connect the soft less fibrous core of the CTO to the patent proximal vessel lumen [3]. The sliding and drilling technique is an effort to explore the cap for these angiographically invisible microchannels. A polymer-jacketed 0.09 mm tapered tip wire (Fielder XT) with a low tip load (0.8 g) is advanced against the cap with gentle tip rotation in a probing fashion to explore the surface of the cap. Torqueing can be performed with or without a torqueing device, realizing that the wire will rotate much faster when the wire is manipulated directly on its shaft rather than through rotation of torqueing device with a larger radius. If the wire visually progresses through the cap via a microchannel, continued forward wire advancement through the mid portion of the occlusion with the same wire and technique is pursued, with efforts not to push the wire too much to avoid forming a knuckle wire or penetrating the sub-intimal plane. The lack of tactile feedback from the wire tip, especially with tapered-tip low-gram wire such as with the Fielder XT family mandates that the operator utilize the expected course of the vessel in multiple angles of view and observe the appearance of the wire to determine whether successful intraluminal progress is being made. In other words, the wire should be guided with fluoroscopic feedback, not tactile feedback. Once the wire is perceived to be across the CTO and in the true lumen, a sliding without rotation technique can be employed, where the wire is simply pushed with the tip away from the wall. The absence of resistance confirms true lumen positioning.

If sliding is initially ineffective or progression halts once entering the fibrous cap, **controlled drilling** is typically the next wire handling technique employed. Drilling is accomplished by controlled relatively quick 90° clockwise and counterclockwise rotations of the tip of a stiffer guidewire. Sometimes, operators will prefer to rotate the wire in the same direction. Speed of the rotation will vary upon the use or not of a torqueing device. In the interest of maintaining a simplified wire escalation algorithm, as exposed in Chap. 5, a Pilot 200 with a moderately stiff tip load (4.1 g) is initially utilized. When drilling, the guidewire is typically not pushed hard into the resistant occlusion, but instead, steady engaged contact is maintained between the fibrous cap and the wire tip. The burrowing quality created by the quick clockwise and counterclockwise quarter turns of the wire allows one to search for a soft zone on the surface of the resistant fibrous cap in order to lift a tissue channel to travel through distally. If progress is not made, rather than pushing harder, a stiffer tip load guidewire (12 g) such as a Confianza Pro 12 should be selected with the same technique. Drilling with a Pilot 200 may result in entering the subintimal space between the media and adventitia, but will rarely result in wire exiting the vessel architecture (wire perforation). In contrast, the stiff tip of the Confianza Pro 12 can penetrate the rubbery barrier of adventitia without difficulty and will often freely pass out of the vessel architecture into the pericardial space. Such wire exits are not uncommon and are most of the time of no clinical consequence, as long as antegrade injection or microcatheter advancement is not performed. Indeed, it is mandatory that the operator accurately identify the wire's distal location, most commonly with contralateral injections, prior to tracking a microcatheter or other equipment over the wire. Failure to accurately do this will convert the usually clinically inconsequential small wire exit perforation into a larger hole that is likely to bleed and result in tamponade.

Not uncommonly, a blunt or heavily resistant calcified cap is encountered and drilling with even the stiffest load tip wires is ineffective at breaching the barrier. In this situation, the operator must transition to a **penetration** wire handling technique (Fig. 4.2, Video 4.1, 4.2, 4.3, 4.4, 4.5 and 4.6). Penetration is accomplished with a Confianza Pro 12, which is the stiffest, highest tip load guidewire (12 g) currently available for coronary intervention. This technique consists of pointing the wire in the desired direction, and advancing it forward without rotation, but instead using the guidewire in a needle-like fashion. The tapered (0.09 mm) stiff tip combined with a hydrophilic coating gives the operator the maximum penetration when attempting to puncture the proximal cap. If the wire stops making progress, gentle drilling will help to track a different tissue plane and a penetration wiring technique can be resumed. In general, most wires will make faster progression with a combination of push and rotation. Keeping the microcatheter close to the tip of the wire when attempting a penetrating strategy can increase the tip load of Confianza Pro 12 to up to 60 g. This maximizes the penetrating power to the occlusion cap, but also increases the likelihood of perforating the vessel sidewall. Multiple angiographic views in order to confirm wire position, or exploring the wire path created by the Confianza Pro 12 with a wire less likely to leave the vessel architecture such as a Pilot 200 (wire 'de-escalation') are necessary prior to safely tracking equipment over the wire.

The fourth wiring strategy is the push and torque, which is quite unique to the Gaia family wires. These wires have a unique internal design and tapered tip that turn them extremely stiff and resistant when torqueing is applied to the wire, but their tip will still deflect when pushed forward. A good analogy is with a watch stainless steel bracelet. Although the bracelet can be bent easily between each link, it is impossible to bend the bracelet laterally, away from its longitudinal axis. With the Gaia wires, a torqueing device should be used, with minimal rotations, limited to 90° in each direction. The wire is pushed in the desired direction. When the tip deflects, the body of the wire enters into a sinusoidal conformation; at this point, the wire is pulled back and its tip redirected. This combination of push and turn is most likely to be successful with this wire (Fig. 4.2, Video 4.1, 4.2, 4.3, 4.4, 4.5 and 4.6).

The proximal cap may be too calcified or fibrotic that even the stiffest wire is unable to penetrate. In such cases, two alternative strategies are available. If suitable interventional collaterals are present, a retrograde strategy can be pursued. Alternatively, if the initial CTO cap entry strategies resulted in the wire entering the subintimal space

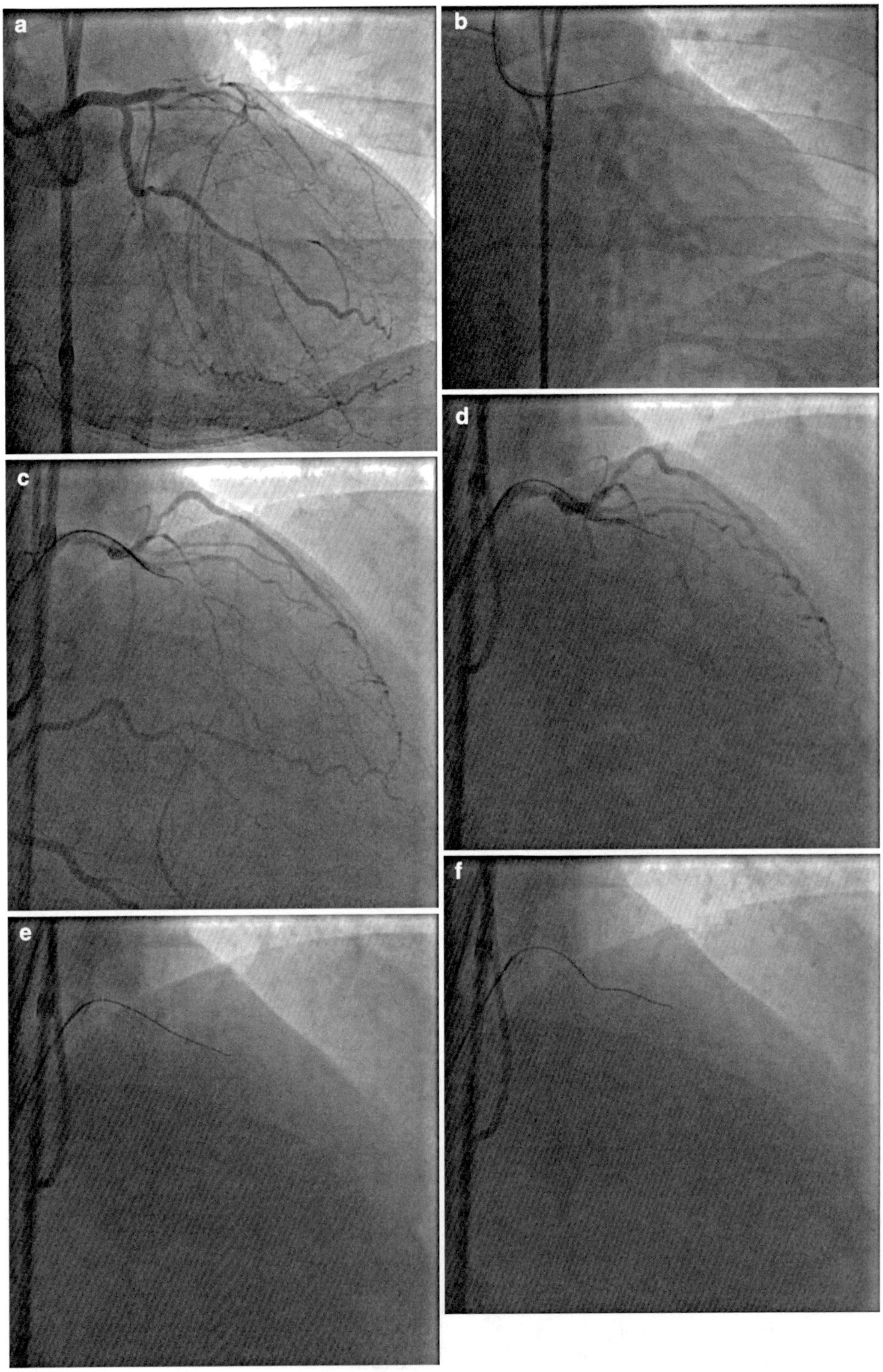


**Fig. 4.2** Tip deflection and torque technique using the Gaia wire. (**a**) Dual angiography showing a non-ambiguous and short CTO (Video 4.1). (**b**) Antegrade approach and puncture of the blunt cap with a Confianza Pro 12 using a penetrating technique (Video 4.2). (**c**) Dual injection showing the wire into the CTO segment (Video 4.3). (**d–i**) Through the Corsair, the wire was exchanged for a Gaia 3rd, and the wire is pushed up to feeling resistance and noticing a tip deflection. The tip is then rotated about 90–180° and the wire re-advanced. Finally, the wire penetrates the distal cap into the diagonal branch with a feel of 'pop and release' (Video 4.4). (**j, k**) Final result after wire exchange and stenting (Videos 4.5 and 4.6)

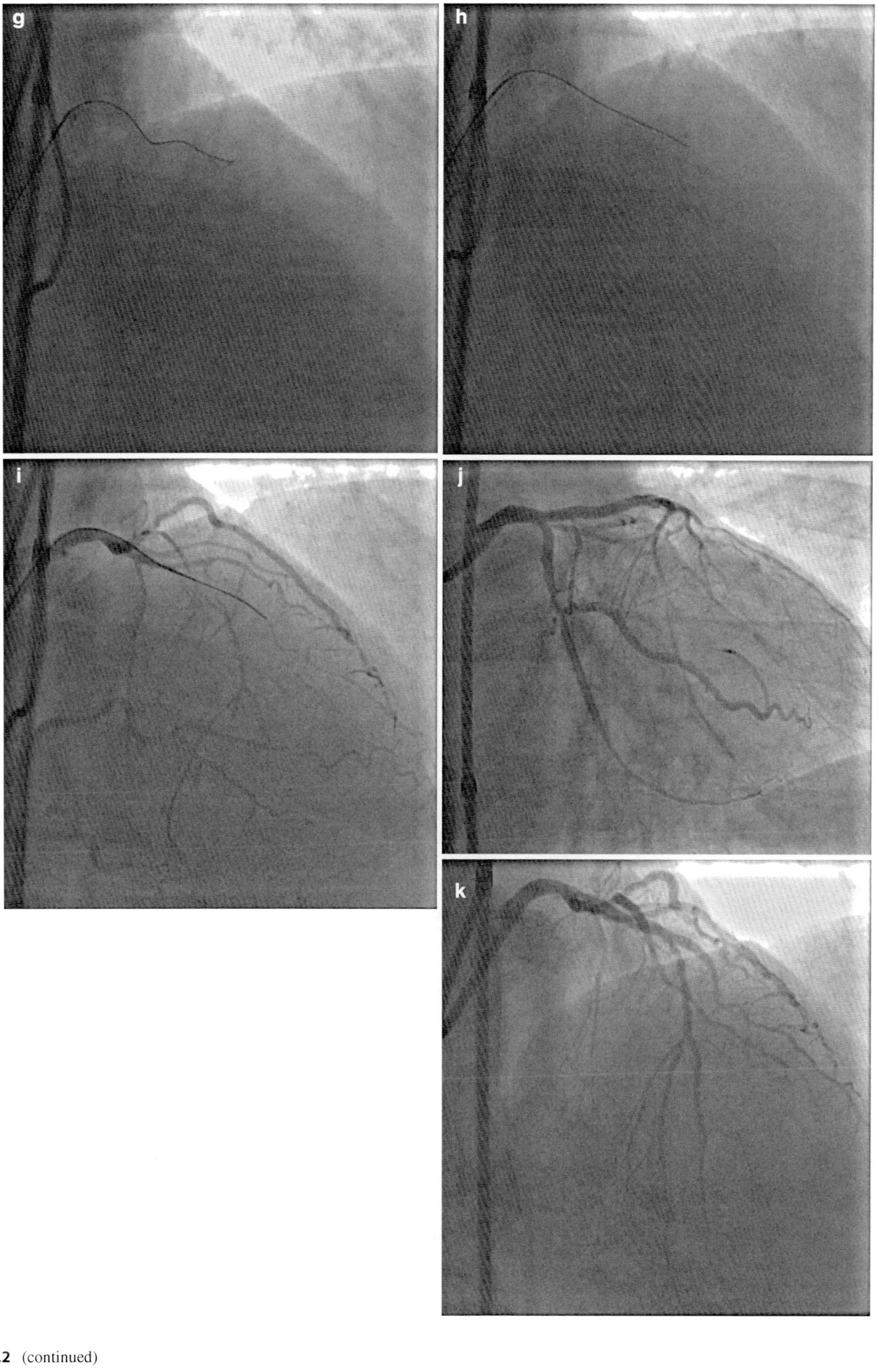


**Fig. 4.2** (continued)

and there is an appropriate distal vessel, antegrade DR can be pursued. Traversing the subintimal space can be accomplished by several methods. Because a stiff tapered guidewire (Confianza Pro 12) may have been the wire that accessed the subintimal space, the operator should be appropriately wary and concerned that the true location of the wire may be outside of the vessel architecture. Overcoming this ambiguity is one of the powerful properties of using a **knuckled wire**. Knuckling a wire is accomplished by pushing a polymer jacketed wire (Fielder XT or Pilot 200) with a typical CTO bend (Fig. 4.3a) out of the end of a microcatheter positioned close to the occlusion. The operator's goal is to have the tip of the wire engage a resistant segment of tissue (Fig. 4.3b). The close proximity of the microcatheter to where the tip of the wire is engaging the vessel resistance supplies the backup to push more wire forward. A rapid pecking technique of the wire tip into the occluded vessel may enhance the likelihood of engaging tissue and forcing the wire to fold upon itself and form a tight loop (Fig. 4.3c–f). After forcing the wire to fold upon itself and enter the subintimal space it is converted into instrument of blunt dissection which can be readily advanced forward (Fig. 4.3g–i). While some operators favor applying a small U-shape or umbrella handle to the tip of the wire to be knuckled, others prefer a typical 1 mm CTO bend to allow the initial tissue engagement to occur. A Fielder XT will typically form a tighter and smaller knuckle than a Pilot 200, but the pushing force through resistant segments of the occlusion may be greater with the Pilot 200.

A knuckle wire possesses several features that other subintimal techniques may lack. Knuckle wires almost never leave the vessel architecture and are therefore excellent tools to resolve vessel path ambiguity. Increasing the size of the loop of knuckled wire, usually by switching to a Pilot 200, is an effective technique in order to increase the likelihood of tracking the main vessel rather than sidebranches. Additionally, knuckle wires can typically traverse long distances of subintimal space in a short period of time. As the knuckle is advanced forward, the microcatheter should be tracked aggressively behind the knuckle to continue supplying the support necessary to continue pushing the knuckle forward (Fig. 4.3j). Many operators will recapture the knuckled segment of wire as the microcatheter is advanced and then re-express the wire in order to "manage" the knuckle's size. Tighter knuckles tend to create less subintimal space and hematoma and make antegrade or retrograde DR more favorable. If being used for retrograde DR, this allows the operator to quickly arrive at the base of operation for reverse CART. If a knuckle wire is used in as for antegrade DR, the large dissection created by the knuckle should be distally extended with a fine dissection device, such as the CrossBoss,

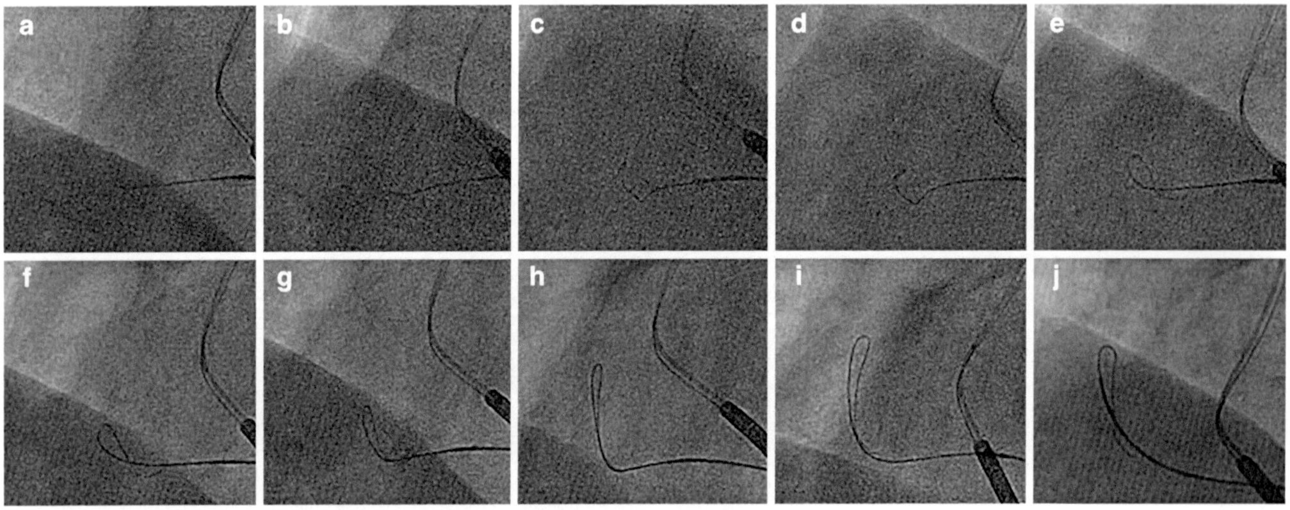


**Fig. 4.3** Series of steps to form and advance a knuckle wire in the subintimal space. Frame (**a**) demonstrates a typical CTO bend tip of a Fielder XT engaging the cap of a CTO (note the close proximity of a microcatheter behind the tip of the guidewire). After the guidewire becomes engaged and forward movement of the tip is impaired (**b**), more guidewire is advanced forward (**c**) creating an initial buckling of the wire. Additional wire is advanced until the guidewire begins to crumple (**d**) and fold upon itself (**e**, **f**). The folded knuckle of wire is pushed forward (**g**) entering the subintimal space, and can then travel via with blunt dissection of the vessel tissue planes past the occluded segment (**h**). Once in the subintimal space, the knuckled guidewire can be advanced rapidly and confidently forward as it will track within the vessel architecture (**i**). Following the knuckled wire with the microcatheter will allow the required pushing force necessary to continue to traverse the subintimal space (**j**)

in order to optimize positioning for successful controlled re-entry into the distal true lumen.

An important rule for the operator to adhere to when using knuckle wires is to avoid spinning or torqueing the knuckle. The looped and bunched segment of knuckled wire is predisposed to forming a knot if the wire is spun or torqued. When this happens, the knuckled wire can become permanently stuck in the subintimal space. Additionally, if a knot is formed, it is larger than the lumen of the microcatheter therefore cannot be withdrawn into the microcatheter. If this occurs during antegrade dissection reentry (ADR), the knotted knuckle wire and microcatheter can be removed as a single unit with the understanding that some vessel trauma may occur. If this occurs with retrograde DR, dragging the knot through a collateral channel used for retrograde access may result in significant collateral channel trauma and perforation. In such a case, one must consider intentionally snapping off the distal tip of knotted wire by pulling hard on the wire through the microcatheter, leaving it permanently behind in the subintimal space rather than risking significant trauma dragging it back through the collateral vessel. Because each of these scenarios and solutions are undesirable, prevention is the best strategy; it is important that the operator avoid spinning or torqueing knuckled wires.

## Trapping Balloon Technique

During CTO PCI it is often desirable to maintain a fixed distal wire position while exchanging the microcatheter for a different over-the-wire device. This occurs most frequently when the operator has either made progress distally within the target vessel or has crossed the CTO. In such scenarios, utilizing a **trapping balloon technique** allows the operator to remove or exchange over the wire equipment when using either a short (180–190 cm) or long (300 cm) guidewire. Trapping imparts both safety and stability to distal wire position. During catheter exchanges, this prevents inadvertent distal movement of CTO guidewires which are particularly susceptible to distal vessel perforation, and can guarantee a guidewire in a favorable position will not be accidentally pulled back. Trapping is achieved by first withdrawing the over-the-wire device on the guidewire several centimeters back into the guide catheter (Fig. 4.4a, b). A balloon is then introduced via the Y-connector directly into the guide, without placing it on a guidewire, but instead advancing it alone next to the equipment already in place within the guide catheter. The balloon is then advanced to the distal end of the guide catheter, past the over the wire equipment that had been partially withdrawn (Fig. 4.4c). Because the balloon is not on a wire, visualization of the balloon catheter can be difficult and careful attention must be given to ensure that the operator does not inadvertently advance the balloon out of the end of the guide catheter and unnecessarily traumatize the proximal coronary artery. Once the balloon is within the guide catheter but distal to the over-the-wire device being removed, it is inflated (Fig. 4.4d) to high pressure. Inflating the balloon will pin the wire to the guide and fix its position, allowing the operator to freely remove the over-the-wire device without needing to observe the now immobilized distal wire position on fluoroscopy (Fig. 4.4e). Once the over-the-wire equipment is removed from the guide catheter, a different over-the-wire device can be placed on the guidewire and advanced within the guide catheter while keeping the trapping balloon inflated. Fluoroscopy is again not necessary as the new equipment can be advanced until it stops due to its abutment into the inflated trapping balloon (Fig. 4.4f). At this point, the guidewire will be available to the operator out of the back end of the over-the-wire device. The trapping balloon is then deflated (Fig. 4.4g, h) and the new over-the-wire device is advanced into the coronary artery to the base of operation. Trapping within the guide invariably entrains air into the guide catheter system. As a result, it is imperative that the operator allows the guide to bleed back by opening the Y-connector until the guide catheter is air free.

The inner diameter of the guide catheter being utilized dictates what balloon size should be used for trapping and limits which equipment can be trapped. Typically, a 2.0 mm rapid exchange balloon is used for trapping in 6 Fr guide catheters. The lower profile of rapid exchange balloons is desirable, but using a 6 Fr system will not provide the catheter space to allow the operator to trap a Stingray balloon, CrossBoss or Coronary Laser Atherectomy catheters. 7 and 8 Fr guide catheters do not limit trapping of the typically utilized CTO equipment. A 3.0 mm balloon is typically chosen for trapping in both 7 and 8 Fr guide catheters. Longer balloons provide the inherent quality of more surface contact with the wire being trapped and 20 mm length balloons are desirable, especially when trapping hydrophilic polymer jacketed wires. The trapping balloon should be inflated to 15–20 atmospheres in order to ensure the wire is adequately pinned. Guide catheter damage resulting from the inflated trapping balloon, even to very high pressure, has never been observed or documented.

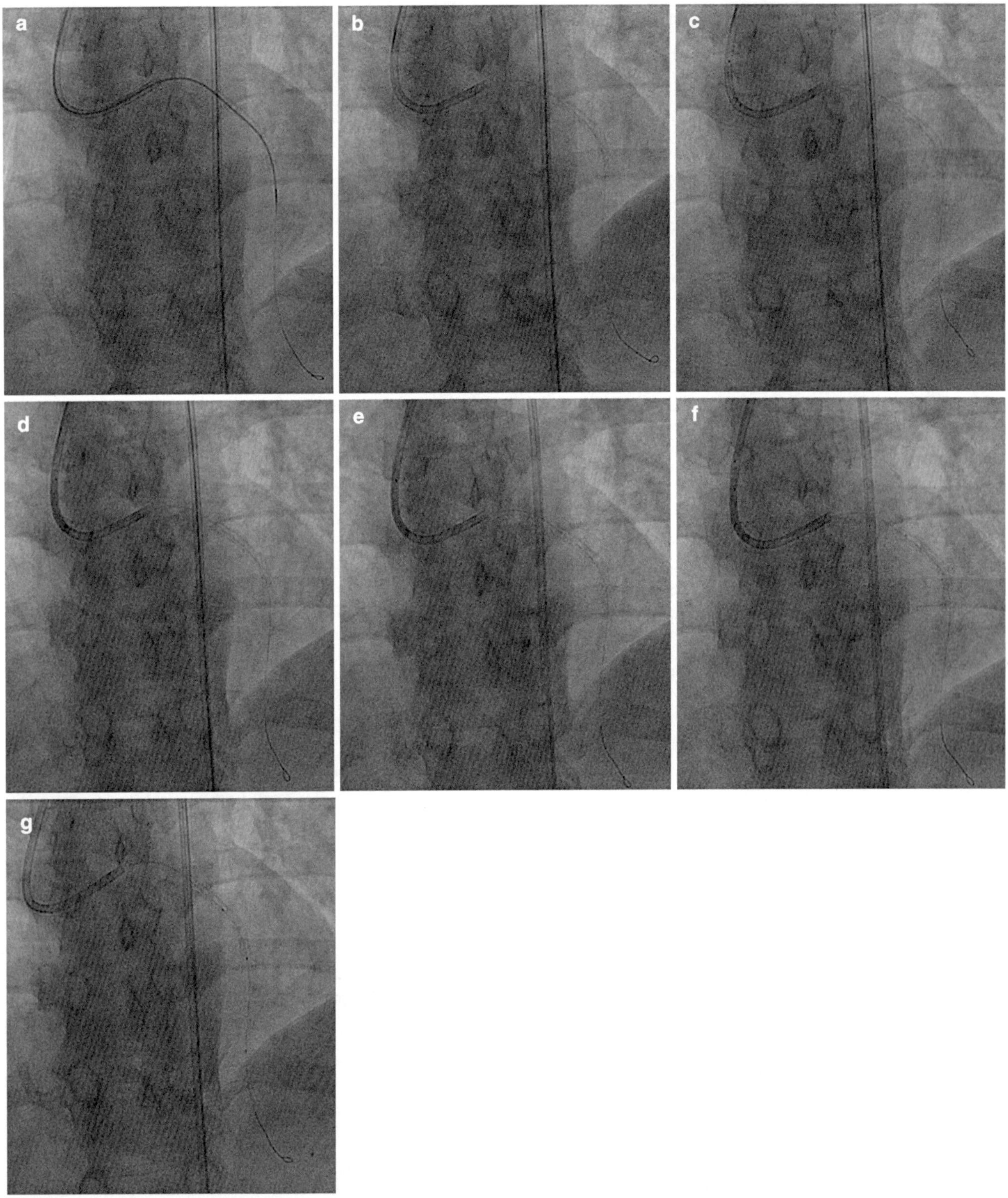


**Fig. 4.4** When removing an over-the-wire device from the coronary artery (**a**), wire trapping for catheter exchanges is accomplished by first withdrawing the over-the-wire device to be removed approximately 5–10 cm into the guide catheter (**b**). A balloon is then inserted and advanced beside the already in place equipment just distal to the over the wire device being removed (**c**). The balloon is then inflated (**d**) and the over-the-wire device is removed while the trapping balloon pins the guidewire to the inside of the guide catheter (**e**). The new over-the-wire device is then inserted on the trapped guidewire and advanced until the inflated trapping balloon impedes further advancement (**f**). The trapping balloon is then deflated and removed (**g**), at which time the Y-connector must be allowed to bleed back to remove any air which has been entrained

## References


1. Morino Y, Kimura T, Hayashi Y, et al. In-hospital outcomes of contemporary percutaneous coronary intervention in patients with chronic total occlusion insights from the J-CTO Registry (Multicenter CTO Registry in Japan). JACC Cardiovasc Interv. 2010;3:143–51.
2. Brilakis ES, Grantham JA, Rinfret S, et al. A percutaneous treatment algorithm for crossing coronary chronic total occlusions. JACC Cardiovasc Interv. 2012;5:367–79.
3. Stone GW, Kandzari DE, Mehran R, et al. Percutaneous recanalization of chronically occluded coronary arteries: a consensus document: part 1. Circulation. 2005;112:2364–72.

# When and How to Perform an Antegrade Approach Using a Wire Escalation Technique

5

James C. Spratt

**Abstract**

Antegrade wire escalation (AWE) represents the most frequent and still the most successful way of chronic total occlusion (CTOs) recanalisation. Its application is optimal within short, well-defined occlusions, where the principles of using increasingly stiff coronary guide wires to penetrate the proximal cap of the occlusion, negotiate through the occluded segment, before penetrating the distal cap into the lumen beyond the occlusion are employed. Wire selection is a decision based on the interactions between the engineering characteristics of the wire, arterial anatomy and wire behavior, with the principles of least possible force being applied. Within the CTO environment guide wires are used selectively and specifically, increasing the rationale for over-the-wire (OTW) equipment and specialty microcatheters. OTW equipment is near indispensable to a successful CTO procedure by facilitating wire exchanges/wire shaping; accessing the proximal CTO cap and crossing resistant plaque. Adjunctive imaging, in the form of cardiac computed tomography angiography (CTA) and intravascular ultrasound (IVUS) can help identify peri-procedural complexity and overcome challenges, such as an unclear vessel course. Although a high success rate can be expected in selected cases with AWE, the common failure modes are due to either failure to address the proximal cap or by inadvertent sub-intimal wire passage. Where the procedure is failing to progress, an alternate strategy should be employed.

**Keywords**

Chronic total occlusion • Proximal cap • Intimal plaque • Microcatheter • Wire escalation • Dual injections • Guide wire

## Introduction

CTO percutaneous coronary intervention (PCI) has evolved from "conventional" PCI, where a coronary guide wire is passed across, but not through, near-occlusive coronary plaque, before balloon dilatation and stent implantation. Fundamentally, with CTO PCI, the objectives remain the same: to connect the proximal true lumen with the distal true lumen, disobliterate the occlusion and scaffold the plaque by deploying a stent. The difference is the presence of an occlusive plaque, which both obstructs and obscures the vessel course. The extent and nature of the obstruction will determine the applicability of these techniques which are most analogous to conventional PCI and which can be termed antegrade wire escalation (AWE).

The majority of CTO cases are still performed successfully by AWE [1], with iterations in techniques that have been informed primarily by advances in wire and microcatheter design [2]. Antegrade wire escalation relies on the principle of least possible force, starting with soft, often polymer-coated wires, before progressing to wires with higher tip loads in the

J.C. Spratt, BSc, MD, FRCP, FESC, FACC
Department of Cardiology, Forth Valley Royal Hospital, Larbert, UK
e-mail: james.spratt@nhs.net



S. Rinfret (ed.), *Percutaneous Intervention for Coronary Chronic Total Occlusion: The Hybrid Approach*,
DOI 10.1007/978-3-319-21563-1_5

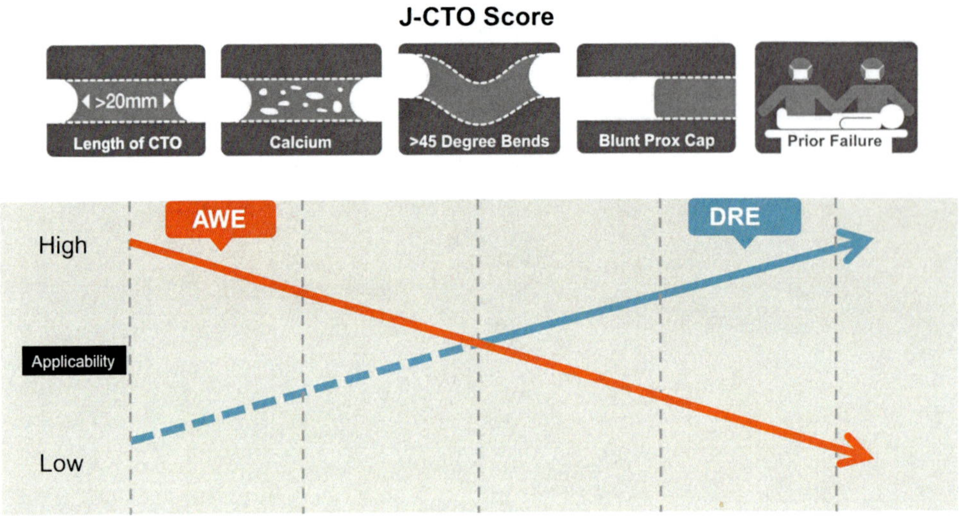


**Fig. 5.1** With increasing lesion complexity there is a decreasing applicability for antegrade wire escalation based strategies and an increasing need for strategies utilizing blunt dissection. *AWE* Antegrade Wire Escalation, *DRE* Dissection-Re-Entry

event of failure to make progress. The intention is to remain within intimal plaque in the CTO segment and thus to enter the lumen of the vessel beyond the distal cap of the occlusion. The development of specialized CTO-specific wires and microcatheters have led to more complex lesion subsets being able to be treated. So although the applicability of AWE remains broad, it is highly dependent on anatomical factors [3]. This chapter builds on concepts and techniques exposed in Chap. 4. The limitations of AWE in more complex anatomy have led to the development of other techniques involving access via the collateral circulation (retrograde) and/or blunt dissection either in an antegrade or a retrograde direction [2, 4].

## Anatomical Subsets that Favor Antegrade Wire Escalation

The applicability of AWE has an inverse relationship with lesion complexity (Fig. 5.1). The most commonly accepted measure of lesion complexity is the J-CTO score [5], where complexity is described by 5 characteristics: lesion length more than 20mm, blunt proximal cap, in-CTO bend of more than 45 degrees, calcified CTO segment, and previous failure. One factor adds 1 point to the J-CTO score, for a maximum of 5 points. CTOs with J-CTO scores of 0 are considered easy, those with 1 point intermediate, 2 considered difficult and those with 3 or more points very difficult.

### Lesion Length

CTO length is a predictor of both case efficiency and chance of inadvertent sub-intimal wire passage [2]. Whilst it is possible to treat longer occlusions by AWE, increasing CTO length functions as a surrogate marker of procedural efficiency, with longer occlusions resulting in longer case times, higher inadvertent rates of sub-intimal wire passage and lower procedural success rates [5]. There is no biological explanation for a binary cut-off in length when deciding what strategy to employ and it may be reasonable for other anatomical features to influence this, not least the feasibility of other strategies.

Lesion length is both a measure of complexity and procedural duration (efficiency), with longer lesions (>20 mm) requiring a longer time to wire and being associated with both a higher chance of inadvertent sub-intimal wire passage and vessel perforation [6]. The argument has been made, therefore, for the prospective use of blunt dissection techniques in longer lesions, with >20 mm having been chosen as the cut-off [7]. It may be, that in the argument for aiming for a more efficient procedure, the development of newer guide wires will result in longer occlusions being treatable efficiently by AWE.

### Proximal Cap Anatomy

For a procedure to be successful from an antegrade perspective, the proximal cap needs to be defined, either angiographically, or by adjunctive imaging (CT coronary angiography or intravascular ultrasound). The morphology of the proximal cap can be described as tapered, blunt or ambiguous (Fig. 5.2), where ambiguity is defined as a lack of clarity as to the subsequen vessel course.

The proximal cap of the occlusion, submitted to diastolic pressure, is usually the area of the most adverse vessel remodeling [8], with higher concentrations of both fibrous and calcific tissue being present. A blunt proximal cap is more likely to be resistant to penetration than a tapered cap, with a higher implied need for coronary guidewires with a high penetration force. There is also a relationship between how "blunt" the proximal cap is and lesion chronicity [9]. If a proximal cap is described as "ambiguous", the term describes a lack of clarity of the subsequent vessel course. The most common causes of

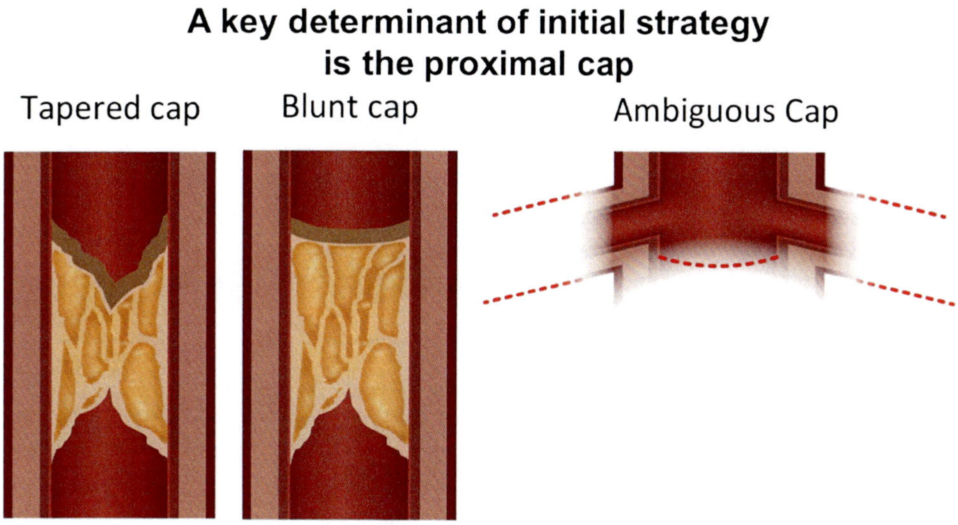


**Fig. 5.2** The proximal cap is a key determinant of procedural strategy and be described as tapered, blunt or ambiguous

"ambiguity" in the proximal CTO cap are either the presence of a (at least moderate sized) side branch or multiple bridging collaterals. Proximal caps associated with significant adverse vessel remodeling and or calcium are more likely to require the early use of highly penetrative wires to advance beyond the proximal cap of the occlusion. The combination characteristics, therefore, of both "bluntness" and ambiguity suggest a requirement for a high penetration wire and a lack of certainty over where it should be directed. It is for this reason that the presence of an ambiguous cap usually implies that a retrograde strategy is best employed and believed to be safer than an antegrade approach. For an AWE strategy to be employed, any ambiguity of the proximal cap must be clarified.

## In-CTO Tortuosity (>45°)

Tortuosity within the CTO segment is associated with both a higher risk of inadvertent sub-intimal wire passage and vessel perforation [6]. This is especially the case when associated with calcium, where the higher resistance to forward progress often necessitates the use of highly penetrative wires, with a consequently higher risk of vessel exit at points of curvature. The presence of in-CTO tortuosity is both a predictor of lesion complexity [5] and a marker of the peri-procedural need to switch strategy [10, 11].

## Presence of Intra-CTO Calcium

The presence of calcium indicates a higher need for penetrative wires and a highly supportive interventional set-up. Where the calcium is very severe, it may not be possible to penetrate with the current generation of wires and blunt dissection strategies may need to be employed to circumnavigate extreme areas of calcification.

## Previous Procedural Failure

As a marker of failure this captures factors associated with lesion complexity, which may be additive, rather than individually predictive, of lesion complexity. In addition factors related to the initial procedure may create difficulties for subsequent procedures, such as the creation of sub-intimal dissection planes.

## Other Factors

So, whilst increasing complexity may predict a decreasing chance of success by AWE, there are specific anatomic considerations that must also be taken into account when deciding the initial choice of strategy:

## Degree of Disease in the "Distal Landing Zone"

The "quality" or degree of plaque burden, of the vessel beyond the distal cap can be referred to as the "distal landing zone". This term largely relates to the feasibility of re-entry procedures, which have negotiated the CTO segment by blunt dissection and aim to "re-enter" the lumen of the distal vasculature from the sub-intimal space. A highly diseased distal landing zone may, however, adversely affect the chances of any antegrade strategy and may favour, if extreme, a primary retrograde procedure.

## Presence of "Interventional Collaterals"

Whilst not directly affecting the feasibility of AWE, the presence of collaterals that can be crossed by interventional equipment (and thus deemed "interventional") will affect the pre-procedure planning in selecting the most appropriate strategy [12].

## Basic Principles of CTO PCI

The fundamental tenets of CTO PCI address the differences between CTO PCI and "conventional" PCI and set the groundwork for a successful procedure regardless of strategy employed.

### Planning

Ad hoc CTO PCI is not recommended, given the critical role planning plays in assessing the anatomical features discussed above. Off-line analysis facilitates detailed analysis of collateral channel pathways enabling a more considered evaluation of the risk/benefit ratio [12].

### Visibility

Occlusive plaque renders the vessel course, in the absence of significant adventitial calcium, invisible. Whilst its course may be inferred, from either previous angiographic films or predictive anatomy, this is inaccurate and difficult to employ within highly mobile coronary vessels. Most CTOs are supplied by the contralateral coronary circulation, so the distal vasculature beyond the occlusion, when viewed by an antegrade injection, is either invisible or only faintly visible. Visualizing the distal coronary bed, via a second guide or diagnostic catheter, is a critical way of ensuring any progress is within the vessel structure. Dual injections also offer an invaluable way of assessing the contralateral collateral circulation, assessing the feasibility of a potential retrograde approach, accurately assessing CTO length and the size and location of the distal target vessel, evaluating whether there is a significant bifurcation at the distal cap, and thus for deciding on the optimal CTO PCI strategy. It is not infrequent to reveal patent microchannels within the CTO segment that were invisible with single catheter injection. The reliance on single catheter visualization for CTO PCI not only reduces distal vessel visibility, rarely adding useful information on wire progress, but also runs the risk of proximal contrast-induced dissection. Dual injection is best performed at low magnification, with prolonged imaging exposure, and without table panning, to allow for optimal delineation of the CTO segment and collateral vessel location and course. The donor vessel (vessel that supplies the territory distal to the CTO) is injected first, followed by injection of the occluded vessel. Bridging collaterals are important to recognize and avoid during both antegrade and retrograde crossing attempts to minimize the risk of vessel perforation, especially when advancing microcatheters and balloons, as their course is invariably outside the CTO artery structure. It is recommended that dual catheter injections are undertaken with interventional guides in both CTO and donor vessel. This will permit a rapid change in strategy if required. However, for operators who are not proficient with the retrograde approach, a diagnostic catheter can be used for contra-lateral guidance of the antegrade work.

### Back-up Support

There is a high need for back-up support within CTO procedures. This is most commonly increased passively by larger French guide catheters, but can also be addressed successfully by "high-support" catheters. Additionally the back up support provided to CTO crossing (either by wires or microcatheters/balloons) can be increased by several methods. For more details, please refer to Chap. 12.

### Use of "Over-the-Wire" Equipment

As CTO procedures use wires for highly selective purposes, there is a high need to either exchange wires or reshape wire tips. The use therefore, of over-the-wire (OTW) equipment enables wire exchange or reshaping without loss of position. OTW equipment will also help increase back-up support for wires, with the weight required to deflect the tip of the wire increasing as the OTW equipment is moved closer to the wire tip. Either OTW balloons or microcatheters can be used; however, OTW balloons are usually less adapted, with balloon tips generally too stiff to deliver co-axial force within tortuous coronary arteries. Moreover, they are more easily kinkable after guidewire removal, in such situation leading to the incapacity to advance a wire though the catheter. Finally, the marker is not at the tip; true position of the distal balloon tip may be uncertain. For all those reasons, we strongly recommend the use of a microcatheter. Such microcatheters are discussed in Chap. 3.

### Wire Selection

There have been considerable advances in wire technology, which have enabled more complex CTOs to be treated. The engineering characteristics of the wire can now be translated with a high degree of precision into clinical characteristics and should inform the operator's choice of wire. While a myriad of choices are available, a more circumscribed choice facilitates a greater understanding of wire handling characteristics, with associated efficiency and economic benefits. A choice of four specific CTO wires will cover most anatomy and can be divided up accordingly:

#### Tapered Polymer-Coated Wires

These are employed to access fine, difficult to visualize angiographically, channels. The polymer coating increases wire lubricity, allowing it to negotiate plaque-dense environments, which otherwise exposed coil wires would be unable to. The low gram weight of the wire, combined with the distal polymer sleeve, means they are rarely associated with vessel exit or inadvertent dissection, as such they are often chosen as the first wire of choice [1]. Examples are the Fielder XT, Fielder XT-A or Fielder XT-R.

#### Medium Weight Wires

There is considerably more diversity within this subset, with variations dependent on tip load, tip coating and torque transmission. Choices are informed on differential ability to transmit torque and the lubricity of either the sleeve or the tip of the wire. Medium gram weight polymer wires are a reliable step-up wire, where low gram weight polymer wires have failed to progress. Again, the presence of the polymer sleeve makes spontaneous vessel exit unlikely at the cost of decreased tactile feel. Examples are the Pilot 150 or 200.

#### High Gram Weight Wires

These highly specified wires are designed to penetrate dense, occlusive plaque and are often tapered at the tip to increase the amount of penetration force that can be applied. The trade-off for the high penetration force is a relative lack of tactile feel which restricts their use to well defined anatomy. Commonly used wires in that family are the Confianza Pro 12, or Progress 200 T.

#### Medium Weight Highly Toqueble Wires

This is the Gaia wire family. These wires have a unique internal design and tapered tip that turn them extremely stiff and resistant when torqueing is applied to the wire, but their tip will still deflect when pushed forward. With the Gaia wires, a torqueing device should be used, with minimal rotations, limited to 90° on each direction. The wire is pushed in the desired direction. When the tip deflects, the body of the wire enters into a sinusoidal conformation; at this point, the wire is pulled back and its tip redirected. This combination of push and turn is most likely to be successful with this wire. Those tapered wires can exit the vessel structure; therefore, care should be applied when using these wires in ambiguous CTO segments.

## The Proximal Cap & How to Assess It

As part of any antegrade procedure, assessment of the proximal cap of the occlusion is perhaps the most important procedural element. Histological data informs us that it is the site of the highest plaque density, with more evidence of calcification and adverse remodeling [8]. Any attempt to wire the distal true lumen of an occlusion may be hampered by early sub-intimal wire passage, as a consequence of eccentric proximal calcification and a failure to appreciate the 3D anatomy of the cap. The proximal cap should be visualized in several (at least 3) orthogonal planes, without radiographic panning. If this is insufficient to define the proximal cap, a selective injection of contrast can be made, via a microcatheter placed just proximal to, but not in, the cap.

The morphology of the cap contributes to defining lesion complexity, and can be described as tapered, blunt or ambiguous (Fig. 5.2). A tapered cap has little or no associated ambiguity and is less likely to require a highly penetrative wire, whereas a blunt cap is a marker of lesion chronicity [8]. If, in the case of an ambiguous proximal cap, the vessel course cannot be clarified this would preclude any antegrade approach and favor a primary retrograde approach.

## Wire Selection: Principles and Rationale

In navigating through a CTO, the wire may have to first penetrate the proximal cap; negotiate in-CTO tortuosity, before penetrating the distal cap and accessing the distal vasculature in a non-traumatic fashion that permits subsequent equipment delivery. It is often not possible for one wire to meet all the engineering challenges inherent with such anatomical heterogeneity. It is from these challenges and the problems encountered when trying to make one wire fit all that the principle of wire selectivity has developed. Modern wires have been engineered to address anatomical challenges, but in delivering certain characteristics, there will inevitably a trade-off with others. Although we refer to antegrade wire 'escalation' the change from one wire to the other, some situations mandate a de-escalation, where the next wire to be used will be softer and more appropriately suited for the next task. It is suggested therefore that wires are chosen, as the course of the CTO is crossed, on the basis of what function is required, with certain key principles adhered to:

### Polymer-Coated Wires

A durable polymer or plastic-jacketed wire causes the wire to be more lubricious, but have less tactile feel. As such polymer wires excel at negotiating hidden (in-CTO) tortuosity, but are less helpful in distinguishing between luminal and sub-intimal wire passage. The lubricity of polymer wires is increased by contact with water; hence they should be wiped before use and the microcatheter flushed. If in contact with a microcatheter for a prolonged period the polymer coat may swell, causing it to interact with the microcatheter and feel "sticky". These wires are mainly advanced by gentle rotation, which reduces the coefficient of friction; they lend themselves less well to fine, torque-dependent movements.

## Penetration Force

The penetration force of a wire is a function of the amount of gram weight required to deflect the wire tip and the surface area of the tip; a tapered-tip on a wire will increase both ease of access to small channels and the penetration force of the wire. The penetration force of a wire can also be further increased by moving a microcatheter (or balloon) nearer to the wire tip. Very high gram weight wires often have less good tactile feel making them a poor choice to negotiate long CTO segments.

## Tactile Feel

The tactile feel of a wire will be improved if the tip is uncoated. Some wires deal with the problem of lesion resistance by having an uncoated tip, but a polymer/hydrophilic sleeve on the shaft. This means that the majority of resistance felt is tip, rather than shaft resistance.

## Newer Generation Wires

Gaia (Asahi Intecc) wires are the latest generation CTO that have an uncoated, distal, flexible coil, a (variable, decreasing from Gaia first to third) tapered tip which is highly flexible and a tip to core design, which provides close to 1:1 torque. This wire is engineered to deflect if it encounters severe resistance and theoretically can be steered through an (relatively non-calcific) occlusion by gentle retraction and rotation when wire tip deflection is encountered.

## Wire Selection

This should be determined by a combination of anatomy and desired function. CTOs with lower markers of lesion complexity will have less need for high gram weight wires and particularly in the presence of a tapered proximal cap, can often be crossed with a combination of a tapered, low gram weight polymer wire and a medium weight wire. Higher levels of adverse remodeling and calcific plaque will necessitate earlier use of high gram weight wires, which should be used highly selectively for penetration only when the vessel course is clear.

## Wire Shaping

CTO wire tip shaping differs markedly from "conventional" PCI, where the goal is to negotiate much larger spaces. The goal of most CTO wires is to negotiate through or penetrate dense intimal plaque; a very distal tip (1–2 mm) is therefore placed on the wire (See Chap. 4, Fig. 4.1). A larger tip is more likely to result in inadvertent sub-intimal wire passage or intra-plaque haemorrhage. The Gaia wires come pre-shaped with this typical CTO bend.

## Confirming Progress and Ensuring Safety

Once the proximal cap has been defined and approached, the goal is to advance a wire past the cap, into the CTO segment, avoiding bridging collaterals, which are fragile and often extra-adventitial. If the cap is tapered, a high probability of progress is expected with a tapered polymer coated wire. This should be confirmed in orthogonal views to exclude advancement into bridging collaterals. If the wire advancement is confirmed to be intra-arterial, the microcatheter should be delivered to just past (1–2 mm) the proximal cap and the initial wire advanced further with reference to orthogonal views.

It is unusual, within the CTO segment, in the absence of significant calcium, to require high gram weight wires. Progress is usually possible with tapered, polymer-coated wires or medium weight wires. If progress stalls, carefully advancing the microcatheter closer to the tip of the wire will often aid advancement, if not, it will facilitate wire escalation without losing wire position. Care should be particularly taken to confirm that advancement is within the CTO and not extra-arterial *prior* to microcatheter advancement.

In most situations, where the collaterals are from the contralateral circulation, angiographic confirmation of correct progress is best obtained from donor vessel injection of contrast. Injection of contrast via the antegrade guide is rarely helpful (in the absence of ipsilateral collaterals) and can be harmful potentially causing a contrast-induced hydraulic dissection, or by enlarging any inadvertent dissection planes created.

Where there is rapid progress of the wire, particularly when accompanied by a sudden drop in forward resistance, correct wire progress must be confirmed. This is especially important with the use of high gram weight wires, where the tactile feedback is often poor and a sudden drop in resistance can either indicate distal true lumen entry or vessel exit. The risk of sub-intimal wire passage is greatest at the proximal and distal caps of the occlusion and these areas are where there is greatest benefit in using high gram weight wires.

## Confirming True Lumen Entry

After penetrating the distal cap of the occlusion, the wire should enter the distal true lumen, but the expected drop in resistance may be subtle, due to lesion resistance and

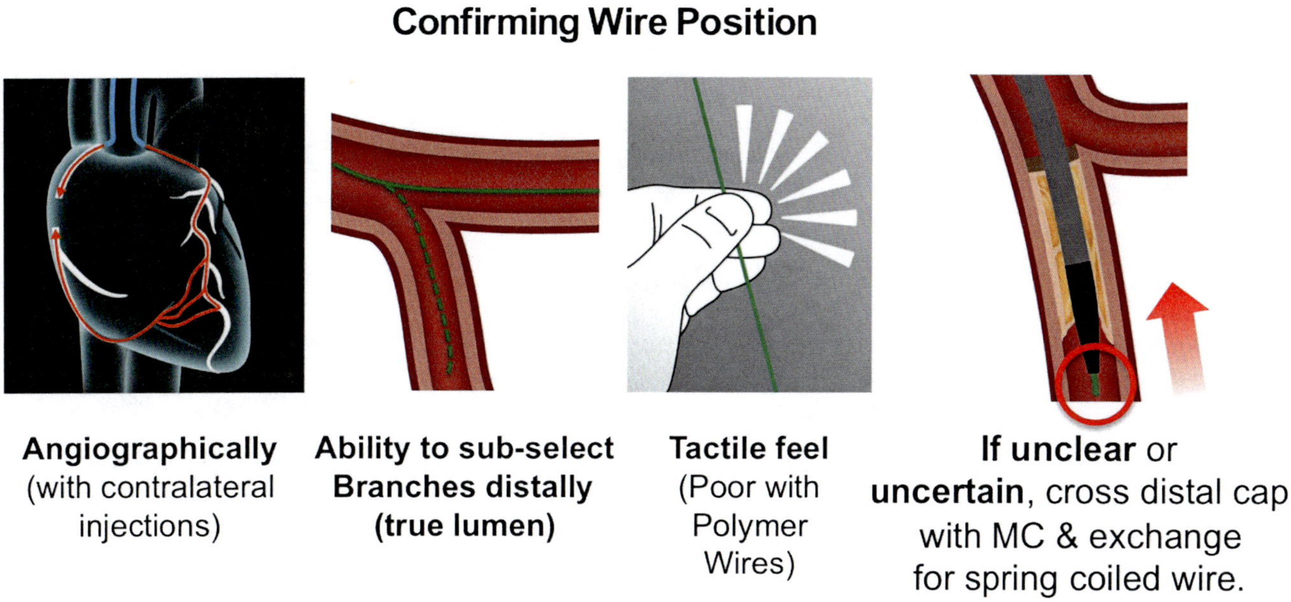


**Fig. 5.3** Where a lack of clarity exists over whether the wire has entered the distal coronary bed within the true lumen it can be clarified by contralateral angiography, ability to sub-select distal branches, the tactile feel of the wire or if doubt persists the use of a spring-coiled wire

confirmation of true lumen position is important before further wire advancement. There are several potential ways of confirming this (Fig. 5.3):

### Angiographically

This should be performed in orthogonal views, with careful attention to the possibility of sub-intimal wire passage. Free rotation of the bended tip tends to confirm true lumen positioning.

### Wire Feel

A sudden drop in forward resistance, accompanied by free wire tip movement is usually sufficient to confirm distal true lumen entry. Care should be taken, however, with medium or heavy weight polymer wires which can advance within the sub-intimal space with only minimal forward resistance. If doubt still exists the microcatheter should be advanced just beyond the distal cap and the CTO wire exchanged for a low gram weight, spring-coiled wire. If this is in the sub-intimal space, it will be unable to be advanced without significant forward resistance and coiling of the tip of the wire. Although commonly performed by some operators, a distal injection via the OTW balloon or the microcatheter is strongly discouraged at this point; if the catheter is rather in a sub-intimal position, the contrast injection will lead to a vessel wall hematoma and sometimes perforation, making subsequent attempts to regain the true lumen very difficult.

### Intravascular Ultrasound (IVUS)

Whilst it is possible to confirm true luminal/sub-intimal wire position with IVUS, practically this may limit the implementation of further strategies if the wire is sub-intimal by enlarging the sub-intimal space further, thereby compressing the true lumen.

## Advancing Equipment

When the wire has accessed the distal true lumen beyond the occlusion, it greatly facilitates subsequent equipment crossing to pass the wire as far as safely possible down the artery – the shaft of almost any wire being considerably more supportive than the tip. In approximately 6 % of cases lesions will be described as "balloon uncrossable", defined as where a standard, low profile balloon is unable to cross without resort to adjunctive measures [13]. A simplified algorithm is illustrated for such eventualities (Fig. 5.4). In such situations the resistance to forward motion of the equipment is high enough to cause the guide catheter to "back-out" or prolapse backwards. This balance between forward resistance and guide catheter support can be redressed by several measures:

### Anchor Balloon

A wire is placed in a proximal side branch and a balloon, sized 1:1 with the side branch, inflated at relatively low atmospheric pressures. This fixes the guide in place and

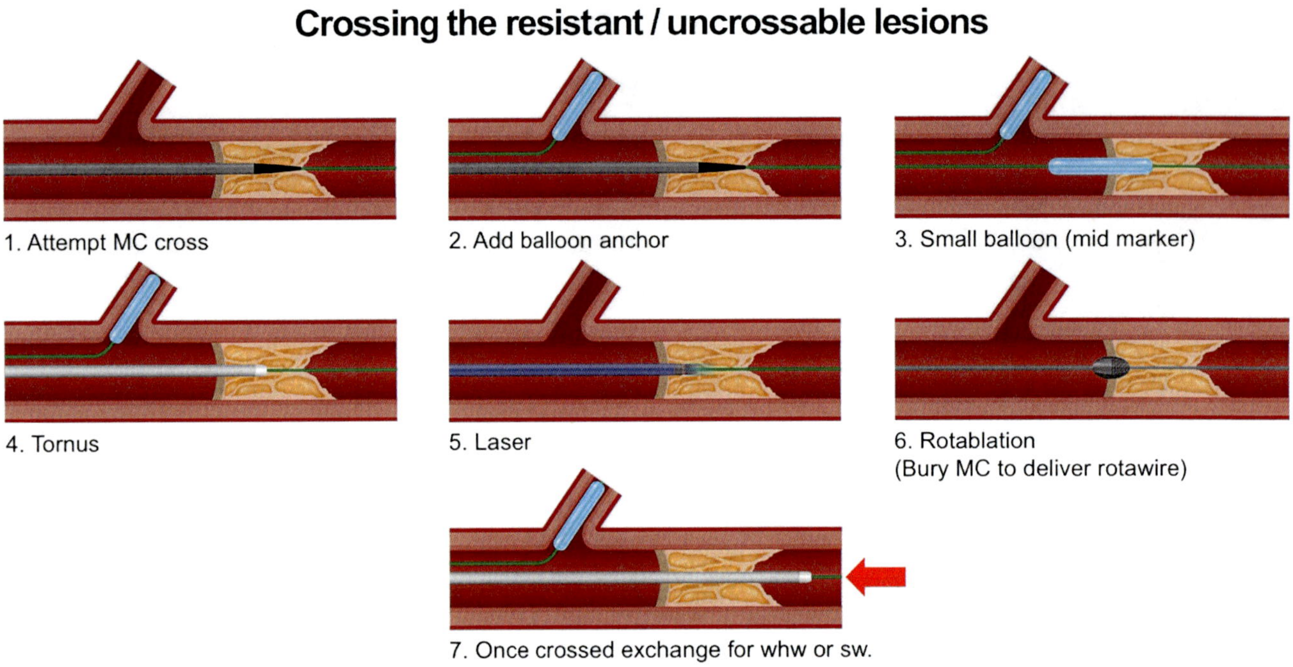


**Fig. 5.4** In cases of balloon-uncrossable lesions, several methods are illustrated for crossing with equipment *MC* Microcatheter, *whw* workhose wire sw=standard wire

allows higher forces to be delivered to the equipment attempting to traverse the occlusion.

## Guide Extension

Delivery of the guide extension such as the GuideLiner (Vascular Solutions, US) or GuideZilla (Boston Scientific, US) to the point of occlusion greatly increases the amount of co-axial force that can be delivered [14].

## Higher Support Microcatheter

The Tornus™ catheter (Asahi Intecc) is a specialty microcatheter, created from wrapped wires, which can be screwed in and out of densely diseased coronary segments and can offer incremental crossing opportunities [15]. It converts rotation forces into forward movement of the catheter. It is advanced by counterclockwise rotations, with a maximum of 20 turns in order not to disrupt the catheter architecture.

*Excimer laser coronary atherectomy* (*ELCA*): the advantage of ELCA in crossing balloon undilatable or uncrossable lesions is that it can be performed on a 0.014″ wire, wire exchange not therefore being necessary [13].

## Rotational Atherectomy

Although highly effective at crossing calcified CTO segments, rotational atherectomy requires a specialized 0.009″ wire. Thus the microcatheter must be delivered and burried as far as possible into the occlusion, before a wire exchange is attempted [16], limiting its usefulness for this indication.

## Indications and Use of Adjunctive Imaging Strategies

The use of adjunctive imaging to test for either ischemia or viability is integral to the CTO PCI pathway, but offers little information to guide a successful recanalisation procedure. The role of echocardiography, CTA and cardiac MRI in the detection and treatment guidance for CTO complications is also vital. Of these modalities, only CTA, however, is able to provide information on lesion complexity and detailed anatomical information, which may favorably alter procedural course.

## CTA

Although the role of co-registration is increasing with CTA, at present the majority of the useful information is obtained pre-procedure and used during planning [12]. CTA is highly sensitive at detecting coronary calcium, true length and path of the occlusion, the degree of plaque beyond the distal cap [17] and to a lesser extent the collateral circulation that supplies the occluded vessel. CTA markers of lesion complexity are consistent with angiographic markers, with calcium, tortuosity and severe tapering of the proximal cap all markers of procedural failure in 110 patients with CTO lesions [18]. Whilst this might not have impacted on the mechanics of procedure, it may serve to identify those patients in whom an AWE strategy is unlikely to be successful. Another area where there is added value in the 3D perspective provided by CTA is the post coronary artery bypass (CABG) patient, where surgical distortion and competing native and graft blood supply can make reconstruction and planning strategy challenging. Finally, in cases where a retrograde approach in impracticable but the proximal cap is ambiguous, the CTA can be used to better understand where wire forces can be applied on the cap while reducing the likelihood of vessel exit (as discussed in Chap. 11).

## IVUS

IVUS is a modality of proven value in the sizing and optimization of stent implantation [19], yet in achieving "true lumen" crossing as part of an AWE approach it really only has one important utility, that of proximal cap identification. A proximal cap is described as ambiguous where the course is unclear after the occlusion. In the presence of a reasonable sized side branch IVUS can help identification, guide wire puncture and assess that the correct (luminal) path has been taken. For simultaneous, "live" IVUS-guided puncture an 8 F guide must be used and the proximal CTO vessel must be large enough to accommodate both the microcatheter and the IVUS catheter. This is most often feasible in ostial left anterior descending (LAD) or circumflex (Cx) occlusions. Alternatively, 2 smaller guides can be used, with one guide used for the antegrade microcatheter and wires, and the other for the IVUS probe. More commonly, angiographic acquisition is used to mark the site of the CTO vessel after it has been identified by IVUS. It is important that this is done in orthogonal projections. After the IVUS has been withdrawn, the angiographic road map is used to guide proximal cap puncture. If necessary repeat IVUS can be used to confirm true course of the wire.

## When to Switch Strategy

A primary objective is for the procedure to be both successful, and efficient. Consideration of a change in strategy should be given if the procedure is failing to progress. At each potential point of difficulty an algorithmic solution should be employed, if failure to progress smoothly. This can potentially occur at several stages: the proximal cap, the in-CTO segment and the distal cap. There are several possible "failure modes" with antegrade wire escalation, but perhaps the most common is *sub-intimal wire passage with failure to re-enter the distal true lumen*. If the wire remains within the arterial structure, this can be utilised positively by switching to an antegrade dissection re-entry (ADR) strategy, in a hybrid perspective [7]. For operators not proficient with the retrograde approach or ADR, stopping the procedure and referring to a specialized operator is likely to save contrast, radiation and complications. Persisting wire-based attempts to re-enter the true lumen (parallel wire, IVUS-guided re-entry) are poorly reproducible and run the risk of exacerbating the problem by enlarging the sub-intimal space at the expense of luminal compression.

**Acknowledgements** The graphic support of Optima education and Adrian Brown (Vascular Perspectives) is gratefully acknowledged. www.optimaskills.com

## References

1. Galassi AR, Tomasello SD, Reifart N, et al. In-hospital outcomes of percutaneous coronary intervention in patients with chronic total occlusion: insights from the ERCTO registry. Eurointervention. 2011;7:472–9.
2. Spratt JC, Wilson WM. The treatment of chronic total occlusions: advances in procedural techniques - antegrade. Curr Cardiol Rev. 2014;31.
3. Rinfret S, Joyal D, Spratt JC, Buller CE. Chronic total occlusion percutaneous coronary intervention case selection and techniques for the non-retrograde operator. Catheter Cardiovasc Interv. 2015;85(3):408–15.
4. Spratt JC, Strange JW. Retrograde procedural planning, skills development, and how to set up a base of operations. Intervent Cardiol Clin. 2012;1(3):325–38.
5. Morino Y, Abe M, Morimoto T, et al. Predicting successful guidewire crossing through chronic total occlusion of native coronary lesions within 30 minutes the J-CTO (Multicenter CTO Registry in Japan) score as a difficulty grading and time assessment tool for the J-CTO registry investigators. J Am Coll Cardiol Intv. 2011;4:213–21.
6. Muhammad KI, Lombardi WL, Christofferson R, Whitlow PL. Subintimal guidewire tracking during successful percutaneous therapy for chronic coronary total occlusions: insights from an intravascular ultrasound analysis. Catheter Cardiovasc Interv. 2012;79(1):43–8. doi:10.1002/ccd.23139.
7. Brilakis ES, Grantham JA, Rinfret S, Wyman RM, Burke NM, Karmpaliotis D, Lembo N, Pershad A, Kandzari DE, Buller CE, DeMartini T, Lombardi WL, Thompson CA. A percutaneous treatment algorithm for crossing coronary chronic total occlusions. J Cardiovasc Interv. 2012;5(4):367–79.
8. Katsuragawa M, Fujiwara H, Miyamae M, et al. Histologic studies in percutaneous transluminal coronary angioplasty for chronic total occlusion: comparison of tapering and abrupt types of occlusion and short and long occluded segments. Am Coll Cardiol. 1993;21:604–11.
9. Irving J. CTO pathology, how does this affect management. Curr Cardiol Rev. 2014;10(2):99–107.
10. Wilson WM, Wilson WM, Hanratty C, Walsh S, Egred M, McEntagert M, Oldroyd K. Strange J, Spratt JC. Outcomes from the UK CTO Hybrid database. Presented @ TCT. 2014.
11. Pershad A, Eddin M, Girotra S, Cotugno R, Daniels D, Lombardi W. Validation and incremental value of the hybrid algorithm for CTO PCI. Catheter Cardiovasc Interv. 2014;84(4):654–9.
12. Spratt JC, McEntegart M. Procedure planning for chronic total occlusion percutaneous coronary intervention. Interv Cardiol. 2013;5(5):549–57.

13. Fernandez JP, Hobson AR, McKenzie D, et al. Beyond the balloon: excimer coronary laser atherectomy used alone or in combination with rotational atherectomy in the treatment of chronic total occlusions, non-crossable and non-expansible coronary lesions. EuroIntervention. 2013;9:243–50.
14. Brilakis ES, Karmpaliotis D, Werner GS, Spratt JC, Uretsky BF, Luna M, Banerjee S. Developments in coronary chronic total occlusion percutaneous coronary interventions: 2013 state-of-the-art update. J Invasive Cardiol. 2014;26(6):261–6.
15. Reifart N, Enayat D, Giokoglu K. A novel penetration catheter (Tornus) as bail-out device after balloon failure to recanalise long, old calcified chronic occlusions. EuroIntervention. 2008;3(5): 617–21.
16. Fairley SL, Spratt JC, Rana O, Talwar S, Hanratty C, Walsh S. Adjunctive strategies in the management of resistant, 'undilatable' coronary lesions after successfully crossing a CTO with a guidewire. Curr Cardiol Rev. 2014;10(2):145–57.
17. Schroeder S, Kuettner A, Leitritz M, et al. Reliability of differentiating human coronary plaque morphology using contrast-enhanced multislice spiral computed tomography: a comparison with histology. J Comput Assist Tomogr. 2004;28:449–54.
18. Ehara M, Terashima M, Kawai M, et al. Impact of multislice computed tomography to estimate difficulty in wire crossing in percutaneous coronary intervention for chronic total occlusion. J Invasive Cardiol. 2009;21:575–82.
19. Kim J-S, Kang T-S, Mintz GS, Park B-E, et al. Randomized comparison of clinical outcomes between intravascular ultrasound and angiography-guided drug-eluting stent implantation for long coronary artery stenoses. J Am Coll Cardiol Intv. 2013;6(4):369–76. doi:10.1016/j.jcin.2012.11.009.

# When and How to Perform an Antegrade Dissection/Re-entry Approach using the CrossBoss and Stingray Catheters

6

Simon Walsh

**Abstract**

Chronic Total Occlusion (CTO) remains the most challenging lesion to treat using Percutaneous Coronary Intervention (PCI). Multiple strategies exist to facilitate lesion crossing and subsequent stenting of the target vessel. The antegrade dissection and re-entry (ADR) technique was developed to provide another option for patients to facilitate a successful CTO PCI procedure. This chapter provides a step-by-step approach to learn the technique.

**Keywords**

Antegrade dissection/re-entry (ADR) • Subintimal wire passage • Subintimal Tracking and Re-entry (STAR) technique • Limited Antegrade Subintimal Tracking (LAST) technique • CrossBoss • Stingray

## Introduction

Chronic Total Occlusion (CTO) remains the most challenging lesion to treat using Percutaneous Coronary Intervention (PCI). Multiple strategies exist to facilitate lesion crossing and subsequent stenting of the target vessel. These are explored in more detail in the chapters detailing antegrade wire-based and retrograde wire-based/dissection re-entry approaches (Chaps. 7, 8, 9, and 11). The integration of the strategic approach to any given lesion will be dictated by the anatomy that is encountered in the case and an overview is provided in the chapter on the hybrid approach to CTO PCI (Chap. 11).

**Electronic supplementary material** The online version of this chapter (doi:10.1007/978-3-319-21563-1_6) contains supplementary material, which is available to authorized users.

S. Walsh, MD, FRCP, FSCAI
Cardiology Department, Belfast Health and Social Care Trust, Belfast City Hospital, Belfast, UK
e-mail: simon.walsh@belfasttrust.hscni.net

Whilst the majority of lesions are still approached with conventional wire escalation strategies (Chap. 5), the success rates with this approach will decline with increasing lesion complexity [1]. This is particularly the case with increasing length of the CTO lesion, where longer lesions are frequently associated with subintimal wire passage [2, 3]. There is an increasing need to use dissection and re-entry strategies for more complex lesions [4]. However, the retrograde approach is also limited, principally by the lack of appropriate interventional collaterals and a failure to pass a guidewire to the patent, collateralized, distal segment of the occluded target vessel (Chap. 9) [5]. Therefore, the antegrade dissection and re-entry (ADR) technique was developed to provide another option for patients to facilitate a successful CTO PCI procedure. This approach has been shown to be highly successful in contemporary practice in cases where other strategies have been attempted and failed [6]. Therefore, the ADR strategy is an important treatment option for patients with CTO lesions and should be one of the strategies that is planned when a CTO lesion is being considered for a PCI.

The ADR approach has evolved over time. The initial description of deliberate use of the sub-intimal space for passing equipment in an antegrade direction was using the



S. Rinfret (ed.), *Percutaneous Intervention for Coronary Chronic Total Occlusion: The Hybrid Approach*, DOI 10.1007/978-3-319-21563-1_6

Subintimal Tracking and Re-entry (STAR) technique [7]. This approach involved folding over a hydrophilic wire (or creating a knuckle) that was pushed into the distal artery. The knuckle could forcibly re-enter the distal lumen, typically at bifurcation points and restore a connection to the distal arterial bed. However, the site of wire re-entry was unpredictable and could result in restoration of flow to a small terminal branch and risked creating no meaningful outflow. This technique was modified to include the use of contrast injections into the subintimal space with the aim of making re-entry more controlled (Chap. 8) [8]. Despite attempts to improve the method, both the STAR and contrast-based STAR techniques remained unpredictable in their acute and long-term outcomes [9, 10] unless they are performed like Carlino describes in a following chapter (Chap. 8). Further attempts were made to improve this method and this resulted in the Limited Antegrade Subintimal Tracking (LAST) technique, whereby after equipment had accessed the sub-intimal space and passed beyond the distal cap, a penetrative wire with a significant bend at the tip was used to immediately attempt to re-enter back into the lumen at this segment of vessel reconstitution. Unfortunately, this technique was also very challenging and unpredictable. Deliberate wire-based re-entry with a stiff tapered wire could be achieved on occasion but failed frequently, mainly because the subintimal space is significantly disrupted when a large knuckle wire is advanced. This creates intramural haematoma with compression of the distal true lumen and results in a low likelihood of successful wire based re-entry. These techniques also fell out of favour due to poor medium term outcomes with high rates of target vessel revascularization and vessel closure [9, 10].

Nevertheless, whilst the previously described STAR, contrast-guided STAR and LAST techniques were unreliable, the concepts behind their development were sound. The main failure mode of antegrade wire escalation for CTO PCI is when wires are passed into the subintimal space and the distal true lumen is not re-entered. While some operators will spend time trying to advance multiple parallel wires into the distal true lumen, this is an unreliable method that is highly dependent on the skill of the individual operator. The CrossBoss and Stingray devices (Boston Scientific, USA) (see Chap. 3) were developed as a system that would create a controlled antegrade dissection plane to facilitate targeted re-entry (Fig. 6.1). The CrossBoss catheter is a blunt dissection device with a 1 mm rounded tip. The CrossBoss will either track through intimal plaque and re-enter the distal true lumen itself or alternatively create a controlled dissection plane that allows the Stingray balloon to be delivered. The Stingray balloon is then inflated to wrap itself around the artery lumen just beyond the distal cap of the occlusion. This allows a purpose-built wire to puncture in a controlled manner towards and then into the distal true lumen. Thus, a targeted procedure can be performed to select the site of re-entry and a reliable and controlled puncture of the distal artery can be achieved in the majority of cases where this technology is used. As opposed to the STAR technique, the use of the CrossBoss and Stingray facilitates re-entry into the artery proximal to all the important distal branches (Fig. 6.2). When the vessel is reconstructed with stents, outflow is guaranteed to multiple branches. This leads to good relief from ischaemia and also leads to medium and long-term outcomes that are more comparable to more traditional wire-based strategies [11].

## Antegrade Dissection and Re-Entry: Basic Principles and the Textbook Case

The goal of any CTO PCI is to achieve revascularization for the patient. Thus, the procedure should be performed in a manner that is safe, results in a complete revascularization with restoration of flow to all distal branches and is performed in a manner that minimizes the patient's exposure to radiation and contrast. It should be recognized and accepted that many lesions will be amenable to a successful procedure that employs any number of different strategies and approaches. Ideally, the safest and most efficient procedure should be performed that leads to a good procedural outcome. Based on the hybrid approach, anatomy should lead an operator towards this scenario and there are a number of features of the occlusion that predispose the lesion for an ADR based approach using the CrossBoss and Stingray system as described in the following chapter on the hybrid approach (Chap. 11) .

Lesions with tapered entries and defined proximal caps with a short course are generally amenable to antegrade wire escalation or a true-to-true approach (Chap. 5). Should this approach fail due to subintimal passage of antegrade equipment, then the lesion may be amenable to an ADR strategy as an immediate bailout. Those lesions that are most suited to ADR are occlusions with defined proximal cap anatomy (either angiographically or by intravascular ultrasound; IVUS), with longer courses (>20 mm, where wire based approaches are less likely to succeed) and where there is a good target vessel to attempt re-entry. When assessing the distal landing zone, areas with a good calibre and without severe calcification or disease are ideal. Most importantly, the landing zone should be remote from and proximal to major side branches and sites of bifurcation in the distal vessel. This factor is crucial to prevent the loss of significant territories after stent deployment. Finally, vessels that have donor arteries providing complex or non-interventional collaterals should also be strongly considered for ADR as a primary strategy.

When an ADR strategy is employed (either as an early bailout after a failed antegrade wire strategy or as a primary manoeuvre) there are a number of key principles that should

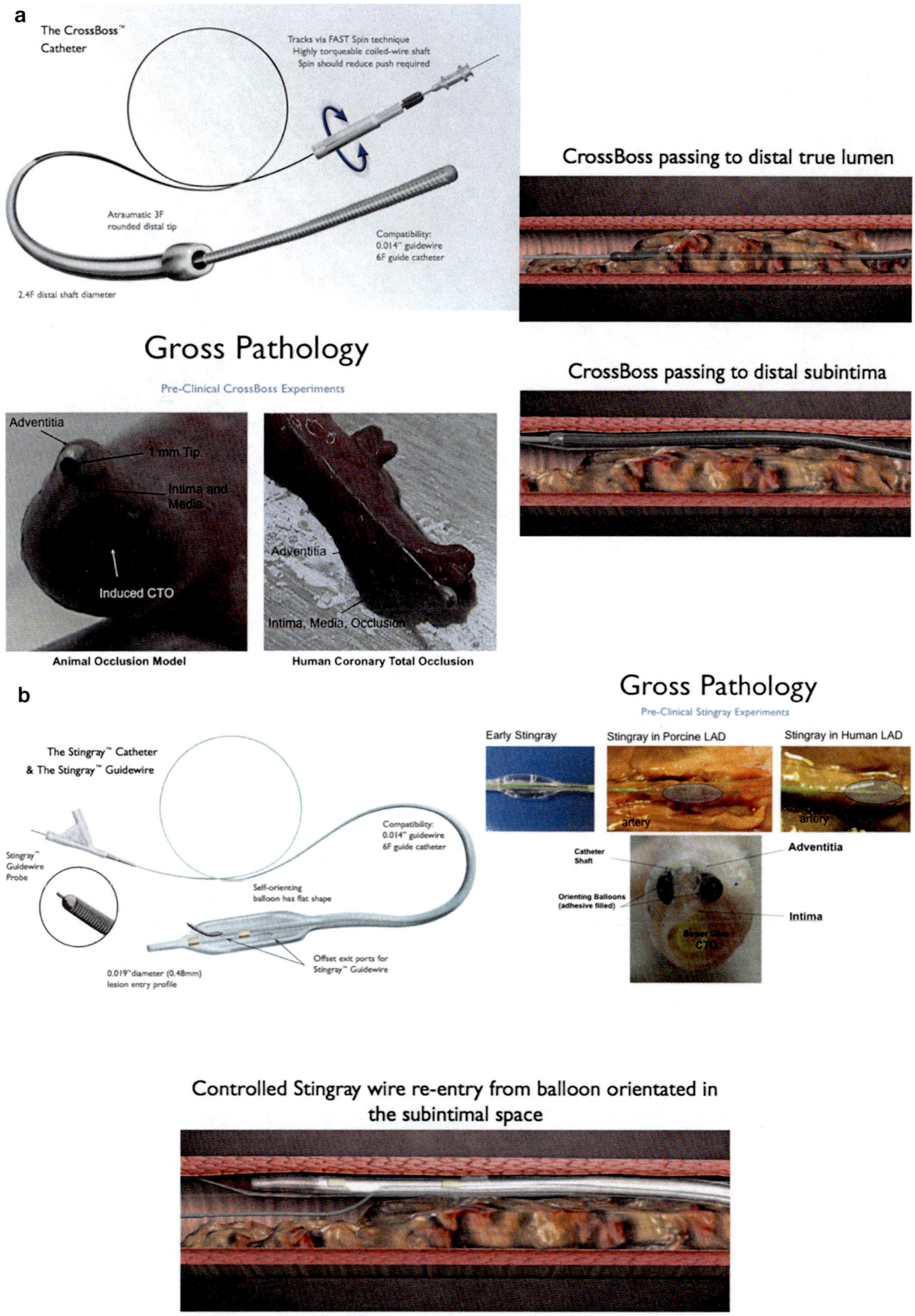


**Fig. 6.1** The CrossBoss and Stingray Dissection and Reentry System. (**a**) The CrossBoss catheter (Courtesy of Chad Kugler and Boston Scientific). (**b**) The Stingray balloon and wire for controlled re-entry (Courtesy of Chad Kugler and Boston Scientific)

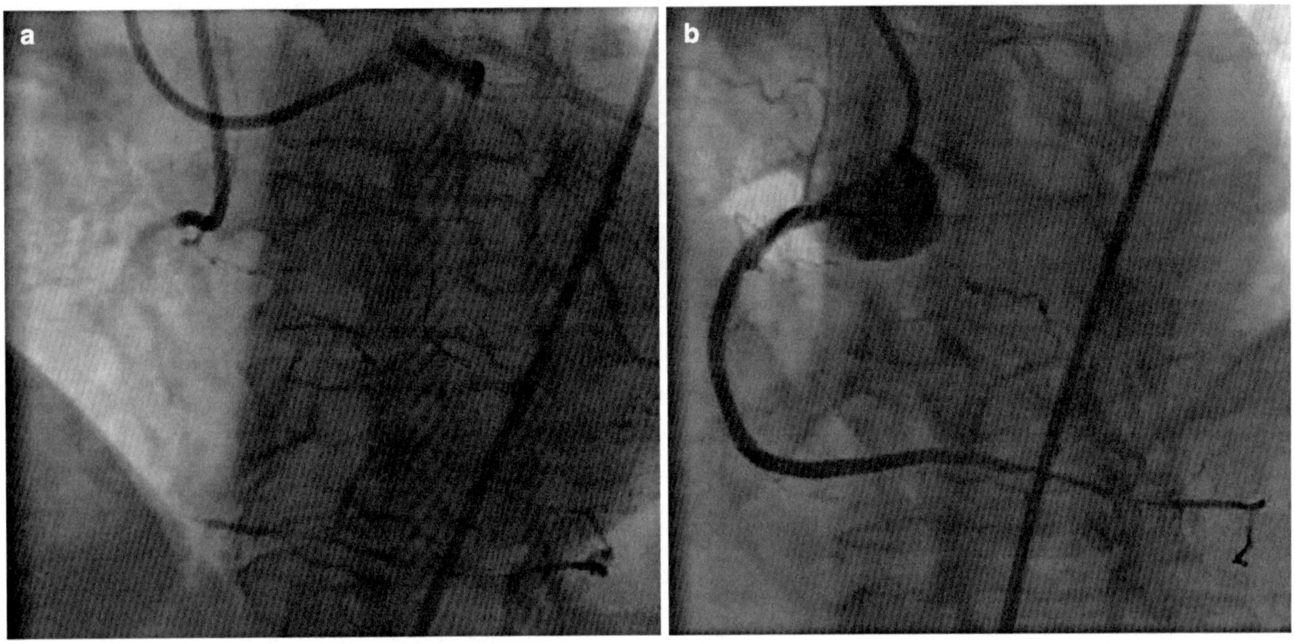


**Fig. 6.2** Long CTO treated with antegrade dissection-reentry (ADR). An occluded right coronary artery (RCA). The CTO is very long, with a clearly defined proximal cap and a landing zone that is visible proximal to the crux of the RCA (Panel **a**). A good result is obtained after an ADR based procedure and stent deployment (Panel **b**)

be adhered to. Ideally, the CrossBoss should be advanced alone with no wire ahead of the device. This is achieved by rapid rotation of the device (Fig. 6.1a) after locking the handle at an appropriate distance from the Y-connector. On occasion, it is necessary to advance knuckled guidewires into the architecture of the occluded vessel. This is usually performed in order to define the anatomy within the CTO segment, particularly in the setting of anatomical ambiguity in the target vessel (Fig. 6.3a). However, knuckle wires will create substantial disruption in the subintimal space. Therefore, as soon as the anatomical course of the vessel is defined, the knuckle should be removed and the CrossBoss advanced alone by rapid rotation. This is particularly important at the landing zone in the distal vessel. "Finishing out" the final few centimeters of subintimal dissection with the CrossBoss will create considerably less disruption in the subintimal space. This will greatly lessen the risk of compressive intramural haematoma and loss of the landing zone and site for re-entry.

Another "golden rule" of ADR is that antegrade contrast injections into the occluded vessel should not be performed. There is a major risk that this will lead to hydraulic dissection in the artery. Again, haematoma in the distal subintimal space is likely to evolve and the landing zone can be lost. When the artery is supplied by auto-collaterals contrast injection from the guide can be avoided by directly injecting contrast into the collaterals or branches that provide them by sub-selecting and siting micro-catheters into these vessels.

The CrossBoss catheter is a stiff device that tends to pass in a straight direction (Fig. 6.3). Therefore, while it will frequently follow the main artery that is the target for recanalization, the device will also track side branches. It is imperative that operators are aware that this can occur during the procedure. Careful radiographic assessment is mandatory and it is advisable to check the position of the CrossBoss in 2 orthogonal views as it makes progress in the vessel. If the CrossBoss tracks a side branch over a short distance, it rarely causes any problems. However, if this situation has not been recognized and the CrossBoss is advanced very distally into a small vessel there is a risk of perforation and this must be avoided. When the CrossBoss has tracked off course into a branch, it should be withdrawn back to the main vessel and a "redirection" manoeuvre is then needed to allow it to track to the landing zone to facilitate Stingray based re-entry. This is usually achieved by advancing a guidewire ahead of the CrossBoss into the architecture of the main target vessel. However, this is done semi-blind and we suggest that the guidewire is advanced for only a short distance beyond the origin of the branch. Once this course is defined, the CrossBoss can be passed beyond the side branch, the wire withdrawn and the CrossBoss advanced on its own as usual.

After the CrossBoss has successfully created a track to the distal landing zone in an area beyond the distal cap of the CTO, but proximal to any significant side branches, then this device must be removed with the Stingray balloon sited in the same segment of the distal vessel. The commonest steps to achieve this exchange (using the trapping-balloon technique, see Chap. 4) of equipment are as follows: Firstly, an 8 F guiding catheter is recommended for the occluded vessel

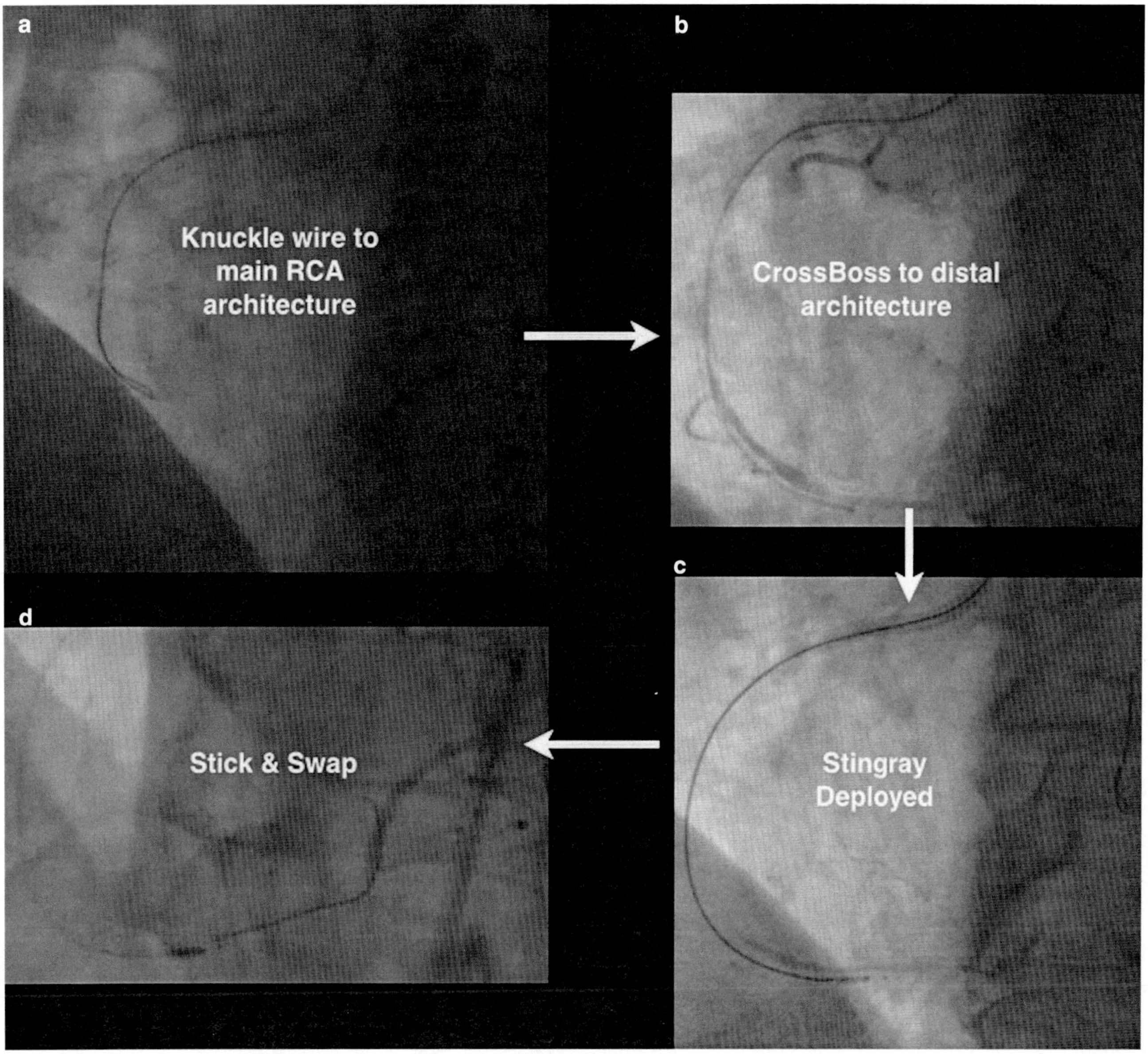


**Fig. 6.3** Step-by-step technique with CrossBoss and Stingray. Steps taken to re-open the RCA in Fig. 6.2. A knuckled wire is advanced via a Corsair (Asahi Intecc, Japan) into the vessel architecture to safely define the anatomy (Panel **a**). The CrossBoss is introduced, advanced over the wire to the mid RCA and then the wire is withdrawn. The CrossBoss is advanced by rapid rotation to the distal landing zone (Panel **b**). The CrossBoss is then swapped out for a Stingray balloon that is inflated at the landing zone with the target vessel noted above the Stingray balloon (Panel **c**). The target vessel is punctured with a Stingray wire and this is swapped out for a hydrophilic wire that is advanced deeply into the target vessel (Panel **d**)

to facilitate the use of trapping balloons in the guide catheter. The CrossBoss is a long, over-the-wire (OTW) device. We usually place a strong hydrophobic wire with a stiff shaft at the tip of the CrossBoss, such as a Miracle Bros 12 (Asahi Intecc, Japan). Taking care not to allow the subintimal wire to drift forwards, the CrossBoss is removed from the artery and brought back inside the guide catheter. At this point, a trapping balloon (3 mm diameter in an 8 F system) is deployed to grip the wire inside the guide catheter and fix the wire's distal position. The CrossBoss can then be removed. Leaving the trapping balloon in place and inflated, the Stingray balloon (also an OTW system) is then advanced into the guide catheter until it reaches the trapping balloon. No fluroroscopy is needed for this step. The operator can feel the Stingray balloon hitting the back of the trapping balloon. At this point the trapping balloon is deflated to allow the Stingray to be advanced into the artery.

Management of the Stingray is a crucial part of the procedure. The preparation and subsequent inflation of the Stingray need to be meticulously performed. The Stingray balloon should be prepared before it is advanced inside the artery while the CrossBoss is still in place, to avoid some unnecessary time during the exchange when blood flow could fill the subintimal space. We recommend the following manoeuvres: The central port (OTW segment) should be flushed with heparinized saline to promote easier balloon advancement. A 3-way-tap should be attached to the side port (balloon segment). A 10 ml Luer-lock syringe should be attached to the 3-way-tap and pulled to "full negative" to create a vacuum. The tap should be closed to the balloon, any air expelled from the syringe and then this manoeuvre should be repeated two or three times to create a substantial vacuum in the shaft of the Stingray balloon. A 2 ml Luer-lock syringe filled with neat contrast should then be attached to the 3-way-tap. All air should be expelled from the system before it is opened to the contrast syringe. Once the tap is opened contrast will be sucked into the Stingray creating a column of contrast from the distal side port to the balloon itself. During advancement of the balloon into the coronary, the small syringe can stay on the side port, while some further suction of contrast into the balloon wings will be achieved with more time. When the balloon is in place, the system should then be closed to the balloon again and an inflation device filled with neat contrast attached. Neat contrast is necessary in the inflation device to allow adequate visualization of the deployed Stingray. Finally, after all air is expelled the tap can be opened between the balloon and the inflation device to allow the balloon to be inflated.

When advancing the balloon, the distal tip of the stiff guidewire that the Stingray is advanced over should not be allowed to drift any further into the target vessel. This will risk disruption and haematoma at the landing zone as well as potentially leading to the unusual possibility of a distal perforation. The Stingray should then be advanced to the landing zone and deployed. The rated burst pressure of the Stingray balloon is 6 atmospheres and inflation to 4 atmospheres is recommended. It is crucial not to inflate the Stingray to high pressure. If the balloon bursts then the subintimal space will be severely disrupted and it is highly unlikely that the procedure will be successful.

Once the Stingray has been successfully deployed, radiographic orientation of the balloon is the next important step of the procedure (Fig. 6.4). Understanding this step of the ADR approach is a key point as this demonstrates the direction that the wire should be advanced in order to achieve re-entry to the true lumen. Advancing the Stingray wire through the wrong exit port and in an incorrect direction risks vessel perforation. The image intensifier and C-arm of the X-ray equipment should be orientated to lay the Stingray balloon out in its longitudinal axis, with minimal foreshortening. In addition, the 2 wings should be overlapped so that only a single line is visible. If both wings of the balloon can be visualized on X-ray then the balloon is en-face and the direction of the attempted re-entry cannot be determined (Fig. 6.4a). When the balloon is laid out correctly, and contrast is injected retrogradely via the donor artery then the direction of the wire re-entry is clearly understood (Fig. 6.4b).

When the target vessel is visualized and the Stingray balloon correctly orientated, then the Stingray wire is advanced to the distal portion of the balloon. At this point, the port that directs the wire towards the lumen must be found and the wire advanced to separate away from the balloon towards the target vessel. When a small separation is demonstrated (<1 mm) the wire should then be advanced in a single motion (without rotating the guidewire) to puncture back into the true lumen. When the Stingray wire has successfully punctured the distal vessel, it is necessary to gain control of the distal artery with the guidewire.

Two manoeuvres are available to achieve this. Where the target vessel is large and disease free, it is often possible to perform a "stick and drive" manoeuvre, carefully advancing the Stingray wire into the distal vessel (Fig. 6.5; Videos 6.1, 6.2, 6.3, 6.4, and 6.5). Once the wire has been passed a sufficient distance distally to maintain safe control of the vessel then the Stingray balloon can be removed from the artery. We would usually use a trapping balloon in the guide catheter to fix the Stingray wire in place. A Corsair or alternative microcatheter can then be introduced into the distal true lumen of the vessel and a workhorse guidewire sited to allow the PCI to be completed. The alternative to "stick and drive" is a "stick and swap" (Figs. 6.3 and 6.6; Videos 6.6, 6.7, 6.8, 6.9, 6.10, and 6.11). This is often performed when there is tortuosity, significant disease or a small calibre of the distal target vessel. Under these circumstances, it is often very difficult to deliver the very stiff Stingray wire sufficiently far into the distal vessel to facilitate completion of the procedure. After successfully puncturing the distal target with the Stingray wire (this puncture is often repeated several times before attempting the swap), the Stingray wire is removed from the balloon. The Stingray balloon is left in position, still inflated and it is imperative that it is not moved. We typically use a medium strength jacketed wire (Pilot 200, Abbott Vascular, USA) for the swap manoeuvre. A 1 mm tip with a similar primary bend to the Stingray wire is then passed out through the same port of the Stingray balloon into the true lumen of the distal vessel. The hydrophilic wire is usually more controllable and can be advanced safely into the distal target vessel. Once again, when enough wire is passed to allow the Stingray balloon to be removed, the same steps should be performed to remove the balloon, swap in a microcatheter and then a workhorse guidewire.

When the distal vessel is controlled with a workhorse wire in the true lumen of the artery, the vessel should be predilated and stented as normal. Care must be taken when deploying stents. It is important that these are appropriately sized to provide a good longterm outcome, but not oversized to risk a perforation. IVUS can be helpful to aid in the choice of stent sizing.

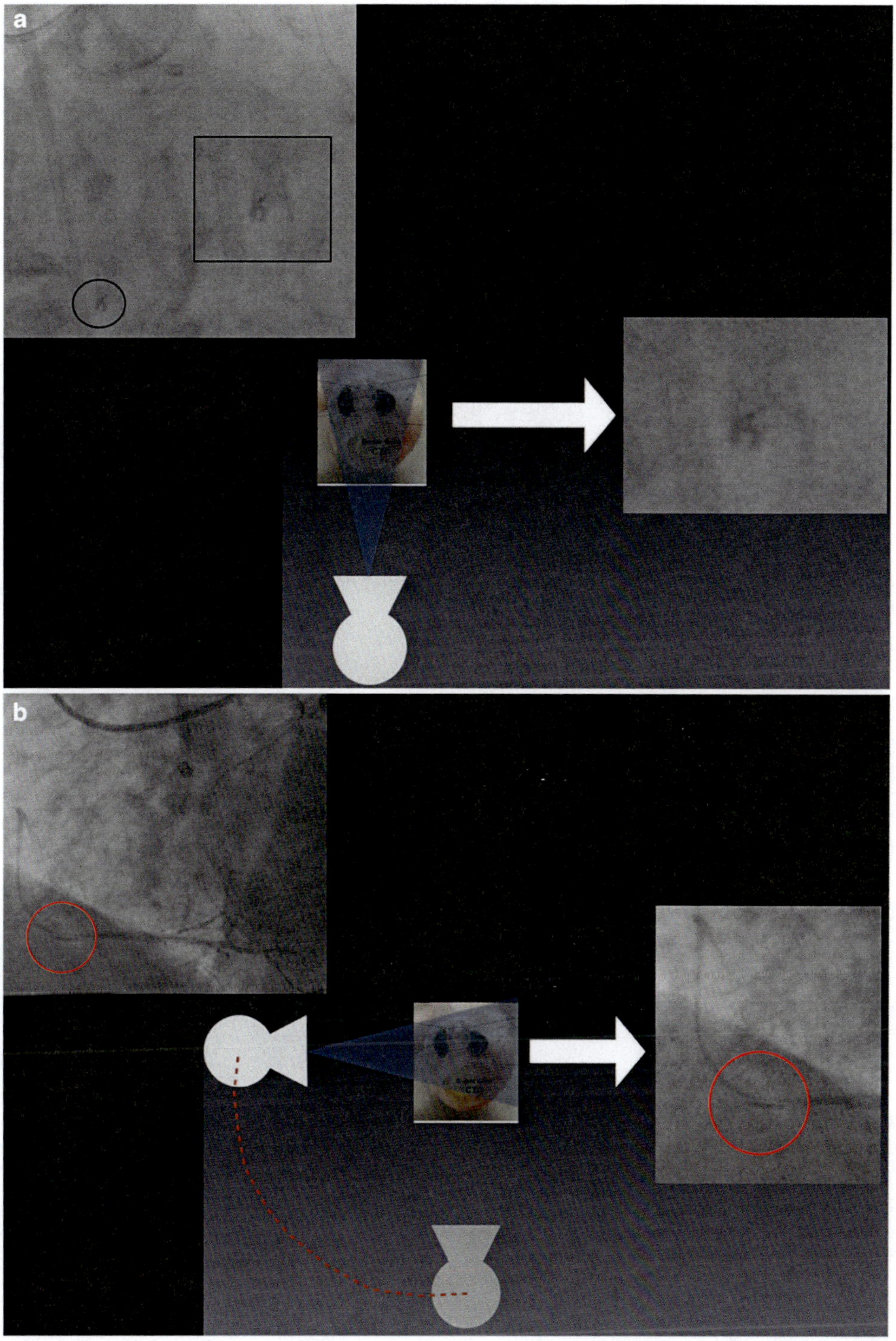


**Fig. 6.4** Orientation of the Stingray balloon for re-entry. (**a**) Incorrect and "en-face" orientation of the Stingray balloon after deployment. (**b**) Correct radiographic orientation of the Stingray balloon. The target vessel is clearly above the Stingray balloon. Therefore, the upper port should be selected for re-entry

## Additional Considerations for ADR that Are Common to Other CTO Procedures

### Vascular Access Site and Guide Catheter Selection

Guide catheter selection is frequently debated for CTO PCI. It is widely accepted that a transradial approach lowers complications compared to transfemoral access for most PCI, including the treatment of ST-elevation myocardial infarction (STEMI). Nevertheless, there are substantial compromises with guide catheter French size and manoeuvres that can be performed during the case that are specific to CTO PCI. A 6 F system is limited in its ability to allow balloon trapping and may not allow an operator to use a Corsair microcatheter (Asahi Intecc, Japan) and a side-branch balloon anchor. In addition, long wire exchanges (using 300 cm wires) will be required if ADR is planned.

A 7 F system will allow some manoeuvres, but will not reliably allow a Stingray balloon and a trapping balloon to be used together. An 8 F system affords a Stingray and trapping balloon in addition to "real-time" IVUS during the procedure. An 8 F system also allows a side-branch anchor balloon, Corsair and trapping balloon to be used in the same guide catheter. Therefore, the operator must be familiar with the equipment and strategies that are likely to be required during the case and should choose their equipment appropriately. Our usual practice is to site a single 8 F system via a transfemoral approach for the occluded target vessel, and improving the support with a long 45 cm introducer.

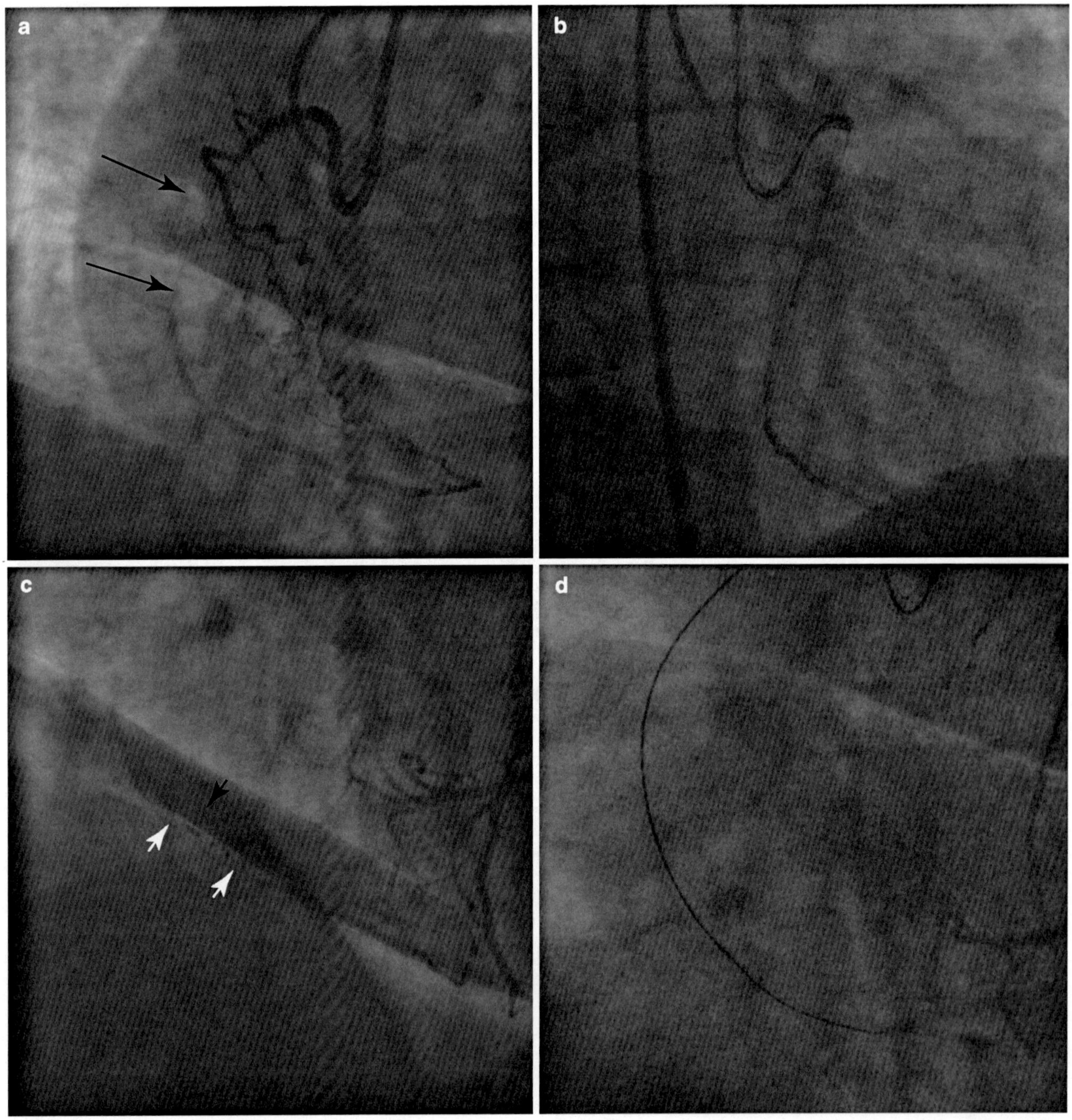


**Fig. 6.5** (Videos 6.1, 6.2, 6.3, 6.4, and 6.5). Classical ADR with a stick and drive technique. (**a**) More than 20 mm RCA CTO without ambiguity of the proximal cap (Video 6.1). (**b**) CrossBoss into vessel structure, into the sub-intimal space at the distal cap (Video 6.2). (**c**) CrossBoss exchanged for Stingray catheter. The Stingray is in place, and both wings of the balloon are superposed (*black arrow*). The true distal lumen can be seen lower than the balloon (*white arrows*). Re-entry will have to be performed through the port pointing inferiorly (Video 6.3). (**d**) Re-entry with the Stingray wire into the distal true lumen, as confirmed with a retrograde injection (Video 6.4). (**e**) Final result post stenting (Video 6.5)

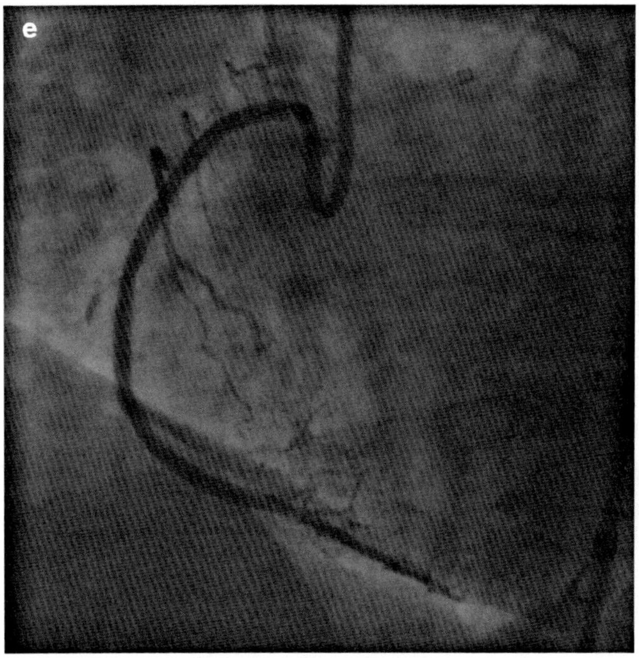


**Fig. 6.5** (continued)

Alternatively, techniques to deliver a standard 8F catheter without a sheath from a transradial approach are explained in a following chapter (Chap. 13). Fluoroscopic guidance is routinely used for the femoral puncture and our experience is that this leads to minimal morbidity related to the transfemoral approach. This will allow an ADR approach in addition to multiple advanced manoeuvres during the case. We usually site a transradial guide catheter in the donor vessel (Fig. 6.5 and 6.6; Videos 6.1, 6.2, 6.3, 6.4, 6.5, 6.6, 6.7, 6.8, 6.9, 6.10, and 6.11). This can be 6 or 7 F depending on the need for retrograde access and/or the need for adjunctive equipment or supportive measures to achieve retrograde access. Individual operators will make their own choices based on the procedural approach, anatomy in the CTO vessel and their skill set. We would simply suggest that physicians are mindful of the compromises that these choices involve and are able to adjust approaches as required subsequent to the evolving progress of the PCI.

## Resolution of Proximal Cap Ambiguity and Crossing "Impenetrable" Proximal Segments

It is important that operators are familiar with a number of key concepts. Defining the anatomy of the proximal cap of the CTO is hugely important for both the safety and likelihood of success of any CTO procedure. Careful angiographic assessment must be undertaken, using multiple views to try to understand where the occluded segment begins. When stiff wires are passed in a blind fashion and the proximal cap or direction of the vessel are not known then perforations can occur commonly. IVUS can be used to help resolve proximal cap ambiguity. When there are multiple small branches around the origin of the CTO, the occluded segment is often visible and can then be entered safely. This approach is explained in the chapter on dealing with difficult antegrade issues (Chap. 7).

In addition, it is a frequent occurrence that the proximal cap is very difficult to penetrate with a wire or that secondary equipment that will not pass beyond this area. CTO operators must be familiar with a variety of manoeuvres to overcome this scenario. There is a hierarchy of steps that will sequentially increase the support available and force employed in order to resolve this scenario. These include using larger calibre guide catheters, using support catheters, guide catheter extension systems and anchor balloons (usually in the side branch, although these can also be deployed co-axially in the occluded vessel as well). Increasingly stiff guidewires offer progressively higher penetration force and are often required to advance beyond the proximal cap. However, additional tools and manoeuvres are often needed to allow secondary equipment to advance into the vessel architecture. These may include: the use of low-profile, small calibre balloons; deliberate balloon rupture at the proximal cap (often referred to balloon-assisted microdissection (BAM) or as "grenade-o-plasty"); use of the Corsair or Tornus devices (both Asahi Intecc, Japan); use of high-speed rotational atherectomy; use of intracoronary laser or combinations of all of the above. A detailed review of these approaches is also described elsewhere [12].

## Techniques to Reduce Ambiguity and Safely Define the Course of the Target Vessel

In addition to resolving proximal cap ambiguity, it is also crucial that the operator understands the course of the occluded segment of the vessel. This is especially the case over longer segments of occlusion where areas of tortuosity will often mislead the operator and the risk of perforation is highest. One of the simplest manoeuvres is to advance a knuckled hydrophilic wire into the occluded segment. This will track the artery or its branches but is extremely unlikely to exit the vessel as it is a blunt dissection tool. Another option is to gently inject contrast into the vessel architecture to outline its course (see Chap. 8). This is also often helpful in altering the compliance of the plaque in the CTO segment and may help to allow other equipment to be advanced after it has been performed.

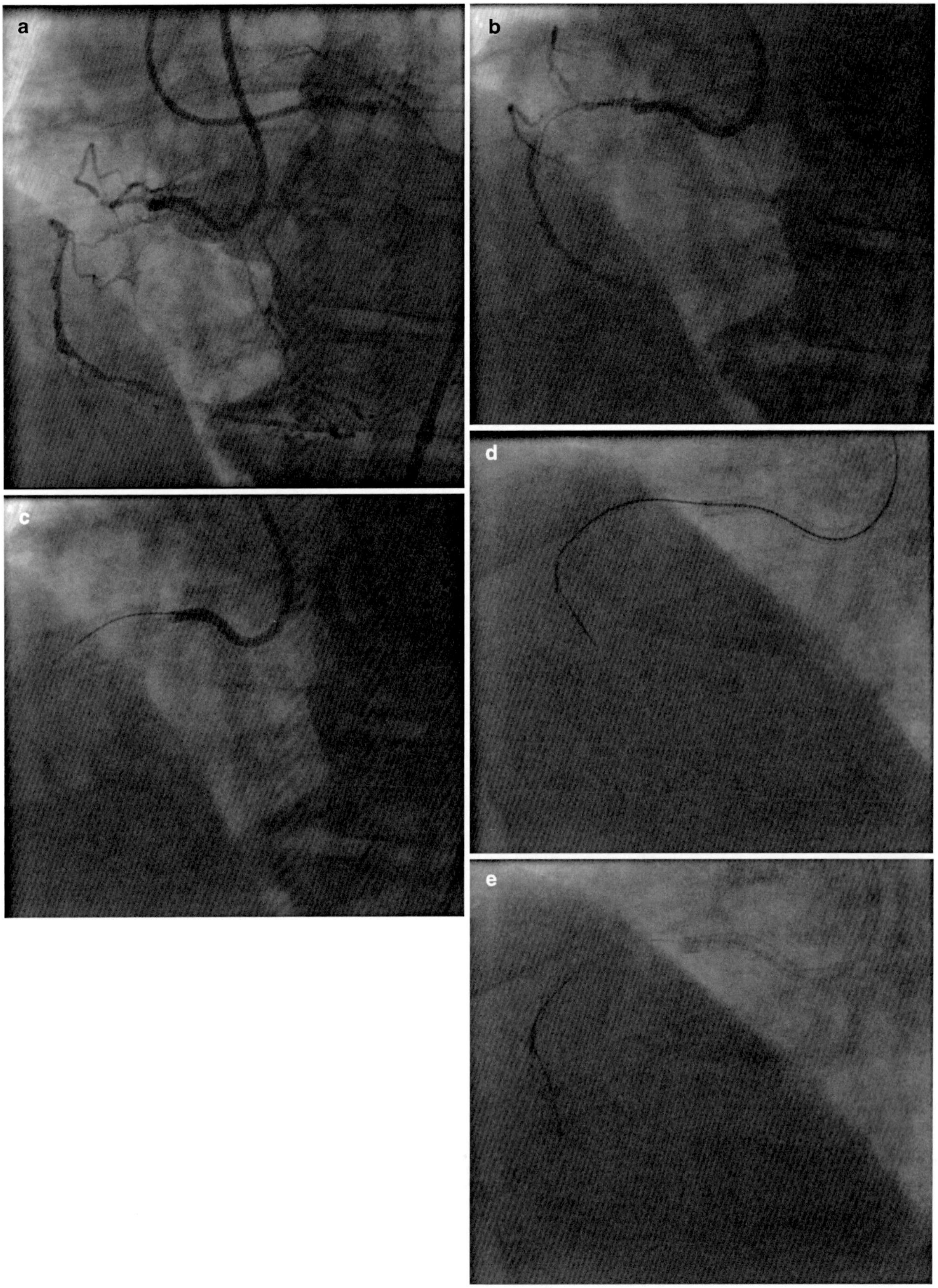


**Fig. 6.6** (Videos 6.6, 6.7, 6.8, 6.9, 6.10, and 6.11). ADR with a 'Stick and Swap' technique. (**a**) 20 mm CTO with a non-ambiguous cap, and a good distal landing zone (Video 6.6). (**b**) Sub-intimal tracking with Pilot 200 guidewire (Video 6.7). (**c**) CrossBoss to distal cap (Video 6.8). (**d**) Stingray balloon in place: Stick with Stingray wire (Video 6.9). (**e**, **f**) Swap with Pilot 200 into distal true lumen, as confirmed with retrograde injection (Video 6.10). (**g**) Final result after stenting (Video 6.11)

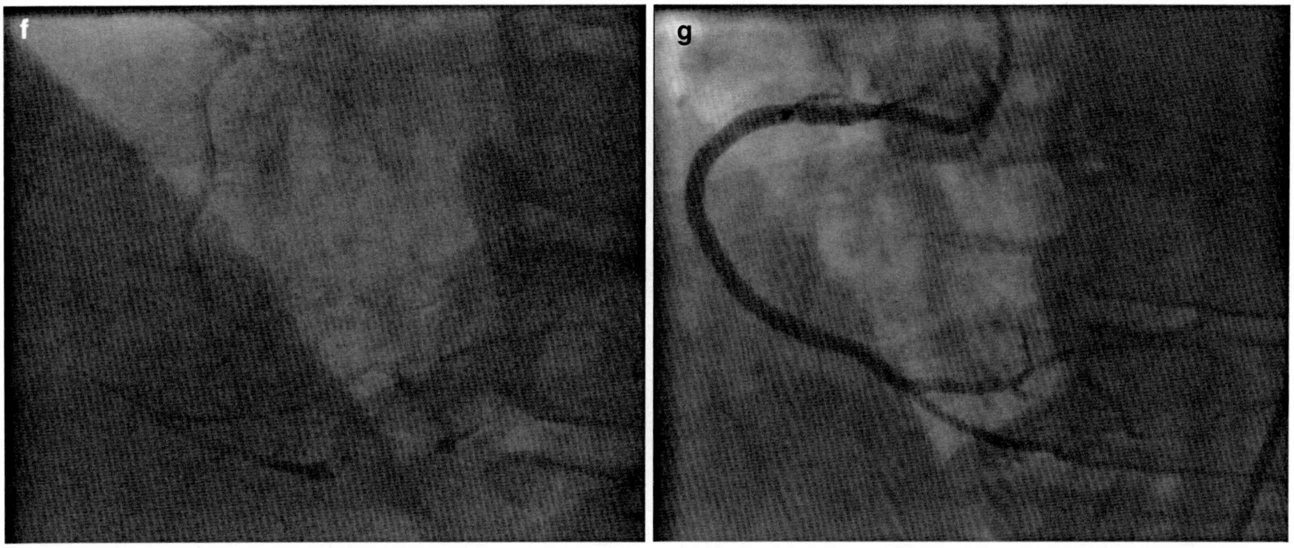


**Fig. 6.6** (continued)

## References


1. Morino Y, Kimura T, Hayashi Y, et al. In-hospital outcomes of contemporary percutaneous coronary intervention in patients with chronic total occlusion. Insights from the J-CTO registry (multicenter CTO registry in Japan). JACC Cardiovasc Interv. 2010;3:143–51.
2. Tsujita K, Maehara A, Mintz GS, et al. Intravascular ultrasound comparison of the retrograde versus antegrade approach to percutaneous intervention for chronic total coronary occlusions. JACC Cardiovasc Interv. 2009;2:846–54.
3. Muhammad KI, Lombardi WL, Christofferson R, Whitlow PL. Subintimal guidewire tracking during successful percutaneous therapy for chronic coronary total occlusions: insights from an intravascular ultrasound analysis. Catheter Cardiovasc Interv. 2012;79:43–8.
4. Daniels D. Hybrid video registry – presented TCT. 2013.
5. Tsuchikane E, Yamane M, Mutoh M, et al. Japanese multicenter registry evaluating the retrograde approach for chronic coronary total occlusion. Catheter Cardiovasc Interv. 2013;82:E654–61.
6. Whitlow PL, Burke N, Lombardi WL, et al. Use of a novel crossing and re-entry system in coronary chronic total occlusions that have failed standard crossing techniques. JACC Cardiovasc Interv. 2012;5:393–401.
7. Colombo A, Mikhail GW, Michev I, et al. Treating chronic total occlusions using subintimal tracking and reentry: the STAR technique. Catheter Cardiovasc Interv. 2005;64:407–11.
8. Carlino M, Godino C, Latib A, Moses JW, Colombo A. Sub-intimal tracking and re-entry technique with contrast guidance: a safer approach. Catheter Cardiovasc Interv. 2008;72:790–6.
9. Godino C, Latib A, Economou FI, et al. Chronic total occlusions: mid-term comparison of clinical outcome following the use of the guided-STAR technique and conventional anterograde approaches. Catheter Cardiovasc Interv. 2012;79:20–7.
10. Valenti R, Vegara R, Migliorini A, et al. Predictors of reocclusion after successful drug-eluting stent–supported percutaneous coronary intervention of chronic total occlusion. J Am Coll Cardiol. 2013;61:545–50.
11. Rinfret S, Ribeiro HB, Nguyen CM, et al. Dissection and re-entry techniques and longer-term outcomes following successful percutaneous coronary intervention of chronic total occlusion. Am J Cardiol. 2014;114:1354–60.
12. Fairley SL, Spratt JC, Rana O, et al. Adjunctive strategies in the management of resistant, 'undilatable' coronary lesions after successfully crossing a CTO with a guidewire. Curr Cardiol Rev. 2014;10:145–57.

# How to Deal with Difficult Antegrade Issues

7

R. Michael Wyman

**Abstract**

Percutaneous revascularization of a chronically occluded coronary artery requires the interventional cardiologist to deal with challenges that are not often met in routine coronary intervention. The Hybrid algorithm provides strategies on how to proceed with initial, secondary and tertiary approaches to CTO PCI, based on anatomy, but within each of these approaches (antegrade, retrograde, dissection reentry, etc.) unique problems can arise that require a set of potential solutions to be considered by the operator (ie, the "algorithms within the algorithm").

In the Hybrid algorithm, there are two potential options for successfully crossing a CTO antegrade (or retrograde): Wire escalation (WE) and with dissection re-entry (DR) techniques. Antegrade challenges can be grouped into two categories: (1) Those that apply to both WE crossing and antegrade dissection and reentry (ADR), and (2) those that are unique to ADR.

**Keywords**

Hybrid algorithm • Wire escalation (WE) • Dissection re-entry (DR) • Antegrade dissection re-entry (ADR) • Proximal cap

Percutaneous revascularization of a chronically occluded coronary artery requires the interventional cardiologist to deal with challenges that are not often met in routine coronary intervention. The Hybrid algorithm provides strategies on how to proceed with initial, secondary and tertiary approaches to CTO PCI, based on anatomy, but within each of these approaches (antegrade, retrograde, dissection reentry, etc.) unique problems can arise that require a set of potential solutions to be considered by the operator (ie, the "algorithms within the algorithm"). In this chapter we will concentrate on challenges encountered during the antegrade approach. Some of those solutions are also discussed in Chap. 11.

In the Hybrid algorithm, there are two potential options for successfully crossing a CTO antegrade (or retrograde): Wire escalation (WE) and with dissection re-entry (DR) techniques. Antegrade challenges can be grouped into two categories: (1) Those that apply to both WE crossing and antegrade dissection and reentry (ADR), and (2) those that are unique to ADR.

It is worth making the following nuances to the WE concept. This technique most of the time involves starting with a softer wire and escalading to stiffer wires. However, hybrid operators will also adapt to the anatomy of the proximal cap for the initial puncture. For example, a blunt and calcified non-ambiguous proximal cap will most likely be successfully engaged with a stiffer wire right from the beginning. However, navigating through the occluded segment with

**Electronic supplementary material** The online version of this chapter (doi:10.1007/978-3-319-21563-1_7) contains supplementary material, which is available to authorized users.

R.M. Wyman, MD
Department of medicine, Torrance Memorial Medical Center, Torrance, CA, USA
e-mail: rmwcor@gmail.com



S. Rinfret (ed.), *Percutaneous Intervention for Coronary Chronic Total Occlusion: The Hybrid Approach*, DOI 10.1007/978-3-319-21563-1_7

softer wires such as the Gaia wire family or the Pilot 200 will be safer and most likely gain access to the true distal lumen. This concept of 'de-escalation' is therefore part of the approach, as discussed in Chaps. 4 and 5.

## Difficult Antegrade Issues That Apply to Both WE and ADR

### Ambiguous Proximal Cap

Ambiguity of the proximal cap is an operator-dependent variable. The simplest way to define this is to pose the question: Are you comfortable with using an aggressive wire (e.g., Confianza Pro 12) to "stick" into what you consider to be the angiographically defined cap? A highly experienced CTO operator may feel confident about doing this in the same anatomical situation that a much less experienced operator would not. In any case, if the cap is felt to be ambiguous, the solutions are:

1. Use of intravascular ultrasound to define the cap and guide entry- this is a very useful technique but requires experience to both recognize the appearance of the cap (Fig. 7.1), and guidewire puncture (Fig. 7.2). In the optimal situation, the IVUS catheter is left in position at the cap while a second microcatheter is introduced, with the appropriate guidewire, to gain entry into the cap under real-time ultrasound guidance. However, proximal disease in the CTO vessel, as well as tortuosity and calcium, frequently hinders the ability to have two catheters side by side in the artery while maintaining a stable position of the IVUS probe. In this situation, the proximal cap can be marked angiographically with the probe, the IVUS catheter withdrawn back into the guide, the proximal cap punctured with the microcatheter and wire, and then the probe brought back down to confirm appropriate entry. With this confirmation, the CTO can then be treated as otherwise guided by the Hybrid algorithm, i.e., with WE crossing if lesion length is less than 20 mm and with ADR if greater than 20 mm with an acceptable reentry zone.
2. It is not uncommon for the anatomy to disallow IVUS interrogation, either because there is no appropriately-sized sidebranch, or proximal disease inhibits passage. In addition, heavy calcification (or the presence of a previously placed stent) can make visualization of the cap nearly impossible. In such circumstances, the ambiguous cap can be "ignored" and the entry performed proximal to the ambiguous cap. This approach has several requirements however: because the subintimal space is purposely entered, an ADR strategy must be committed to. This in turn requires the presence of an adequate reentry zone, as well as no significant sized branch (e.g. a diagonal) between the newly formed proximal entry and the body of the CTO (as the branch would not be perfused following successful reentry). Assuming these conditions are met, the two strategies for making a new proximal entry in the coronary are *Scratch and Go*, and BASE (Balloon Assisted Subintimal Entry).

*Scratch and Go* (Fig. 7.2) involves gaining entry into the subintimal space proximal to the ambiguous cap by using a

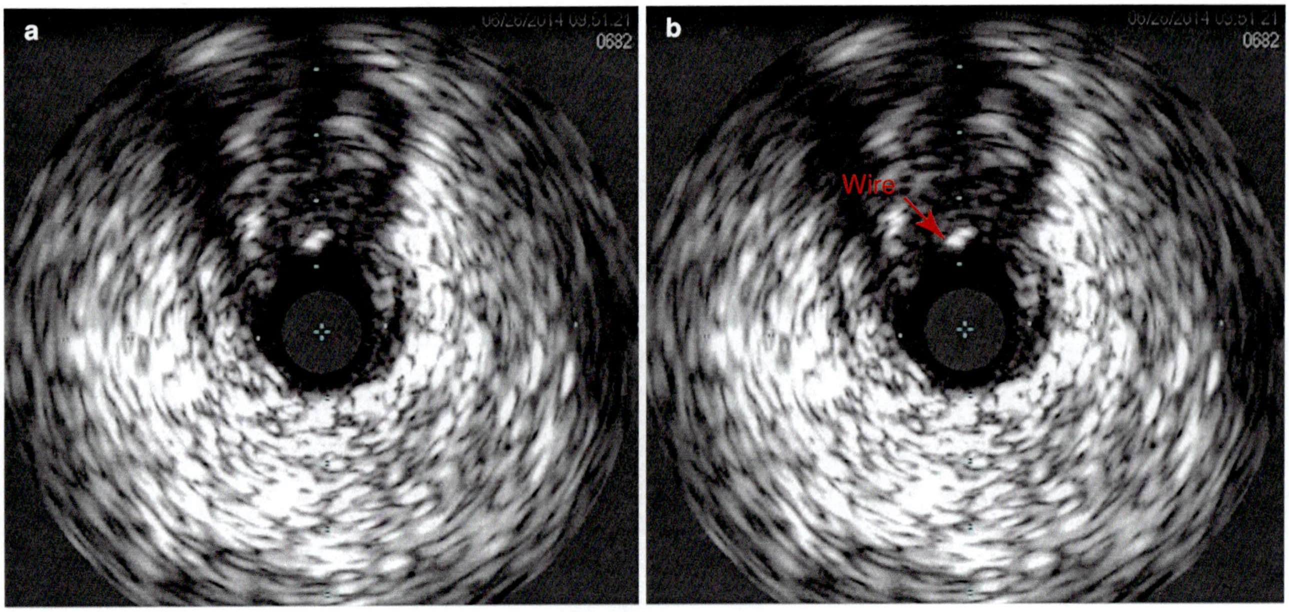


**Fig. 7.1** IVUS-guided proximal cap puncture. (**a**) IVUS of proximal cap. (**b**) Guidewire entering into proximal cap

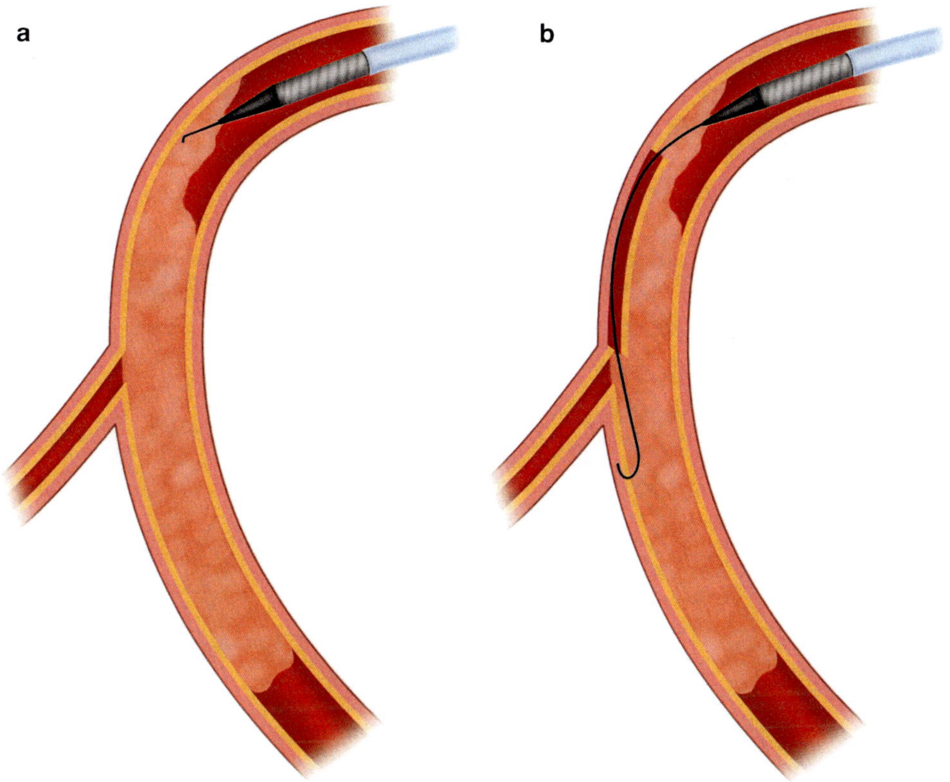


**Fig. 7.2** (**a**, **b**) Scratch and go technique

Corsair microcatheter and Confianza Pro 12. A long (3–4 mm), sharply angulated bend is made on the wire, which is then used to puncture into the subintimal space over a very short distance (5 mm). This technique will be easier to perform in the presence of a plaque that can be targeted with the wire. The tip of the Corsair is then carefully advanced (rotated) over the wire, which is then exchanged out for a plastic-jacketed wire (usually a Fielder XT, also with an exaggerated bend). The Fielder XT is then purposely knuckled into the subintimal space, and advanced into the body of the CTO, but not beyond the distal cap. The dissection is completed using the CrossBoss catheter, as described in other chapters, with reentry using the Stingray balloon and wire. The manipulation of the Corsair and Confianza Pro 12 in this technique is technically difficult and requires considerable previous experience with both, to prevent excessive wire penetration and/or loss of position. In addition, there are several anatomical characteristics that can render this technique nearly impossible, specifically a large proximal vessel with heavy calcification.

BASE is a more user-friendly version of the same concept (Figs. 7.3 and 7.4, Videos 7.1, 7.2, 7.3, 7.4, 7.5, 7.6, 7.7, 7.8, 7.9, 7.10, and 7.11). A balloon (sized about 1:1) is brought into the CTO artery, proximal to the presumed ambiguous cap, and dilated up to high pressures, with the goal of making several dissection planes. Again, this technique is easier to perform when a plaque, even when non-significant, is present. A Corsair is then brought into the artery, again with a plastic jacketed wire (Fielder XT or Pilot 200), and the wire is knuckled into the subintimal space, with advancement and subsequent exchange for the Crossboss as noted above. This is an easier (and somewhat safer) technique to master, but can also be limited by large vessels that are heavily calcified.

Ultimately, if these approaches fail, or if the anatomy is not conducive to start with, a retrograde strategy should be applied, if possible.

## Impenetrable Cap

This is defined as an inability to gain wire entry into a defined (i.e., non-ambiguous) proximal cap. The solutions include: (1) Maximizing support- this can include the use of anchor balloons and guide extensions. A Corsair should be utilized as the microcatheter of choice, as it will be able to get closer to the tip of the wire (and thus enhance penetration power) than other alternatives. In some situations, a "power position" of the Corsair can be obtained by inflating an appropriately sized balloon in the artery next to the Corsair, thus pinning it and providing even more support for the wire. (2) Use of the stiffest wires available-Confianza Pro 12 is the preferred coronary wire in this scenario, but other wires, including the Stingray wire, the Progress 200 T and peripheral options (if available in one's lab) can also be successful. (3) If the cap is well defined, and the operator is experienced

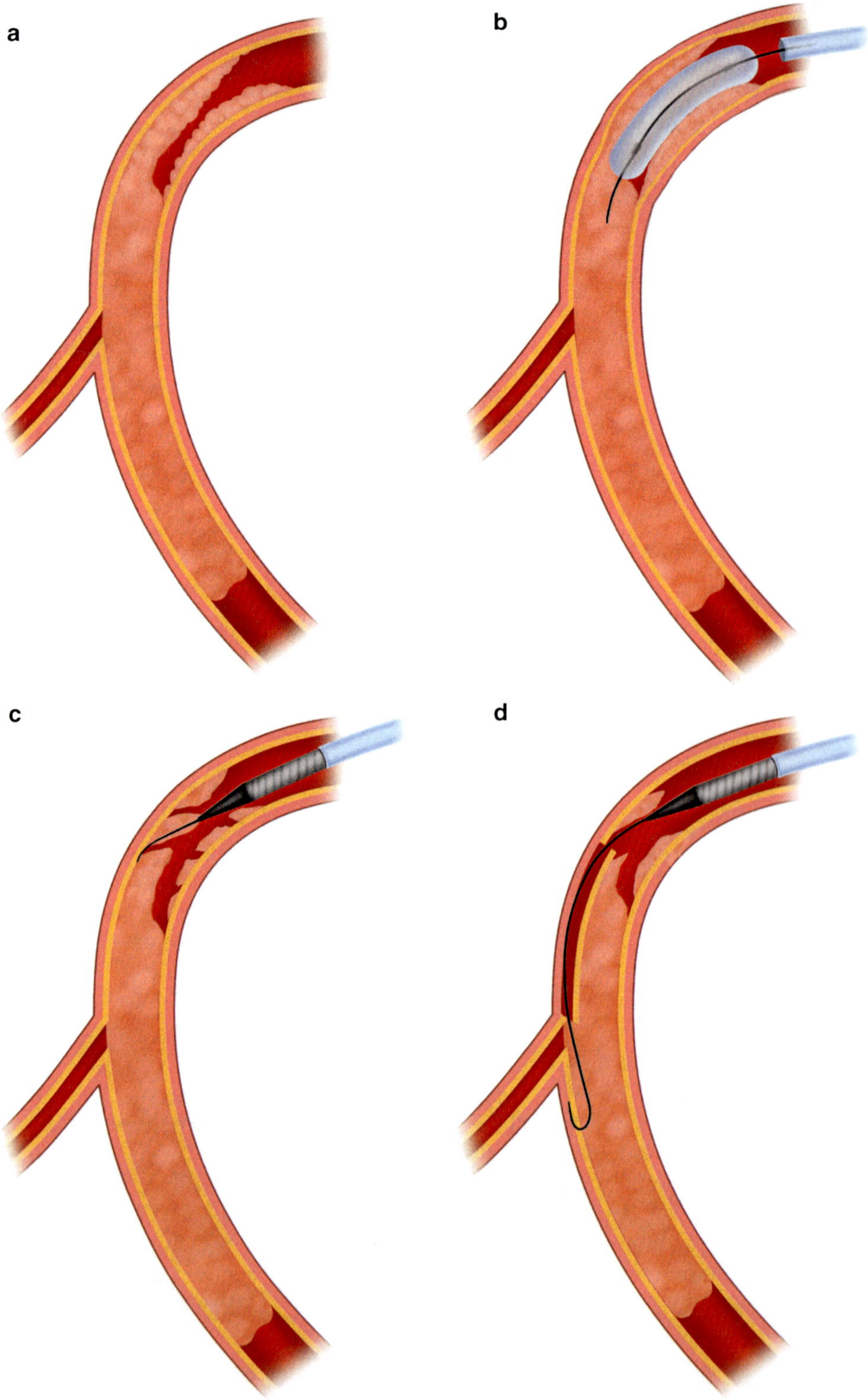


**Fig. 7.3** (**a–d**) Balloon-assisted subintimal entry (BASE)

with use of coronary laser, a 0.9 mm laser catheter can be brought down to the tip of wire and energy applied (without catheter advancement) to allow for modification of the cap and subsequent wire entry. (4) Similarly, hydraulic cap modification can be performed (see Chap. 8): The Corsair catheter is advanced as far as possible over the wire, with the tapered tip hopefully "buried" into the cap. The wire is removed and a small volume of contrast is carefully injected (using a 3 cc syringe), under fluoroscopic guidance. Care must be taken to avoid a large dissection and/or "mushroom cloud" formation. The guidewire is then reintroduced and the modified cap entered.

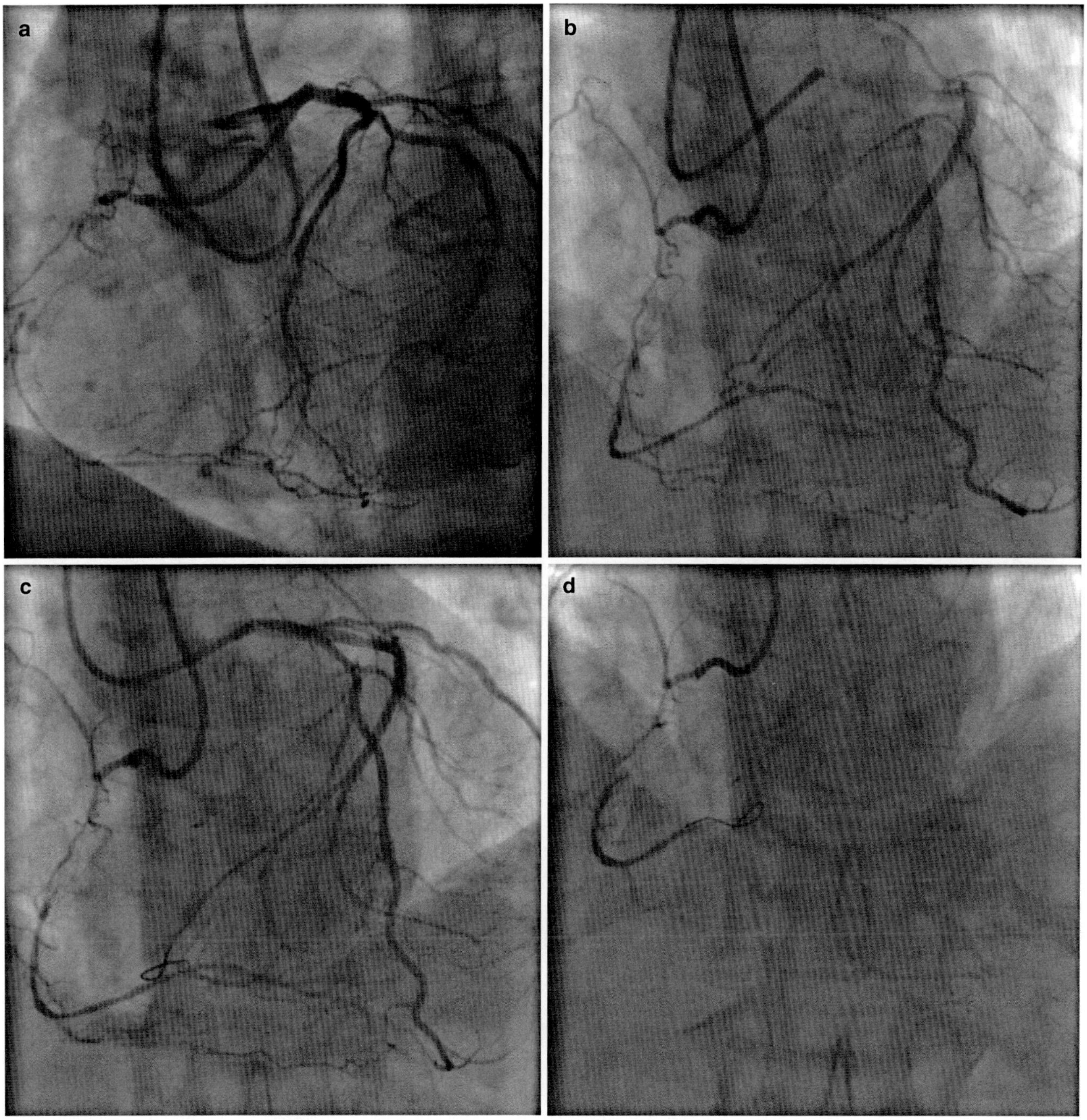

**Fig. 7.4** (Videos 7.1, 7.2, 7.3, 7.4, 7.5, 7.6, 7.7, 7.8, 7.9, 7.10, and 7.11). Balloon-assisted subintimal entry (BASE) and blind stick techniques. (**a**, **b**) More than 20 mm RCA CTO with a very ambiguous proximal cap, with many ipsilateral bridge collaterals (Videos 7.1 and 7.2). (**c**) Retrograde approach with a Sion through the large epicardial CC from the LCX to the PLV (Video 7.3). (**d**) Failure to connect into the distal RCA, with subintimal tracking in the last few mm (Video 7.4). (**e**) Antegrade bailout with the BASE (balloon-assisted subintimal entry). After dilating the proximal RCA segment with a 3.0 mm balloon, a very tiny injection was performed with 1 cc of contrast, showing a dissection plane (Video 7.5). (**f**) A Fielder XT in knuckled into the dissection plane, with the support of a CrossBoss (Video 7.6). (**g**) The CrossBoss is advanced to the distal RCA for re-entry (Video 7.7). (**h**) A Stingray is in place (*Circle*), but an antegrade hematoma is compressing the true lumen. Suction of blood from the Stingray ports did not improve visualization (Video 7.8). (**i**) A first stick is performed through the port pointing upward, as the common position of a Stingray following a CrossBoss is following the great curvature of the artery (Video 7.9). (**j**) Successful "swap" with a Pilot 200 shaped as the Stingray wire (Video 7.10). (**k**) Final result after DES deployment (Video 7.11)

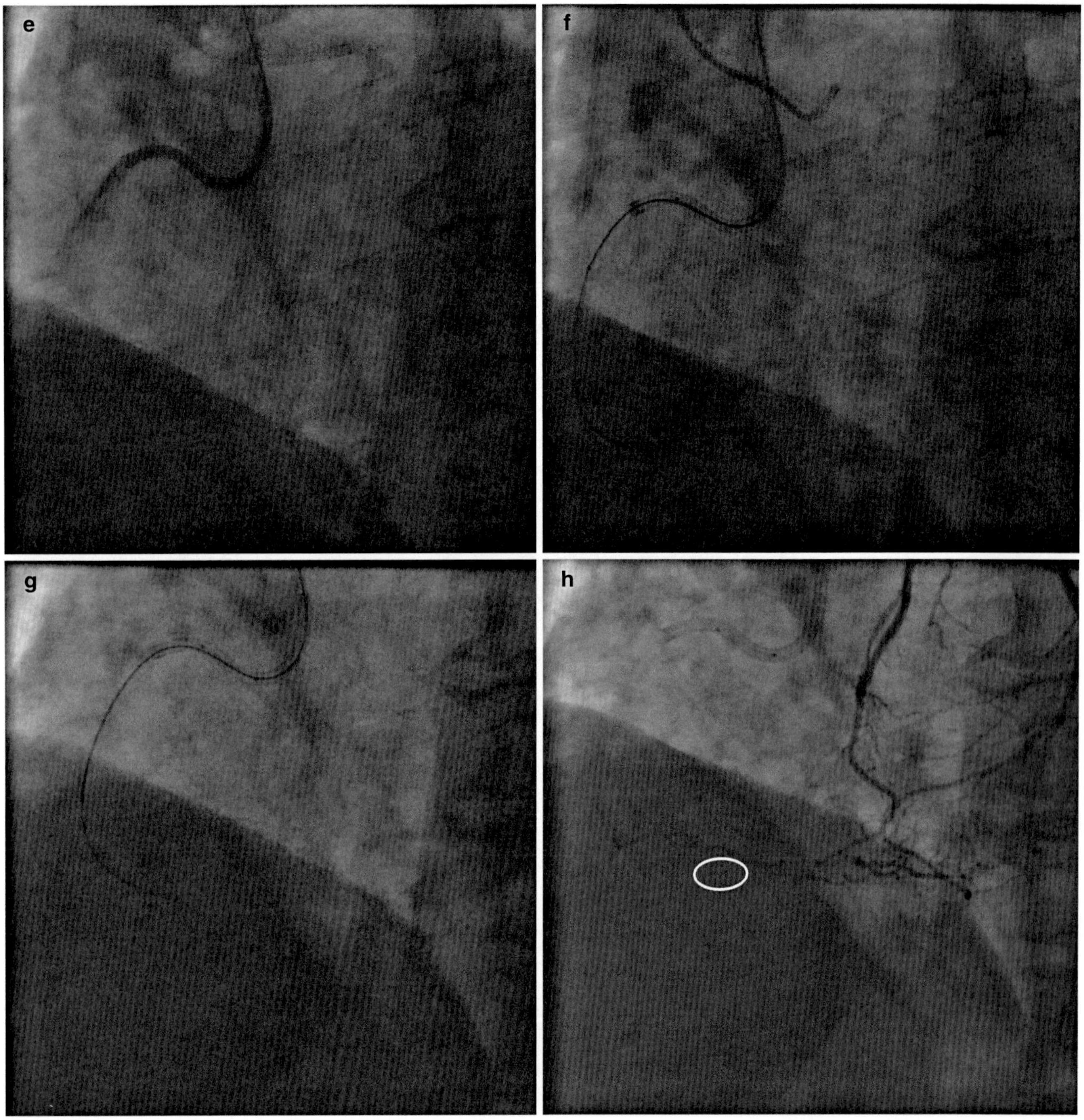


**Fig. 7.4** (continued)

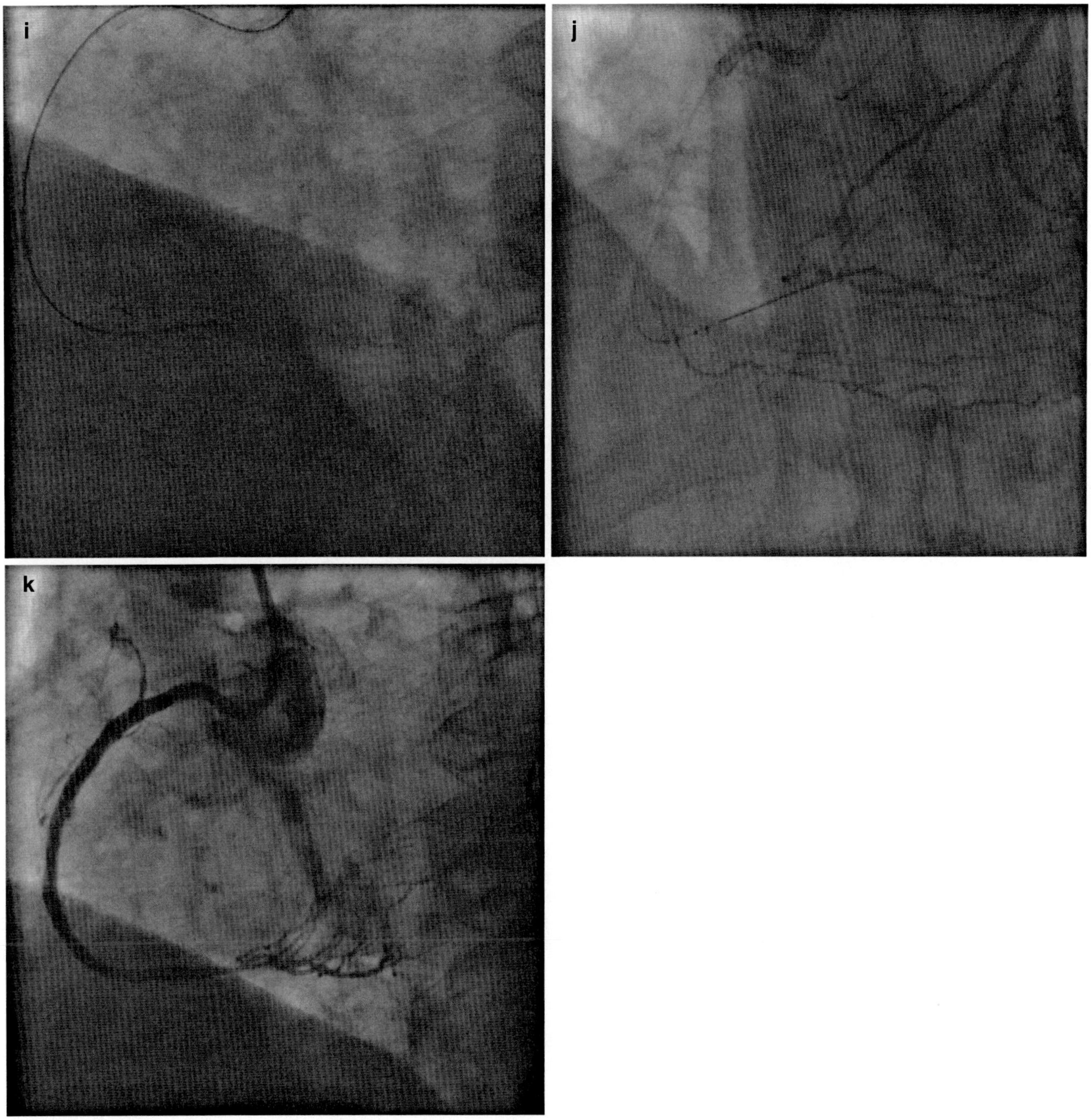


**Fig. 7.4** (continued)

Any of the previous techniques can be successfully used to proceed with either WE or ADR. However, in many instances, the difficulty in crossing the proximal cap with a wire becomes a predictor of continued significant challenges in advancing all other gear (microcatheters, CrossBoss, Stingray, balloons, etc.). Because of this, it is frequently advantageous to once again ignore the existing cap and utilize Scratch and Go, and BASE to make a new and more proximal entry. As noted above, this requires a commitment to using ADR (with the aforementioned anatomical requirements). However, moving equipment through the subintimal space is often much easier than advancing through a very resistant cap.

Again, if these techniques are unsuccessful, or cannot be applied because of anatomical constraints, then a retrograde approach is necessary. A retrograde wire (knuckled) is also an effective way of modifying the proximal cap and allowing for subsequent antegrade wire and catheter advancement for retrograde dissection reentry.

## Uncrossable Lesion

This scenario differs from an impenetrable cap in that the wire has successfully crossed and is either within the true lumen, or within the architecture of the vessel (subintimal or otherwise), but no gear can cross over the wire. The solutions for this are: (1) Again, maximizing support using anchors or guide extensions, and using a Corsair as the microcatheter of choice (a Tornus can also be attempted in this situation), (2) exchange out for a 1.5 or smaller monorail balloon, 15–20 mm length. The balloon is advanced as far as possible, then inflated up to rated burst pressure. If, on deflating, the balloon is able to advance even a short distance, then inflations and advancement are repeated. If however, the balloon does not advance, then BAM (Balloon Assisted Microdissection) is performed by inflating the balloon rapidly up to very high pressure with subsequent rupture. As soon as this occurs, maximal negative pressure should be applied to avoid pinhole high pressure jets of contrast into the artery. Frequently, this technique will result in subsequent successful passage of other catheters. (3) If laser is available, it is wise to begin warming up the console as the first two steps are being applied. If they are unsuccessful, then the laser is ready to be introduced. A 0.9 mm catheter is slowly advanced, at maximal settings, until the lesion is crossed. (4) Another way to modify the lesion is via an "external cap crush". This involves knuckling a second wire and microcatheter into the subintimal space proximal to the resistant lesion (see Scratch and Go and BASE above), then exchanging the microcatheter for a 2.5 mm balloon. The latter is inflated next to the resistant lesion, usually modifying it from the outside sufficiently to allow for subsequent gear passage over the initial wire. If still unsuccessful, then the second wire can be utilized to proceed with ADR. (5) Finally, if all else fails, the microcatheter can be buried as far as possible into the lesion (Finecross is at times more effective for this maneuver), the wire removed, and a floppy Rotablator wire advanced. This usually requires that the radiopaque tip of the RotaWire be shortened by 10–20 mm in order to allow for sufficient working length of the radiolucent portion past the lesion (as the burr will not advance over the .014 radiopaque portion). A 1.25 mm burr at high rotational speeds (over 180,000 rpm) is then carefully advanced through the lesion, virtually guaranteeing subsequent advancement of gear.

## Difficult Antegrade Issues That Are Unique to Antegrade Dissection Reentry

Antegrade dissection reentry in the Hybrid Algorithm is dependent on the use of the dedicated CrossBoss and Stingray device. The indications for, and basic utilization of, the device are well described in the previous chapter. However, as with all CTO PCI, there are unique challenges that can be encountered with this approach, and a working knowledge of solutions is crucial to ensure a high likelihood of success.

## Principles with Sub-intimal Dissection Planes and Management

The various dissection techniques that are currently used to gain access and control of the sub-intimal space are associated with different levels of vessel trauma and potential for sub-intimal hematoma formation. In increasing order of induced sub-intimal vessel trauma; (1) a straight sub-intimal wire positioned near a distal true lumen creates the least disruption and remains associated with minimal hematoma usually, unless simultaneous wires are used (parallel wire); (2) this is followed by CrossBoss dissection when advanced in the last few mm distally close to the re-entry point; (3) the use of knuckled guidewires will however lead to more extensive dissection planes, increasing the likelihood of the sub-intimal layers to be filled with hematomas and hinder subsequent re-entry. The Fielder XT is usually associated with smaller dissection planes than those caused by the Pilot 200, which is more powerful and creates larger loops when pushed; and finally (4) the injection of contrast in the sub-intimal planes leads to the largest vessel trauma in our experience.

When attempting a true-to-true lumen crossing, if a straight wire ends up near the distal true lumen in the sub-intimal plane, it can be considered the least traumatic situation. In such instance, a Corsair can be advanced to the tip of the wire, creating a 1 mm channel that will be large enough for the Stingray catheter to follow. Alternatively, a quick wire-based re-entry attempt with a Confianza Pro 12 wire can be performed, keeping in mind that it may lead to some hematoma formation. It is wise not to commit to a longer dissection and attempt re-entry more proximal if possible, as the re-entry zone can always be moved more distally if needed. If a knuckled wire was however necessary to gain access to the sub-intimal space, the CrossBoss should be used to finish the dissection plane prior to re-entry attempts. Finally, if contrast was used to dissect the sub-intimal planes, a wire-based reentry strategy will usually be required, using knuckled or straight wires (contrast-guided STAR technique, see Chap. 8).

## Crossboss Challenges

The CrossBoss catheter is at times unable to advance through the body of the CTO, even with optimal rapid spinning techniques. The first response to this should be to advance a Pilot 200 wire beyond the resistant area, and then to spin the Crossboss catheter over the wire. If this is unsuccessful, the Pilot 200 (or, as above, a Fielder XT) can be knuckled past the resistance, followed by advancement of the CrossBoss, often referred to as the *Knuckle-Boss* technique (Fig. 7.5). Care should be taken not to advance the knuckled wire too far, especially beyond the distal cap, in order to avoid the formation of a large subintimal space which would hinder reentry. Finally, a Confianza Pro 12 wire may be necessary to advance beyond a particularly resistant lesion. In this situation, it is strongly recommended that the CrossBoss catheter be exchanged out for a Corsair, the Confianza Pro 12 advanced over a short distance, the Corsair advanced (as described with Scratch and Go above), and then a knuckle wire used to proceed further. Once the operator is comfortable that the knuckled wire is within the vessel architecture, the CrossBoss is then exchanged for and used to complete the dissection beyond the distal cap. In summary, the CrossBoss is often a poor dissection starter, but always a good finisher. If the sub-intimal space is finally engaged successfully, care should be made to finish the dissection plane with the CrossBoss, as it will usually create a dryer virtual space ideal for the Stingray.

If the wire advances with any of these techniques, but the CrossBoss still will not advance, then the "uncrossable lesion" algorithms (BAM, laser, Rotablator, etc.) can be applied.

It is not uncommon for the Crossboss catheter to veer into a sidebranch as it is being spun through the CTO. It is important to recognize this as quickly as possible, as continued advancement of the Crossboss into a small sidebranch can lead to vessel perforation. This is especially the case with RCA CTO; the CrossBoss is a stiff catheter and tends to track the greater curvature of the vessel, where the right ventricular side branches take off. Frequently assessing orthogonal views as the CrossBoss makes forward progress is crucial, especially in one's early experience. If the CrossBoss is noted to be exiting into a branch, the solutions are similar to those noted above. Initially one should try a "wire redirect", usually with a Pilot 200 (Fig. 7.6). If successful, this has a potential benefit over knuckling in that a smaller

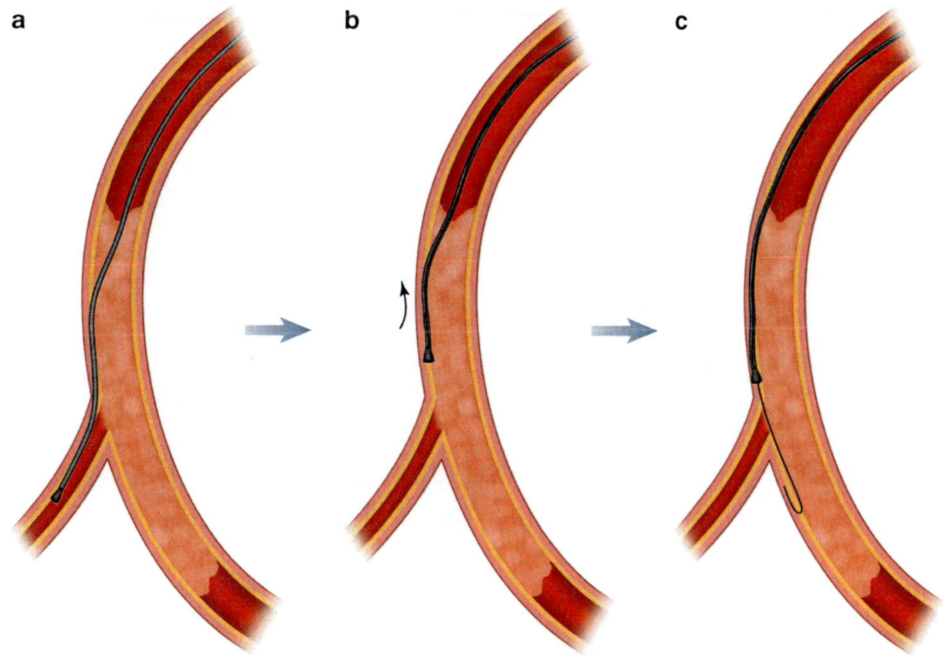


**Fig. 7.5** (a–c) Knuckle-Boss technique

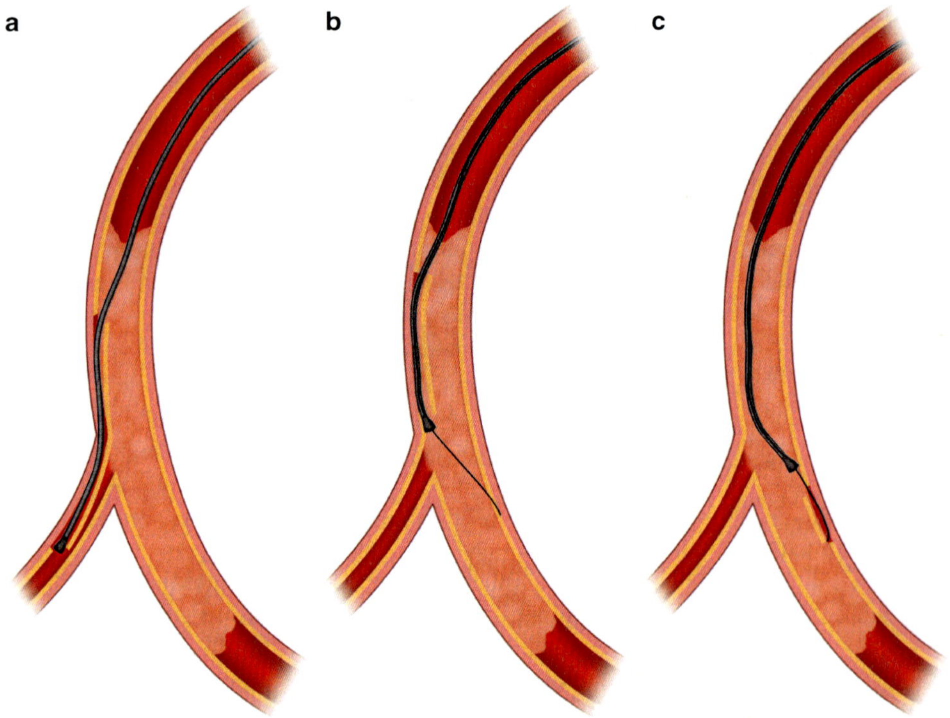


**Fig. 7.6** (a–c) Wire redirect of CrossBoss

subintimal path is created, based on the principles discussed above. However, at times, the knuckled wire is the only potential mechanism to avoid recurrent passes into the sidebranch (Fig. 7.5), as the size of the knuckle will facilitate advancement down the main vessel, rather than the smaller diameter branch. As always, finishing the dissection with the Crossboss is mandatory to lead to a dryer re-entry spot. In certain circumstances the knuckled wire will continue to direct only into the sidebranch as well, and in these situations the Confianza Pro 12 may again be necessary for redirection, with the usual caveat that it is best to first exchange the Crossboss out for a Corsair microcatheter during those maneuvers. When redirected, the CrossBoss should be taken back again. Finally, if all else fails, a new dissection plane can be utilized by entering a space more proximal to that already used. This is best accomplished by leaving the existing gear in place and advancing a second microcatheter and knuckled wire in alongside, to minimize the chance of entering the same space.

## Reentry Challenges

The Stingray balloon and wire were purposefully engineered to successfully reenter the true lumen from a subintimal position. Initial experience with the device demonstrated potential failure modes due to anatomical challenges such as diffusely diseased distal vessels (i.e., poor reentry zones) and enlarging subintimal hematomas. Technique iterations were subsequently developed to deal with these dilemmas: (1) The most frequently applied solution is that of the Stick and Swap technique (Fig. 7.7, Videos 7.12, 7.13, 7.14, 7.15, 7.16, and 7.17). Because the Stingray wire was developed as a puncturing device, its ability to negotiate through diseased distal vessels, after reentry into the true lumen, is limited. "Swapping" out for a much more maneuverable wire, usually a Pilot 200, will frequently allow for successful distal vessel access. The Stingray wire is used to make the initial puncture across the intimal layers to the true lumen (demonstrating adequate wire separation from the balloon in the appropriate view is key) and is then removed. The Pilot 200 wire is then introduced with a very small (<1 mm) distal tip angulation of at least 45°. The wire is exited out the same port that the Stingray wire had punctured, and is then advanced into the distal vessel. The wire should move freely, with minimal resistance. Care should be taken to avoid multiple unsuccessful passes, with wire buckling, as this will continue to enlarge the subintimal space and inhibit subsequent reentry attempts. (2) The Stingray wire is sometimes unable to puncture across the subintimal atheroma and across the true lumen. In this situation, making a more angulated tip on the wire can be helpful. Sometimes the Stingray wire distal probe can be damaged and bended with attempts to reenter. We therefore advocate the use of other more penetrating wires including a Confianza Pro 12 or the Progress 200 T wires. If penetration is still unsuccessful, or the Stick and Swap technique has failed, then the Stingray balloon should be moved to a different position (either backwards or forwards) for reentry. Optimally, this would be in the least calcified portion, and at the position that is closest to the true lumen. (3) An enlarging and compressive subintimal hematoma can at times seriously hamper reentry attempts. The most effective means of dealing with this is prevention. As noted previously, minimizing the size of the antegrade subintimal dissection depends on limited and careful use of knuckled (and also non-knuckled) wires, maximizing use of the Crossboss, and assiduously avoiding antegrade injections. However, if distal vessel visualization becomes limited, due to compression, several solutions are available. First and most simply, the lumen of the Stingray balloon should be aspirated using a 3 cc syringe while exchanging for the Stingray wire. This can lead to a successful, although transient, decompression and distal vessel visualization with retrograde injection. If not, the STRAW (subintimal tracking and withdrawal) technique can be applied in one of two ways: A second wire is advanced into the subintimal space next to the Stingray balloon, and a Corsair microcatheter is brought

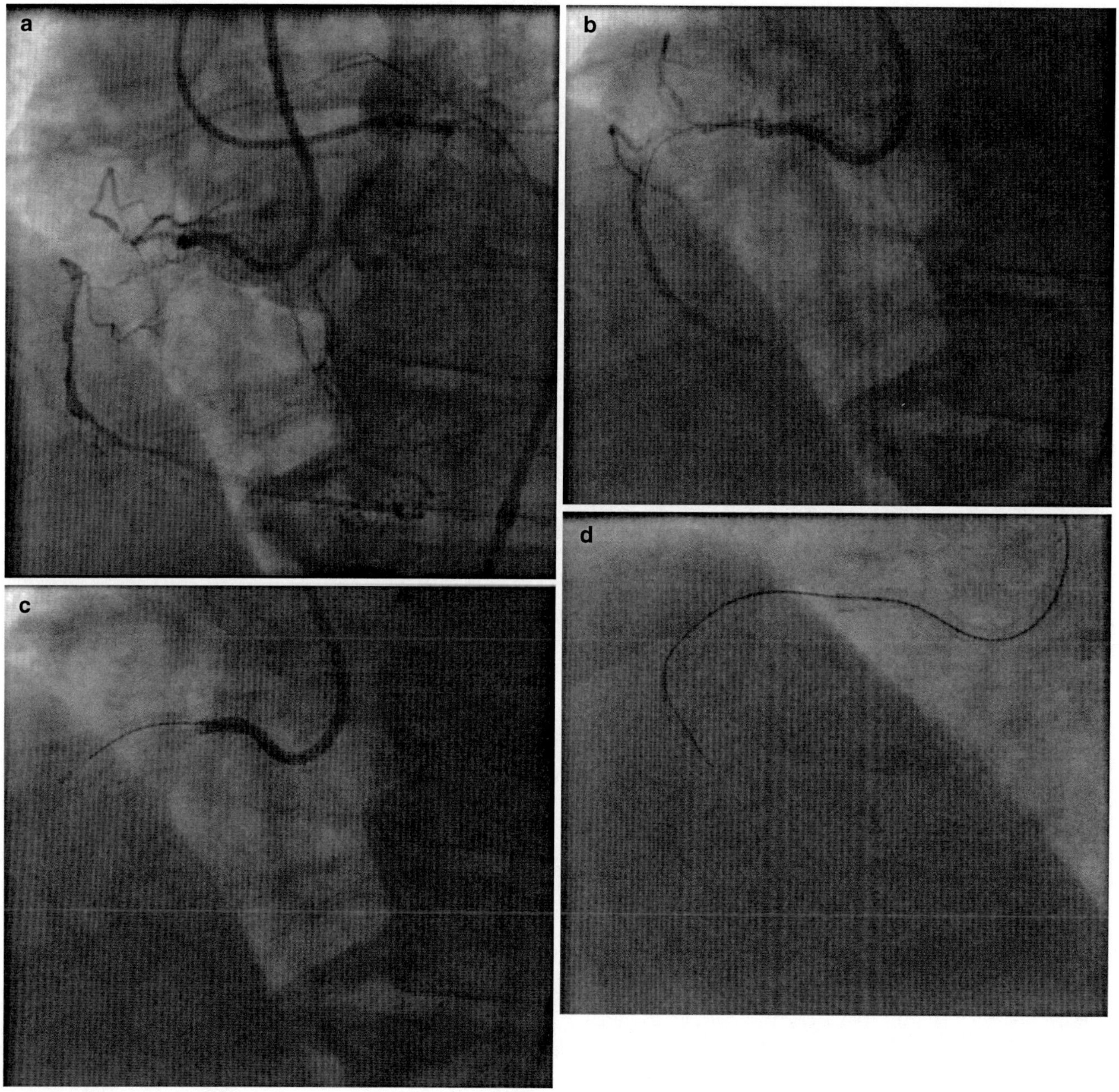

**Fig. 7.7** (Videos 7.12, 7.13, 7.14, 7.15, 7.16, and 7.17). ADR with a 'Stick and Swap' technique. (**a**) 20 mm CTO with a non-ambiguous cap, and a good distal landing zone (Video 7.12). (**b**) Sub-intimal tracking with Pilot 200 guidewire (Video 7.13). (**c**) CrossBoss to distal cap (Video 7.14). (**d**) Stingray in place: Stick with Stingray wire (Video 7.15). (**e**, **f**) Swap with Pilot 200 into distal true lumen, as confirmed with retrograde injection (Video 7.16). (**g**) Final result after stenting (Video 7.17)

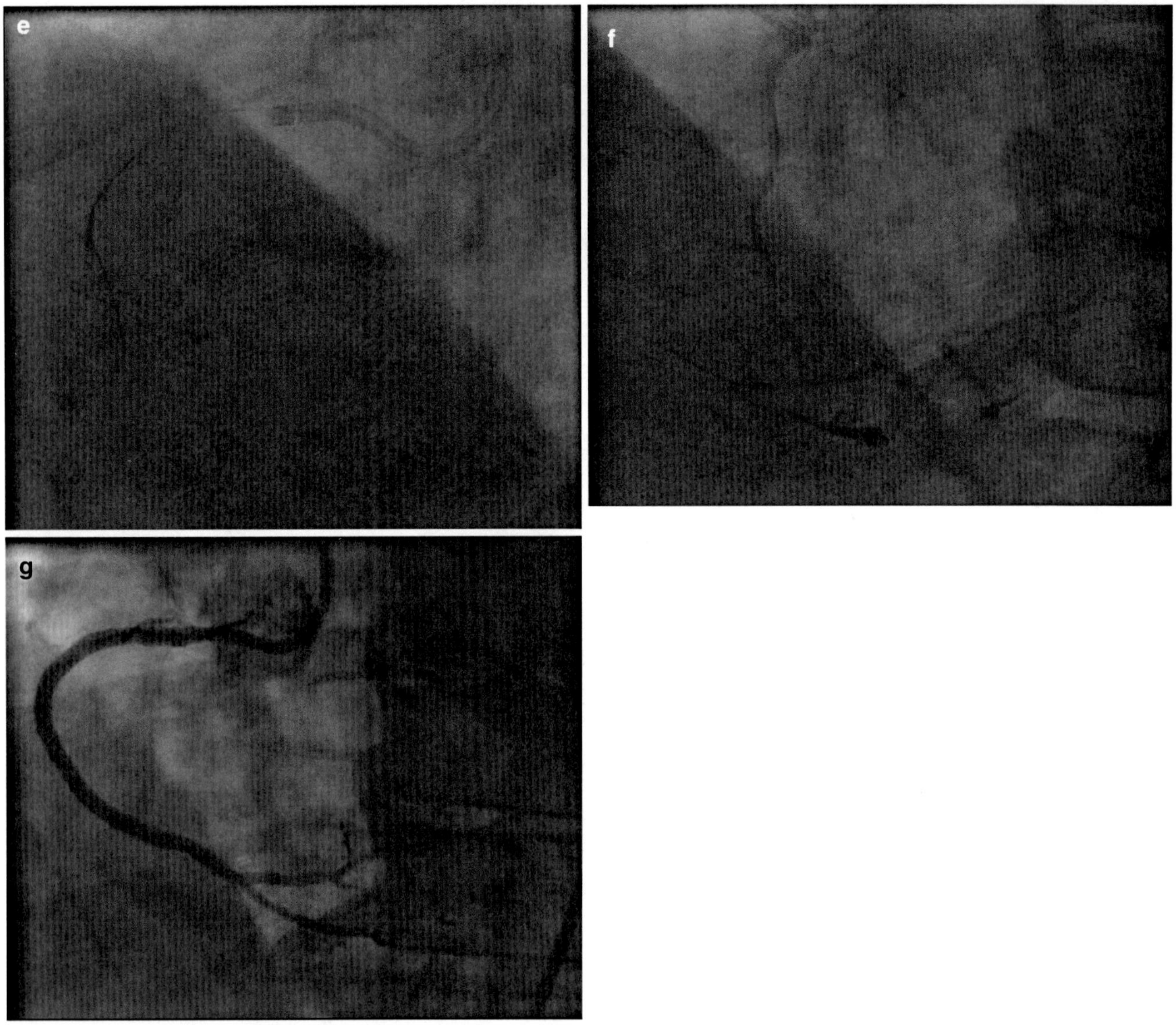


**Fig. 7.7** (continued)

into the space, with removal\of the wire and subsequent aspiration through the Corsair. This is relatively simple but is potentially limited by continued proximal inflow. To deal with this, an over the wire balloon (usually 2.5 mm) can be utilized instead, with inflation of the balloon to block inflow, and continued aspiration through the distal tip. This technique, however, is limited by the available space within an 8 Fr guiding catheter, which will only allow for a limited number of commercially available over the wire systems (Emerge balloon, Boston Scientific, UC or Ryunjin outside US) alongside the somewhat bulky Stingray catheter. Whichever aspiration technique is applied, a contralateral injection will often demonstrate reconstitution of the distal vessel and allow for successful reentry. Finally, a Blind Stick technique can be used when poor distal vessel reentry site persists (Fig. 7.8, Videos 7.18, 7.19, 7.20, 7.21, 7.22, 7.23, 7.24, 7.25, 7.26, and 7.27). This technique involves sticking both holes of the Stingray balloon with the Stingray wire, and using a "modified" Stick and Swap technique. With this technique, the proximal hole is probed gently with the Pilot 200, in search of a path of least resistance, followed by the same maneuvers through the distal hole. When the Stingray successfully fenestrate the intimal plane to the true lumen, the Pilot 200 usually follows with ease. Sticking the Stingray guidewire towards the adventitial wall is usually benign as tissue recoils and prevents subsequent passage of the Pilot 200. If reentry continues to be challenging despite application of the above, and especially if there is no suitable retrograde option, then a new dissection plane can be attempted, as described previously in the Crossboss section, leaving the initial gear in place and aiming for a different position that is more suitable for successful reentry.

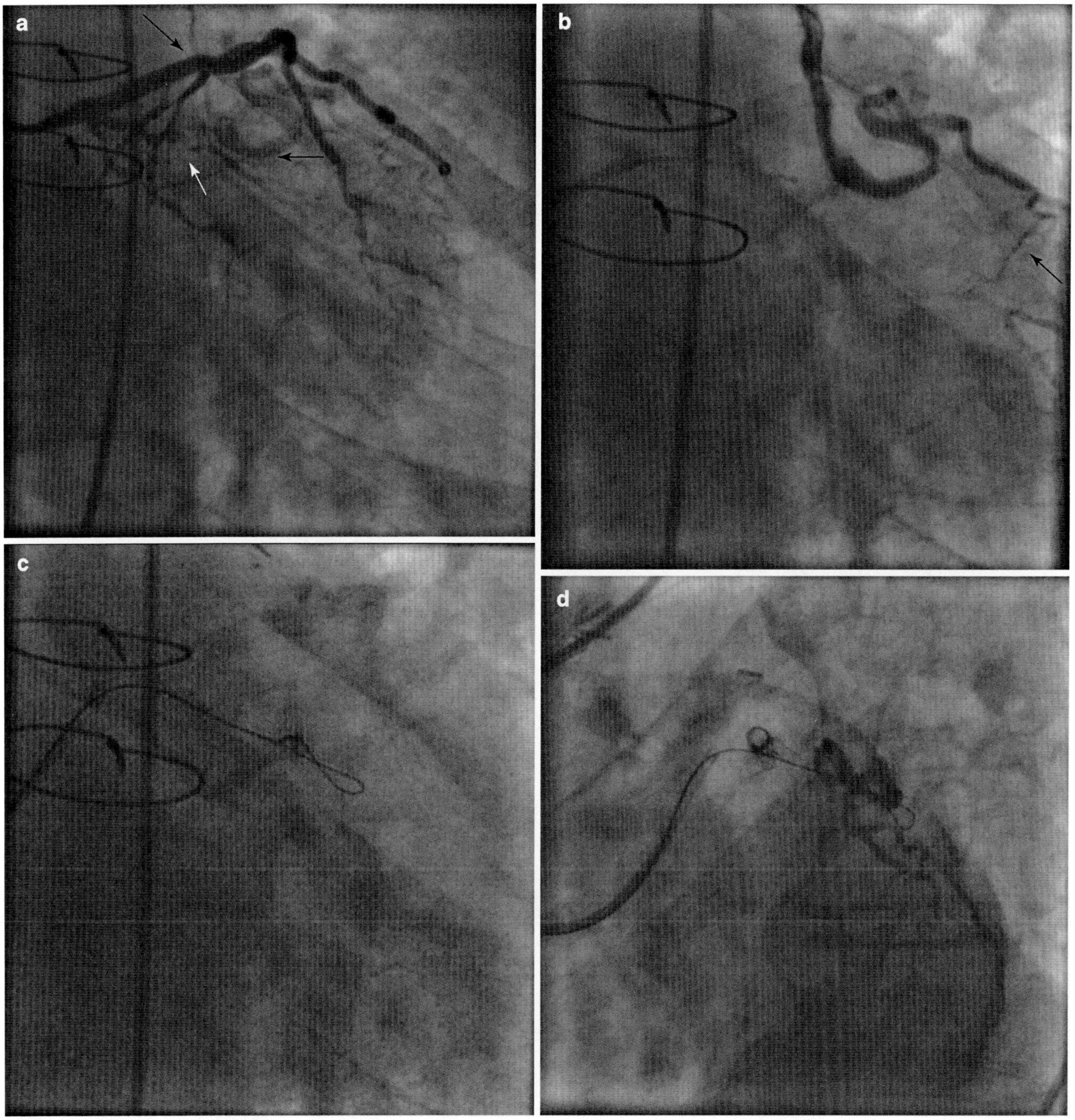


**Fig. 7.8** (Videos 7.18, 7.19, 7.20, 7.21, 7.22, 7.23, 7.24, 7.25, 7.26, and 7.27). Knuckle-Boss and Blind Stick and Swap technique using the CrossBoss and Stingray Antegrade dissection re-entry system. (**a**) Angulated but short CTO of the OM (*white arrow*), that used to be grafted by a sequential SVG to one OM and one diagonal, which was stented in the past, with occlusion of the first latero-lateral anastomosis (*bold black arrow*) (Video 7.18). (**b**) CrossBoss at the proximal cap; failure to start the dissection. The distal OM is irrigated by distal epicardial collateral channels from the diagonal branch (*black arrow*) (Video 7.19). (**c**) Knuckled Pilot 200 to start the dissection (Video 7.20). (**d**) The knuckled wire is in the vessel structure, and the CrossBoss is then advanced to create a dryer dissection plane (Video 7.21). (**e**) Poor retrograde filling of the OM branch, likely from an hematoma caused by the knuckled wire; the Stingray is visualized in a wrong view (Right Anterior Oblique) (Video 7.22). (**f**) Both wings of the Stingray balloon are overlapped in the Left Anterior Oblique view. Because of poor distal vessel filling, the direction of the stick is ambiguous (Video 7.23). (**g**) A blind stick technique is performed; first, the port pointing upward is punctured; a strong resistance is encountered (Video 7.24). (**h**) Then, the port pointing downward is punctured; a 'pop and release' sensation is felt (Video 7.24). (**i**) A Pilot 200 (swap technique) is used to track the second hole created by the Stingray; it advances without resistance (Video 7.25). (**j**) Retrograde injection that confirms that the Pilot 200 is in the true lumen (Video 7.26). (**k**) Final result post dilation and stenting (Video 7.27)

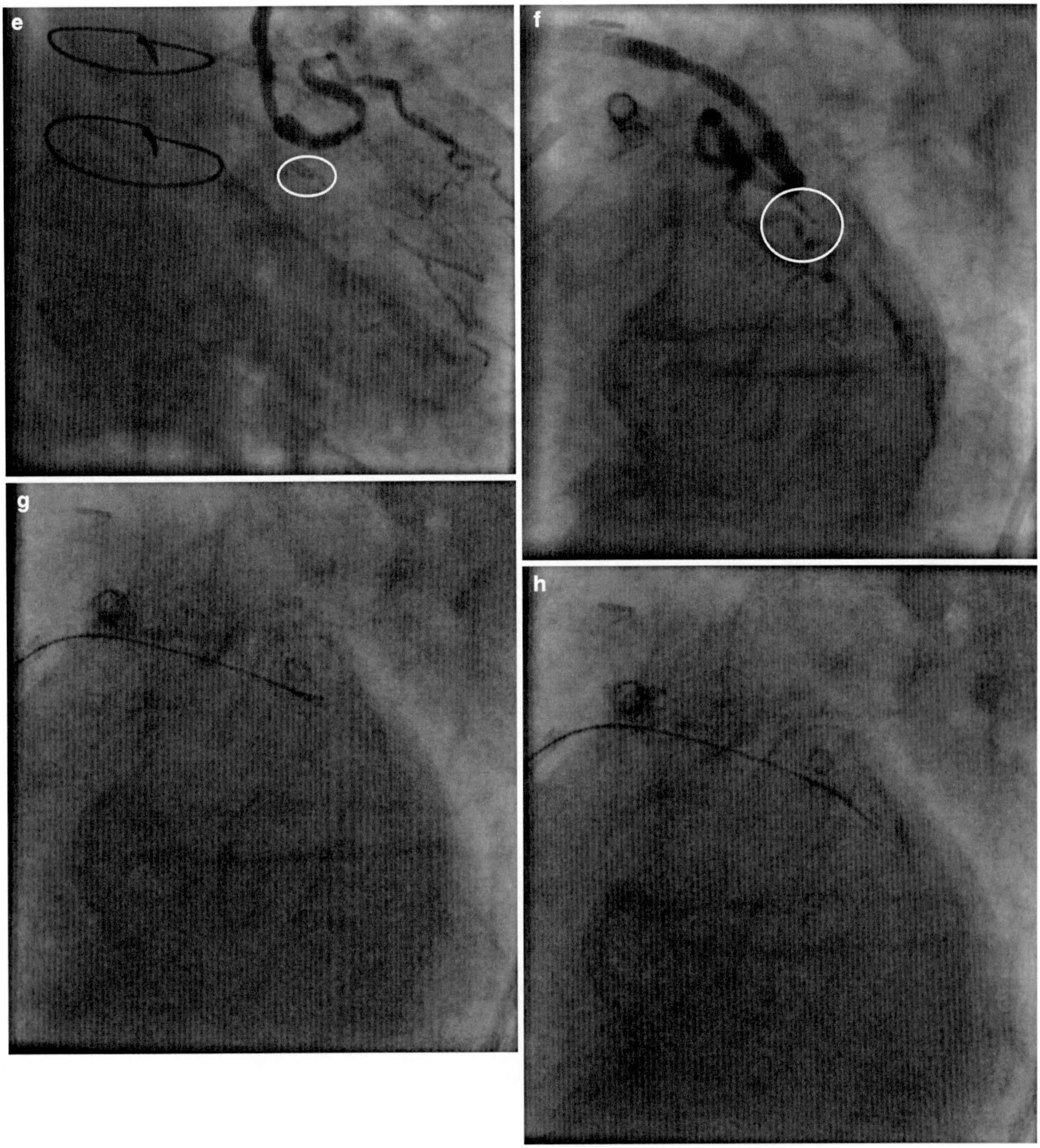


**Fig. 7.8** (continued)

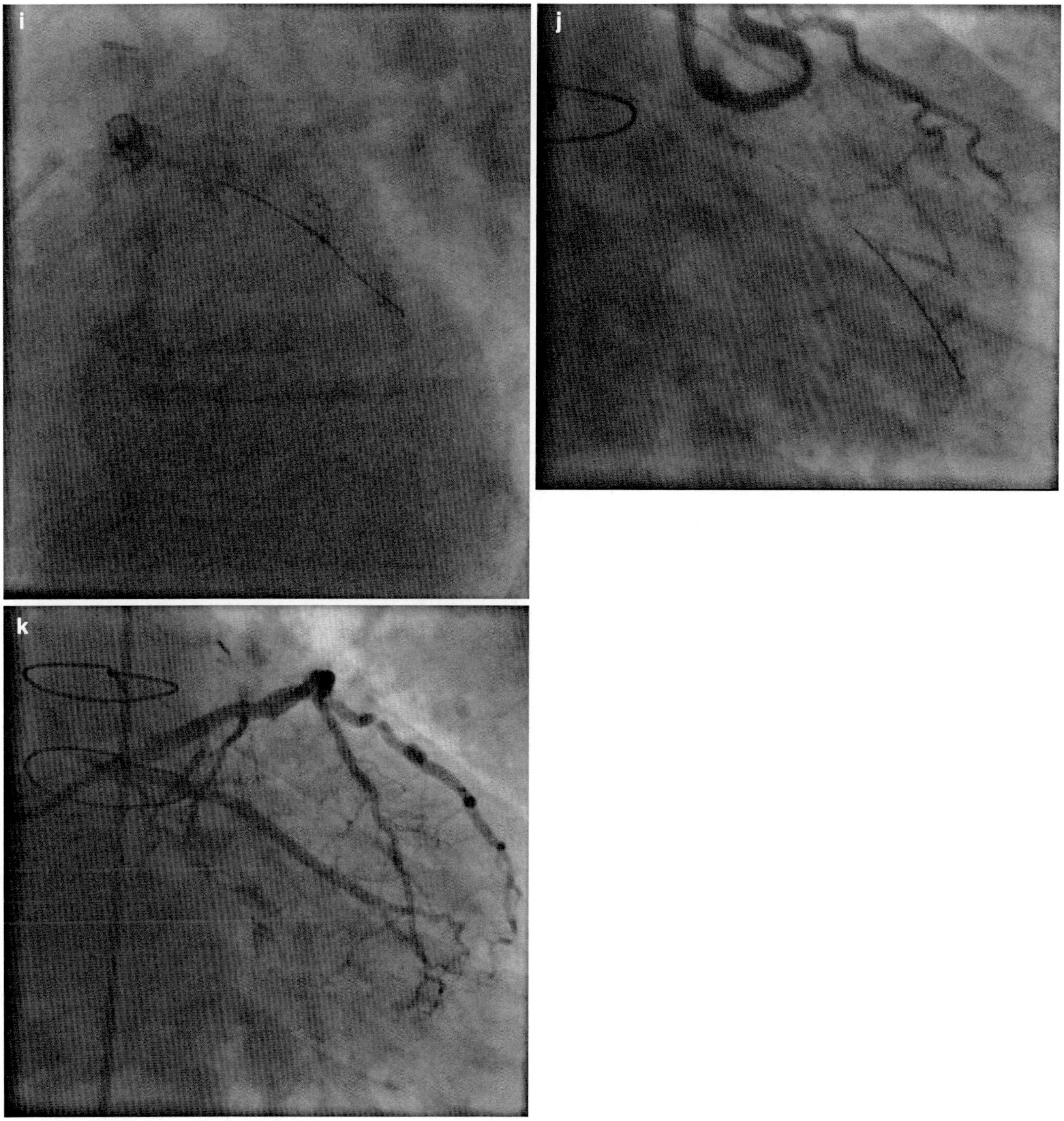


**Fig. 7.8** (continued)

In summary, a wide variety of solutions have been developed within the Hybrid algorithm to deal with specific procedural obstacles encountered during CTO PCI. Familiarity with these techniques, many of which are not generally employed in routine coronary intervention, can markedly improve the interventional cardiologist's chances of success in this challenging lesion subset.

# Intra-occlusion Microinjection of Contrast: When, Why and How

# 8

Mauro Carlino

**Abstract**

The STAR technique was an important advance in the history of percutaneous treatment of the CTO as it demonstrated that the subintimal space could be used therapeutically to recanalize the vessel. A subsequent refinement of this technique has been the introduction of the injection of a relatively large volume of contrast (up to 5 ml) with the aim of providing a 'road map' of the occluded segment, which was particularly useful for long and tortuous segments facilitating the safe advancement of a "knuckled" wire in the subintimal space, increasing operator confidence in tackling difficult CTOs. Occasionally this injection could also facilitate re-entry into the true lumen. The technique was limited however by a high rate of restenosis, unpredictability of the reentry site and the potential for coronary perforation.

A further evolution of this technique has been the adoption of a modified microinjection manoeuvre involving a gentle injection of a small volume of contrast (<1 ml). The purpose of the microinjection is to modify the compliance of the plaque by softening the loose tissue of the occluded segment facilitating CTO crossing with a dedicated coronary guidewire.

Moreover this microinjection could resolve ambiguity of the CTO fibrous cap or ambiguity of the vessel course and it is applicable to both anterograde and retrograde approaches.

**Keywords**

Subintimal Tracking And Re-entry (STAR) technique • Intra-occlusion injection of contrast • Dissection and re-entry technique (DR) • Tubular dissection • Storm cloud dissection

The treatment of coronary chronic total occlusions (CTO) with the Subintimal Tracking And Re-entry (STAR) technique, was developed based on a similar technique for the treatment of peripheral arterial CTOs.

The STAR technique, described by Colombo et al. in 2005 [1], was the first reported antegrade dissection and re-entry technique (DR), also discussed in Chaps. 4, 6, 7, 9, and 11. It involves the creation of a subintimal plane of cleavage by advancing a 0.014 knuckled polymeric guide wire which dissects the different layers of the arterial wall with the aim of re-entering the true lumen distal to the occlusion. As mentioned in Chap. 6, the classical STAR technique is limited by lack of control over the location of re-entry, often resulting in long dissections into the terminal branches and occlusion of more proximal branches. However, the STAR technique did effectively demonstrate that blunt dissection through the subintimal space could traverse occlusion segments rapidly, without perforation of the adventitia.

Moreover, this manoeuvre can be performed without a "road map" of the occluded artery. Prior to the advent of the

M. Carlino, MD
Department of Interventional Cardiology, San Raffaele Hospital Milano, Milan, Italy
e-mail: Carlino.Mauro@hsr.it


S. Rinfret (ed.), *Percutaneous Intervention for Coronary Chronic Total Occlusion: The Hybrid Approach*, DOI 10.1007/978-3-319-21563-1_8

STAR technique, wire advancement and progression through long segments of occlusion was based on the presumed anatomical distribution of the occluded vessel, on the presence of calcium and on the resistance encountered by the guide wire, and would sometimes lead to vessel perforation.

In 2008, we reported the "Contrast Guided-STAR technique" [2] where we introduced for the first time the concept of contrast injection into the subintimal space. This technique was aimed to simplify the original STAR technique and make it safer, more straightforward and more widely applicable. Once the operator enters the subintimal space with the guidewire (intentionally or not), an over-the-wire (OTW) balloon or a microcatheter is advanced over it. Then, after removing the wire, a small amount of pure contrast is injected delineating the subintimal anatomy of the occluded segment.

The main goal of the contrast injection is to provide a "road map" of the occluded artery, which is particularly useful for very long and tortuous segments, facilitating safe advancement of a knuckle wire in the subintimal space. In the early days of the technique, use of contrast injection increased operator confidence in tackling difficult CTOs, not approachable with other techniques available at that time. The amount of contrast injected in the subintimal space, in order to obtain a roadmap of the occluded segment, was however much larger (5–10 mls) compared to the amounts used in current practice (1–2 mls). Occasionally, injection of larger amount of contrast would dissect into the distal true lumen. When a liquid (in this case contrast) is injected in a confined space (in this case the area between the media and the adventitia), the forces exerted by the contrast are homogenously distributed over the entire surface. The adventitia provides greater resistance compared to the subendothelial layers favouring overstretching of the latter, sometimes creating a direct communication with the true lumen without the use of a guidewire (hydrodynamic recanalization). However, the smaller volumes of contrast used in current practice that are injected to guide the next strategy do not usually result in recanalization.

If the injection of contrast does not achieve re-entry, mechanical recanalization can be attempted by advancing a knuckled polymeric guidewire in an attempt to create a communication between the false and true lumen. The resistance exerted by the subendothelial layers is variable along the length of the vessel and is lower in areas where the atherosclerotic disease is particularly advanced, often leading to the re-entry into the true lumen in these areas. Alternatively, if the knuckle wire keeps extending the dissection further distally, a hard and straight wire such as the Confianza Pro 12 can be used to limit dissection and preserve distal branches.

The intra-occlusional contrast injection allows operators to differentiate between two different types of dissection, according to their angiographic appearance: a "tubular" or a "storm cloud" dissection.

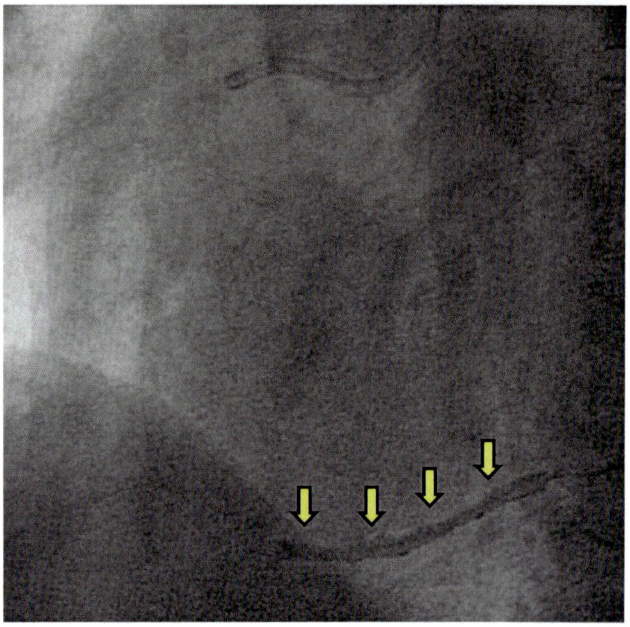

**Fig. 8.1** One case of tubular dissections. *Arrows* indicate the contrast-induced dissection

The tubular dissection (Fig. 8.1) shows a linear morphology consistent with the vessel outline, likely because the contrast lies between the media and the adventitia or between the intima and the media, while the storm cloud dissection appears like a diffuse staining of contrast media with a heterogeneous and irregular morphology. The latter type of dissection could be easily confused with a perforation. Figure 8.2 illustrates recanalization after storm cloud dissection and illustrates the true nature of this dissection, which is spilling of contrast between the media and adventitial layers. In most cases, the "storm cloud" appearance is rapidly reversible, likely due to transient alteration of the vessel permeability due to an over-stretching caused by excessively generous injection of contrast compared to the true size of the vessel, and not a perforation as demonstrated in Fig. 8.2.

The principle information we can obtain from this dissection classification is regarding the location of the microcatheter or the OTW balloon within the vessel architecture. A tubular dissection suggests that the distal tip of the over the wire (OTW) balloon is in the subintimal space of a main branch or a big side-branch and the contrast is homogenously distributed over a wide area between the media and the adventitia. This type of dissection is associated with a higher chance of re-entry into the true lumen. The following step is breaking hydrodynamically or mechanically the flap of the occlusive dissection in order to connect the false with the true lumen.

On the other hand, a storm cloud dissection, suggests that the distal tip of the OTW balloon is pointed towards the subintimal space of a small side-branch: the storm cloud angiographic appearance is probably caused by an injection of contrast in a branch so small that it is not capable to contain even a very small amount of contrast. When a storm cloud appears, it is mandatory to stop the injection as any further amounts of contrast can cause a perforation.

A storm cloud dissection needs to be converted to a tubular one using appropriate manoeuvres: the OTW balloon should be pulled back in order to position it in the main vessel, in a more favourable and wider spot capable of containing a greater amount of contrast. Once this is confirmed with a small injection (showing a tubular dissection), and the course of the main branch is delineated, the operators can insert an appropriately shaped guidewire in the OTW balloon (or microcatheter), steering it towards the direction of the main vessel, avoiding the small side-branch.

Hence, by analysing the characteristics of the dissection operators can make informed decision about when and how to continue with the procedure.

## Alternative Uses of the Intraocclusional Injection of the "Carlino Technique"

With the increase of our experience and confidence we discovered other utilities of the subintimal contrast injection manoeuvre. Failure to cross a lesion with a guidewire or a balloon is most often due to severe calcification at the occlusion site that can be quite challenging to overcome. Several strategies have been proposed [3], and can be summarized into two categories: (1) strategies that increase guide-catheter support and (2) strategies that provide lesion modification. Strategies that increase guide-catheter support include (i) deep guide intubation, (ii) use of guide-catheter extensions, such as the Guideliner catheter (Vascular Solutions) and the Guidezilla (Boston Scientific), and (iii) use of various anchor techniques (such as side-branch anchor and distal anchor). Those techniques are described in Chap. 12 of this book.

Strategies that involve lesion modification include (i) "rupturing" small balloons, advanced as far as possible into the lesion in an attempt to modify the proximal cap (a technique often called balloon-assisted microdissection (BAM) or also "grenadoplasty"), (ii) use of various microcatheters, such as Tornus (specifically designed to "screw into" resistant lesions, creating a channel), Corsair or Finecross, and (ii) use of laser or the Crosser catheter (Flowcardia, Inc) or rotational atherectomy.

Injecting contrast into the occlusion is an alternative strategy that can lead to lesion modification. Soft plaque consists of cholesterol-laden cells and foam cells with loose fibrous tissue and a network of neovascular channels and is more frequent in younger occlusions (<1 year old) [4]. Soft plaque is more likely to allow wire passage either directly through tissue planes or via neovascular channels into the distal lumen. Conversely, hard plaques are more prevalent with increasing CTO age and are characterized by dense fibrous tissue and often contain large fibro-calcific regions without neovascular channels [5]. Areas of calcification frequently occur even in CTOs <3 months of age, although the extent and severity of calcification increase with occlusion duration. Older (>1 year) occlusions are more likely to deflect guide-wires into the subintimal area, creating dissection planes. This age-related increase in calcium and collagen content of CTOs in part explains the progressive difficulty during PCI in crossing older occlusions.

The typical CTO may be classified as "soft," "hard," or a mixture of both. The so-called resistant or uncrossable CTO lesions have a high content of harder intimal plaque and dense calcium formations. Such lesions are approached using a different type of injection compared to the one used in the STAR technique. This technique was refined over time by reducing volumes of contrast injected and minimizing the level of force applied during the injection. The rationale behind the minimal volume of contrast and reduced injection forces lies in the generation of hydraulic forces in an anterograde direction along the longitudinal axis of the involved vessel. If hydraulic forces are applied through a solid occlusion by a selective injection of a small volume of contrast, the contrast will follow the path of least resistance, represented by the loose tissue segments in the occlusion.

If the amount of contrast or the injection pressure used is increased, the presence inside the occlusion of areas of high-resistance (fibro-calcific plaques) will divert hydraulic forces to a radial direction involving the subintimal space, which is usually softer than the intraluminal obstructing material, and lead to contrast extravasation. The purpose of this microinjection is to modify the compliance of the plaque by softening the loose tissue of the occluded segment through an injection of viscous liquid (in this case contrast). This technique subsequently facilitates the CTO crossing with a polymer coated coronary guide wire or, in the case of failure, can guide the operator where to pursue with antegrade contrast-guided STAR or other antegrade DR.

From the technical point of view, the injection should be performed gently with a very small amount of contrast in order to delineate a vague localized "blush" of contrast with a "patchy" distribution inside the occluded segment. This "patchy" distribution of the contrast could indicate the presence of islands of fibrotic tissue and/or loose fibrous tissue in the context of a very high calcific occlusion (Fig. 8.2). In order to prevent dissection, the microinjection must be performed in a controlled manner, under fluoroscopic guidance. This enables tailoring the amount of contrast administered along with the force of injection to each individual case, as these parameters depend on the anatomic characteristics of the occlusive

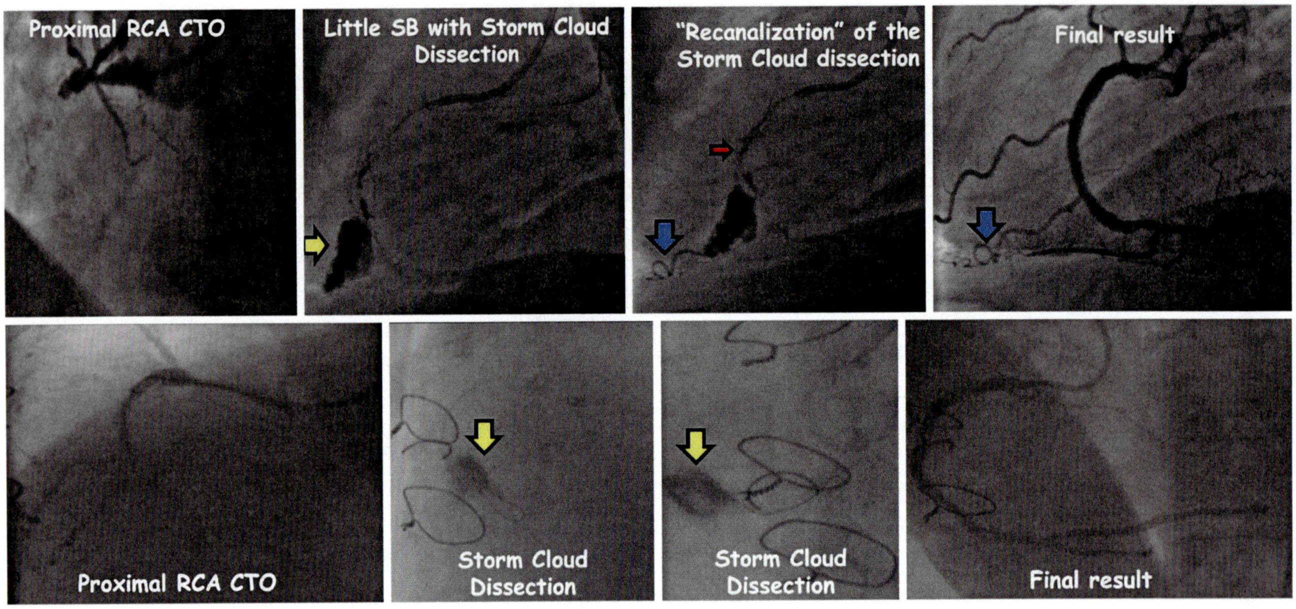


**Fig. 8.2** Two cases of storm cloud dissections. *Line A*: here a proximal CTO of a right coronary artery treated using the contrast-guided STAR technique. Being in the sub-intimal space, the operator applied the contrast guided STAR technique, injecting contrast and producing a storm cloud dissection (*yellow arrow*). At this point he slightly pulled back the balloon, adjusting the position of its tip and identified the course of the vessel but a small amount of contrast continued towards the dissection and increased the storm cloud effect. However, at the same time, it surprisingly produced a re-entry into the true distal lumen. This demonstrates that the storm cloud dissection is not a perforation, because otherwise the contrast would have gone into the pericardial space, which is a low-pressure chamber by comparison with the resistance offered by the vessel. But what is even more interesting and surprising is that following stent implantation the side branch appears to be absolutely healthy, with no evidence of perforation or residual contrast staining. In the line below we can see a Storm Cloud dissection appeared during a CTO treatment using the contrast guided STAR technique. This picture could be confused with a perforation. But an orthogonal image of the storm cloud dissection compared to the previous one shows a peri-adventitial distribution of the contrast excluding the perforation one might have suspected looking at the previous picture. Both cases illustrate recanalization after storm cloud dissection and excellent final angiographic result after stenting with drug eluting stents

plaque. Because microcatheters have radiopaque markers or segments at their tip, we strongly advocate their use for this specific purpose over a small over-the-wire balloon, where the tip position is definitely harder to define angiographically.

Finally, another opportunity offered by the microinjection of contrast is to better define the anatomy of an ambiguous proximal fibrous cap (PFC) of a CTO. The presence of a clearly defined PFC of a CTO, even if it is blunt rather than tapered, means it can be approached with confidence as the CTO entry point and the initial vessel course is clear. An ambiguous PFC refers to one where there are multiple branches, often bridging collaterals, and there is a "flush" proximal occlusion with uncertainty with regards to the initial vessel course [6]. In these cases, an early microinjection of contrast could show a storm cloud dissection or a 'tubular filling' which would suggest that the micro-catheter is pointed towards a little small side-branch or the main course of the occluded vessel, respectively. Finally, microinjection of contrast is increasingly used during the retrograde approach for distal cap modification, or to better delineate vessel anatomy. As flow is opposed to the retrograde direction, such technique is usually well tolerated and rarely result in vessel perforation when small amount of contrast are used.

In conclusion, the use of dissection and re-entry techniques, either antegradely or retrogradely have improved the success rates of CTO PCI. The ability to understand, negotiate, and manipulate the subintimal space has been the key step in improving success in contemporary CTO PCI, whether operating antegradely or retrogradely. Using tricks obtained from the early experience of the STAR technique can help tackle challenging CTOs [7].

## References

1. Colombo A, Mikhail GW, Michev I, Iakovou I, Airoldi F, Chieffo A, et al. Treating chronic total occlusions using subintimal tracking and reentry: the STAR technique. Catheter Cardiovasc Interv. 2005;64(4):407–11.
2. Carlino M, Godino C, Latib A, Moses JW, Colombo A. Subintimal tracking and re-entry technique with contrast guidance: a safer approach. Catheter Cardiovasc Interv. 2008;72(6):790–6.
3. Michael TT, Papayannis AC, Banerjee S, Brilakis ES. Subintimal dissection/reentry strategies in coronary chronic total occlusion interventions. Circ Cardiovasc Interv. 2012;5(5):729–38.

4. Srivatsa S, Holmes Jr D. The histopathology of angiographic chronic toral coronary artery occlusion and changes in neovascular pattern and intimal plaque composition associated with progressive occlusion duration. J Invasive Cardiol. 1997;9(4):294–301.
5. Srivatsa SS, Edwards WD, Boos CM, Grill DE, Sangiorgi GM, Garratt KN, et al. Histologica correlates of angiographic chronic total coronary artery occlusions: influence of occlusion duration on neovascular channel patterns and intimal plaque composition. J Am Coll Cardiol. 1997;29(5):955–63.
6. Brilakis ES, Grantham JA, Rinfret S, Wyman RM, Burke MN, Karmpaliotis D, et al. A percutaneous treatment algorithm for crossing coronary chronic total occlusions. JACC Cardiovasc Interv. 2012;5(4):367–79.
7. CTO fundamentals website: http://ctofundamentals.org/.

# How and When to Perform the Retrograde Approach

9

Stéphane Rinfret and Dimitri Karmpaliotis

**Abstract**

The retrograde approach is a cornerstone technique of the hybrid chronic total occlusion (CTO) percutaneous coronary intervention (CTO) portfolio. Mastering the retrograde approach substantially improves treatment options and success rates. This chapter will provide the reader with a framework on how to select cases for the retrograde approach based on the angiographic analysis, will review the techniques to be used in a step-by-step fashion, and offer solutions to common problems that may be encountered during the several stages of the procedure.

**Keywords**

Retrograde approach • Collateral channels (CC) • Surgical grafts • Septal collateral channels (CC) • Epicardial Collateral channels (CC) • Intra-myocardial non-septal collateral channels (CC) • Patent surgical grafts • Occluded surgical grafts

The retrograde approach is a cornerstone technique of the hybrid chronic total occlusion (CTO) percutaneous coronary intervention (CTO) portfolio [1–4]. Mastering the retrograde approach substantially improves treatment options and success rates [5]. This chapter will provide the reader with a framework on how to select cases for the retrograde approach based on the angiographic analysis, will review the techniques to be used in a step-by-step fashion, and offer solutions to common problems that may be encountered during the several stages of the procedure.

**Electronic supplementary material** The online version of this chapter (doi:10.1007/978-3-319-21563-1_9) contains supplementary material, which is available to authorized users.

S. Rinfret, MD, SM (✉)
Multidisciplinary Department of Cardiology, Quebec Heart and Lung Institute, Quebec City, QC, Canada

Laval University, Quebec City, QC, Canada
e-mail: Stephane.Rinfret@criucpq.ulaval.ca

D. Karmpaliotis, MD, PhD, FACC
Department of Cardiology, NYPH/Columbia University Medical Center, New York, NY, USA

## When to Select the Retrograde Approach: How to Analyse the Coronary Angiography

Based on the hybrid CTO algorithm [4], the retrograde approach should be preferred in the case of a CTO with an ambiguous proximal cap, in the presence of distal vessel disease or of a major bifurcation at the distal cap. A proximal cap can be considered ambiguous if it is blunt, if the trajectory of the coronary is not clear, if a major side branch arises at the level of the cap, or if there are numerous bridging ipsilateral collaterals at the level of the cap that makes the identification of the actual entry unclear. Practically, the operator can conclude that the cap is ambiguous if it would be hazardous to puncture it with a stiff wire such as the Confianza Pro 12 (Asahi Intecc, Japan) and follow the course of the wire by advancing gear, because of fear of perforation by exiting the vessel structure. A diffusely diseased distal vessel with small lumen and a distal cap at a major bifurcation are also anatomic variations that favor the retrograde approach. Finally, although long lesions can be approached with antegrade dissection and re-entry (ADR), very long and calcified lesions can also be managed successfully with the retrograde dissec-



S. Rinfret (ed.), *Percutaneous Intervention for Coronary Chronic Total Occlusion: The Hybrid Approach*,
DOI 10.1007/978-3-319-21563-1_9

tion and re-entry (DR) as well. This is obviously conditional to the identification of a retrograde path that is suitable to be crossed safely to deliver gear to the distal cap of the occlusion. It should be emphasized that what actually constitutes an "interventional collateral" depends to a great extent upon the skill and experience of the operator. These considerations will be discussed in the next section. Dual angiography should be performed as usual. For the proximal cap of the occlusion, magnified views can help to identify small stumps that may change the approach.

## How to Set up the Procedure

The procedure set up is similar to any hybrid procedure, keeping in mind some general principles. Retrograde CTO PCI is not just "CTO PCI going backwards". Several points should be considered in order to allow for an effective, safe and efficient retrograde CTO PCI. First, an 8F guide is better for the antegrade side, as it improves support and allows for the use of alternative techniques that could be necessary in the case of a failure to connect from the retrograde side. Under these circumstances alternative approaches, such as ADR or IVUS-guided proximal cap puncture can be applied (see Chap. 11). Moreover, a larger antegrade guide provides a larger target lumen for the retrograde wire, after crossing the lesion during the process of externalization. For the retrograde side, most operators nowadays are comfortable using 6F guides, to reduce contrast administration, and the likelihood of donor artery dissection, especially after externalization, as described later. Smaller 6F guides usually provide enough support and space for the retrograde equipment, which needs mostly to be rotated instead of being firmly pushed. Use of a 90 cm version of the catheter on the retrograde side is useful especially when contemplating to use a graft or an epicardial collateral, as it allows for the retrograde microcatheter to reach the antegrade guide after the CTO crossing. However, as discussed later, the use of an antegrade mother-and-child (MAC) catheter such as the GuideLiner (Vascular Solutions, USA) can help to reduce the distance from the tip of a retrograde catheter to the antegrade system. Rotation of retrograde microcatheters such as the Corsair (Asahi Intecc, Japan), or the Turnpike (Vascular Solutions, USA) is converted to forward movement, and therefore necessitates less support (Fig. 9.1, Video 9.1). Operators have published favorable experience with 6F guides on the retrograde side [6, 7]. However, for maximum support, the use of an 8F guide on the retrograde side can be advantageous, and is still preferred by many operators. Both catheters can be delivered either from the femoral or the radial arteries. A detailed review of the techniques on how to perform transradial CTO PCI, even with 8F guides (Fig. 9.2, Video 9.2), is provided in Chap. 13. As a general principle, early on in the operator's learning stages, two 8 French guides are recommended, with the use of long 45 cm sheaths if delivered from the femoral artery, to improve the support. When performing a retrograde procedure, the heparin is the

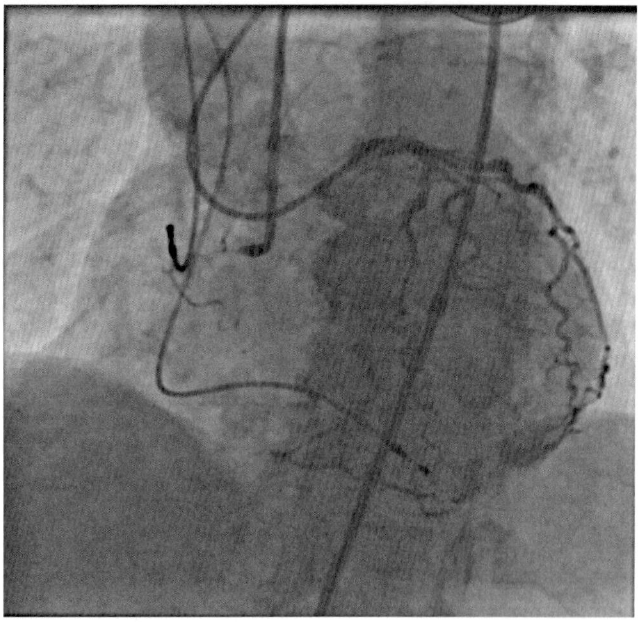

**Fig. 9.1** (Video 9.1). Dual injection showing a long RCA CTO, with the distal cap at a major bifurcation, and good septal collateral channels from the left system. A 6F XB 3.5 90 cm in used from the right radial into the left main, and an 8F JR 4 from the femoral approach into the RCA. A long 45 cm introducer is used from the femoral

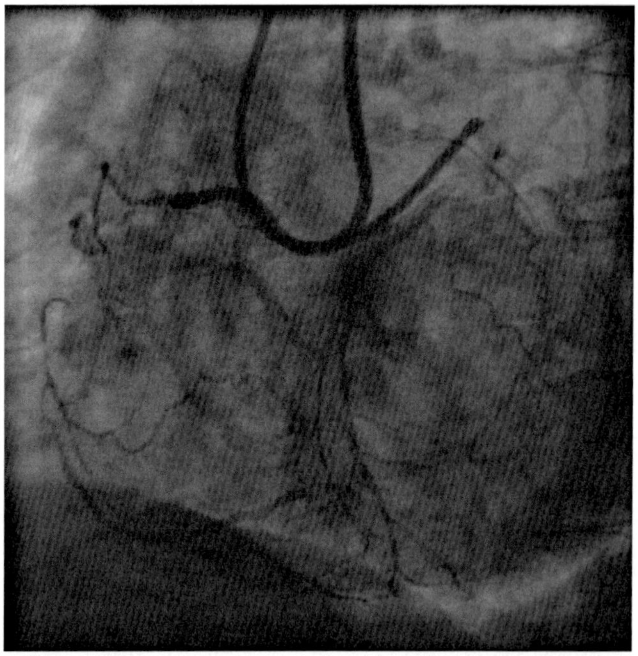

**Fig. 9.2** (Video 9.2). Dual injection using a bilateral transradial approach. An 8Fr AL1 is inserted from the left radial, using a sheathless technique, and an XB 3.5 90 cm from the right radial

anticoagulant of choice, and the ACT should be kept higher than 300–350 s as long as the equipment is present in the retrograde donor artery. Also, meticulous flushing of the retrograde catheters to avoid thrombus should be performed.

## Pathways to the Distal Cap (Table 9.1)

There are two types of conduits that can be used to deliver retrograde wires and microcatheters to the distal cap: collateral channels (CC) and surgical grafts. While CCs can be divided into *septal* CC, *epicardial* or *intra-myocardial non-septal* CC, surgical grafts can be divided into *patent* or *occluded*. The following section provides general principles with both conduits.

## Collateral Channels

Septal channels are clearly the most commonly used CCs for the retrograde approach. They are safer than epicardial CCs, as a perforation usually fenestrates into a ventricular chamber or lead to benign septal hematomas, or arteriovenous fistulas. An exception to this general rule is that occasionally very proximal septal CC will communicate with one right postero-lateral (RPL) branch, or distal septal CC can emerge at the free wall of the RV and thus become by definition epicardial at some point during their course; perforation of such channels at these areas may lead to tamponade. The septal channels are best evaluated in the straight right anterior oblique (RAO) view, or the RAO cranial view (typically 30° right, 30° cranial) (Figs. 9.3 and 9.4, Videos 9.3, 9.4, and 9.5). Occasionally an RAO caudal view is useful to assess

**Table 9.1** Retrograde pathways to the distal cap of the CTO

| | Septal CC | Epicardial or intra-myocardial non-septal CC | Patent graft | Occluded graft |
|---|---|---|---|---|
| Skill required to cross with wire | + | +++ | – | ++ |
| Risk as a conduit | + | +++ | – | + |
| Better if | Straight, numerous | Large, not too tortuous, previous cardiac surgery | Severely diseased SVG, several in-stent restenosis | Surgical clips to delineate trajectory, aortic stump |
| Able to dilate? | Yes | No | Yes | Yes |
| Higher risk if | Single tortuous CC | In the atrio-ventricular groove, intact pericardium | Internal mammary artery, especially if tortuous | Stump less occlusion, absence of clips |

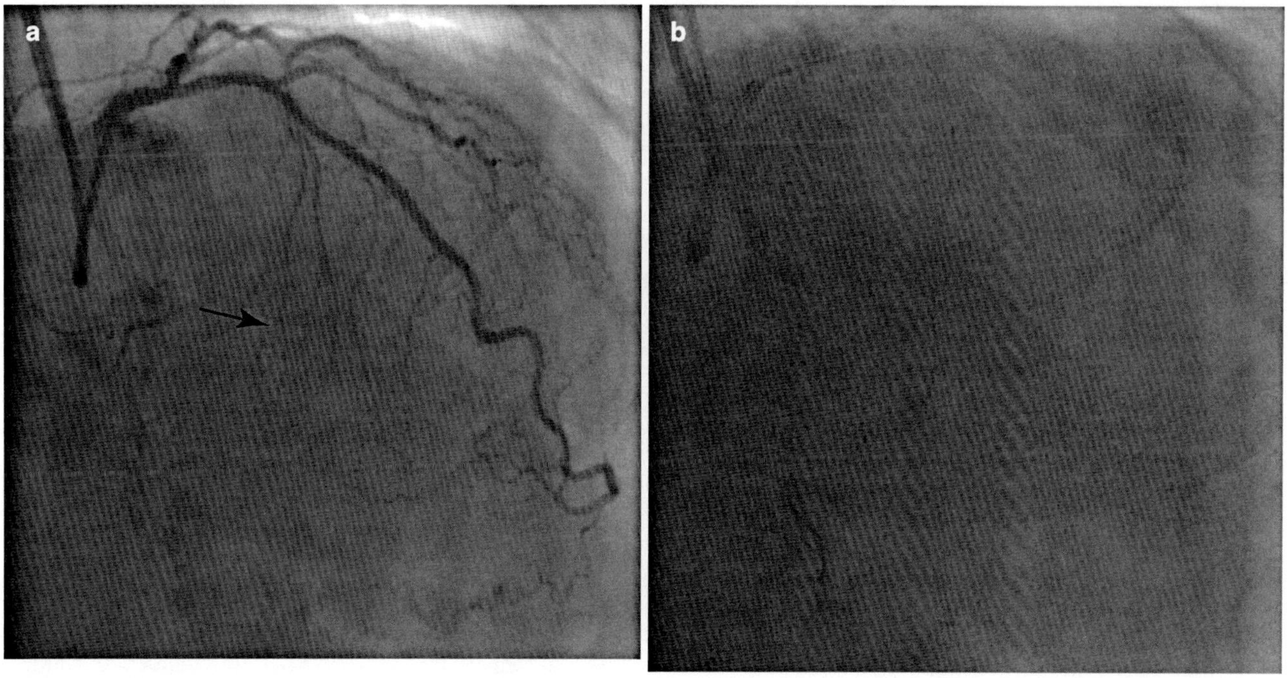


**Fig. 9.3** (Videos 9.3 and 9.4). Crossing septals using the surfing technique. (**a**) Presence of several septal collateral channels (*CC*), most CC1 and CC0, with possible connection to the recipient vessel indicated by the *arrow* (Video 9.3). (**b**) Finecross in proximal septal trunk. Connection with a Sion wire into the PLV branch after surfing (Video 9.4)

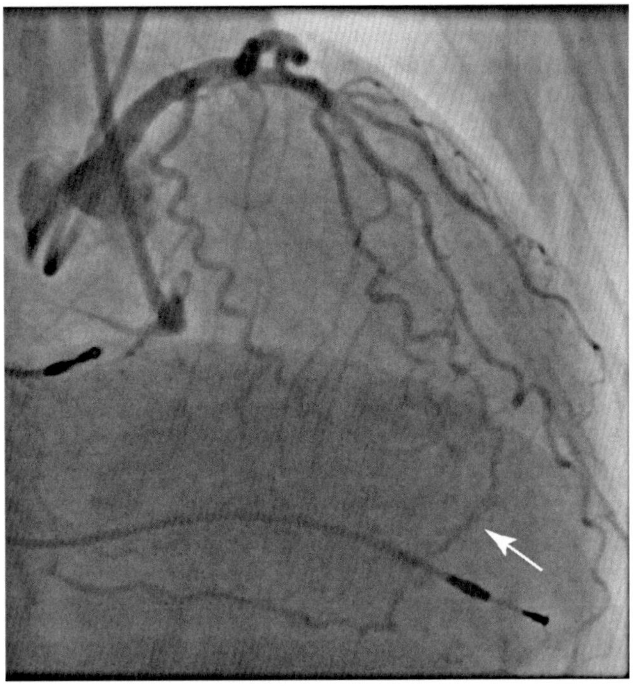

**Fig. 9.4** (Video 9.5). Presence of several septal collaterals and one epicardial collateral. Dual injection showing several CC0 and CC1 connections to the PDA. However, there is also a non-interventional collateral from the distal OM branch to the tip of the PDA. This epicardial and very tortuous CC is dominant and non-interventional (*arrow*)

the collateral channel anatomy at the base of the heart, as they enter, or exit the PDA. The operator should look for the presence of connections from the donor vessel to the receiving vessel. Typically, septal CCs will collateralize a right coronary artery (RCA) CTO to the posterior descending artery (PDA) from the left anterior descending (LAD) artery, or an LAD CTO from the PDA. In the left dominant system, the septal CCs will collateralize an LAD CTO from a left PDA, or vice versa.

The Rentropp score has been used to evaluate the efficiency of collateral flow to the occluded vessel, but is less useful to identify collaterals that can be used for the retrograde approach [8]. There are methods to analyse which CC is most effective in providing flow to the receiving vessel. When looking at the angiography and analyzing it frame-by-frame, it is often clear to see where the receiving vessel first lights up with contrast. With this information, by playing the cine-angiogram frame-by-frame, forwards and backwards, we can identify the channel that provides this preferential flow to the vessel. It is usually the largest CC, but not necessarily the one that is the best to be crossed. Indeed, we usually prefer to attempt crossing other septal CCs to allow for the largest to provide flow to the target vessel during the intervention, when possible.

The Werner classification identifies collaterals as either invisible (CC0), as thread-like tinny vessels (CC1) or as small vessel-like channels (CC2) (Fig. 9.5, Videos 9.6, 9.7, 9.8, 9.9, and 9.10) [9]. This classification has been shown to be helpful to predict success in crossing a septal CC when using a Japanese-style technique with selective tip injection [10]. However, when using a different technique such as the septal surfing, this classification is much less useful. We will discuss this technique and how to cross collaterals in the next section. It is also important to look if there is a large septal vessel trunk leading to the CCs. This is often the case with LAD to PDA CCs. However, as the branching of collaterals increases with distance from the LAD towards the PDA, the septal CCs are often very small and invisible close to the PDA (Figs. 9.4 and 9.5, Videos 9.5, 9.6, 9.7, 9.8, 9.9, and 9.10). This doesn't mean that they don't exist or connect however. As a general principle, CCs are most likely to be crossed easily if larger and straighter. Tortuosity of a septal CC is an issue and may preclude crossing with the wire. However, invisible collaterals, if straight, can be crossed with a surfing technique as explained later. Sometimes, challenges may arise at the entry of the septal CC, because of severe angulation or calcification. Despite connecting, such collateral may be very difficult to engage.

The epicardial collaterals are a separate subset of connections and pose a completely different set of challenges and considerations (Fig. 9.6). They typically arise from the postero-lateral (PL) to the obtuse marginal (OM) or diagonal branches, from the distal LCX to the PLVs, from diagonals to OM or *vice-versa*. They can also arise from the apical LAD or posterior descending artery (PDA) and feed any CTO vessel with a course on the surface of the heart. Also, epicardial CC are common from the RCA on the surface of the right ventricle, connecting or arising from the conal branches (with the LAD) or the acute marginal branches. They tend to be friable and by their location, they are at a higher risk of rupture following wire or microcatheter crossing. Larger collateral are the ones to prefer. Tortuosity is less significant issue with those collaterals. Patients who underwent prior cardiac surgery are at a much lower risk of complication in the case of an epicardial CC perforation, especially if the CC course is not basal, but rather run on the mid ventricular or apical portion of the left or right ventricles. Epicardial CC that are present in the atrio-ventricular (AV) groove of the heart are not trivial to cross, even in post-CABG patients; in case of perforation, the blood can accumulate posterior to the atria, leading to a contained hematoma and focal tamponade (Fig. 9.7). However, if a more apical collateral is perforated in a patient who underwent cardiac surgery in the past, such an event usually does not lead to tamponade, as the pericardium is adherent to the heart (Fig. 9.6, white arrow Video 9.11). In summary, epicardial channels can be considered good interventional routes if large, especially if not too tortuous, and if used in patients with prior cardiac surgery. An exception to this rule is the

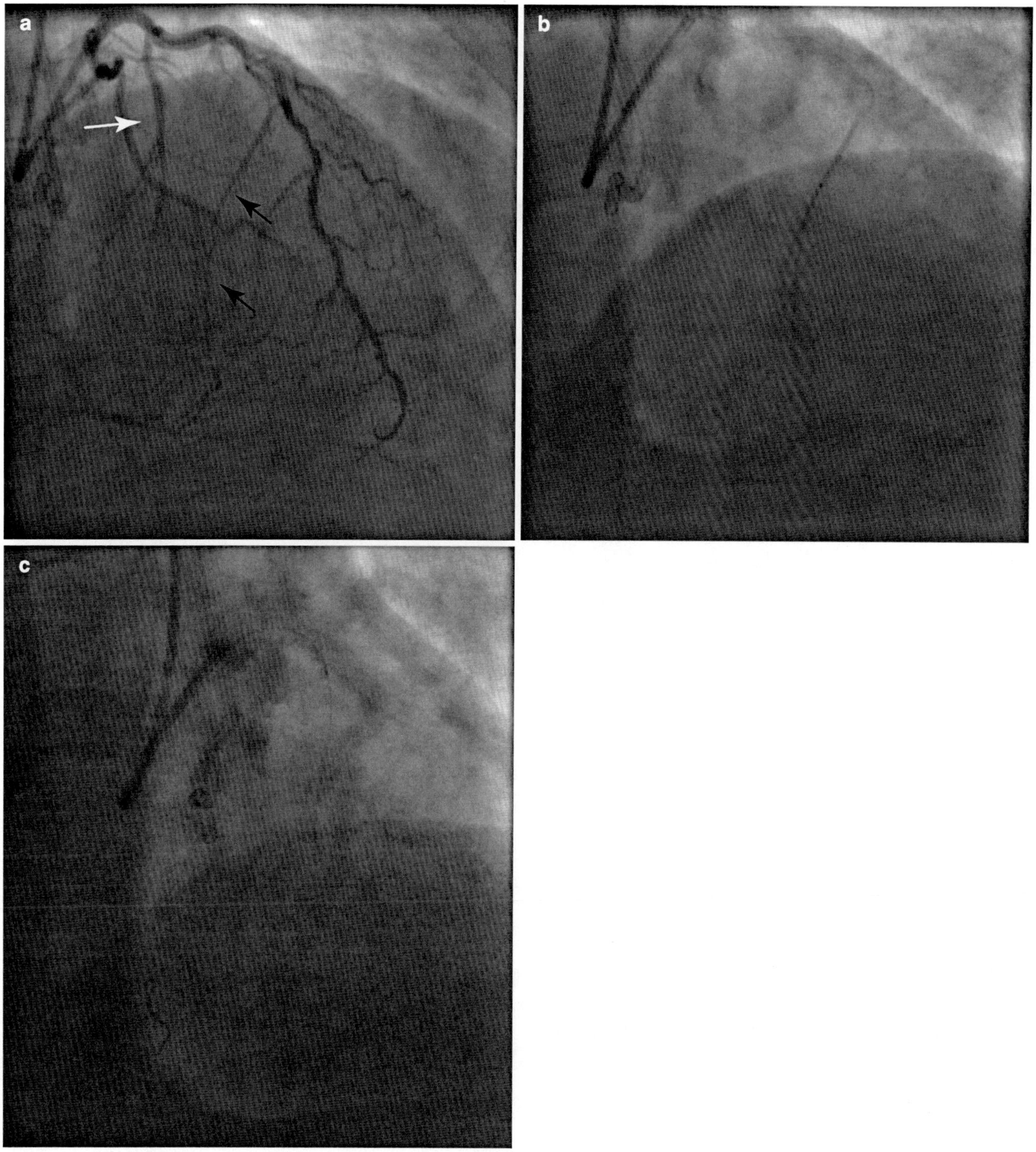


**Fig. 9.5** (Videos 9.6, 9.7, 9.8, 9.9, and 9.10). CC0, CC1 and CC0 channels. (**a**) *Black arrow* indicates a large but tortuous CC2 septal channel. However, the first septal (S1) provides small CC1 channels and even CC0 channels (*white arrow*) (Video 9.6). (**b**) Selective injection with FineCross shows how tortuous the largest collateral is (Videos 9.7, 9.8, and 9.9). (**c**) After a failed crossing attempt through the CC2, successful crossing was achieved using a surfing technique from S1, though an invisible CC0 connection (Video 9.10)

presence of AV groove collaterals that can lead to tamponade if perforated, both in patients with or without an intact pericardium. An additional point requiring special attention is the possibility that by occluding a dominant large epicardial collateral, the sole blood supply to the target vessel may be severely compromised and thus can lead to severe chest discomfort, hemodynamic and electrical instability. In such cases this collateral should be abandoned and alternative col-

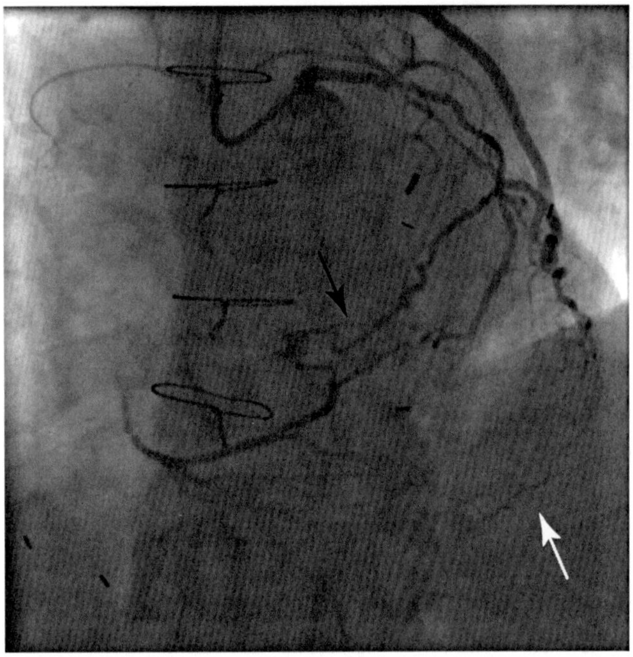

**Fig. 9.6** (Video 9.11). Interventional vs. non-interventional epicardial collateral channels. A post CABG RCA CTO receives very large but tortuous epicardial collateral (*back arrow*) from the native distal LCX to the PLV and also a straighter interventional epicardial CC from the OM branch (grafted with a LIMA) to the PDA (*white arrow*)

lateral channels should be explored. Only experienced operators should attempt crossing of tortuous and small epicardial collaterals, especially in patients with an intact pericardium.

A sub-category of non-septal collaterals are the intramyocardial collaterals (Fig. 9.8, Video 9.12). They tend to be present more often when there is a connection between the RPL and the OM branches, of from the OM to a distal PDA. They sometimes have the angiographic appearance of a network, they are occasionally compressed during systole; they pose unique challenges as they are often difficult to wire because of acute angulations as they dive into the myocardium and exit back to the epicardial surface. Advancing microcatheters can be also challenging and applying more forward pressure should be avoided since they may be rended along with the near-by myocardium leading to catastrophic tamponade. Instead very meticulous spinning of the microcatheter should be applied. These collaterals are best used in patients with prior cardiac surgery. Extreme care should be applied in patients with an intact pericardium (Fig. 9.8, Video 9.12). If still difficulties are encountered, then these collaterals should be abandoned and a different approach should be undertaken.

With all collaterals, it is also important to analyse the relationship between the connection to the distal vessel and the distal cap of the CTO. If the CC connects too close to the distal cap, entry into the occlusion can sometimes become very difficult or even impossible. Regarding this point, the best collaterals are the ones that connect at a distance from the distal cap to allow for the microcatheter to engage the CTO without a steep angle.

Typical collateral patterns are depicted in Figs. 9.9, 9.10 and 9.11. For RCA CTOs, the most common dominant collaterals are septals (Fig. 9.9). For LCx CTOs, a frequent pattern of collateralization is from the diagonal branches (Fig. 9.10). Finally, for LAD CTOs, septals from the PDA are most often providing the collateral flow (Fig. 9.11).

## Surgical Grafts

Surgical grafts can serve as effective routes to the distal CTO vessel. Arterial grafts can sometimes be used to deliver gear to the distal cap. This is the case, for example, of a severe ostial diagonal disease filled with retrograde flow from the left internal mammary artery (LIMA) to the LAD, in the presence of a proximal LAD CTO. This common situation, which often arises after the occlusion of a saphenous vein graft (SVG) to the diagonal, can be dealt with opening the LAD CTO towards the diagonal, restoring antegrade flow to the anterolateral wall. In such a case, the LIMA can serve as a route to the distal LAD CTO cap. Another situation is the presence of a RIMA to the PDA, an RCA CTO, and severe disease in a large PL branch. Treating the PL branch from the right internal mammary artery (RIMA) is sometimes impossible because of the presence of two acute angulations. However, a retrograde recanalization of the RCA followed by stenting towards the PL will be most effective and efficient. Finally, the LIMA can be used to access the LAD which provides septal collaterals to the PDA, in the presence of an occluded native LAD. When considering the use of an arterial graft as a retrograde donor vessel, the following principles should be considered: (1) caution should be applied in the presence of severe loops. After advancing a microcatheter to the distal vessel and prior to attempting the retrograde recanalization, the operator should assess flow into the arterial graft. If flow is impaired with the retrograde microcatheter in place into the LAD, the procedure should be aborted and an alternative retrograde route or an antegrade approach selected instead. (2) Caution should be applied to arterial grafts that serve as the last conduit of blood supply to the heart; a donor artery complication would be disastrous. Caution should be applied while manipulating the guide and equipment in the LIMA since ostial guide dissection can occur with any movement of the gear. 6F guides are recommended to minimize this risk. Moreover, the selective cannulation of the LIMA with a 6F or 5.5F MAC catheter can really help to stabilize the catheter in place, while reducing the risk of ostial dissection. The ostial LIMA guide should be maintained in the field of view whenever possible. In general, we would lean towards having a higher threshold in using the LIMA as a retrograde conduit, compared to other grafts, or alternative routes.

SVGs can also be used. They can either be patent or occluded. Patent SVGs can be used for the same reasons as

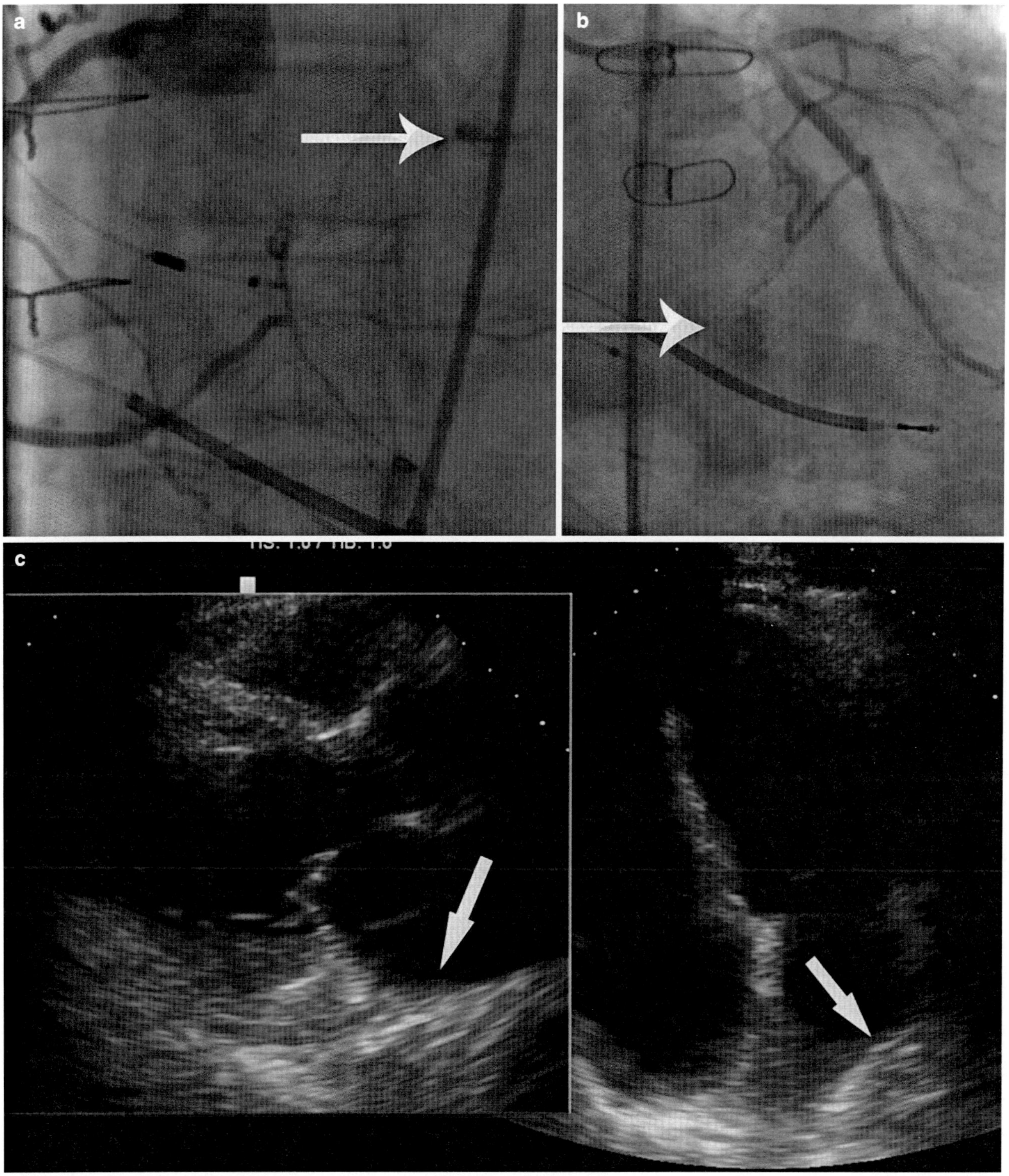

**Fig. 9.7** Perforation of an epicardial collateral in the atrio-ventricular groove in a post-CABG patient leading to a contained hematoma. Panels (**a**) and (**b**). The *arrow* indicated the perforation with contrast spilling (type 3 perforation). Panel (**c**). Echocardiogram showing a contained hematoma being to the left atrum (*arrow*) (From Spratt [14] with permission)

the ones cited in the previous section. In addition, the presence of severe disease in a degenerated SVG can raise the option of opening the native instead of treating the SVG, since long-term SVG patency may be limited despite the use of several DES (Fig. 9.12). Moreover, stenting degenerated grafts can lead to acute complications, such as no-reflow, especially if distal protection cannot be used. Another situation is the presence of recurrent restenotic lesions in an SVG, which is a prelude to occlusion of the graft in a near future. It is therefore wise to consider opening the native artery instead of keeping treating the diseased SVG.

SVGs can also be used even if occluded. This is best performed if the occlusion is recent, as crossing a thrombosed graft is relatively easy (Fig. 9.13). However, instead of treating the graft, the native artery CTO will be addressed with a retrograde approach. This can also be performed in SVGs that have been occluded for several weeks, even years. The ostial graft occlusion morphology should be taken into consideration since blunt/stumpless occlusions are harder to cross compared to tapered ones. We will discuss the techniques on how to perform these approaches in the next section.

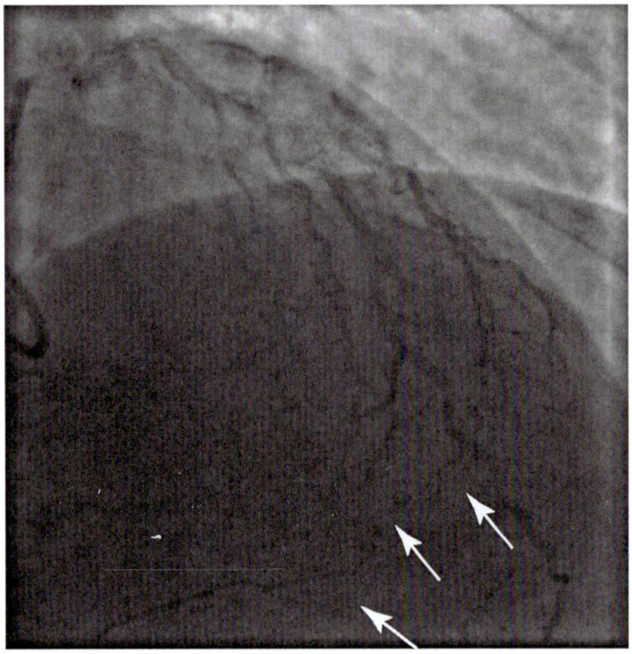

**Fig. 9.8** (Video 9.12). Intra-myocardial collateral channel from the OM to the PDA. During systole, the collateral disappears

In summary, there are multiple ways to get to the distal cap (Table 9.1). If the algorithm favors the use of the retrograde approach, it should be attempted in the presence of collateral channels or grafts that are suitable for the approach. Even tiny or even invisible septal CC can be crossed with a surfing technique; therefore, in the case of an RCA or an LAD CTO with septal CCs, an attempt to cross the CC should be made before concluding that the collaterals are not suitable or a retrograde approach impossible.

## Step-by-Step Approach

### Crossing the Collateral Channel or the Graft with a Wire and a Microcatheter

#### Crossing a Septal CC with the Wire

Initially, the technique involves the use of a microcatheter advanced on a workhorse wire. In the case of LAD to PDA CCs, the operator should target the collateral that is most likely to connect. Additional anatomic considerations when choosing the CC to cross include the tortuosity of the donor vessel, the angle of the take-off of the septal (a retroflex septal is obviously challenging to engage), and the point of insertion

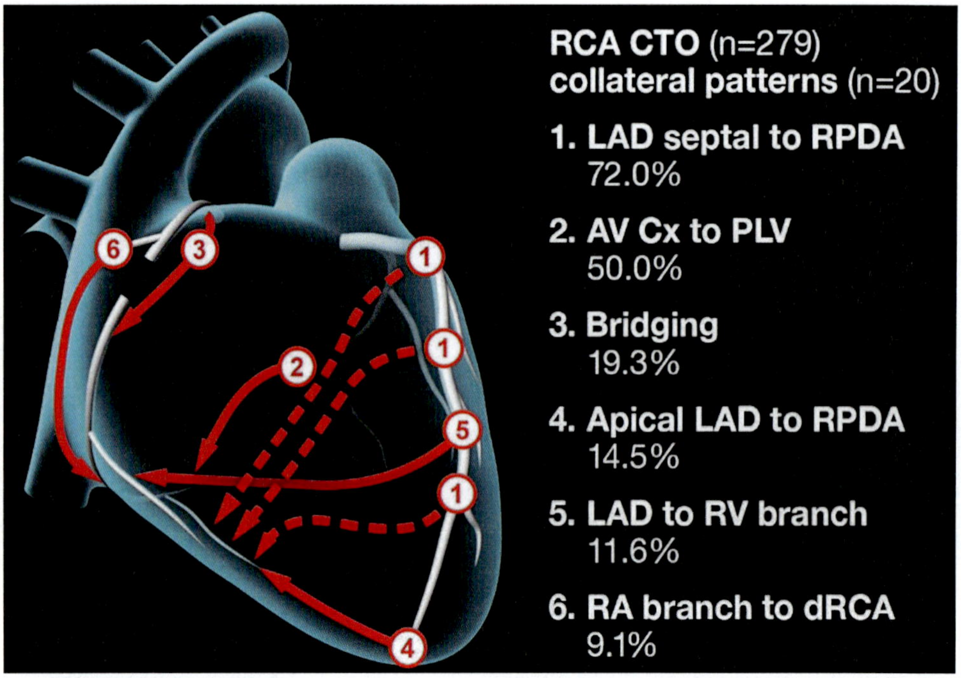


**Fig. 9.9** RCA CTO collateral patterns (From Spratt [14] with permission)

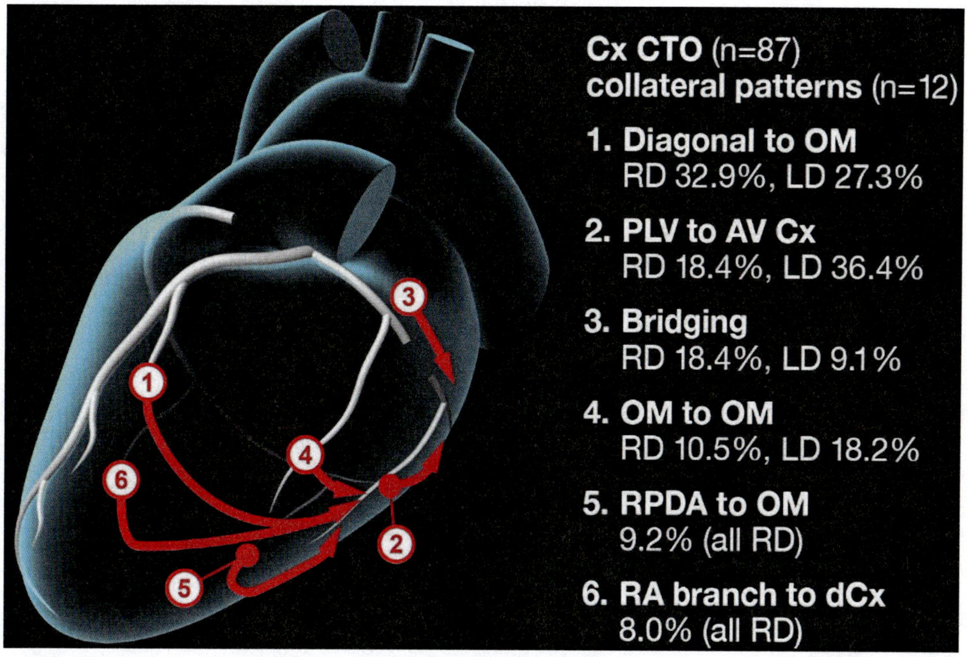


**Fig. 9.10** LCx CTO collateral patterns (From Spratt [14] with permission)

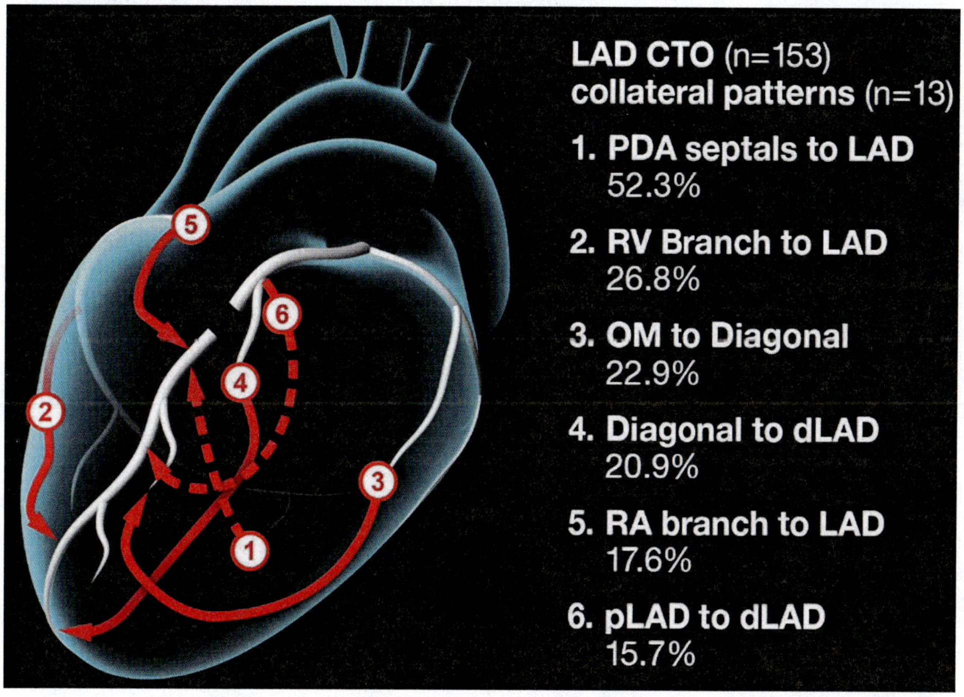


**Fig. 9.11** LAD CTO collateral patterns (From Spratt [14] with permission)

into the target vessel on relation to the distal cap, (insertion of the collateral very close, or at the distal cap is suboptimal). Usually, we will attempt to cross the largest and straightest one. However, other septal channels can be crossed also, even if there is no visible connection (CC0) (Fig. 9.14). If a large septal trunk is present, the Corsair catheter should be delivered on a workhorse wire shaped properly to engage into the proximal portion of the septal, followed by advancement of the catheter. The wire should be then be exchanged for a Sion wire (Asahi Intecc, Japan), with a small 30–45° bend at 1 mm from the tip. Alternatively, a Fielder FC wire can be used, although the Sion wire has clearly become the dominant wire for that task. This wire will be advanced in the CC in the search of a low resistance connection. We call this technique the *surfing technique* (Fig. 9.3, Videos 9.3 and 9.4). The wire is quickly advanced and pulled back when feeling a resistance, and redirected in a different channel. Once feeling some buckling, drilling of the wire can lead to passage into

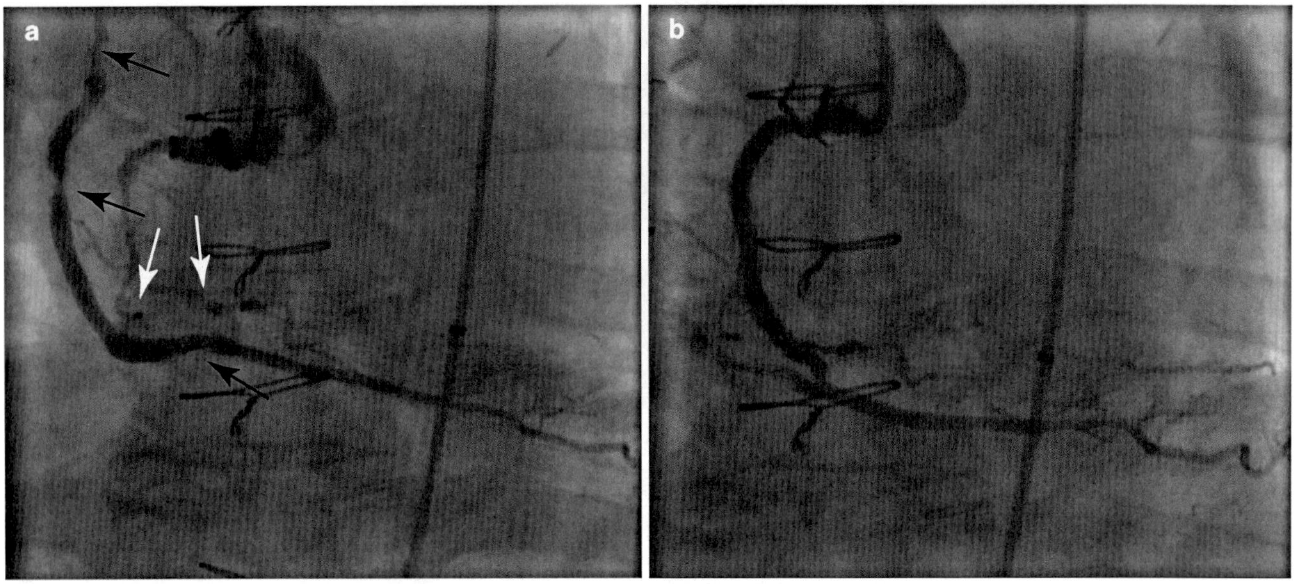


**Fig. 9.12** Treatment of a native artery CTO instead of a diseased graft. (**a**) Severely degenerated SVG to PDA with several stenoses (*black arrows*), and an RCA CTO (*white arrows*); (**b**) Post retrograde CTO PCI of the RCA via the SVG graft

the recipient vessel. This technique offers the advantage to test several options of crossing from one proximal septal trunk. If the operator fails to connect from a given septal, the Corsair should be pulled, a different one is then engaged with the workhorse wire shaped appropriately for the proximal septal angulation. After advancement of the Corsair, the new septal branch with its CCs are "surfed" again with the Sion. It is common to see the wire entering into a ventricular cavity. The wire will then loop and will seem to float freely into a large cavity. It will then be simply pulled and re-advanced into a different direction. Entering a cavity is benign as long as the microcatheter is not advanced. A good septal track to the recipient vessel can be identified when a repetitive course of the wire is noticed with sequential pulling and pushing on the wire; if the wire keeps on making the same turns, it likely tracks a vessel structure that may finally connect. Therefore, it is advanced to the point of resistance, and drilled at this level, seeking a release into the recipient vessel. The feeling is often of a free wire that tracks nicely the PDA or LAD, and engage branches at the distal CTO cap. A wire that successfully crossed a septal will be free; with the heart beats, a too-an-fro movement of the wire can be seen and the wire often track side branches. Otherwise, the wire is probably not into the recipient vessel. A retrograde angiography should be performed to confirm that the distal wire tip is at the distal cap before advancing the Corsair through the CC.

If the septal surfing technique fails, it may be necessary to perform a tip injection of contrast from the Corsair. This technique involves pulling out the wire, aspirating back blood from the Corsair, and then injecting 2–3 cc of contrast using a small syringe, to assess the course of the collateral channel. Such a technique is useful especially in the case of large but tortuous CC2 collaterals that offers resistance to passage of the guidewire (Fig. 9.5, Videos 9.6, 9.7, 9.8, 9.9, and 9.10). A distal tip injection can help to identify bends in the CC that was not identified with non-selective injections. It is often very useful to use a straight left anterior oblique (LAO) projection to better assess the collateral with the tip injection. This second injection can be performed with only saline into the Corsair, flushing the remaining contrast out of the Corsair and providing information from another view before reinserting the wire. The tip injection technique carries the risk of septal dissection, or perforation, which will preclude subsequent use of this route. However, septal surfing can also lead to septal perforation. They are usually smaller and appear as small stains in the septum (Fig. 9.15). They are for the vast majority benign.

If the septal branches are tiny, it is often helpful to start surfing with a microcatheter that has a smaller tip. The Finecross (Terumo, Japan) can be very helpful to follow a workhorse wire that was advanced into a small septal CC at its origin; then, the wire can be exchanged for the Sion and septal surfing performed (Fig. 9.3, Videos 9.3 and 9.4). If the wire connects into the recipient vessel, an attempt to cross the collateral with the Finecross can be done. The Finecross can be manipulated with the same rotations as for the Corsair. If it crosses, this catheter will be adequate for less complex CTOs that are likely to be traversed with a retrograde true-to-true (TTT) crossing strategy. However, if a long CTO is attempted, switching for a Corsair will tremendously improve the support from the retrograde side for subsequent wire manoeuvers, especially involving knuckled wires. This is because of the screwing pattern of the Corsair that stabilize the catheter in its position, providing additional back-up support that will be lacking with the Finecross. Exchanging the Finecross for a Corsair or a Turnpike (Vascular Solutions,

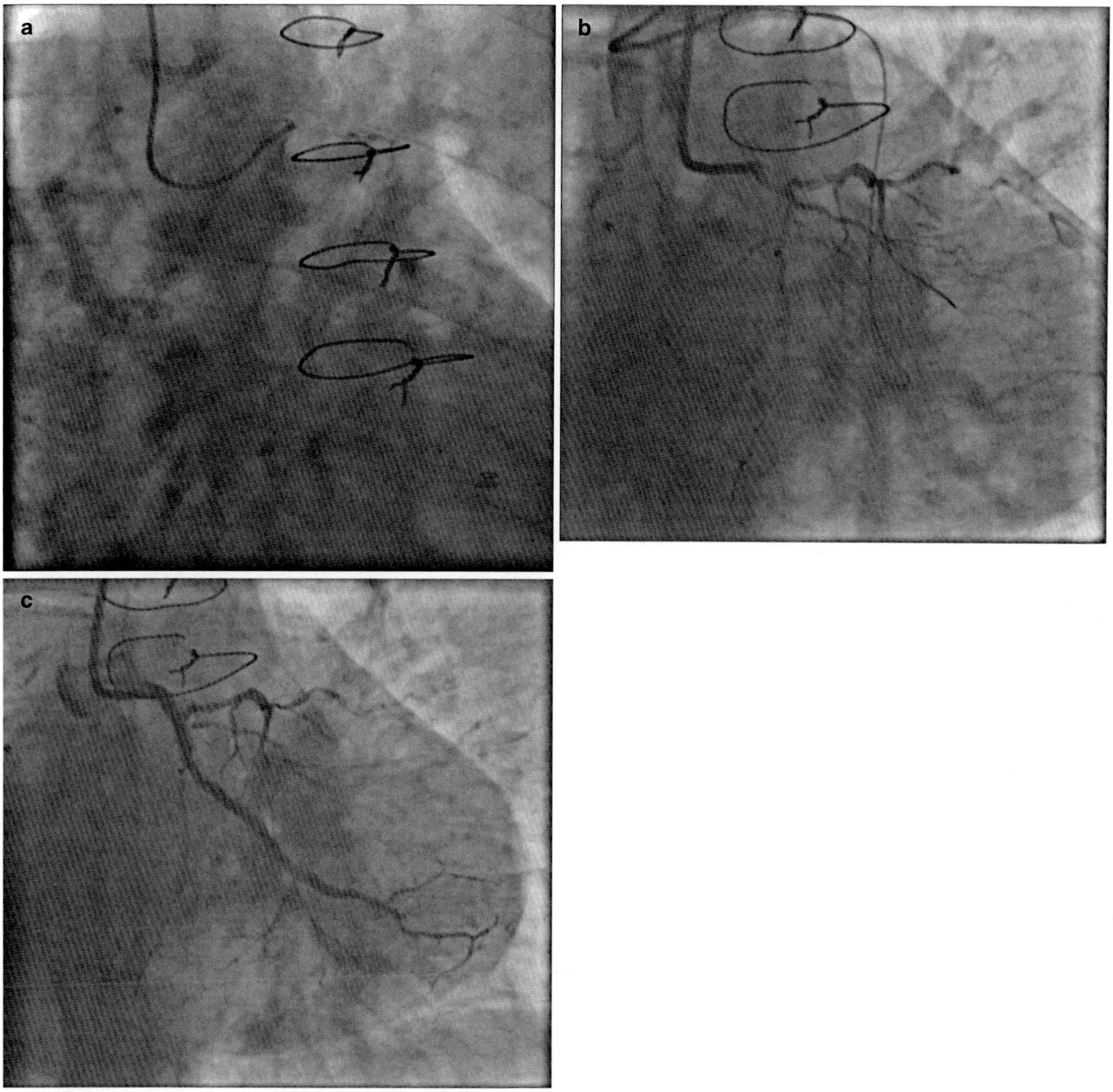


**Fig. 9.13** Using an occluded graft as a route to the distal cap. (**a**) Sub-occluded severely degenerated old SVG to OM. (**b**) Access to the distal cap of the OM occlusion from the old graft. (**c**) Final result after rotational atherectomy and stenting

US) can be done with a trapping technique, even in a 6F guide, using a 2.0 mm balloon. The trapping technique is explained in Chap. 4.

When performing septal surfing in the case of a PDA providing septal collaterals to the LAD, the same principles apply. One major nuance if that the septal CCs are often very tiny or even invisible close to the PDA, as branching increases towards the inferior septum. However, if the wire successfully engages a connecting collateral, its advancement becomes easier as it moves towards the LAD, with the wire navigating progressively into larger vessels. It is therefore unusual to be able to deliver a Corsair in a septal branch to start surfing (Fig. 9.16, Video 9.13). The best technique is the leave the Corsair in the PDA, and to start surfing from the PDA, leaving the wire tip as free as possible as it engages several little septal branches. If one offers minimal resistance, the wire can be pushed further and directed into the LAD. If a larger CC is present and seems to connect, it should be first targeted. Once the wire advances freely, engages branches in the recipient vessel, and when a to-and-fro movement of the wire is visualized, it is safe to follow with the microcatheter. A retrograde injection should however be performed to confirm the location before advancing the microcatheter in case of doubt.

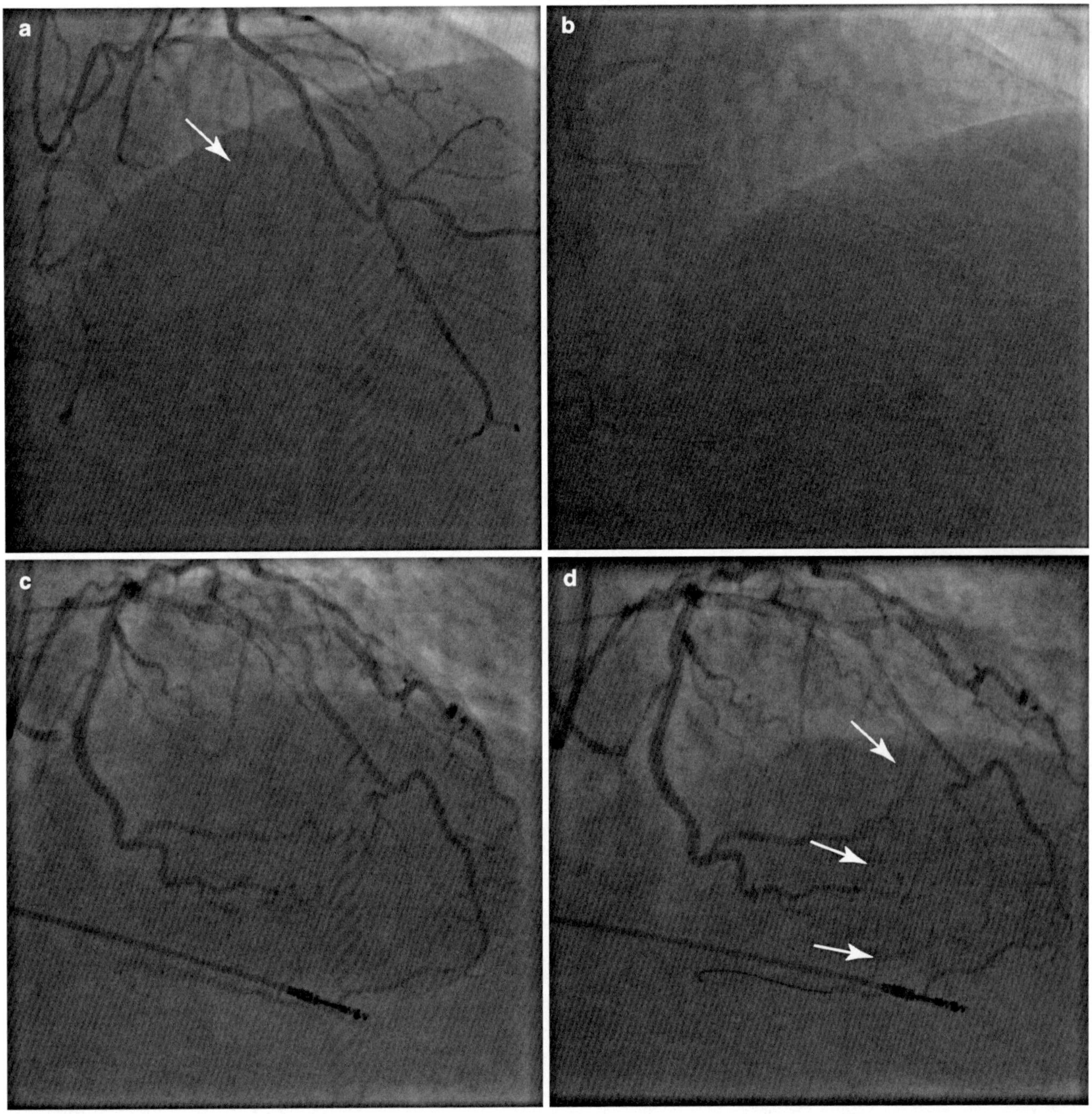

**Fig. 9.14** Crossing invisible septal collateral channels. (**a**) Retrograde injection showing no clear evidence of connection from the septal branches, especially from the first septal. (**b**) Connection through an invisible septal channel into the PDA with the surfing technique. (**c**) Another case showing several CC1 connections from the LAD to the PDA. (**d**) Connection to the PDA through an invisible septal channel

## Advancing the Microcatheter to the Distal Cap Through the Septal CC

If a FineCross was used to surf the septal CCs, crossing of the collateral can be attempted with this catheter. However, the FineCross is not a septal dilator, and sometimes will not be as efficient in crossing a collateral. Alternative clockwise and counter clockwise rotations can be applied to help deliver the catheter to the distal cap. However, the FineCross provides much less support for retrograde crossing of the CTO. It should therefore be reserved for simpler and shorter CTOs where a true-to-true crossing is likely to be successful. In all the other situations, the Corsair is the preferred catheter. If a FineCross was first used, it can be exchanged for a Corsair using the trapping balloon technique as explained in Chap. 4. As described in Chap. 3, it is engineered as a septal dilator. It will be advanced with alternative clockwise and counter-clockwise rotations to the distal cap. It will often stop advancing at the inferior portion of the sep-

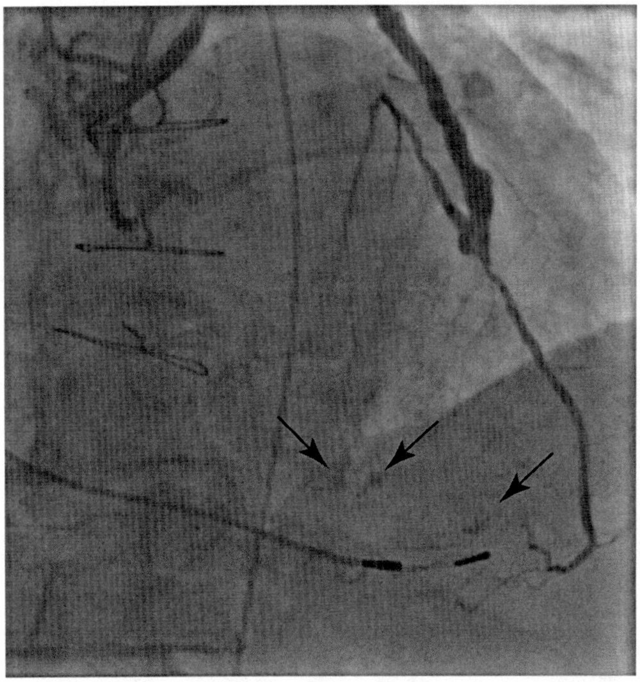

**Fig. 9.15** Failed attempt to connect retrograde from the LAD with some benign septal stains of contrast (*arrow*)

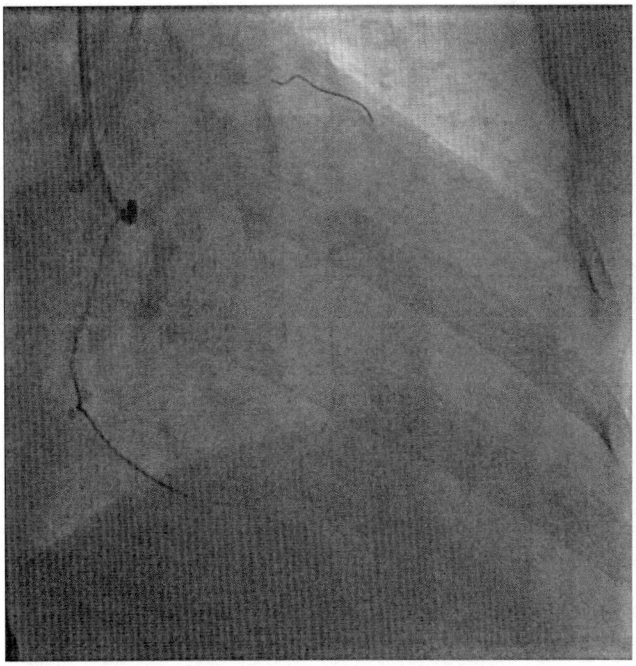

**Fig. 9.16** (Video 9.8). Septal surfing from the PDA to the LAD. The Corsair is positioned into the PDA, and the wire manipulated to engage septals and complete the course up to the LAD

tum, where the septal CC is smaller and angulated. If is often necessary to apply 5–10 turns in one direction followed by a change of direction to help the catheter advance. If that step fails, the Corsair can be withdrawn and a 1.25 or 1.5 balloon used to dilate the septal at the point of resistance (Fig. 9.17, Videos 9.14, 9.15, 9.16, 9.17, 9.18, 9.19, 9.20, and 9.21). Then, crossing with the Corsair is attempted again. Occasionally using the 135 cm version of the Corsair to dilate a resistant part in the septum is more effective, followed by the exchanged for a long Corsair to complete the procedure. Alternatively, especially if already on the table, the reattempt can be done with the FineCross. Lack of support is also one of the common cause of absence of progression of the Corsair into the septal. It is possibly more frequent with 6F than with 8F guide catheters, although it can be encountered with the latter. The Corsair can be withdrawn, and a MAC technique used to increase the support. We like to use the 5.5F version of the GuideLiner that offers adequate inner lumen size to accommodate the Corsair, but also has a smaller outer diameter when delivered deep into the donor vessel, thus reducing the risk of donor artery dissection (Fig. 9.17d, Video 9.17). The GuideLiner can sometimes be pushed to the level of the septal and the Corsair re-advanced. However, once the Corsair is successfully delivered to the distal cap, the GuideLiner should be retrieved into the guide to minimize donor artery trauma. Alternatively, an anchoring balloon technique (see Chap. 12) can be used to improve support. Finally, the Corsair can sometimes dry through the septal, or even get "fatigued" after several clockwise and counter-clockwise rotations. The Corsair should be left alone for a few seconds, and movements re-applied after this short rest. Otherwise, it is wise to simply take it out, flush it and rewet the outer surface of the hydrophilic coating of the catheter as well as the wire. If this steps fails to help crossing the collateral with the Corsair, use of a new Corsair (or a TurnPike, Vascular Solutions, US) can be necessary. Flushing the lumen of the Corsair with Rotaglide (Boston Scientific, US) can help reduce the friction and minimize the occurrence of Corsair fatigue. This phenomenon should be recognized early on during the procedure to allow for a timely change for a new Corsair before the wire gets entrapped into the Corsair, in which case the whole system has to be removed as a unit. If all those steps failed, which is very unusual, the retrograde wire should be left in place and an antegrade approach attempted, using the retrograde wire as a target (kissing wire technique).

## Crossing an Epicardial CC with the Wire and the Microcatheter

Surfing has no role in wiring the epicardial collaterals. Wiring epicardial collaterals is a very controlled and meticulous technique that relies on detailed definition of their course using frequent tip injections in different angiographic projections, as single projections frequently are inadequate to delineate their complex three-dimensional course. Furthermore, epicardial collaterals can change configuration as wires and microcatheters are introduced and advanced, a factor that should be taken into consideration while performing this most technically demanding maneuver.

Many operators prefer to use the FineCross when crossing an epicardial collateral for the following reasons: (1) the outer diameter of the FineCross is smaller and less likely to occlude the vessel; (2) there is no need to dilate an epicardial collateral; and (3) the tip is more flexible—if the wire is pulled to be reshaped, the tip of the FineCross is less likely

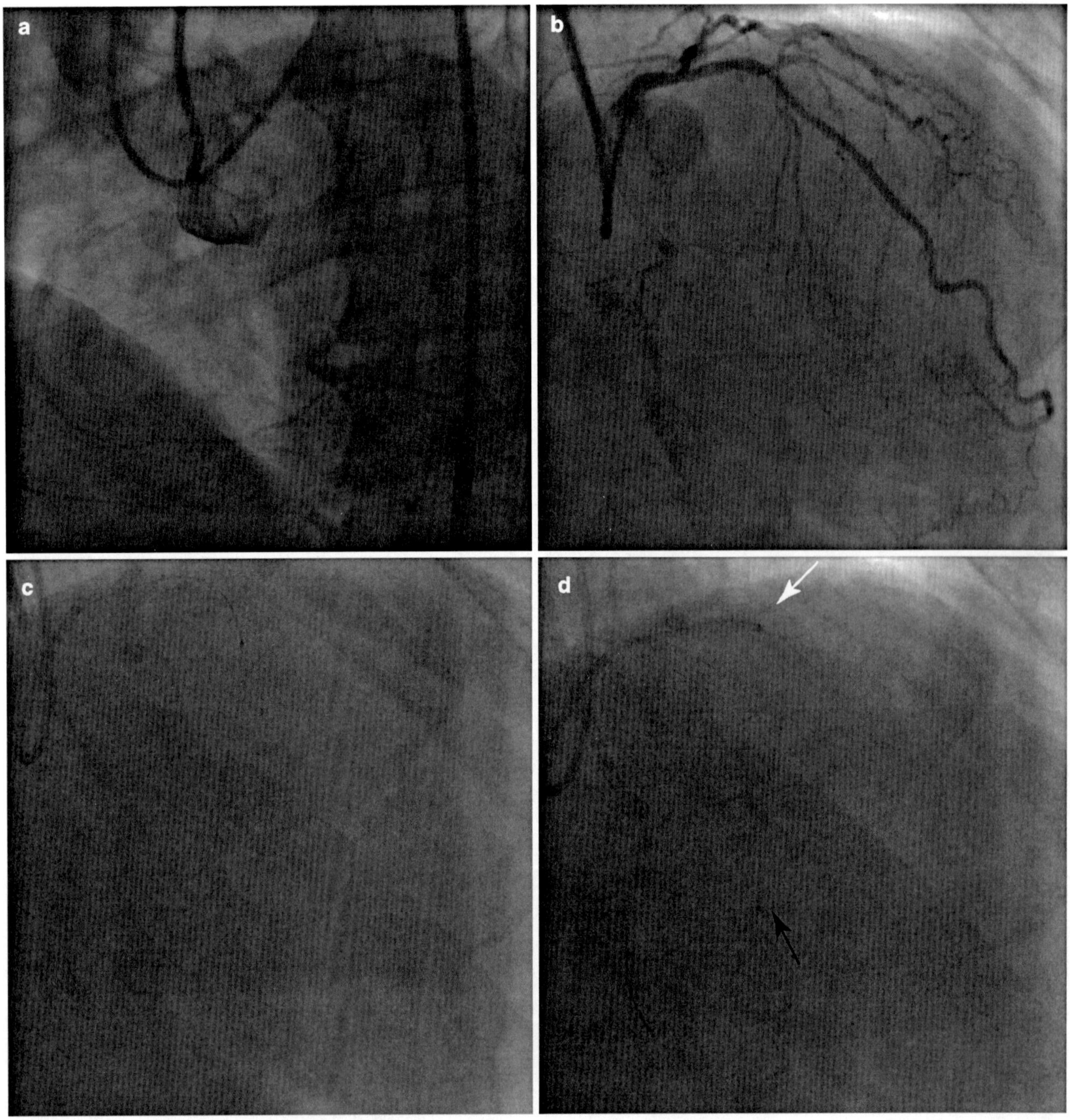


**Fig. 9.17** (Videos 9.14, 9.15, 9.16, 9.17, 9.18, 9.19, 9.20, and 9.21). Aorto-ostial RCA CTO treated with the retrograde approach. (**a**) Flush aorto-ostial RCA CTO, with septal collaterals, mandating a retrograde approach (Video 9.14). (**b**) Small septal channels connecting to PDA and PLV (Video 9.15). (**c**) One small invisible septal was crossed into a PLV with a surfing technique (Finecross and Sion wire), through a stent that jailed the first septal (Video 9.16). (**d**) After a failed attempt to deliver a Corsair through the septal CC (after dilating the stent struts at the ostium of the septal with a 1.5 mm balloon), a septal balloon dilation is performed at the point where the Corsair failed to progress with a 1.25 balloon at 12 atm (*black arrow*), with the support of a 5.5 F GuideLiner into the LAD (*white arrow*) (Video 9.17). (**e**) Corsair successfully delivered to the distal CTO cap (Video 9.18). (**f**) A true-to-true CTO crossing into the aorta was done (Video 9.19). (**g**) After snaring a long retrograde wire, balloon dilation and stenting with DES on the externalized guidewire (Video 9.21). (**h**) Final result (Video 9.21)

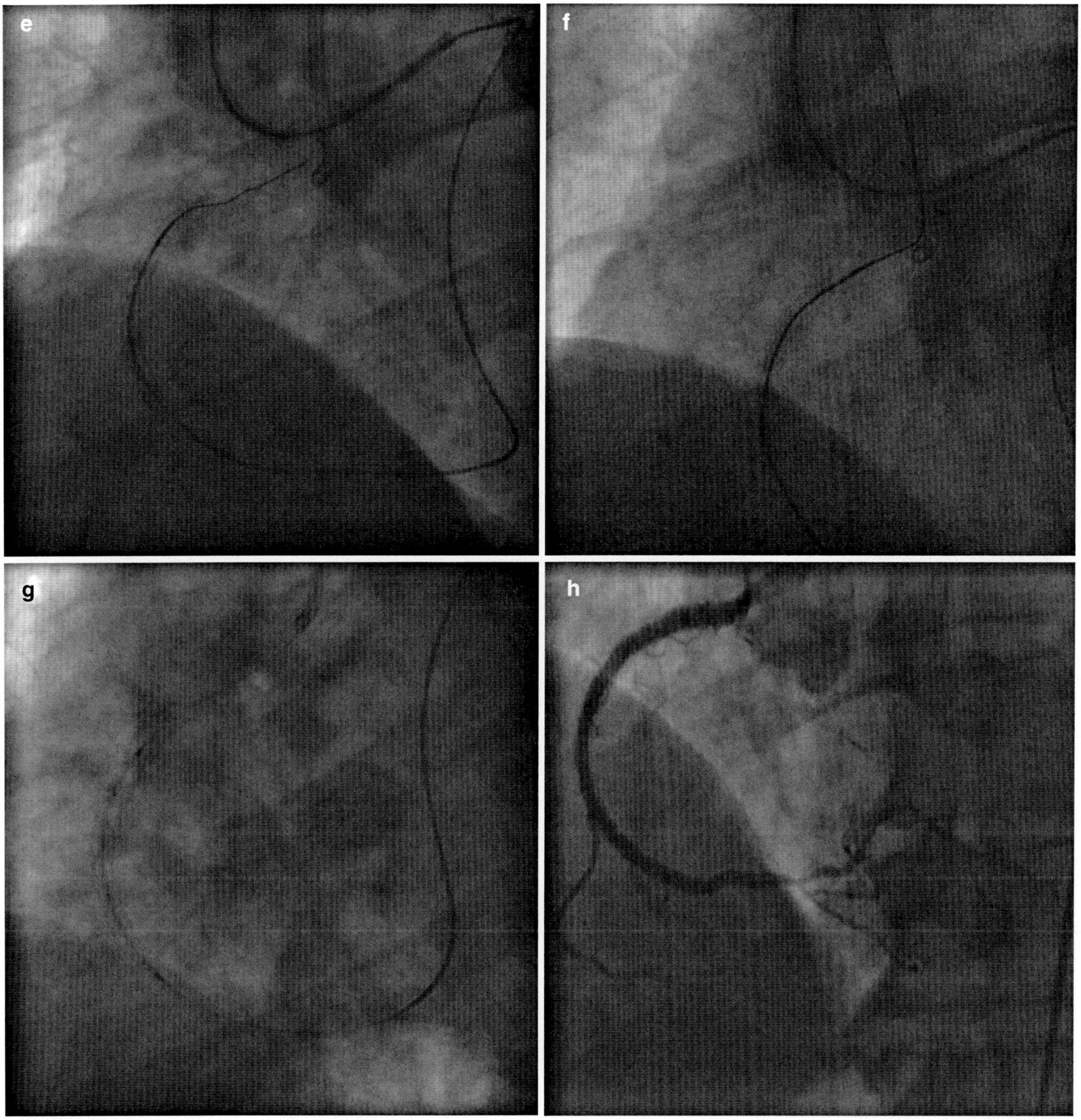


**Fig. 9.17** (continued)

to damage the CC compared to the Corsair. However, in some larger epicardial vessel, the Corsair offers the advantage of being more easily advanced with rotation (Fig. 9.18, Videos 9.22, 9.23, 9.24, 9.25, 9.26, 9.27, and 9.28). Once the microcatheter is delivered into the donor vessel over a workhorse wire, the latter is exchanged for the Sion wire. No other wire than the Sion wire should be used for this challenging task. The same bend should be applied as the one described for the septal channels. However, it is sometimes helpful to add an additional bend 2 mm from the tip to help crossing tortuous collateral. Then, the Sion should be manipulated with care, keeping the tip free all the time. Progression into the epicardial CC is often "jumpy"; once the Sion crosses a bend, the CC becomes straightened, pushing the wire forward. There is often significant vessel motion on the surface of the heart, which makes wire control extremely difficult. Again, surfing has no role in wiring epicardial collaterals. We recommend distal tip injections in multiple views to fully understand the course of the channel before attempting to wire it. Once the wire seems free, and its intraluminal position at the target distal vessel in confirmed by angiography, the microcatheter can be advanced with rotations to the distal cap. If a FineCross fails to progress, it can be exchanged for a Corsair.

## Crossing a Graft with a Wire and a Microcatheter

Patent SVGs are easy to cross, even with a workhorse wire, to the distal cap. They provide the operator who is new to the retrograde approach a safe environment to first attempt

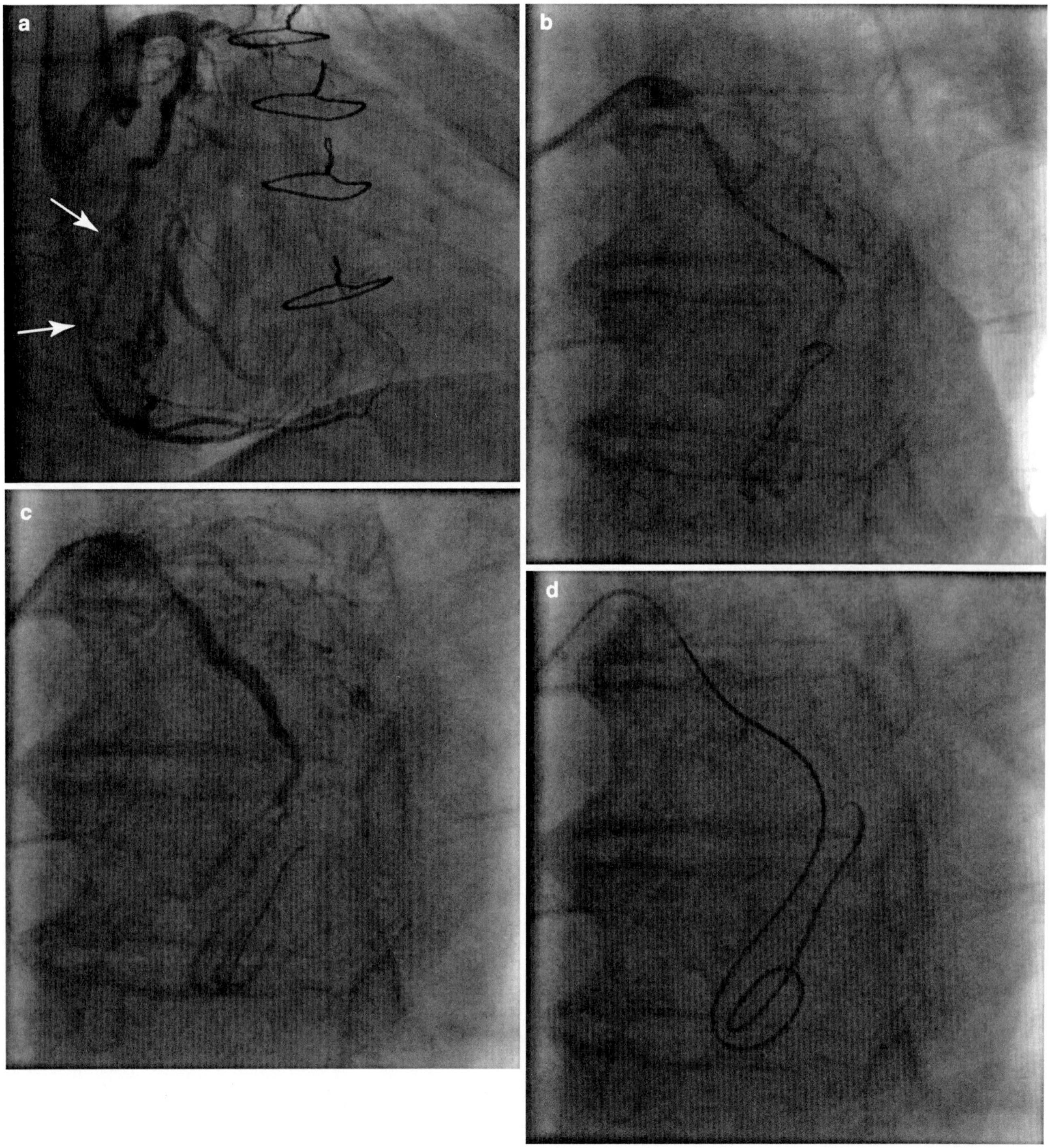


**Fig. 9.18** (Videos 9.22, 9.23, 9.24, 9.25, 9.26, 9.27, and 9.28). Retrograde approach through an epicardial collateral with a Ping-pong catheter technique. (**a**) Post CABG LCX CTO, which is collateralized by a large but tortuous ipsilateral epicardial CC (*arrow*). A catheter was used in the RCA (Video 9.22). (**b**, **c**) Higher-risk retrograde approach with a Sion wire advanced with controlled drilling (Videos 9.23 and 9.24). (**d**) Corsair delivered at the distal CTO cap (Video 9.25). (**e**) Reverse CART with ping-pong catheters. Note that the collateral is straightened by the Corsair (Video 9.26). (**f**) Stenting on an externalized guidewire (Video 9.27). (**g**) Final result after stenting, with the collateral that recovered its tortuous appearance (Video 9.28)

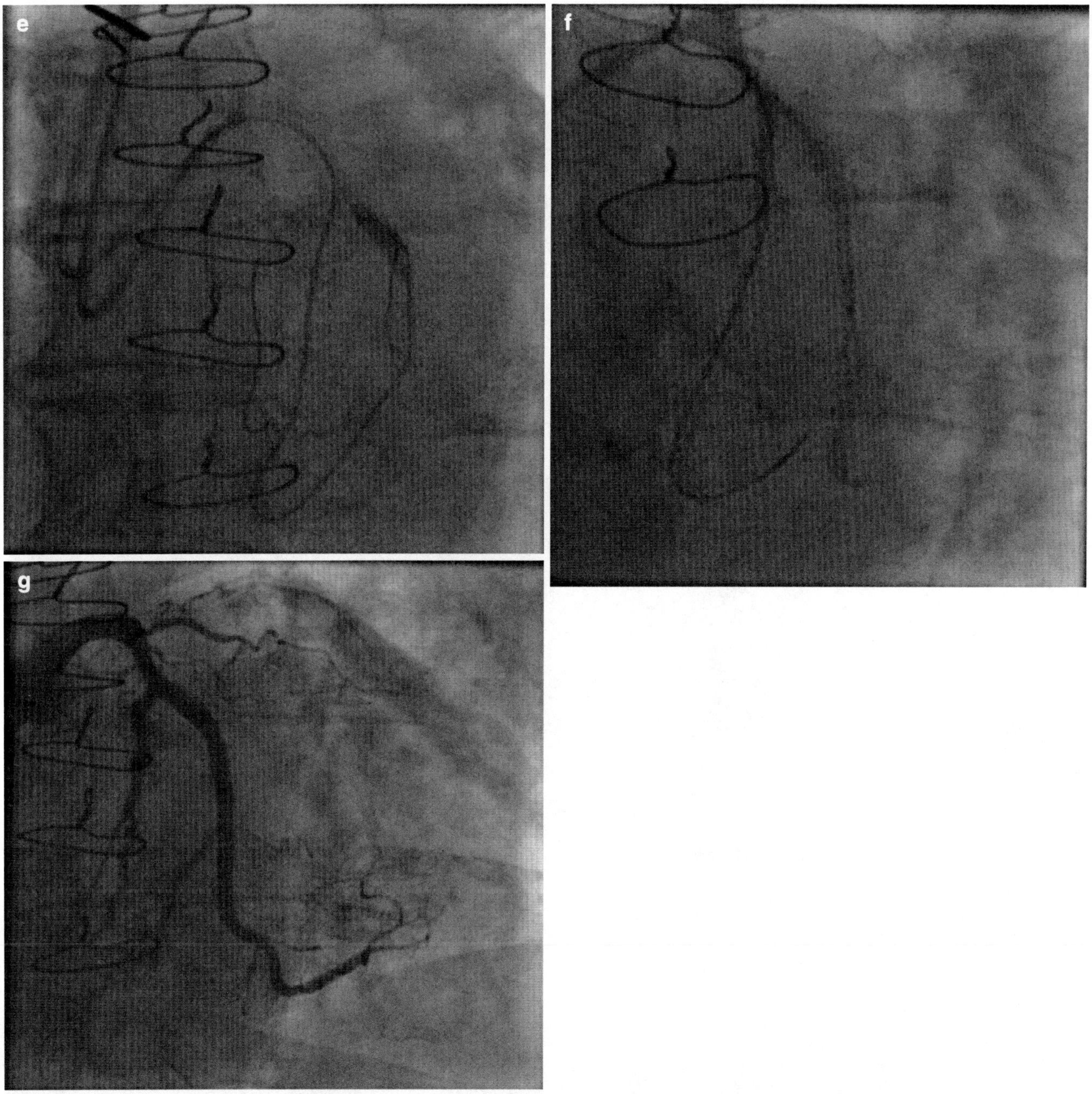

**Fig. 9.18** (continued)

crossing a CTO from the distal edge. Good cases include those SVGs that are severely diseased, old and degenerated, because of the poor short [11] and long-term outcomes [12] of those grafts after PCI despite the use of DES, with target-vessel revascularisation rates in up to 28 % of patients (Fig. 9.12). Also, patients presenting with recurrent in-stent SVG restenosis are good candidates for the recanalization of their native coronary instead. SVGs with recurrent in-stent restenosis are safer than de-novo degenerated SVGs to wire, since the risk of distal embolization is minimal. Once the distal cap is reached, the principles with crossing the CTO exposed later should be applied. Use of a microcatheter is strongly encouraged, and we advocate the use of the Corsair. Usually, it is easier from an SVG to the PDA, or an SVG to the LAD to access the proximal vessel and then the CTO distal cap. However, SVG to OM distal surgical anastomosis are often performed at a more acute angle, making the turn backward towards the proximal OM and circumflex more challenging in some cases (Figs. 9.12 and 9.19, Videos 9.29, 9.30, 9.31, 9.32, and 9.33). There are two options if the workhorse or a Sion wire cannot navigate from the graft towards the proximal OM segment: first, use of a Venture catheter (Vascular Solution, USA), which has a deflectable tip that can be oriented towards the proximal OM can be very useful. Second, use of a supportive wire such as the Miracle 12 wire can be essential. Such wire, when preformed with a round shape, can be oriented towards the proximal OM direction, and can support the delivery of the microcatheter without prolapsing towards the distal OM. Once the microcatheter engages the proximal OM segment, this wire is exchanged for an appropriate wire based on the anatomy and the preferred crossing strategy.

Occluded SVGs can also be crossed with a wire and a microcatheter, especially if they have been occluded for less than 1 year, although we have had several successes with grafts that had been occluded for a longer period of time, even years (Figs. 9.13 and 9.19, Videos 9.29, 9.30, 9.31, 9.32, and 9.33). Usually, the trajectory of the graft can be guessed by the presence of surgical clips, and the distal anastomosis can also be seen from collateral filling from another

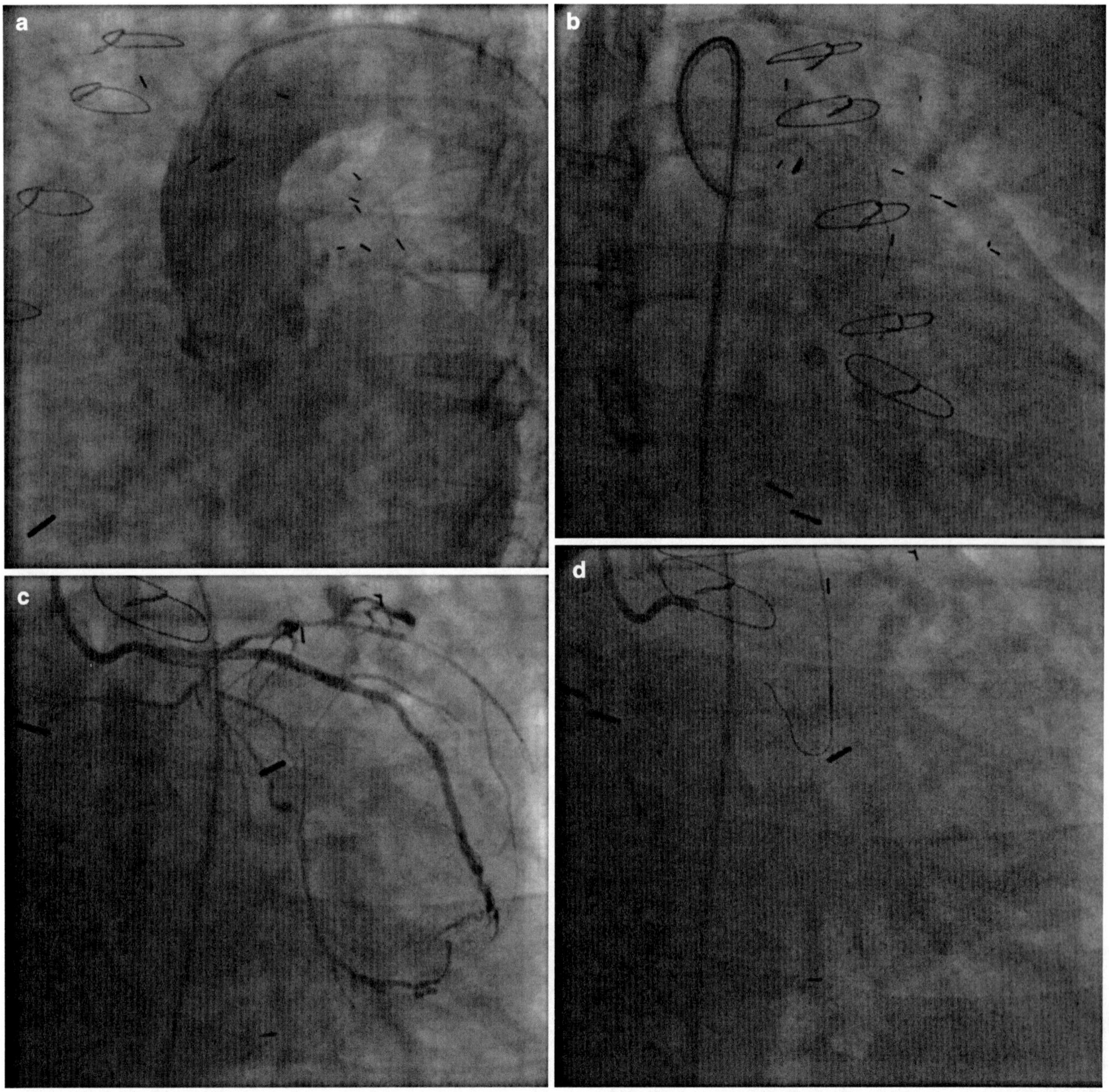


**Fig. 9.19** (Videos 9.29, 9.30, 9.31, 9.32, and 9.33). LCx CTO PCI through an occluded graft. (**a**) A flush ostial graft occlusion is documented with an aortogram. (**b**) An 8F JR4 catches a stump, close to surgical clips. A Pilot 200 is advanced with drilling, guided by the surgical clips (Video 9.29). (**c**) The injection from the left main with an 8F AL guide shows the OM filled by a very tortuous epicardial collateral that would have been very risky to cross. It also shows that the Pilot 200 navigated to the OM true lumen (Video 9.30). (**d**) A Sion wire navigates retrograde to the distal cap, followed by the Corsair (Video 9.31). (**e**) Connection into the antegrade guide after reverse CART (Video 9.32). (**f**) Final result after stenting (Video 9.33)

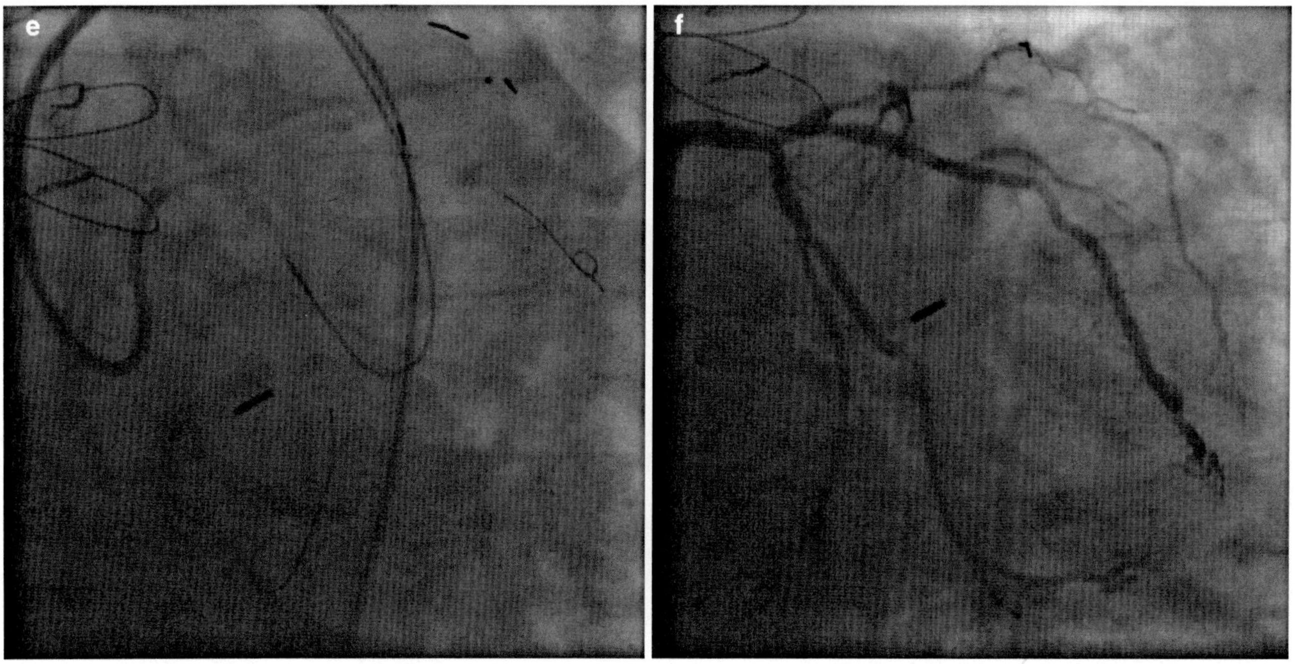


**Fig. 9.19** (continued)

source (Fig. 9.19, Videos 9.29, 9.30, 9.31, 9.32, and 9.33). When an occluded graft can be used instead of a single epicardial collateral, we prefer such an approach because it avoids ischemia caused by the inevitable transient occlusion of the collateral, and because of a much lower risk in case of perforation.

Technically, a good supportive guide catheter should be selected. Use of the femoral approach vs. the radial approach is left to the operator; however, if a radial approach is used, and especially if a 6F catheter is preferred, the use of a GuideLiner or GuideZilla (Boston Scientific, USA) to follow the microcatheter can be very helpful. The preferred microcatheter for this task is again the Corsair. The proximal cap should be punctured with a Pilot 200 (Abbott, USA) and drilling should be performed with a straight tip, avoiding to 'knuckle' the wire down the path of the graft. Usually, the occluded material, composed of old thrombus, is relatively soft and the wire can easily progress to the distal vessel. If the Pilot 200 fails to puncture proximally, a Confianza Pro 12 (Asahi Intecc, Japan) can be used, the Corsair advanced, but this sharp wire should be quickly exchanged for the Pilot 200, as perforation is easier in such friable and thin-walled grafts. In the case of SVG course ambiguity, it may be helpful to deliver the Corsair in the proximal segment and perform a tip injection with few ccs of contrast, that may highlight the course of the graft. Then, the Pilot should be used again, with care to drill and keep its tip straight down the highlighted path. It should be followed by Corsair advancement, with the same clockwise and counter clockwise technique used for retrograde channel crossing. Once the Corsair is in the distal native vessel, a Sion or a Miracle 12 wire can be used to re-direct the catheter towards the distal cap of the native coronary CTO (Fig. 9.19, Videos 9.29, 9.30, 9.31, 9.32, and 9.33). Once the CTO is opened, a small injection in the graft should be performed. If the graft appears to be patent, coiling of the graft can ensure the absence of competitive flow and potentially minimize the risk of subsequent thrombosis of the newly deployed stents in the native coronary. This is especially important if the SVG that was crossed was widely patient (but restenotic for example). In such cases, some operators will prefer to deliver coils to sacrifice the graft, therefore ensuring that all the flow to the distal bed comes from the native vessel; this strategy however remains understudied and controversial.

## Crossing the CTO; True-to-True or Dissection and Re-entry

This section assumes that the operator was able to deliver the microcatheter to the distal cap. If the wire could be delivered, but not the microcatheter despite all the solutions exposed earlier, the procedure can be converted to an antegrade approach with "kissing wires", with the distal wire helping to target with a true-to-true (TTT) antegrade approach, or even with an antegrade dissection and re-entry (ADR) as a bailout.

If the microcatheter is positioned to the distal cap, the operator has to select one of the two crossing strategies; TTT or DR. In general, retrograde wire escalation or use of other retrograde wire strategies such as knuckles follow the same principles as with the antegrade approach. TTT will be favored in the case of a short (<20 mm) CTO, especially if there is no severe bending in the CTO segment or ambiguity in the vessel course. The preferred wire for this task is the Pilot 200. The Fielder XT (Asahi Intecc, Japan) can be tried, but its lack of tactile feedback make its manipulation more difficult from the retrograde approach when the intention is to keep it straight for TTT crossing. If the Pilot 200 fails, a Confianza Pro 12 can help crossing to the true lumen proximally. This approach can be assisted with a use of a mother-and-child (MAC) catheter such as the GuideLiner or the Guidezilla from the antegrade side, which shortens the working distance with the stiff guidewire (Fig. 9.20). The Gaia wire family, especially the Gaia 2nd and 3rd (Asahi Intecc, Japan), can be very useful for this task, because of their superior torque control.

It is important to highlight nuances about the location of the CTO to be crossed. RCA CTOs, the most common CTOs to be referred to CTO PCI, are much less at risk in case of sub-intimal tracking of the retrograde wire, even when pushed back in the aortic or sinus wall (Fig. 9.21, Videos 9.34, 9.35, 9.36, 9.37, 9.38, 9.39, 9.40, 9.41, and 9.42). However, when dealing with a proximal LCX or a proximal LAD CTO, a failed retrograde TTT crossing tracking the sub-intimal plane can lead to a hematoma of the left main and subsequent occlusion of a patent LCX or LAD. Therefore, if a TTT attempt is performed in the case of an LAD or an LCX CTO, we strongly encourage the use of a mother-and-child (MAC) catheter such as the GuideLiner or the Guidezilla, which can be delivered passed the carina of the left main, into the vessel with the CTO close to the proximal cap (see Fig. 9.20). Then, retrograde attempts should target the MAC catheter, with care not to track sub-intimally in the left main.

That brings the concept of the ***base of operations***. This corresponds to the CTO segment where most of the efforts are performed to connect and cross. Traditionally, we advocated the proximal cap to be the base of operation for retrograde CTO PCI, especially when a retrograde DR was employed. However, the advent of MAC catheters have substantially changed our way to perform re-entry (Fig. 9.22, Videos 9.43, 9.44, 9.45, 9.46, 9.47, 9.48, 9.49, 9.50, 9.51, and 9.52).

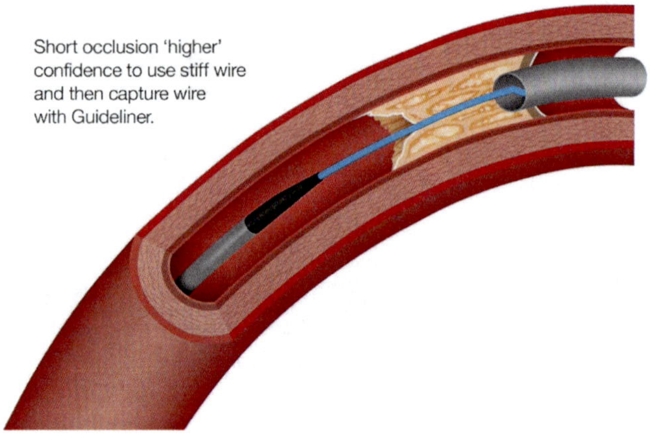


**Fig. 9.20** Retrograde true-to-true crossing using a mother-and-child catheter from the antegrade side (From Spratt [14] with permission)

If a TTT approach fails, or if the CTO is long and the course is ambiguous, a retrograde DR strategy should be employed, as a dissection created with proper techniques is less likely to cause vessel perforation (Fig. 9.23). When such a DR strategy also involves the use of an antegrade balloon to enlarge a dissection plane, it is usually referred to reverse-controlled antegrade and retrograde sub-intimal tracking or reverse-CART (Fig. 9.24).

A retrograde DR involves distal cap puncture with a Pilot 200 (or a Confianza Pro 12 if very hard), followed by Corsair advancement to the tip of the wire. It is very common to puncture with a hard wire to start tracking the vessel, especially if the distal cap is calcified. Then, a knuckled wire should be pushed to the proximal cap of the occlusion. If there seems to be some ambiguity of the location of the distal cap (which is far less common than proximal cap ambiguity), a tip injection from the microcatheter can really help to delineate some features of the distal cap, such as branches or microchannels. Sometimes, to soften the distal cap, it may be necessary to inject few cc of contrast from the microcatheter advanced few mm into the distal CTO extremity to create hydraulic dissection to help starting the retrograde dissection (also called the modified Carlino technique, see Chap. 8). We prefer to use the Fielder XT that creates smaller knuckles. However, for more powerful knuckles, especially in a sub-adventitial space beside heavy calcifications, the Pilot 200 is the preferred tool. To create a knuckle, the wire can simply be taken as is, with no bend, and pushed hard into the vessel. A knuckle wire should be pushed and never torqued, to avoid knotting its tip (see chap. 4). Once the knuckle reaches the proximal cap, the Corsair should follow as far as possible, and the knuckled wire should be retrieved. Then an antegrade injection should be performed to locate the relationship of the Corsair to the proximal cap. In the case of a short distance, a Confianza Pro 12 can be used to re-enter into the proximal vessel (or the aorta). In such instance, this sharp wire should be shaped with a longer 2 mm 45° bend. Otherwise, if such a strategy fails, it is time to perform reverse-CART.

Reverse CART (R-CART) is a retrograde DR that is facilitated with an antegrade dilation, to help the retrograde equipment to cross into the antegrade true lumen (Fig. 9.24). The ideal situation, especially when a retrograde wire was pushed into a sub-intimal plane, is to advance an antegrade wire into the sub-intimal space as well. It will be much easier to perform such a step with the retrograde Corsair or knuck-

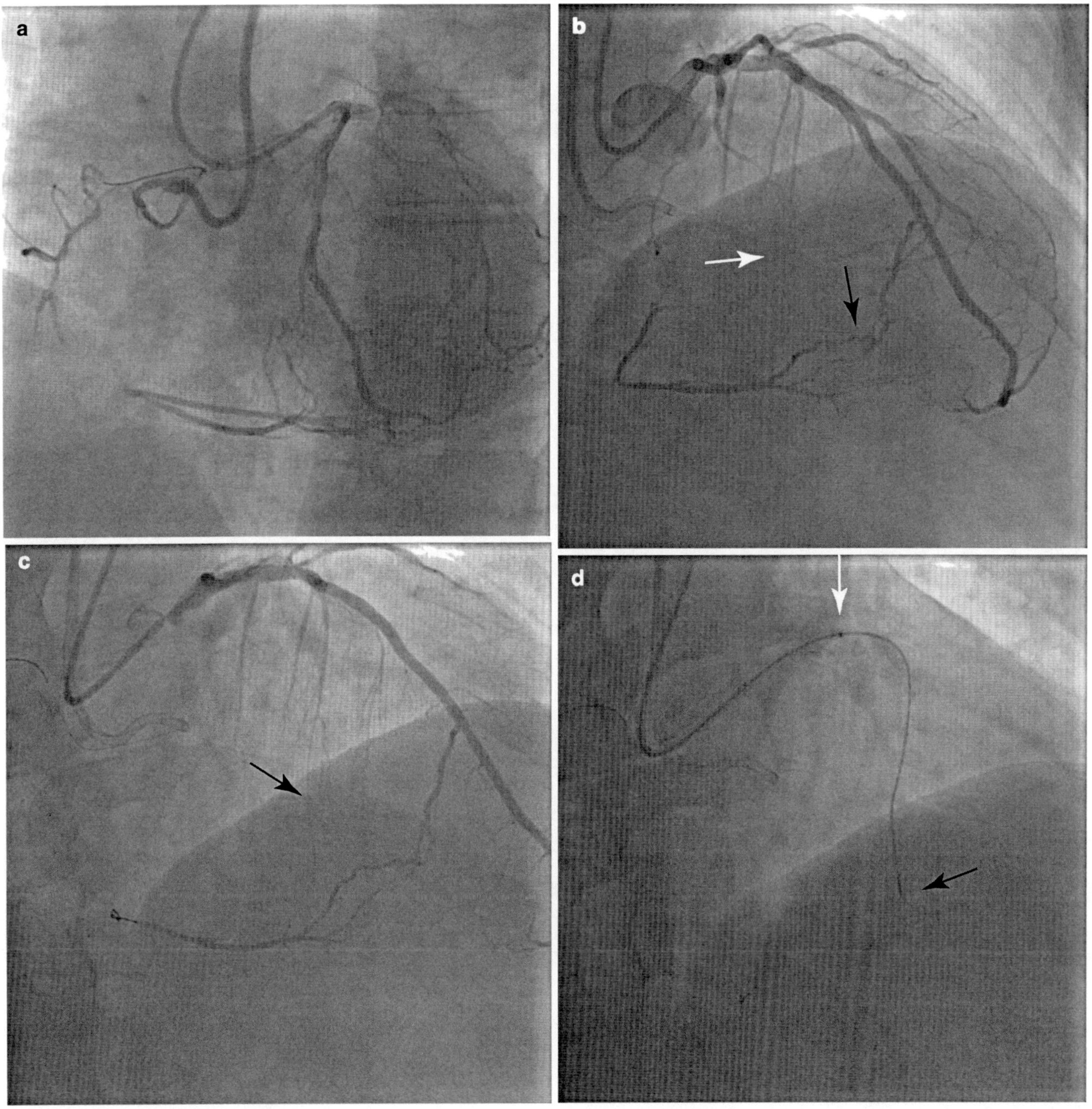


**Fig. 9.21** (Videos 9.34, 9.35, 9.36, 9.37, 9.38, 9.39, 9.40, 9.41, and 9.42): Retrograde dissection and re-entry of a long RCA CTO through an invisible septal channel. (**a**) Long RCA CTO with an island of patent RCA in the mid segment, with an ambiguous proximal cap, and a distal cap at the crux bifurcation, mandating a retrograde approach. An 8F catheter is used antegrade from the left radial, and a 6F is used on the retrograde side from the right radial. A guidewire is placed in the auricular branch to stabilize the antegrade guide (Video 9.34). (**b**) Very large but tortuous CC2 septal CCs are visualized from the LAD to the PDA (*black arrow*). There are other septal branches that give CC0 collateral channels (*white arrow*) (Video 9.35). (**c**) After 5 min of surfing one of the most proximal septal with a Sion through a Finecross, a connection to the PDA was achieved (Video 9.36). (**d**) The Finecross is exchanged for a Corsair (*black arrow*), which is advanced through the septal CC with the support of a 5.5F Guideliner MAC catheter (*white arrow*) (Video 9.37). (**e**) A Pilot 200 is used to create a retrograde dissection up to the proximal cap. The *arrow* indicates the tip of the knuckled wire (Video 9.38). (**f**) An anchoring balloon technique (using a 2.0 mm balloon) is used to stabilise the antegrade guide, and to improve support (*black arrow*). A Pilot 200 is advanced targeting the retrograde knuckled wire and subsequently also knuckled beside the retrograde system. Both the antegrade and the retrograde wires are in the sub-intimal space. A 3.0 mm balloon in used to connect both system together (reverse CART) (Video 9.39). (**g**) The balloon is moved more proximally (reverse CART). There is a very close contact of the antegrade balloon with the retrograde Corsair (Video 9.39). (**h**) A straight Pilot 200 is used to navigate through the dissection plane, up to the aorta (Video 9.39). (**i**) After advancing the Corsair to the RCA ostium, a soft workhorse wire is redirected into the antegrade guide. (Alternatively, snaring could have been performed) (Video 9.40). (**j**) Control angiography of the donor artery (Video 9.41). (**k**) Final result, showing preserved distal branches, but also some few side branches of the RCA in the mid segment, despite a dissection-re-entry technique used. Please note that there remain a small channel above the stent from previous retrograde re-entry attempt (*arrow*). It will close within days after the CTO PCI (Video 9.42)

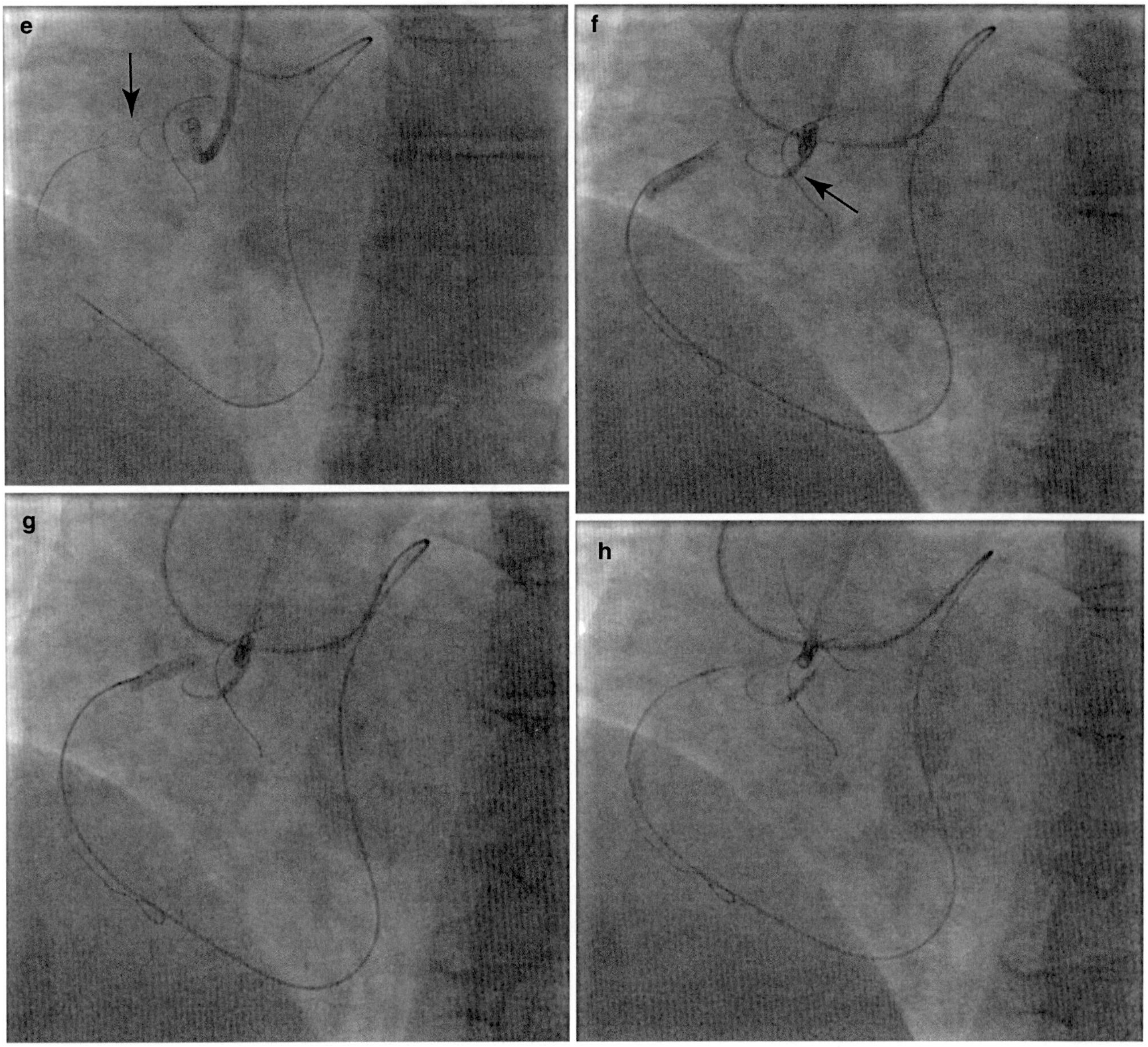


**Fig. 9.21** (continued)

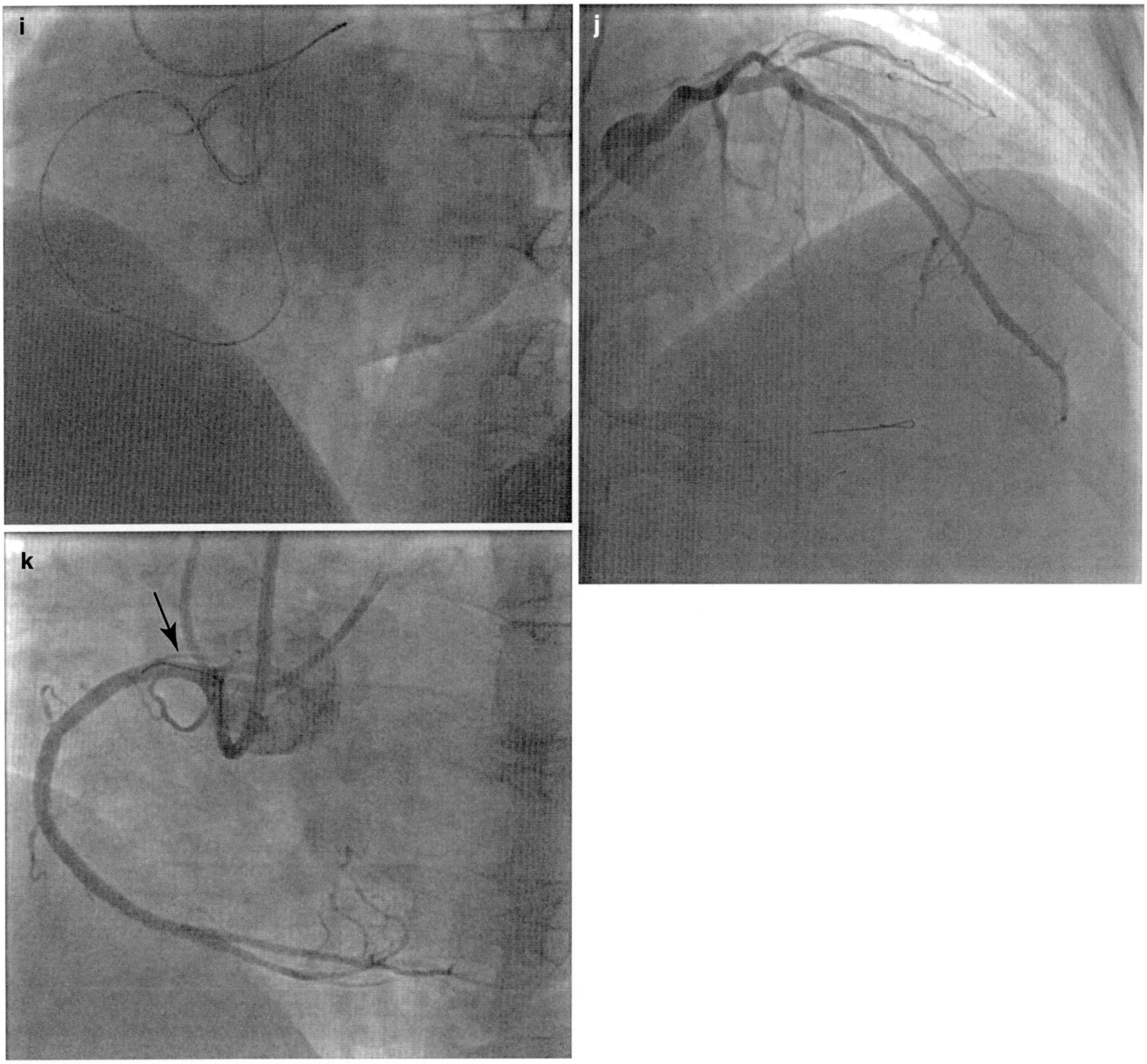


**Fig. 9.21** (continued)

led wire in place, that provide a clear target for the antegrade wire to puncture and advance into the same virtual space. A Confianza Pro 12 guidewire can be used for the antegrade puncture, if on a short distance, or a Pilot 200. As soon as the wire penetrates and tracks along the retrograde gear, several views should be assessed to make sure that both systems are in parallel, and 'dance with each other' (Fig. 9.22h, i, Videos 9.48, and 9.49). Then, an OTW or another microcatheter can be advanced, and the wire exchanged for a polymer-jacketed wire that can be knuckled beside the retrograde system, to gain an antegrade control of the artery. Care should be applied not to push the antegrade knuckled wire too far down into the vessel, which could lead to significant side-branch occlusion resulting from hematoma formation. Then, a rapid exchange balloon will be delivered into the CTO segment, and inflated. The size of the balloon should be selected based on the presumed size of the vessel. The size of the knuckled wire, from one side to the other side of the loop, can help give a gross idea of the size of the vessel. Alternatively, the use of IVUS can help to determine the true size of the vessel, and select an appropriate balloon to make the connection. The most common reason for a difficult R-CART is under sizing of the antegrade balloon. Once the inflation is performed, the balloon is deflated, and the retrograde wire is advanced with the intention to track the antegrade wire towards the antegrade MAC catheter, guide or aorta (Fig. 9.21, Videos 9.34, 9.35, 9.36, 9.37, 9.38, 9.39, 9.40, 9.41, and 9.42). We like to use the Pilot 200 for this task, as

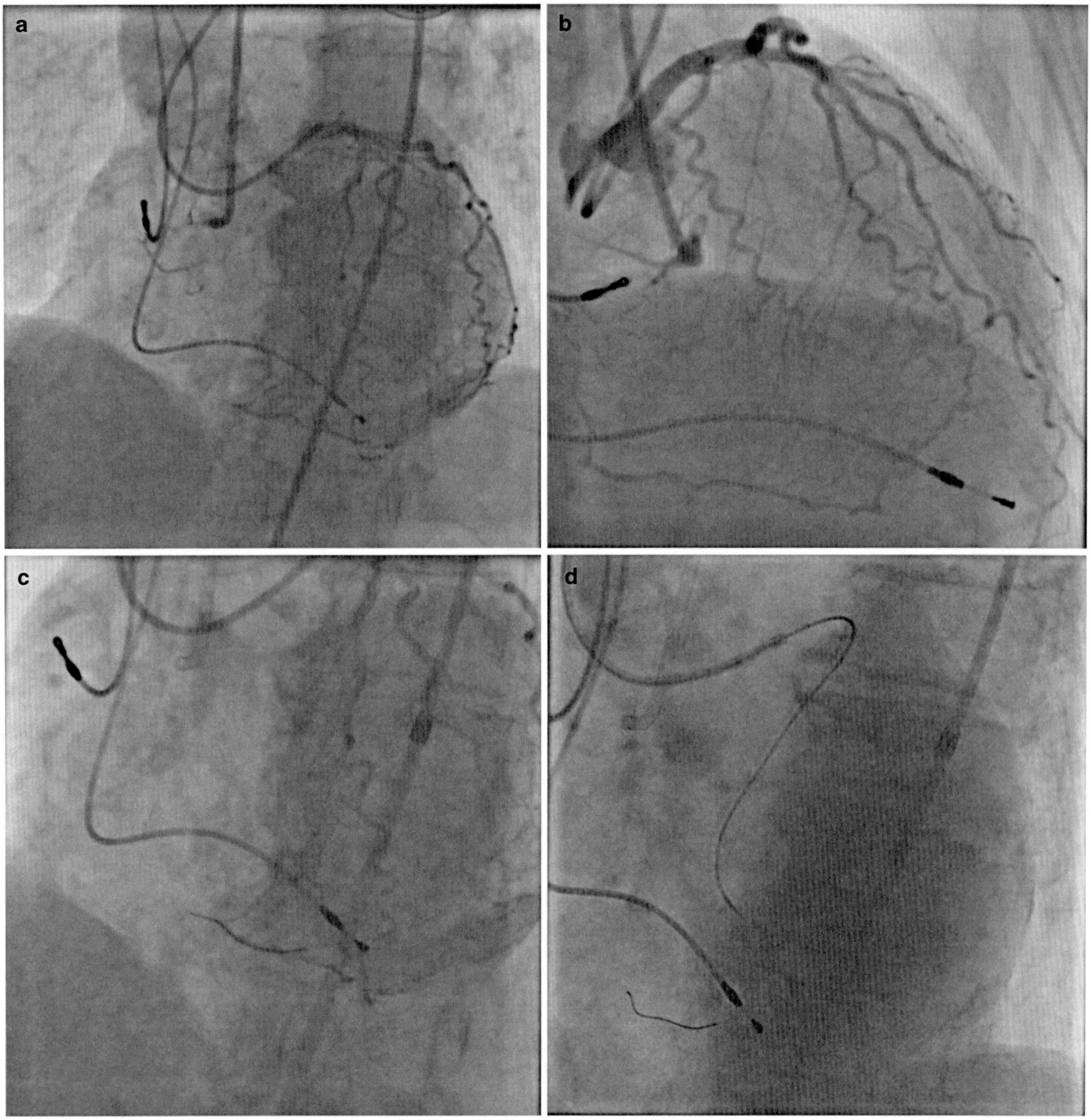


**Fig. 9.22** (Videos 9.43, 9.44, 9.45, 9.46, 9.47, 9.48, 9.49, 9.50, 9.51, and 9.52). Retrograde dissection and re-entry technique facilitated by the use of an antegrade mother-and-child catheter. (**a**) Dual injection showing a long RCA CTO, with the distal cap at a major bifurcation, and good septal CCs from the left system. A 6F XB 3.5 90 cm in used from the right radial into the left main, and an 8F JR 4 from the common femoral artery into the RCA (Video 9.43). (**b**) Dual injection showing several CC0 and CC1 connections to the PDA. However, there is also a non-interventional collateral from the distal OM to the tip of the PDA. This epicardial and very tortuous CC is dominant and non-interventional (Video 9.44). (**c**) Sion wire at the distal cap, after surfing septals. (**d**) Corsair advanced through the septal channel. (**e–g**) Retrograde dissection with a knuckled Feilder XT. The size of the loop indicates that the vessel is likely larger than 4.0 mm (Videos 9.45, 9.46, and 9.47). (**h**, **i**) Antegrade knuckled wire (Fielder XT) to gain control of the artery. Both the antegrade and the retrograde system are aligned in the sub-intimal space, moving together with heart beats, ready to perform reverse CART (Videos 9.48 and 9.49). (**j**) MAC-assisted reverse CART: antegrade dilation is performed, where both systems cross. Please note how far the retrograde Corsair is from the antegrade balloon shaft, highlighting again that the vessel is likely close to 4.0 mm in diameter. A 6F GuideLiner is used (*black arrow*) (Video 9.50). (**k**) The MAC catheter is advanced over the inflated antegrade balloon, anchored into the CTO segment, where the intention is to make the connection (base of operation). After deflation of the balloon, a retrograde Pilot 200 is directed into the MAC, which prevents recoil from balloon dilation (Video 9.51). (**l**) Final injection, after externalization of a long wire, stenting on this wire, and removal of the retrograde system (Video 9.52)

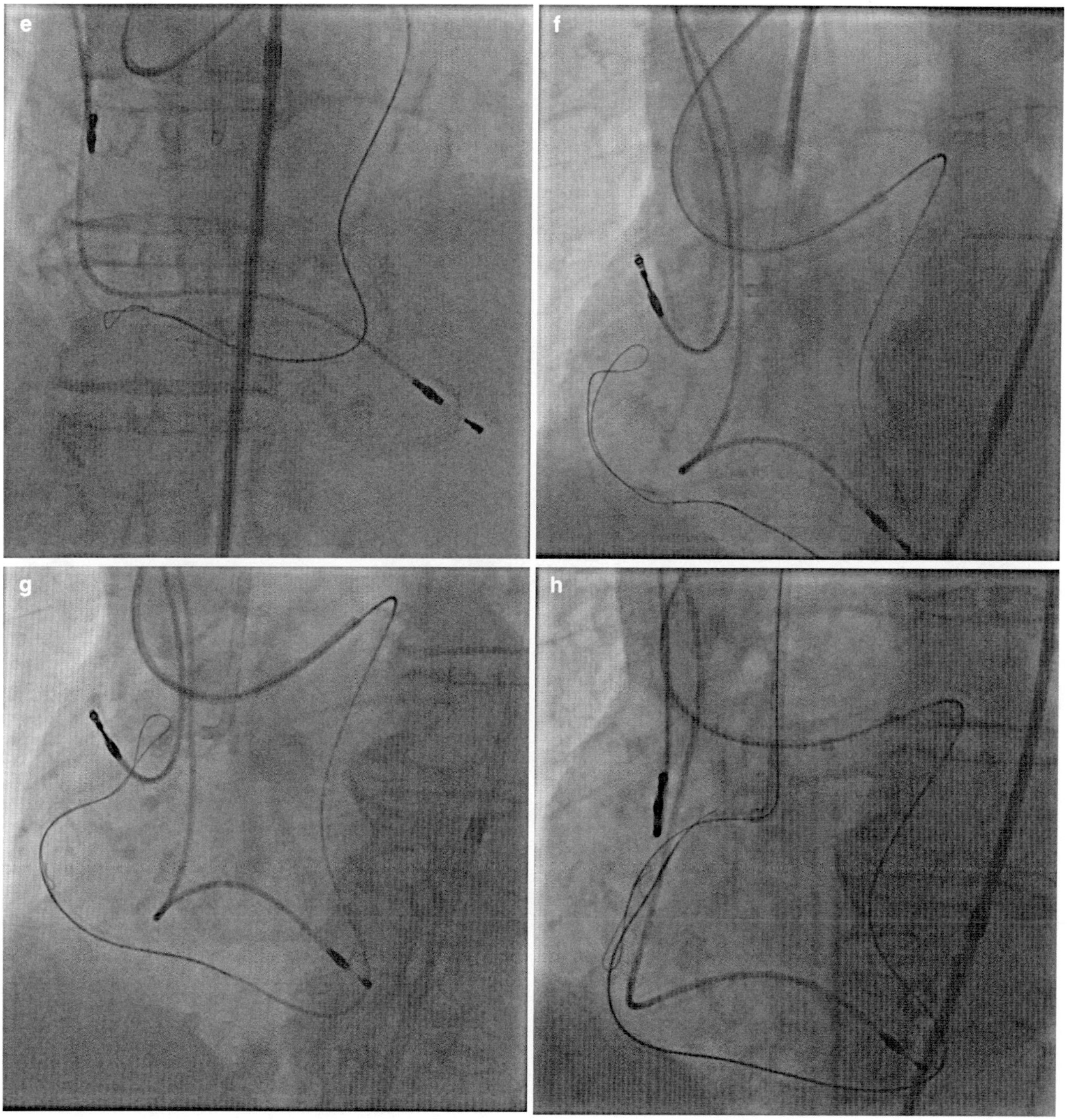


**Fig. 9.22** (continued)

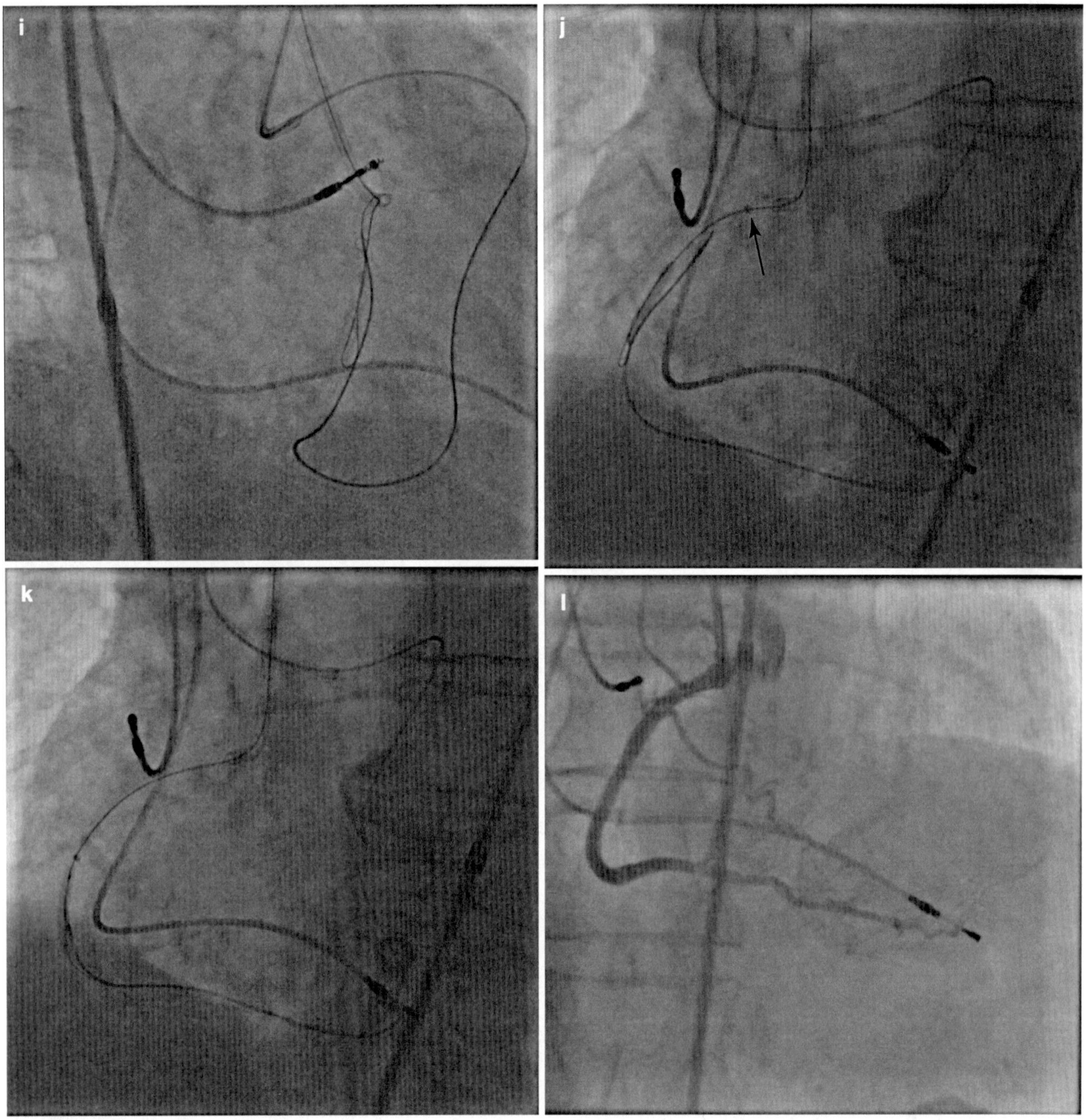


**Fig. 9.22** (continued)

it tends to stay within the track created with the antegrade balloon, and is less likely to re-enter into a new sub-intimal channel that does not connect. Gaia 2nd or Gaia 3rd wires are also very effective. If the operator fails to connect into the proximal vessel, a Confianza Pro 12 shaped the same way as previously exposed for re-entry can be used to penetrate the few remaining tissue planes that still offer resistance to connection (Fig. 9.25, Videos 9.53, 9.54, 9.55, 9.56, 9.57, 9.58, 9.59, 9.60, 9.61, 9.62, 9.63, 9.64, and 9.65). Sometimes, use of a bigger balloon will help to make the connection.

There are four possible combinations for the antegrade and retrograde wires into the CTO segment or at the base of operation. (1) Antegrade into the plaque, retrograde into the plaque; (2) Antegrade into the plaque, and retrograde in the sub-intimal space; (3) antegrade into the sub-intimal space and retrograde into the plaque, and; (4) antegrade into the sub-intimal space and retrograde in the sub-intimal space (Fig. 9.26). In the first situation, both wires are into the same structure, and antegrade dilation, with dissections, should create enough space for the retrograde wire to

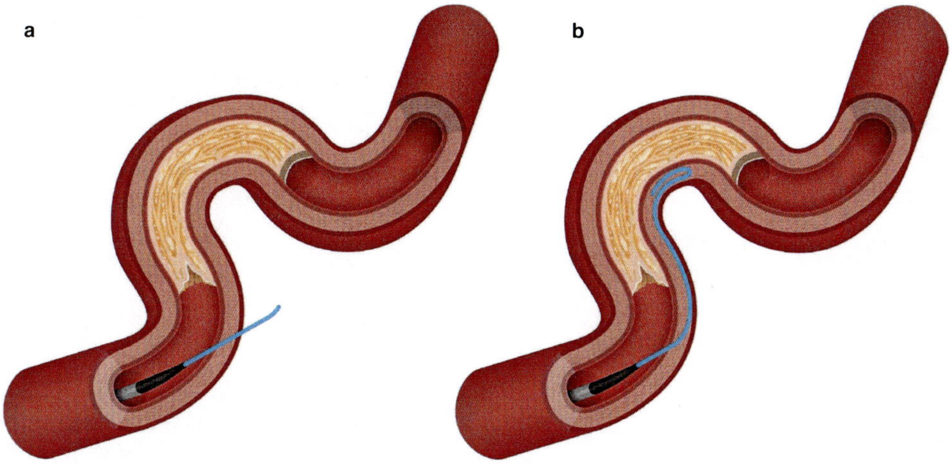


**Fig. 9.23** Tortuous and long CTO crossed with a retrograde dissection technique. Panel (**a**) shows how a stiff wire can easily exit the vessel structure when facing ambiguity in the vessel course. Panel (**b**). A knuckled polymer-jacketed guidewire is advanced in the natural cleavage plane between the adventitia and the atheroma, without exiting the vessel structure (From Spratt [14] with permission)

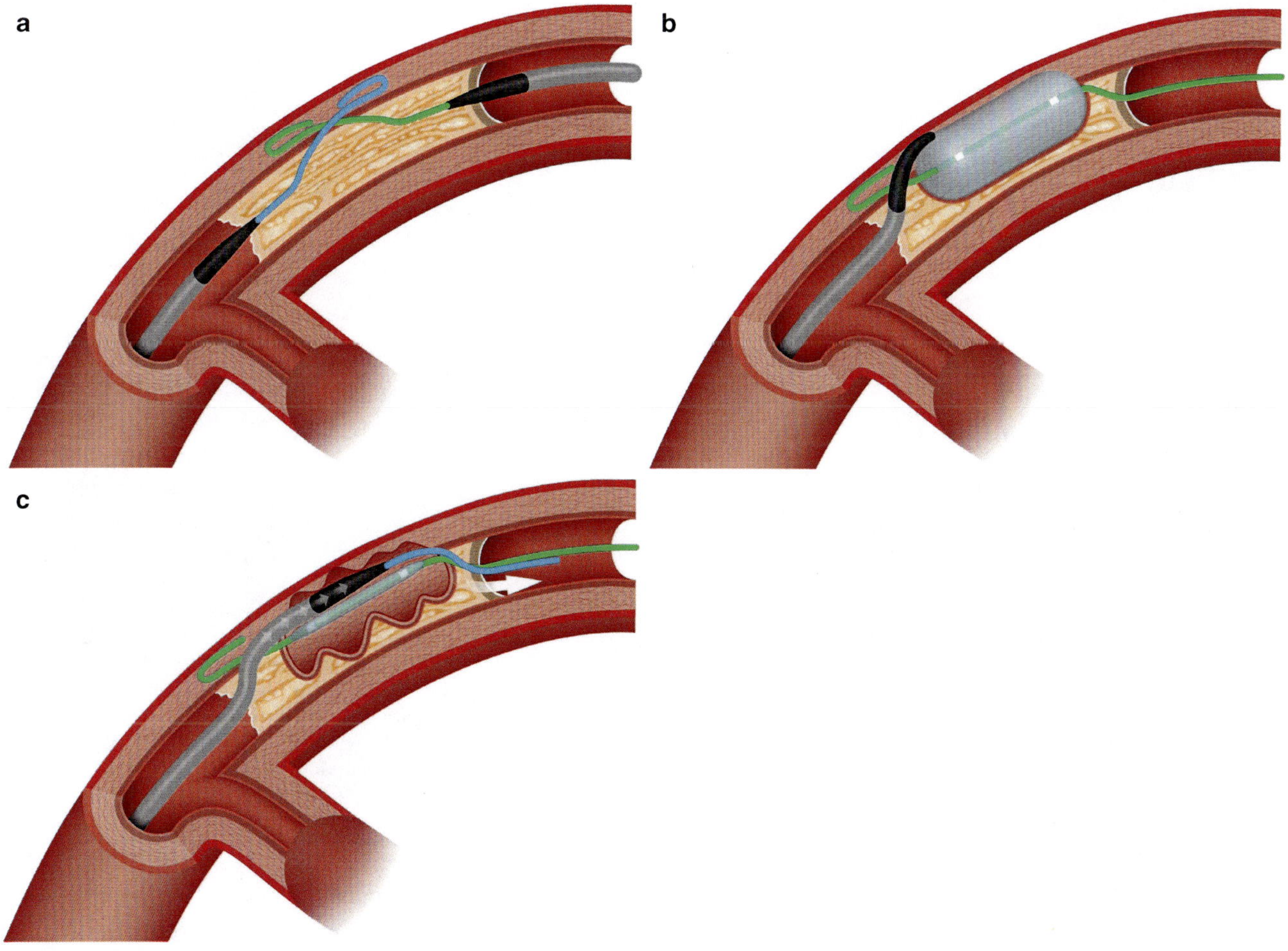


**Fig. 9.24** Reverse CART. Panel (**a**). A guidewire is knuckled from the retrograde side into the subintimal space, and an antegrade wire is also knuckle in the same space. (**b**) An antegrade balloon is inflated to enlarge the space. (**c**) The retrograde wire connects with the antegrade system, and crosses into the antegrade true lumen (From Spratt [14] with permission.)

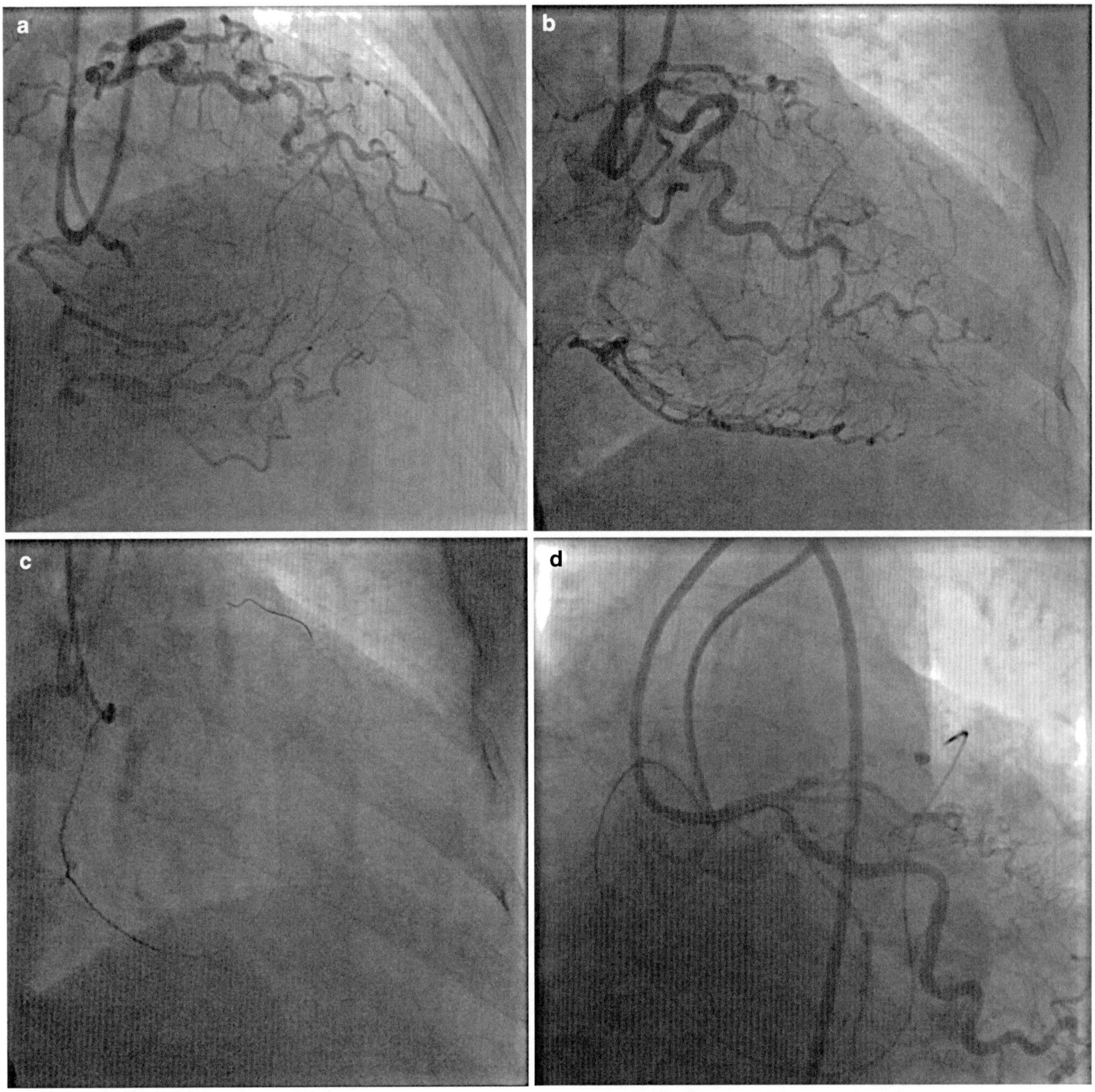


**Fig. 9.25** (Video 9.53, 9.54, 9.55, 9.56, 9.57, 9.58, 9.59, 9.60, 9.61, 9.62, 9.63, 9.64, and 9.65). LAD CTO treated with MAC-assisted reverse CART. (**a, b**) Proximal LAD CTO with nice septal CCs from the RCA (Video 9.53 and 9.54). (**c**) Successful septal surfing (Video 9.55). (**d**) Corsair at the distal cap; the proximal LAD shows a partially recanalized segment (Video 9.56). (**e**) Distal injection from the antegrade Finecross to better define the proximal cap and potential channel (Video 9.57). (**f, g**) Antegrade dissection with knuckled Fielder XT (Videos 9.58 and 9.59). (**h**) Distal injection from the Corsair showing the tip of the antegrade knuckle close to the distal cap (Video 9.60). (**i**) MAC (GuideLiner)-assisted reverse CART; a 2.5 mm balloon is inflated over the knuckled wire (Video 9.61), and (**j**) the MAC catheter is advanced into the LAD CTO segment to scaffold the dissection planes (Video 9.61). (**k**) The Fielder XT is withdrawn and a Pilot 200 is advanced from the retrograde Corsair, targeting the antegrade GuideLiner catheter, but stays sub-intimal (Video 9.62). (**l**) Successful connection into the GuideLiner with a Confianza Pro 12 (Video 9.63). (**m**) Stent placement over an externalized R350 guidewire (Video 9.64). (**n**) Final result (Video 9.65)

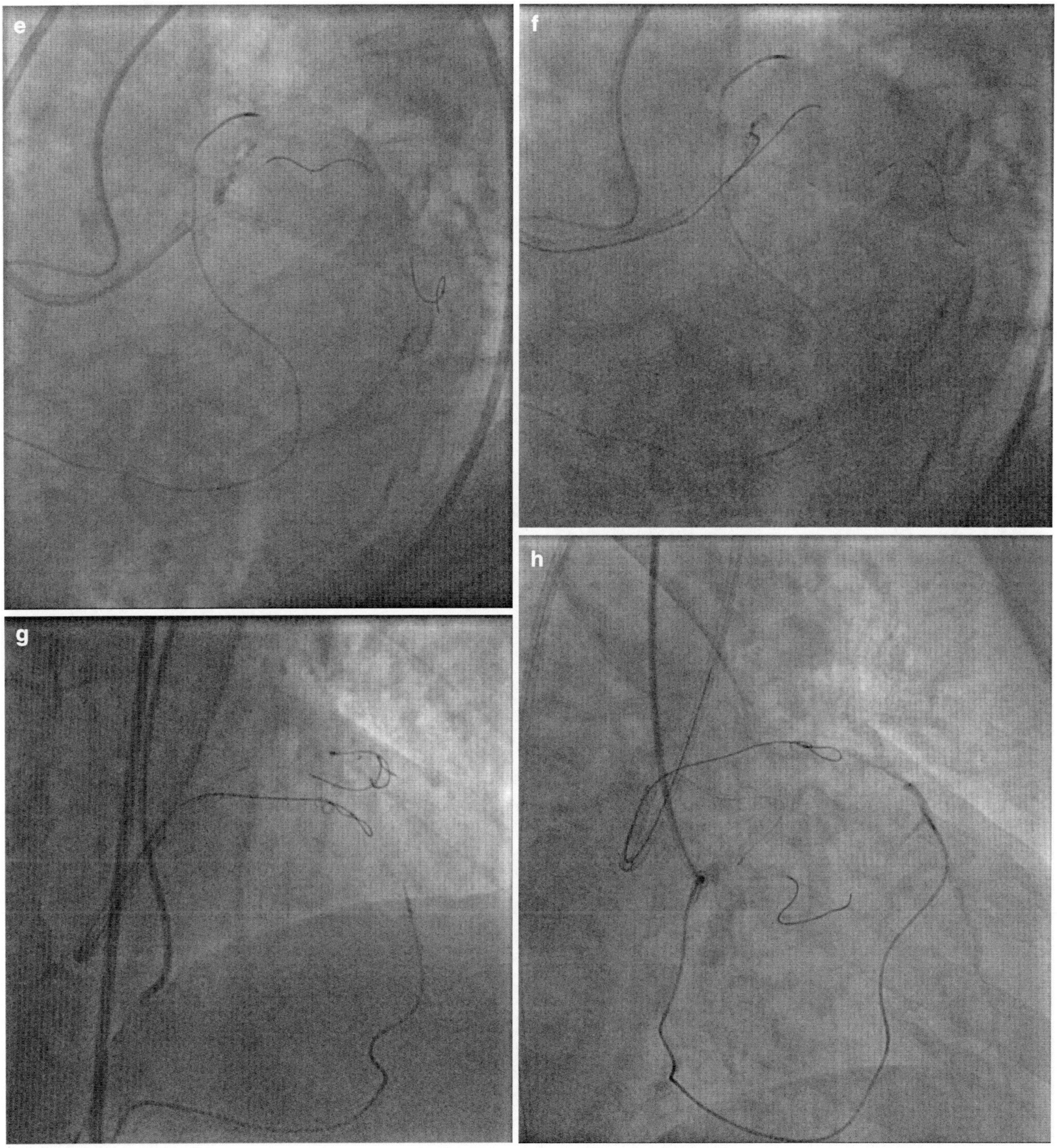


**Fig. 9.25** (continued)

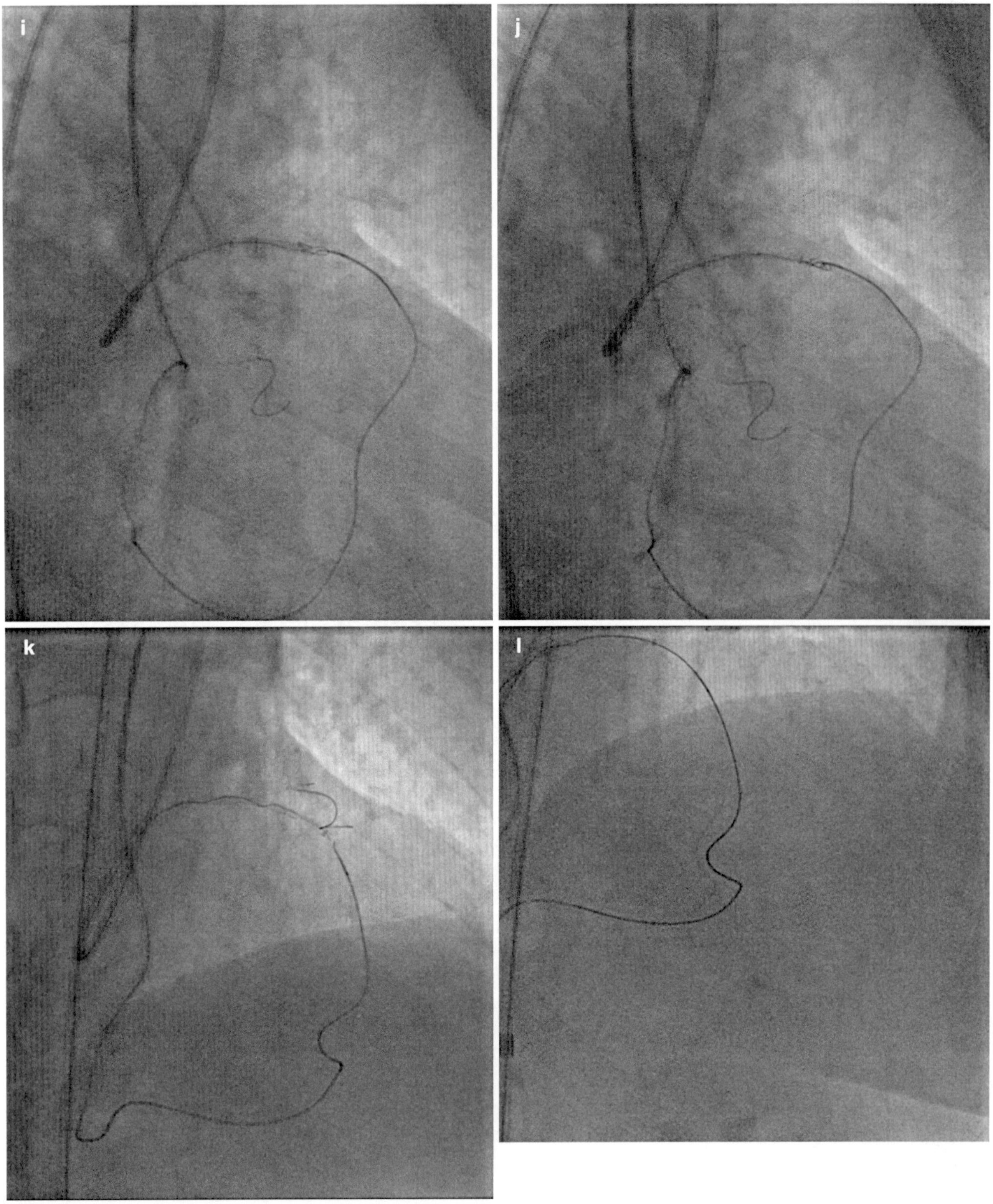


**Fig. 9.25** (continued)

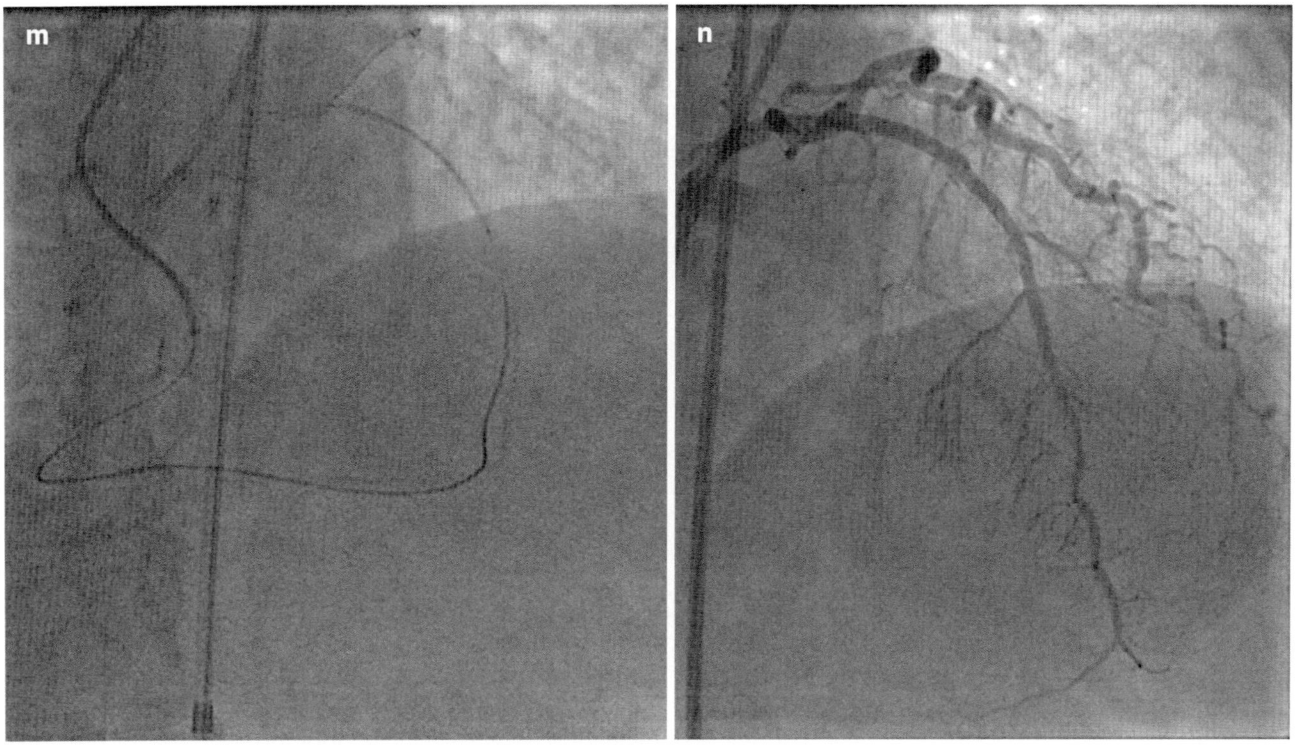


**Fig. 9.25** (continued)

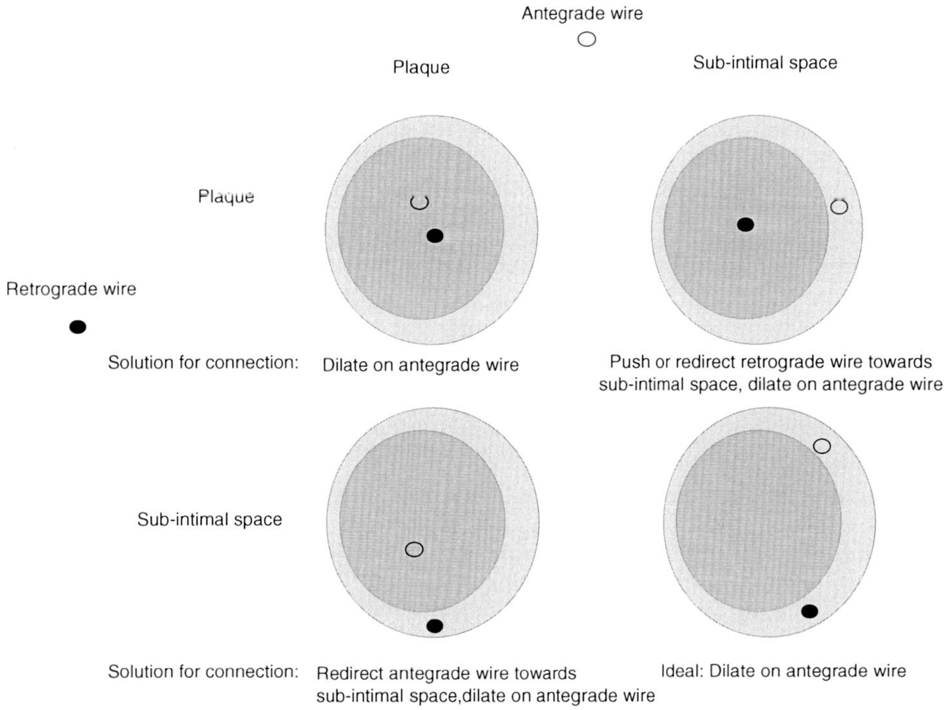


**Fig. 9.26** The four possible combinations of retrograde and antegrade wire in the base of operation and solutions for connection

track to the proximal vessel. This is also the case for the last situation, which is ideal, where both wires are sub-intimal. Enlarging the space enough with a properly sized antegrade balloon will lead to a connection of the retrograde wire and even the microcatheter with the antegrade space (Figs. 9.21 and 9.22, Videos 9.34, 9.35, 9.36, 9.37, 9.38, 9.39, 9.40, 9.41, 9.42, 9.43, 9.44, 9.45, 9.46, 9.47, 9.48, 9.49, 9.50, 9.51, and 9.52). The other two situations are more problematic. When the antegrade wire is into the plaque, but the retrograde is in the sub-intimal space, aggressive antegrade dilation will be required to create enough connection and dissection planes to reach the sub-intimal level. This is often impossible to perform. It is therefore better to redirect the antegrade wire to the sub-intimal plane as well, and then perform antegrade balloon dilation in this new space. When the antegrade wire is into the sub-intimal plane but the retrograde wire is into the plaque, it is usually because the retrograde wire has not been pushed hard enough to penetrate the sub-adventitial layer. Applying this solution will help for a subsequent connection. New operators are encouraged to use IVUS to better understand the wire relationships prior to performing R-CART.

An alternative to R-CART (antegrade balloon with a retrograde wire connection), is the classical CART approach, which involves the use of a retrograde balloon into the segment, and an antegrade wire manipulation into the enlarged space. Such an approach has fallen out of favor in the majority of cases since the advent of Corsair. First, it may be laborious to deliver a retrograde balloon, although a previous septal dilation with the Corsair is usually sufficient to allow for a retrograde balloon to cross. Second, the technique does not involve externalization, which is inconvenient in some cases; an externalized wire provides the best support for subsequent stent delivery and placement. Finally, CART carries the risk of distal side branches dissection or occlusion, which is less likely with reverse CART. The operator should convert to CART in the rare situation where the Corsair fails to navigate to the proximal vessel. In such cases, a retrograde dilation, followed by Corsair advancement can also be done, and reverse CART resumed. Otherwise, CART can be attempted.

As explained earlier, there is a significant difference between reverse CART performed in the RCA vs. when done in the LAD or the LCx (Fig. 9.25, Videos 9.53, 9.54, 9.55, 9.56, 9.57, 9.58, 9.59, 9.60, 9.61, 9.62, 9.63, 9.64, and 9.65). One of the potential advantages of the retrograde DR is that the dissections are limited within the CTO segment of the vessel. In RCAs, this is less important since the RCA is a conduit vessel without significant branches until the crux; occlusion of RV branches by dissection flaps have very minimal consequences for the vast majority of patients. This is not the case in LADs since there are multiple important branches, both septals and diagonals that need to be preserved. Keeping the length of the dissections as short as possible is crucial in CTO PCI of LAD and LCX. Furthermore, the technique to connect the retrograde wire into the proximal true lumen often involves many sequential attempts with multiple wires up to a point that the wire enters into the proximal true lumen. Such attempts, with sub-intimal tracking, can lead to left main dissection and dramatic complication if not enough care is applied to keep the base of operation distal to the left main carina. Therefore, we strongly advocate the use of a MAC catheter, delivered passed the carina, to avoid such dissections and isolate the base of operation. With a MAC catheter in place, the balloon dilation can be performed through it, and once performed, the retrograde wire can simply target the MAC catheter for connection. Once entering the MAC catheter, the retrograde wire is therefore also into the antegrade guide catheter, and the retrograde microcatheter can be advanced to reach the MAC catheter, followed by externalization of a long wire (Fig. 9.25, Videos 9.53, 9.54, 9.55, 9.56, 9.57, 9.58, 9.59, 9.60, 9.61, 9.62, 9.63, 9.64, and 9.65). For RCA, it is less of an issue, as there are no major bifurcation in the proximal segment. It is therefore easier to make the connection, either into the guide catheter or the aorta (Fig. 9.21, Videos 9.34, 9.35, 9.36, 9.37, 9.38, 9.39, 9.40, 9.41, and 9.42). However, we strongly advocate for the use of MAC catheters even in the RCA (Fig. 9.22, Videos 9.43, 9.44, 9.45, 9.46, 9.47, 9.48, 9.49, 9.50, 9.51, and 9.52), for the following reasons: (1) First, the MAC catheter can be advanced into the antegrade channels that were created with the balloon, preventing the newly created dissection plane to collapse or recoil, and thus helping the retrograde wire to connect through it. (2) Second, the MAC catheter can be advanced into the coronary to change the base of operation. Traditionally, before the advent of MAC catheters, reverse CART performed in long RCA CTOs with the balloon inflated in the mid or distal segments were very difficult. It was common for the retrograde wire to connect, but subsequently track another plane not connecting into the proximal RCA true lumen. Now with MACs catheters, it is wise to select the base of operation based on the relationship between the retrograde and antegrade wires. It is where the wires seem to be closest to one another (or seem to cross) that the connection is most likely to be successful (Fig. 9.27). Therefore, antegrade dilation, followed by MAC catheter intubation over an anchored balloon at the base of operations can be performed at the level where both retrograde and antegrade wires seem to "cross" followed with retrograde connection with a wire (Pilot 200 usually, or Confianza Pro 12, with a small CTO bend) into the MAC catheter (Figs. 9.22 and 9.28, Videos 9.43, 9.44, 9.45, 9.46, 9.47, 9.48, 9.49, 9.50, 9.51, and 9.52). This approach can also be very helpful in case if the retrograde wire tracks an old SVG anastomosis. It is sometimes very difficult to redirect the wire into the native vessel structure. However, if an antegrade knuckled

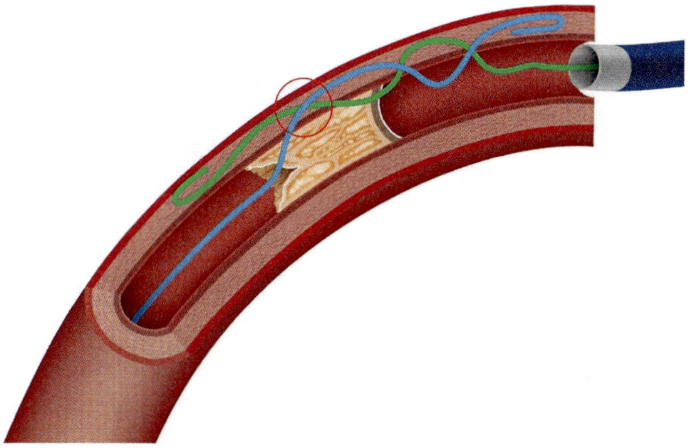

**Fig. 9.27** When using a MAC catheter, the most likely connection spot is where the antegrade and retrograde wires seem to cross (From Spratt [14] with permission)

wire is advanced passed this point, followed by a MAC catheter intubation, the connection can be made easier (Fig. 9.29, Videos 9.66, 9.67, 9.68, 9.69, 9.70, 9.71, 9.72, 9.73, and 9.74). It should be emphasized that as soon as antegrade balloon dilation has started, no antegrade injection should be performed, in order to avoid perforation or hydraulic dissection. This is especially true when using a MAC catheter, especially if the pressure damps. We recommend disconnecting the syringe from the antegrade manifold once antegrade preparation of the vessel has started, to avoid accidental injection of contrast in the intentionally created dissection planes that may shut the distal vessel down and terminate the procedure.

## Connecting the Retrograde Wire into the Native Vessel, the MAC Catheter, the Guide Catheter or the Aorta

Once the CTO is crossed with the wire, the latter will either sit into the proximal vessel, navigate into the MAC catheter or the antegrade guide catheter, or flow freely into the aorta. However, it is not unusual to notice that the antegrade wire finally re-entered successfully into the distal true lumen after reverse-CART. In such instance, the procedure should be converted to an antegrade procedure.

If a stiff retrograde wire with an acute bend crosses the CTO, but there is significant disease to navigate up to the antegrade guide, it is wise to advance the Corsair and exchange for a softer wire to engage the guide (Fig. 9.21, Videos 9.34, 9.35, 9.36, 9.37, 9.38, 9.39, 9.40, 9.41, and 9.42). Otherwise, if the wire penetrates into the MAC or guide catheter, the next step will be to follow with the microcatheter up until it reaches the antegrade guide. During this step, it may be helpful to pin the retrograde guidewire into the antegrade guide with a balloon. We will use a 3.0 mm balloon in an 8F, a 2.5 mm in a 7F, and a 2.0 mm in a 6F guide. If anchoring is performed into a MAC catheter, the size of the balloon will depend on the size of the MAC catheter, keeping in mind that the actual inner diameter of the MAC catheter is one French smaller that the corresponding guide size. Once few cm of Corsair or Finecross are into the antegrade guide or MAC catheter, the wire used to cross the CTO will be pulled out and externalization performed with a dedicated long wire. The RG3 (Asahi Intecc, Japan) is a long 330 cm 0.010″ wire especially made for that task. Alternatively, the R350 (Vascular Solutions, USA), which is 0.013″ in diameter, can serve for the same purpose. A RotaWire can also be used, although it can more easily kink. Finally, if the retrograde or the antegrade guide is 90 cm long, a simple 300 cm Pilot 200 can serve for the purpose. We like to administer 2–3 cc of pure RotaGlide into the microcatheter to ease wire externalization, especially when the R350, the RotaWire or the Pilot 200 are used. With the RG3, this step is not needed. Pushing the wire all the way back to the antegrade guide valve takes time; it is shorter with the RG3. Care should be made not to kink the wire. When externalizing, the antegrade valve connector is unhooked, and the proximal hub of the antegrade catheter occluded with a finger, to avoid back bleeding. As soon as the operator (or assistant) feels the retrograde wire pointing out on the finger, a wire introducer is inserted into the valve connector, and the wire tip inserted into the wire introducer tip. The hemostatic valve is then connected again to the guide catheter, and the retrograde wire pushed and pulled at the same time to externalize the long retrograde wire. Alternatively, if a MAC catheter was used, the hemostatic valve can stay connected, and the MAC simply be pulled to the level of the valve when the wire is ready to exit the guide. Also, a balloon can be inflated in the MAC catheter next to the tip of the long wire used for externalization (especially if a 0.014′ wire was used) and the MAC pulled out, pulling out the wire at the same time. It should be emphasized that serious complications can occur during the retrograde procedure when gear (wires, catheters, balloons) is pulled. This is because significant tension can be stored in the system and cause "squeezing" of the heart, resulting in hypotension, brady-arrhythmias and chest discomfort. Also, pulling on the gear will lead to deep intubation of the retrograde guide, which can lead to donor artery dissection. The solution to those problems is to stop pulling and let the system equilibrate. We recommend against pulling hard on the externalized wire but rather "walking it out" while it is pushed from the retrograde guide. Once the wire is externalized, the MAC catheter can be reinserted to the coronary, or simply taken out, as support is rarely an issue with an externalized guidewire. Few cm out the valve is enough to deliver antegrade rapid exchange gear, as the wire is coming from inside the patient's body, not the reverse, and cannot be lost. A torque-

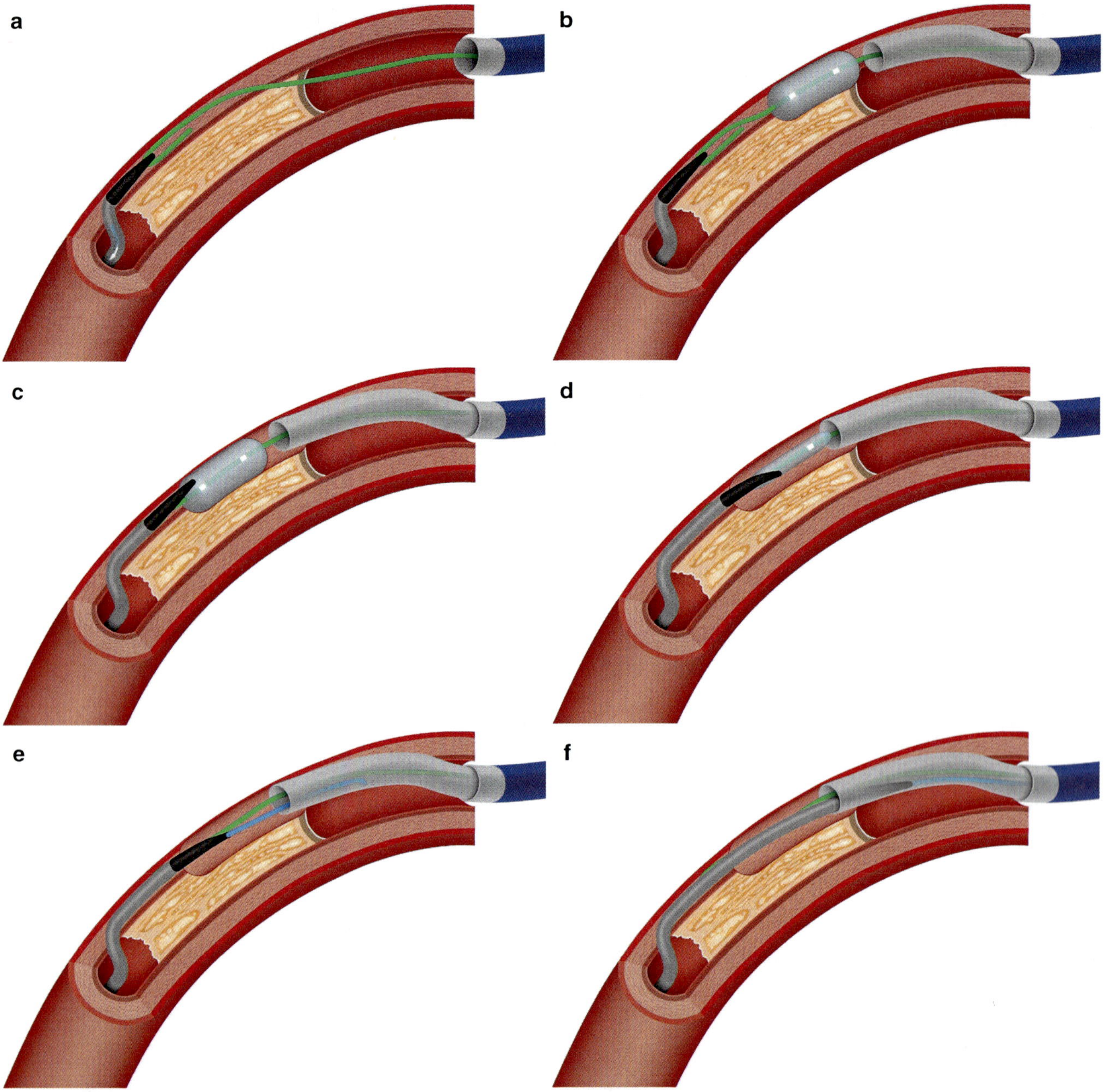


**Fig. 9.28** MAC-assisted reverse CART. (**a**) An antegrade polymer-jacketed guidewire is knuckled into the sub-adventitial plane. The retrograde Corsair is also is the same space. The retrograde wire has been removed. (**b**) An antegrade balloon is inflated to enlarge the space. (**c**) The MAC catheter is delivered over the inflated balloon to scaffold the dissection planes. The antegrade balloon is inflated close to the Corsair. (**d**) The Corsair tip moves with balloon inflation and deflation, which indicates that connection is most likely to occur. (**e**) A straight retrograde wire is directed into the MAC catheter. (**f**) The Corsair is advanced into the antegrade MAC, and a long wire externalized (From Spratt [14] with permission)

ing device should be placed on the proximal end of the long wire, especially if only 300 cm long, to avoid an inadvertent loss of the proximal wire position into the Corsair or Finecross. Before externalizing a wire, care should be applied not to lose the antegrade guide position. Also, during externalization or once the wire is externalized, any back tension on that wire will lead to deep intubation of the retrograde guide. Therefore, it is necessary to pull the retrograde guide outside the coronary before applying back tension on an externalized wire or on the Corsair.

If the wire tracks out of the vessel into the aorta, it should be left there, unless the proximal vessel is not diseased; in the latter situation, the microcatheter can be advanced close to the antegrade guide tip and the wire exchanged for a softer wire to engage the antegrade guide (Fig. 9.21, Videos 9.34, 9.35, 9.36, 9.37, 9.38, 9.39, 9.40, 9.41, and 9.42). Otherwise,

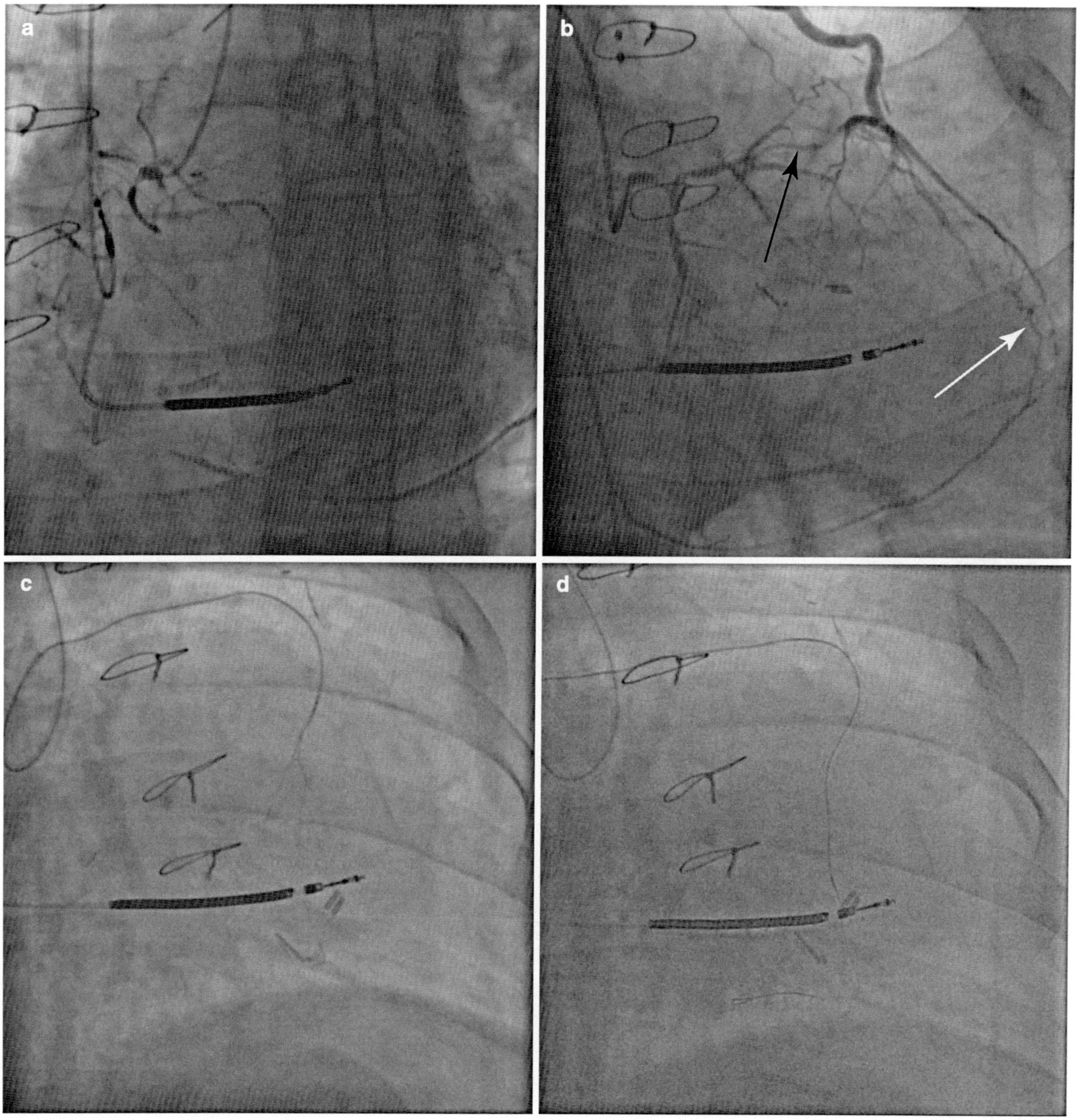


**Fig. 9.29** (Videos 9.66, 9.67, 9.68, 9.69, 9.70, 9.71, 9.72, 9.73, and 9.74). Retrograde RCA recanalization from the native LAD, guided by the LIMA. (**a**) Long post-CABG RCA CTO, with an ambiguous proximal cap and collaterals from the LIMA to the LAD and PL branch (Video 9.66). (**b**) Patent native LAD despite the presence of a LIMA graft (*black arrow*). Faint septal CC to PDA and tortuous non interventional epicardial collateral CC to PLV (*white arrow*) (Video 9.67). (**c**) Through the native LAD, a Corsair is delivered in a septal CC (with guidance from LIMA injections), with distal tip injection after failed septal surfing (Video 9.68). (**d**) Connection with a Sion wire (Video 9.69). (**e**) Distal injection through Corsair that confirms a connection from the PDA to the PLV, and injection from the RCA, confirming the very long length of the CTO (Video 9.70). (**f**) Knuckled wire tracks an old graft; it is impossible to redirect into the native RCA structure. The *arrow* indicates a graft surgical clip (Video 9.71). (**g**, **h**) Antegrade knuckled wire to move the base of operation distal to the occluded graft anastomosis (Video 9.72). (**i**) A MAC catheter is delivered on an inflated balloon distal to the anastomosis to the base of operation to perform reverse-CART (Video 9.73). (**j**) Final result after externalization and stenting on the externalized wire (Video 9.74)

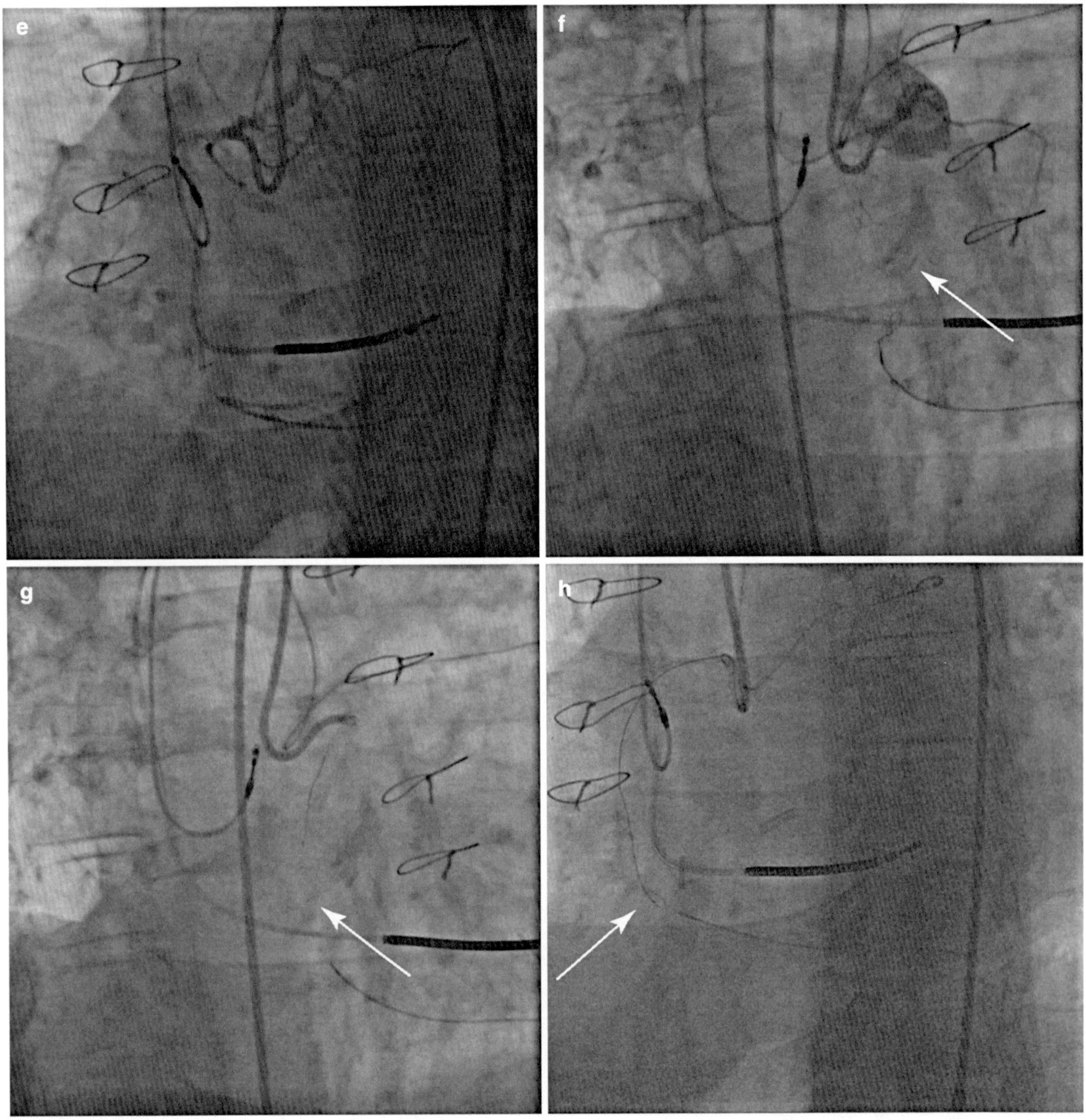


**Fig. 9.29** (continued)

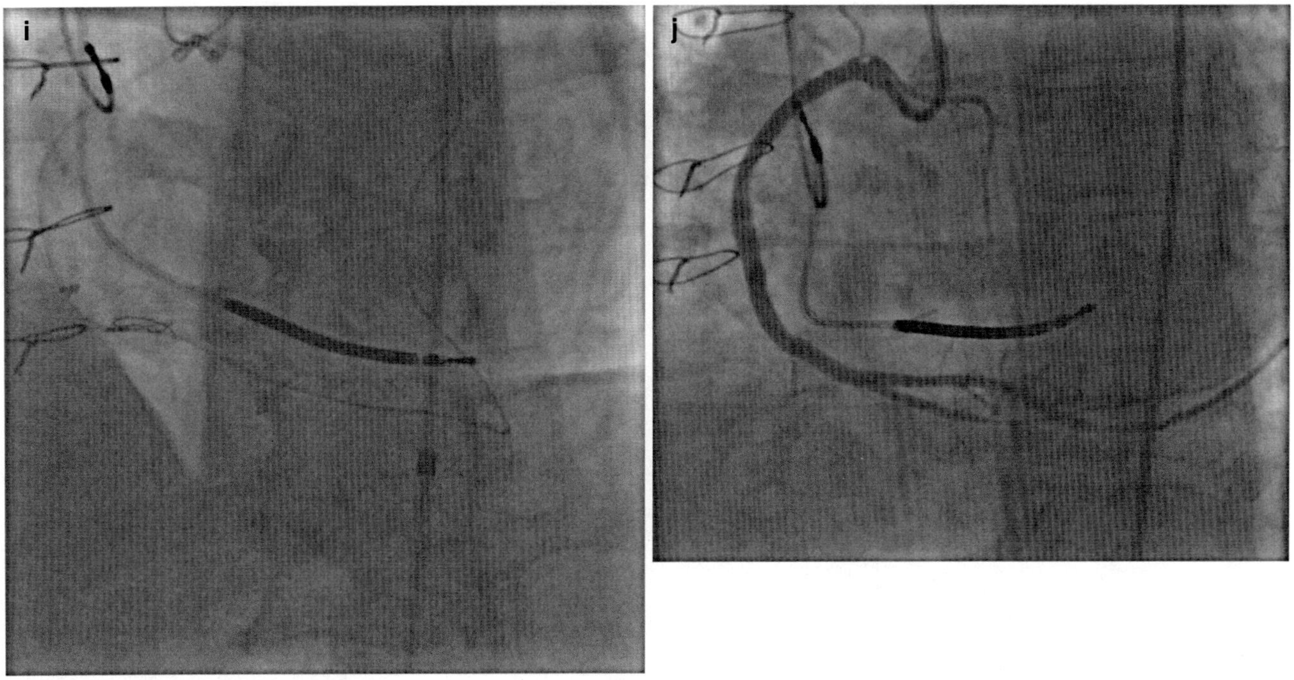


**Fig. 9.29** (continued)

the simplest approach, especially if the disease was located at the ostium, is to follow with the microcatheter into the aorta. Then, snaring will be performed to externalize the wire (Fig. 9.30). Only long wires should be snared from the antegrade guide. Typically, the long wire is advanced through the retrograde microcatheter. An antegrade snare is advanced into the antegrade guide. We prefer En-Snare 18–30 mm snares with three loops that substantially ease wire catching. The operator will simply use the metallic snare part of the kit, and not the white plastic sheath, with the snare directly inserted through the hemostatic valve into the guide. A 6–8 French 90 cm JR 4 guide is recommended. Snaring can be performed in several locations. We recommend snaring in the brachiocephalic artery (Fig. 9.30c, d, Video 9.75), but it can also be done at the right or left coronary cusp or in the ascending or descending aorta. Once the retrograde wire seems to go through one of the three loops, gentle tug on the snare will confirm the wire position. Snaring is not a benign maneuver. Meticulous technique is required and pulling hard on the snare should be avoided. It is better to maintain mild constant tension on the snare to keep the wire locked in the snare, while simultaneously pushing the wire from the retrograde guide. When pulling the wire with the snare, the retrograde guide tends to be sucked into the vessel at the same time. It is therefore important to pull out the retrograde guide into the aorta when an externalization with a snare is performed. Once the wire exists the valve, the bended portion of the wire is cut with a scissor, in order for the antegrade rapid exchange gear to be inserted on this wire.

Alternatively, if the microcatheter cannot cross the CTO segment despite anchoring the retrograde wire into the antegrade guide, or if the short retrograde wire is in the aorta but the microcatheter cannot cross the CTO, a retrograde PCI should be performed with a small balloon, followed by a reattempt to advance the microcatheter through the occlusion. Exchanging the Corsair for a Finecross can help.

## Opening and Stenting the CTO

Once the long retrograde wire is externalized, it will serve as an antegrade rail to deliver balloons and stents to the CTO segment. The Corsair is pulled with continuous clockwise rotations to the distal vessel, making sure that it still covers the whole length of the collateral vessel. Failing to cover the CC with the microcatheter can lead to slicing of the small channel and perforation. An externalized wire provides the ultimate support experience for device and stent delivery. Caution should be applied to keep the retrograde catheter outside or partly outside the donor vessel, to avoid deep seating with back tension on the wire or microcatheter. Such deep seating can lead to donor artery dissection, which can be catastrophic. Use of 6F instead of larger bore catheters on the retrograde side is likely safer and also provides enough support, even from the radial approach. If the stent catches on calcium or other stents in the CTO segment, a gentle traction on the tip of the externalized wire, with or without a torqueing device, will help to deliver the stent to its wanted location.

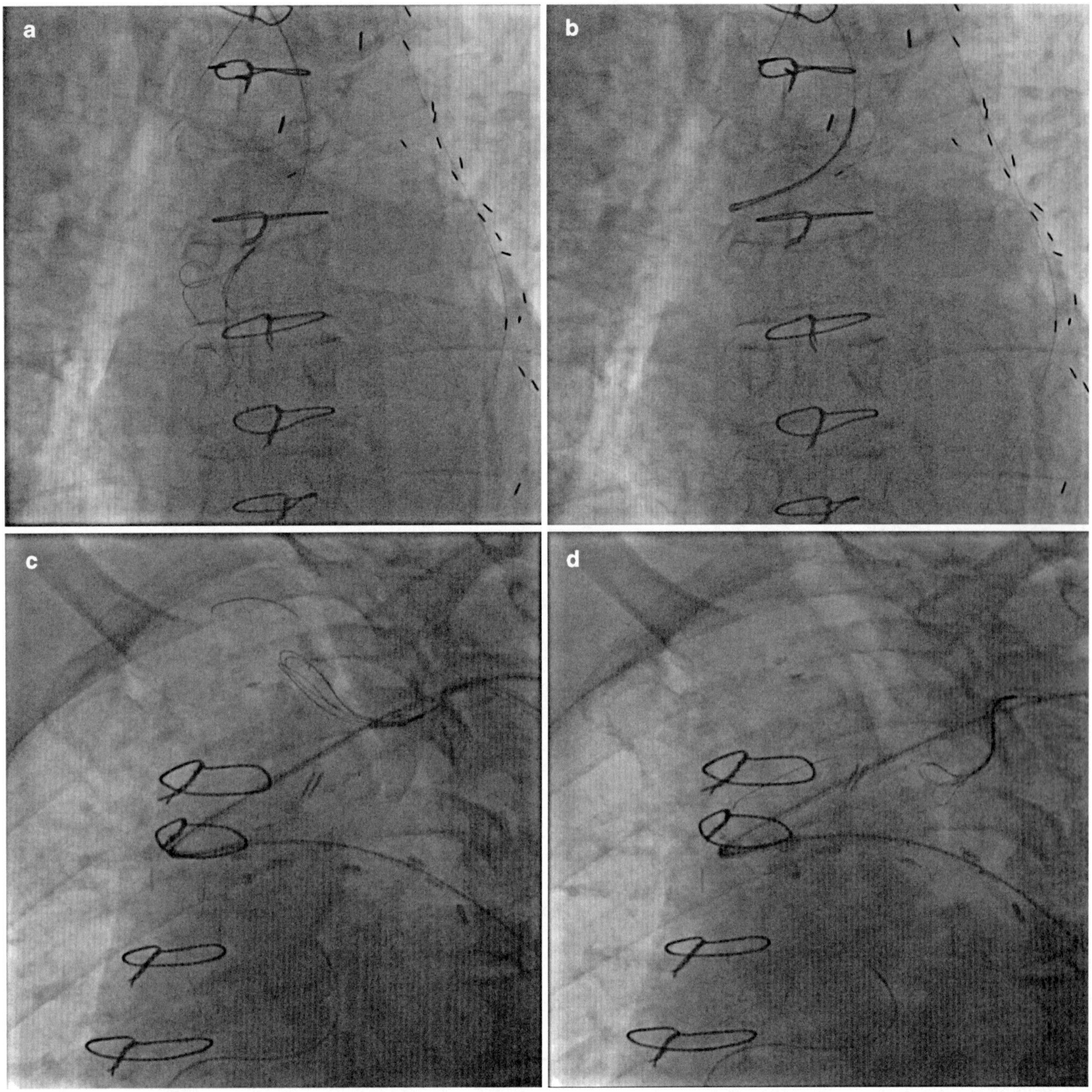


**Fig. 9.30** Snaring a long retrograde wire. (**a**, **b**) A retrograde 300 cm Pilot 200 is snared with an En-Snare 18–30 mm advanced into the antegrade guide. (**c**, **d**) (Video 9.75). One convenient location to perform snaring is in the brachio-cephalic trunk

If too much resistance is encountered during stent delivery, it is recommended that further balloon pre-dilatation be performed, or alternatively to use a MAC catheter. This is important given the excellent support that the externalized wire provides; too aggressive pushing of a stent may lead to shearing of the stent from the stent delivery system. Also, if too much force is applied to the wire, the shortening of the externalized wire can lead to squeezing of the heart by the wire, causing vagal-like reactions. Therefore, as soon as the stent crosses, tension on the full system should be released.

It is wise not to over treat the CTO vessel distal to the occlusion, as negative remodelling and under filling of the distal vessel is the rule rather than the exception in CTOs [13]. Therefore, stenting the occluded segment with properly placed and sized DES, with or without IVUS guidance, and leaving distal narrowing alone if not associated with impaired flow is our preferred approach.

When the last stent is delivered, the retrograde gear needs to be removed. This is one the most critical steps of the retrograde PCI procedure, since many catastrophic complications can occur if it is not done carefully. In order to do so, the Corsair is first advanced to the antegrade guide or MAC catheter, or alternatively into the recently stented segment of the target vessel. Then, the retrograde externalized wire is pulled from its proximal end, the wire enters into the antegrade guide and finally exists out from where it was inserted initially. Then, the Corsair or Finecross is pulled with clockwise rotations. These steps should be performed in a slow manner and under fluoroscopic visualization. Disengaging the retrograde guide and keeping it in the ascending aorta is critical to avoid ostial coronary dissections. There are however two different techniques to apply whether the crossed collateral was a septal channel or an epicardial channel. In the case of a *septal channel* (or a graft), the microcatheter can simply be pulled to the proximal donor vessel segment, and a small injection performed from the retrograde catheter to rule out any donor artery damage or thrombosis. If a suspected problem is visualized, a workhorse wire can be inserted through the microcatheter to the distal donor vessel, the microcatheter pulled into the guide, and a better injection performed. Sometimes, the use of an LAD to PDA septal branch can lead to proximal plaque rupture, or distal vessel dissection at the bifurcation of the LAD and the septal branch carina. In such instance, it should be treated appropriately and promptly with stenting. If thrombosis is noted, thrombo-aspiration should be performed. In order to avoid donor artery thrombosis, it is crucial to keep the ACT higher than 300 as long as a retrograde gear remains in place. In the case of an epicardial *channel*, the microcatheter should first be pulled back proximal to the channel, but close enough to the channel so that a therapy can be applied if a perforation is noticed, leaving the wire distally. If no issues are identified, the Corsair is re-advanced past the collateral, the wire is removed and then the Corsair is finally remove by gentle pull and clockwise rotations. Treatment of a perforated epicardial channel is discussed in Chap. 15 and includes embolization with coils, thrombus or fat.

Sometimes, the retrograde gear has to be taken out prior to finishing the CTO stenting. Few examples that require to shorten the period with retrograde equipment in place include when a donor artery problem is suspected, such as thrombosis or dissection, or simply when it is desirable to restore flow through a single collateral because of ischemia. After balloon dilation has been performed, an antegrade guidewire can be delivered to the distal vessel, and the retrograde gear pulled out. If there is concern about potential difficulties in crossing dissection planes from the antegrade side, before stenting, a TwinPass (Vascular Solutions, US) dual lumen catheter can be used. Its rapid exchange lumen will be inserted on the retrograde wire so that the catheter is delivered distally. Then, through the over-the-wire lumen of the TwinPass, a workhorse wire will be delivered to the distal bed. PCI can then be performed from the antegrade side as usual.

## Special Situations and Considerations

### Post CABG RCA CTOs with Ambiguous Connection of the PLB to the PDA at the Level of the Crux

This anatomy is frequent. Most of the time, the PLB vessels are filled from epicardial channels from the native LCx, whereas the PDA are supplied by septal CCs, usually from the LIMA to the LAD. Therefore, at the beginning of the procedure, a dual retrograde injection with the left main and the LIMA should be performed, to adequately fill the RCA distal bed and assess if the PL and the PDA are still connected with a patent lumen at the level of the distal RCA bifurcation (Fig. 9.31, Video 9.76). Such a dual retrograde injection can serve to plan the retrograde approach. Both catheters can be maintained in their position during the retrograde crossing, either from the native left system or from the LIMA to the LAD. Once the retrograde wire and the microcatheter is at the distal cap, an antegrade catheter can be placed into the RCA from the access site that did not serve for the retrograde approach, and the procedure continued.

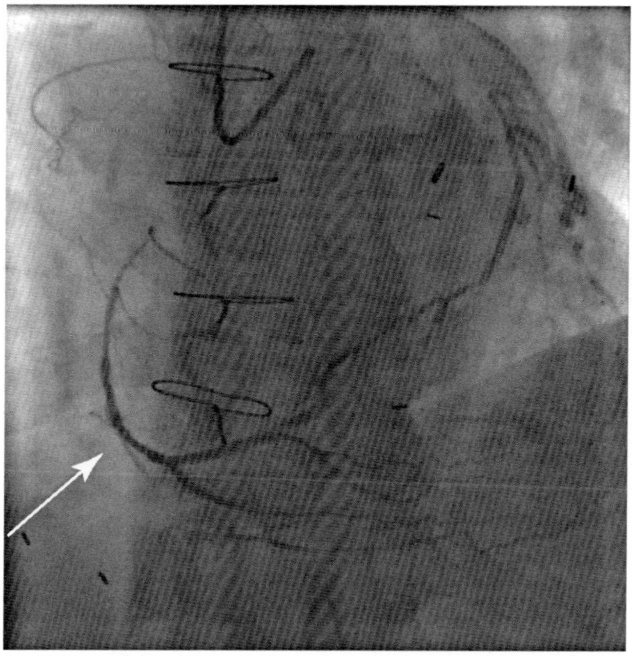

**Fig. 9.31** (Video 9.76). Dual retrograde injection at the start of the CTO PCI to evaluate if all distal RCA branches connect together. Dual retrograde injection with LIMA to OM which gives CC to an early take-off PDA and the left main, that provides collateral from the LCX to the PLV. There is a patent connection between the PDA and the RCA

## Using an Internal Mammary Artery as a Retrograde Route

Post-CABG RCA CTOs are frequent target for the retrograde approach. Sometimes, only septal CCs from the LAD can be identified. RIMAs are sometimes anastomosed to the RCA that provide collaterals to the LAD or the LCx system. Extreme care should be applied when using the IMA as a retrograde route, especially given the dramatic consequence of a donor artery dissection. If the native LAD is patent, it should be used instead (Fig. 9.29, Videos 9.66, 9.67, 9.68, 9.69, 9.70, 9.71, 9.72, 9.73, and 9.74). In the case of tortuous IMAs, it is important to verify if antegrade flow to the distal native vessel is maintained despite the presence of a microcatheter, before attempting to cross a collateral channel. If flow is interrupted, a different approach should be selected. Also, use of MAC catheters to engage the IMA clearly help to protect its ostium and provide excellent support for the advancement of the microcatheter. The Corsair will fit adequately into 6F GuideLiner or Guidezilla, and even into the 5.5F version of the GuideLiner. As mentioned previously, operators should have a high threshold to attempt retrograde PCI via the LIMA.

## LAD or LCX CTOs

As explained earlier, the operator should be careful not to extend a retrograde dissection into the left main when attempting retrograde TTT crossing, or after reverse CART. The use of MACs to 'isolate' the LAD or the LCx can help to protect the left main from dreaded dissection (Fig. 9.25, Videos 9.53, 9.54, 9.55, 9.56, 9.57, 9.58, 9.59, 9.60, 9.61, 9.62, 9.63, 9.64, and 9.65).

## LAD or LCX CTOs in a Dominant Left System or When There Are Only Ipsilateral Collaterals

In such situation, both the donor artery and the CTO are stemming from the left main trunk. Therefore, an 8F 90 cm guide catheter should be used to allow for the Corsair to come back to the guide in the case of a retrograde approach. However, any injection performed from this single guide to visualise the retrograde channels carries the risk of extending an antegrade dissection as well. Alternatively, a ping pong technique, using two guides in the left main, one for the retrograde gear and one for the antegrade devices can be used (Fig. 9.18, Videos 9.22, 9.23, 9.24, 9.25, 9.26, 9.27, and 9.28). Once the channel has been crossed with the wire and microcatheter, the retrograde guide catheter can be pulled out into the aorta, to leave more space for the antegrade guide. A MAC catheter can be used from the retrograde catheter to selectively intubate the donor artery, and minimize antegrade flow to the CTO segment. In the case of a dominant LCx CTO for example, a MAC catheter inserted into the LAD will ensure that contrast injection from the retrograde guide is selective into the LAD therefore reducing the risk of extending an antegrade dissection in the LCx. Such a technique can be used with antegrade DR as well.

## Post CABG CTOs; Using the Easiest Route to the Distal Cap

Typically, there are several collaterals leading to the distal vessel in a post-CABG CTO. However, if there is a simpler solution of going through a graft to open the CTO in a 2-step fashion, it should be considered. For example, as depicted in Fig. 9.32 (Videos 9.77, 9.78, 9.79, 9.80, 9.81, 9.82, and 9.83), a long LCx CTO is targeted for CTO PCI. There is a blunt proximal cap. The collateral connecting to the distal LCx is crossable, but it runs on the atrial wall and therefore the risk of tamponade is high in case of perforation. Moreover, the distal connection of the collateral is close to the distal cap, and taking a very steep angulated curve with the wire and microcatheter would have been difficult. In this case, three catheters were used: one in the RCA to visualize the distal LCx, one in the OM graft, and one in the left main. A triple-injection helped to understand some of the ambiguity. We elected to recanalize the proximal LCx into the left main from the OM SVG (much easier), snared and externalized a long guide wire; then, on this guidewire, after balloon dilation, we delivered a Twin-Pass in the LCx to use a second wire (Pilot 200) to recanalize the distal LCx. In summary, post-CABG anatomies are opportunities for creative solutions to make the procedure safer and more efficient.

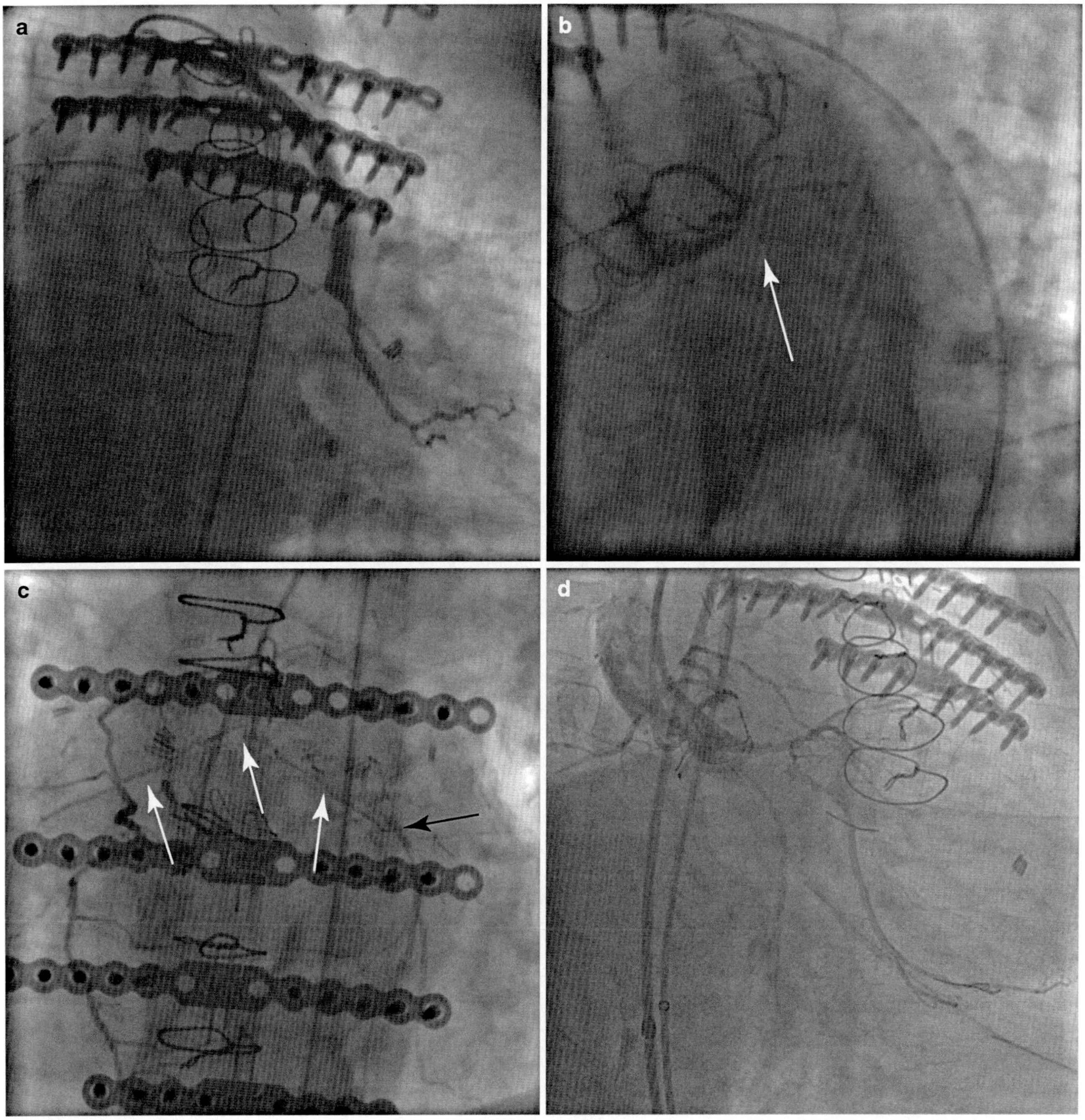

**Fig. 9.32** (Videos 9.77, 9.78, 9.79, 9.80, 9.81, 9.82, and 9.83). Complex 3-guide recanalization of a post-CABG distal LCX CTO. (**a**) Patent SVG to OM. (Patient had a previous cure of sternal dehiscence). (**b**) Ostial and very ambiguous stumpless LCX CTO (*arrow*). (**c**) Distal LCx collateralized by an epicardial collateral from the proximal RCA (*white arrow*) that connects very close to the distal CTO cap (*black arrow*). (**d**) Triple-injection at time of PCI (two femoral accesses, and one radial access) (Video 9.77). (**e**) Retrograde access to the proximal LCX from the OM graft with a Corsair, supported by a 5.5F GuideLiner (Video 9.78). (**f**) Successful retrograde crossing into the aorta with a Confianza Pro 12 (Video 9.79). (**g**) Snaring a 300 cm Pilot 200 (Video 9.80). (**h**) Balloon dilation of proximal LCX. (**i**) Twin-Pass delivered into the graft (*arrow*) and Pilot 200 advanced into the OTW port. (**j**) Twin-Pass pulled back into the proximal segment and RCA injection to guide antegrade wiring of the LCx. (**k**) Pilot 200 directed into distal LCx (Video 9.81). (**l**) After exchanging the Pilot 200 with an OTW balloon and dilating the distal cap, stenting if performed. (**m**) Final result on graft: no damage. (**n**, **o**) Final result after LM and LCX stenting (Videos 9.82 and 9.83)

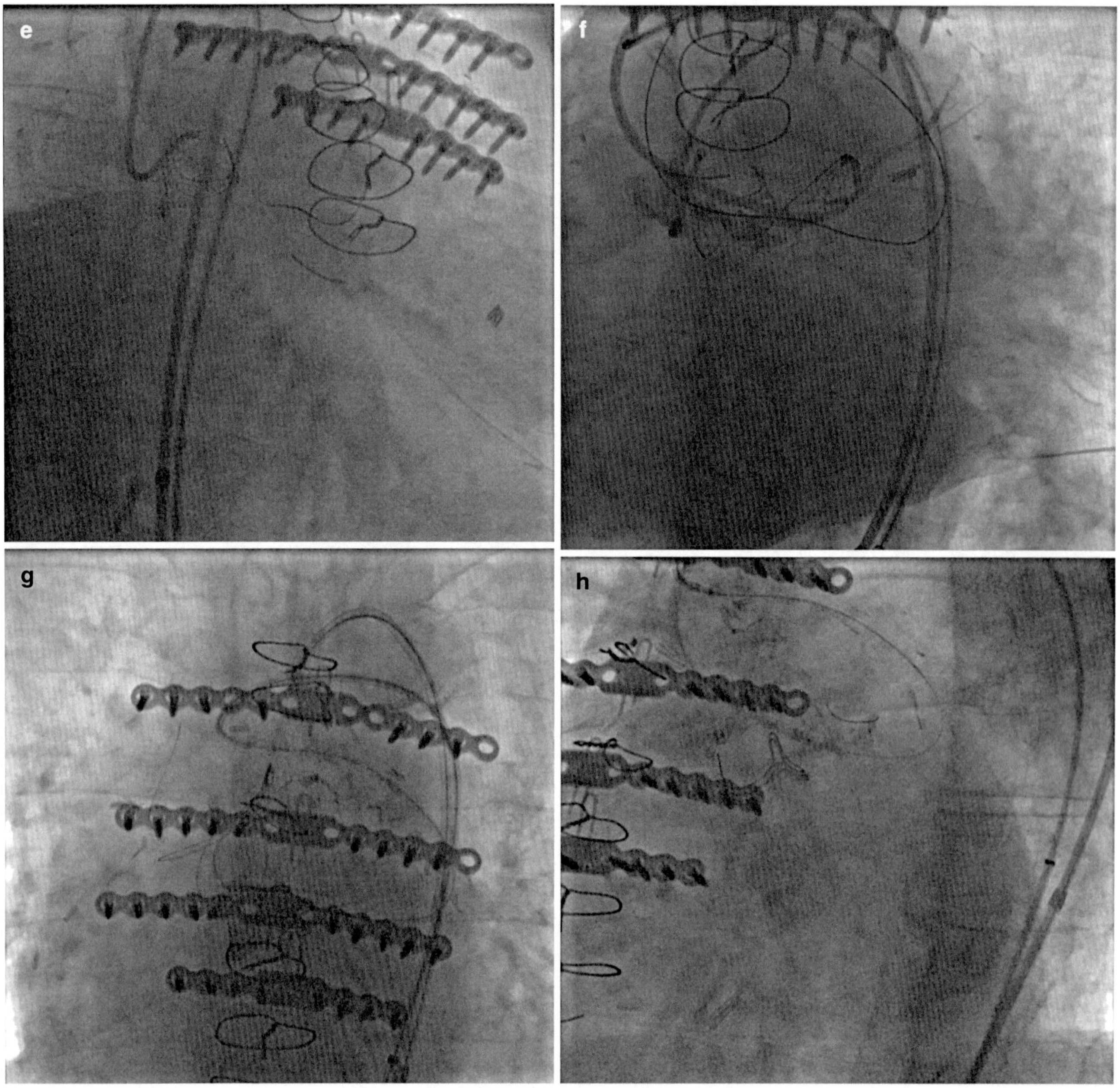


**Fig. 9.32** (continued)

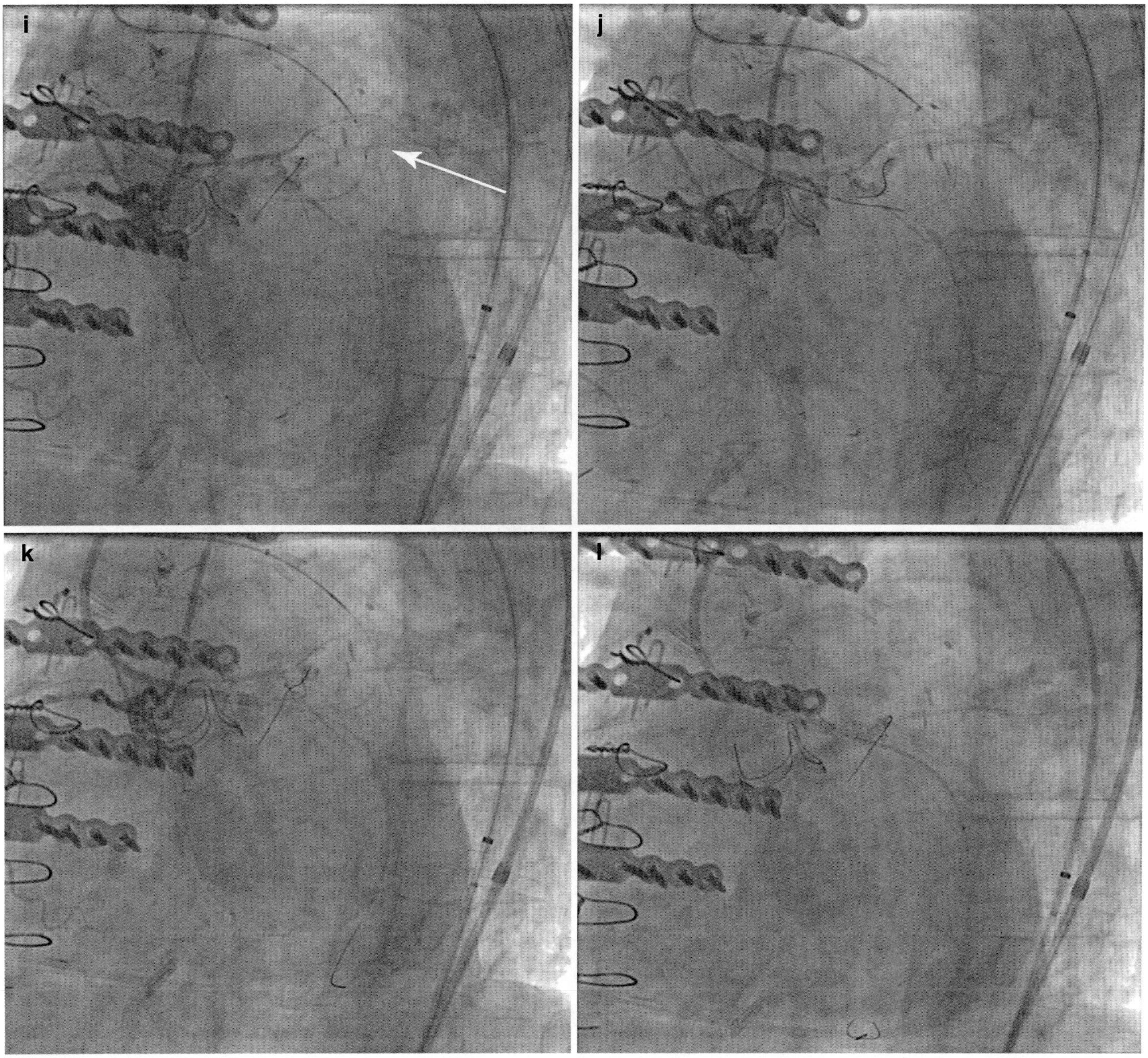


**Fig. 9.32** (continued)

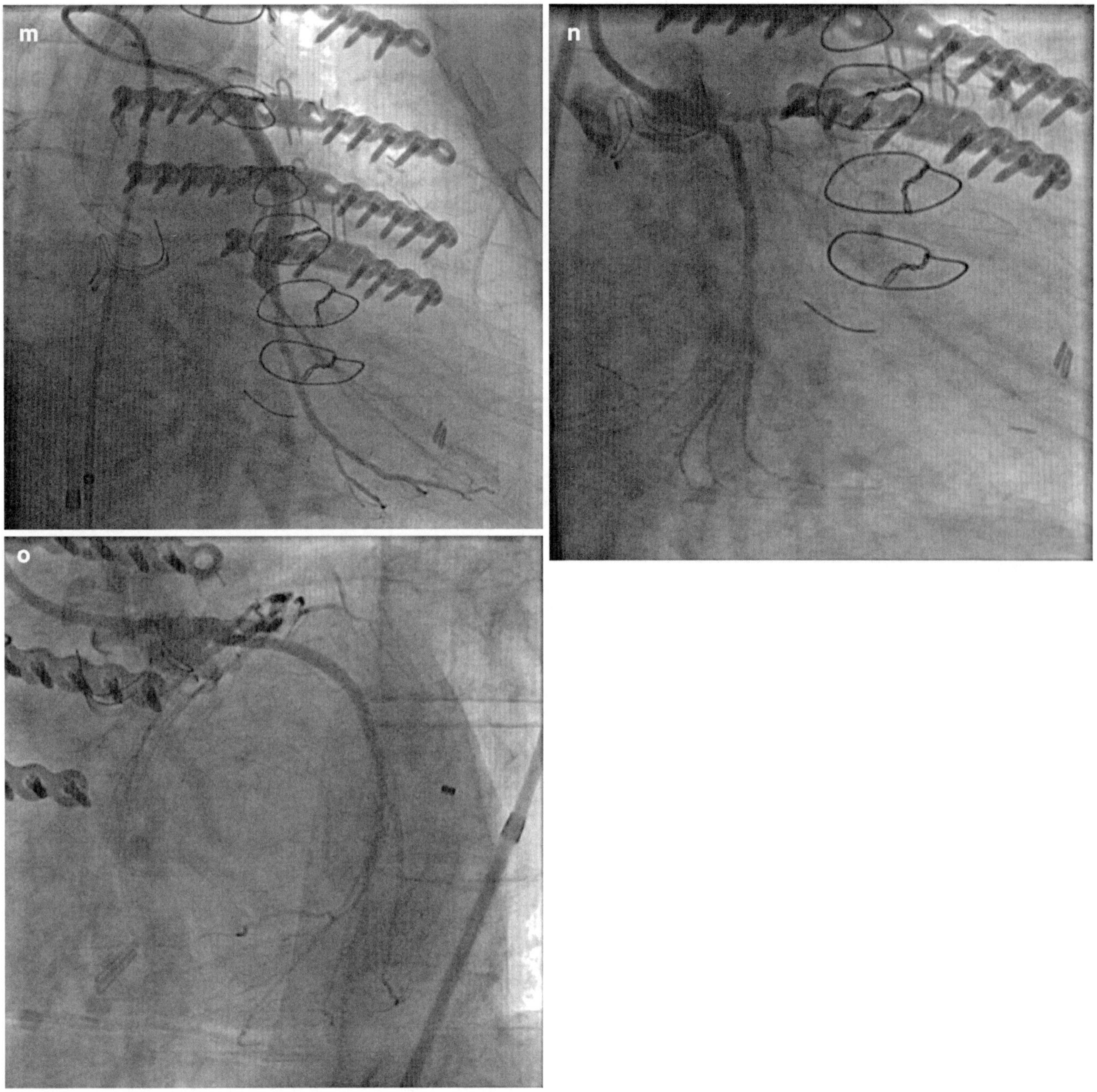


**Fig. 9.32** (continued)

## References


1. Michael TT, Papayannis AC, Banerjee S, Brilakis ES. Subintimal dissection/reentry strategies in coronary chronic total occlusion interventions. Circ Cardiovasc Interv. 2012;5:729–38.
2. Karmpaliotis D, Michael TT, Brilakis ES, Papayannis AC, Tran DL, Kirkland BL, Lembo N, Kalynych A, Carlson H, Banerjee S, Lombardi W, Kandzari DE. Retrograde coronary chronic total occlusion revascularization: procedural and in-hospital outcomes from a multicenter registry in the united states. JACC Cardiovasc Interv. 2012;5:1273–9.
3. Joyal D, Thompson CA, Grantham JA, Buller CE, Rinfret S. The retrograde technique for recanalization of chronic total occlusions: a step-by-step approach. JACC Cardiovasc Interv. 2012;5:1–11.
4. Brilakis ES, Grantham JA, Rinfret S, Wyman RM, Burke MN, Karmpaliotis D, Lembo N, Pershad A, Kandzari DE, Buller CE, DeMartini T, Lombardi WL, Thompson CA. A percutaneous treatment algorithm for crossing coronary chronic total occlusions. JACC Cardiovasc Interv. 2012;5:367–79.
5. Thompson CA, Jayne JE, Robb JF, Friedman BJ, Kaplan AV, Hettleman BD, Niles NW, Lombardi WL. Retrograde techniques and the impact of operator volume on percutaneous intervention for coronary chronic total occlusions an early U.S. experience. JACC Cardiovasc Interv. 2009;2:834–42.
6. Rinfret S, Joyal D, Nguyen CM, Bagur R, Hui W, Leung R, Larose E, Love MP, Mansour S. Retrograde recanalization of chronic total occlusions from the transradial approach; early Canadian experience. Catheter Cardiovasc Interv. 2011;78:366–74.
7. Nombela-Franco L, Urena M, Jerez-Valero M, Nguyen CM, Ribeiro HB, Bataille Y, Rodes-Cabau J, Rinfret S. Validation of the j-chronic total occlusion score for chronic total occlusion percutaneous coronary intervention in an independent contemporary cohort. Circ Cardiovasc Interv. 2013;6:635–43.
8. Rentrop KP, Thornton JC, Feit F, Van Buskirk M. Determinants and protective potential of coronary arterial collaterals as assessed by an angioplasty model. Am J Cardiol. 1988;61:677–84.
9. Werner GS, Surber R, Ferrari M, Fritzenwanger M, Figulla HR. The functional reserve of collaterals supplying long-term chronic total coronary occlusions in patients without prior myocardial infarction. Eur Heart J. 2006;27:2406–12.
10. Rathore S, Katoh O, Matsuo H, Terashima M, Tanaka N, Kinoshita Y, Kimura M, Tsuchikane E, Nasu K, Ehara M, Asakura K, Asakura Y, Suzuki T. Retrograde percutaneous recanalization of chronic total occlusion of the coronary arteries: Procedural outcomes and predictors of success in contemporary practice. Circ Cardiovasc Interv. 2009;2:124–32.
11. Brilakis ES, Rao SV, Banerjee S, Goldman S, Shunk KA, Holmes Jr DR, Honeycutt E, Roe MT. Percutaneous coronary intervention in native arteries versus bypass grafts in prior coronary artery bypass grafting patients: a report from the national cardiovascular data registry. JACC Cardiovasc Interv. 2011;4:844–50.
12. Garg N, Hakeem A, Gobal F, Uretsky BF. Outcomes of percutaneous coronary intervention of chronic total saphenous vein graft occlusions in the contemporary era. Catheter Cardiovasc Interv. 2014;83:1025–32.
13. Galassi AR, Tomasello SD, Crea F, Costanzo L, Campisano MB, Marza F, Tamburino C. Transient impairment of vasomotion function after successful chronic total occlusion recanalization. J Am Coll Cardiol. 2012;59:711–8.
14. Spratt JC. A guide to mastering retrograde CTO PCI. Online: Optima Education Ltd.; 2015. www.ctoibooks.com.

# How to Recanalize In-Stent Chronic Total Occlusions

10

Benjamin Faurie and Stéphane Rinfret

**Abstract**

In-stent chronic total occlusions (IS CTOs) remain one of the most difficult and challenging subset of lesions in the field of CTO interventions. In a modern practice, this is not a rare situation and the prevalence has been reported between 5 and 25 % of all CTOs. Given that patients with CTOs caused by in-stent restenosis (ISR) are usually excluded from clinical trials, little published data exists to guide coronary intervention in this setting.

The clinical impact of IS CTO is fairly significant and most patients will present with recurrent stable angina at the time of repeat angiography (60 %), while a minority of these patients present with unstable syndrome.

These procedures have traditionally been associated with low success rate mainly due to wire crossing difficulties. The pathophysiology of these specific occlusions is perceived by CTO operators to play a role in the behavior of wires and subsequent success. In this chapter, we will discuss the specificities that makes in-stent occlusions challenging to re-open. Then, we will discuss how angiographic appearance can guide our strategies and how the hybrid algorithm apply to this specific entity. Finally, we will discuss different bailout techniques to avoid failing the intervention.

**Keywords**

In-stent chronic total occlusion (IS CTO) • In-stent restenosis (ISR) • Hybrid algorithm • Prevalence of CTO due to ISR • In-stent occlusive restenosis

## Introduction

In-stent chronic total occlusions (IS CTOs) remain one of the most difficult and challenging subset of lesions in the field of CTO interventions. In a modern practice, this is not a rare situation and the prevalence has been reported between 5 and 25 % of all CTOs [1–4]. Given that patients with chronic total occlusions (CTOs) caused by in-stent restenosis (ISR) are usually excluded from clinical trials, little published data exists to guide coronary intervention in this setting.

The clinical impact of IS CTO is fairly significant and most patients will present with recurrent stable angina at the time of repeat angiography (60 %), while a minority of these patients present with unstable syndrome [5].

These procedures have traditionally been associated with low success rate [2, 3] mainly due to wire crossing difficulties. The pathophysiology of these specific occlusions is perceived by CTO operators to play a role in the behavior of wires and subsequent success. In this chapter, we will discuss the specificities that make in-stent occlusions

B. Faurie, MD (✉)
Institut Cardiovasculaire, Groupe Hospitalier Mutualiste de Grenoble, Grenoble, France
e-mail: b.faurie@ghm-grenoble.fr

S. Rinfret, MD, SM
Multidisciplinary Department of Cardiology, Quebec Heart and Lung Institute, Quebec City, QC, Canada

Laval University, Quebec City, QC, Canada


S. Rinfret (ed.), *Percutaneous Intervention for Coronary Chronic Total Occlusion: The Hybrid Approach*, DOI 10.1007/978-3-319-21563-1_10

challenging to recanalize. We will further discuss how angiographic appearance can guide our strategies and how the hybrid algorithm applies to this specific entity. Finally, we will discuss different bailout techniques to optimize the intervention whilst minimizing failure rates.

## Prevalence

The prevalence of CTO due to ISR was 10.9 % in the Christopoulos et al. registry [1]. In a study of 78 patients, Abbas et al. reported a 25 % prevalence of CTOs due to ISR [2], whereas Wilson et al. reported a 14.9 % prevalence of ISR in 349 CTO PCIs [4]. Following literature and personal database review, Werner et al. estimated that 5–10 % of all CTOs were due to ISR [3]. However, the true incidence of in-stent occlusion following PCI remains largely unknown. While Shah et al. reported a 1.6 % rate of bare metal stent total occlusion in 955 native coronary lesions at 6-month angiographic follow-up [5], the occlusion rates following DES are much lower.

## What Is Unique to In-Stent Occlusions?

First of all, in-stent CTO can be a consequence of in-stent restenosis (ISR) or stent thrombosis (ST). The proportion of these two entities remains unknown although stent thrombosis is probably less frequent due to a clinical presentation that tends to be more often acute than chronic. In addition to a large tissue burden, there will be, after successful crossing of an IS CTO, at least two layers of stent struts, resulting in higher stent recoil and the need for higher inflation and post dilatation pressures with adequately sized balloons. To counteract the expected higher lesion recurrence, one needs to consider the adverse synergistic consequences of a CTO ISR lesion. Therefore, optimal stent apposition and expansion is required, which can be best achieved by intravascular ultrasound guidance. This may, then, also minimize the potentially higher late stent thrombosis risk resulting from multi-stent layers [3].

## Pathophysiology

### In-Stent Occlusive Restenosis

As for other types of in-stent restenosis, those resulting in complete vessel occlusion may result from stent recoil, underdeployment or fracture that lead to smooth muscle cells ingrowth (neointima proliferation). This phenomenon was frequent with BMS but dramatically decreased with drug eluting stents (DES). Christopoulos et al. [1] underlined the role of diabetes mellitus for in-stent restenotic CTO genesis. Diabetes was present in 56.1 % and 39.6 % ($p = 0.02$) respectively for in-stent CTOs and de novo CTOs. The other differences between the two groups were the occlusion length which was greater in the in-stent CTO group: (38 mm (29–55) vs. 30 mm (20–51), $P = 0.04$) and the calcifications were less important than the de novo CTO group: 5.3 % vs. 16.2 %, $P < 0.001$. Indeed, CTOs that result from in-stent restenosis are most commonly composed of a hypocellular matrix made up primarily of hard and resistant collagenous material, and therefore differ from other CTOs because of a relative absence of in-plaque microchannels, thus explaining the lower success rates evident with soft, tapered wires [6]. However, in some cases, the restenosis process is spotty and leave some areas of patent "islands" within the stent, likely highlighting a different proliferative process. In some cases, it is presumed that the restenosis process was concentric, therefore leaving a central area of looser tissue in the centre of the occluded stents. Penetrative wires with high tip loads are sometimes required in this setting but often result in wire passage through the stent struts, precluding subsequent device delivery, even if the distal true lumen has finally been successfully wired.

### In-Stent CTO as a Result of Previous Thrombosis

As said, there are two pathophysiological mechanisms proposed stimulating for the occurrence of CTOs following stent implantation; neo-intimal proliferation; acute thrombosis leading to an organized CTO, or a mixture of both. Some stents are occluded likely as a result of a previous stent thrombosis, a condition that was more likely to occur with the earlier DES generations, and when mechanical factors such as poor expansion, distal dissection and poor outflow were overlooked when the stent was first placed. The proportion of in-stent occlusion that result from an earlier thrombosis is however unknown.

## Angiographic Appearance of In-Stent CTOs

Usual angiographic predictors of successful percutaneous coronary intervention (PCI) for de novo CTOs play a limited role in patients who have IS CTO, and the mechanisms of failure are different.

IS CTOs can have different angiographic appearance depending on the restenosis or thrombotic phenomenon and time of occlusion. When the CTO results from a restenotic process, the proximal cap tends to be more frequently tapered than if a previous thrombosis caused the occlusion (Fig. 10.1). These will frequently present with in-stent patent lumen islands that interrupt the occlusion length. But overall, in-stent occlusions are more frequently blunt at the proximal cap compared with de novo CTOs [2]. Sometimes, a microchannel is visible in portion of the stent occlusion especially

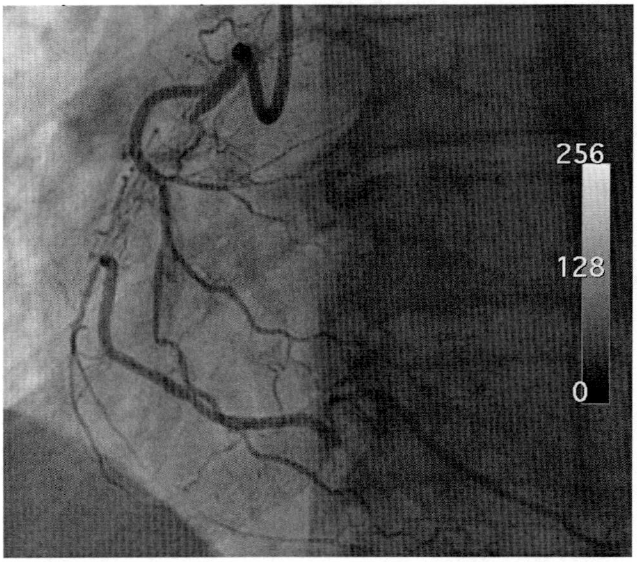


**Fig. 10.1** IS CTO due to restenosis with a tapered proximal cap

when islands of patent coronary artery are present. This aspect suggest restenosis as the most likely mechanism and is easier to cross with CrossBoss (CB) catheter (Figs. 10.1 and 10.2).

On the other hand, in-stent chronic thrombosis are more likely associated with poor initial angiographic results with residual dissections or heavy disease at the proximal or distal edge of the stent. They often are associated with completely occluded stents, showing no patent islands, with the proximal cap starting proximal to the entrance of the stent (Fig. 10.3). The original post PCI result can actually give an idea as to why the stent occluded in the first place. If a per fect result was documented, and the patient presents with progressive symptoms, a restenotic process was the most likely the culprit phenomenon. However, if stents were placed as a result of dissections, if poor outflow was present at the end of the procedure, thrombosis might have occurred, especially when considering an angiographic appearance such as depicted in Fig. 10.3.

## Treatment Algorithm Applied to This Entity

Low success rates with conventional antegrade wire-based approach even in very skillful and experienced hands have been reported. There is limited published data on the success of IS CTO PCI. Werner et al. reported a 70 % primary success in IS CTOs compared to 85 % in de novo lesions [3]. Abbas et al. reported 63 % procedural success in patients with CTOs due to IS restenosis [2]. These lower success rates occur despite the presence of previously placed stents serving as a "road map" of the course of the occluded artery as well as providing some protection against vessel perforation. Failure usually results from the inability to cross the lesion with a guidewire, with a hard proximal cap making lesion engagement and penetration difficult. It can also result in sub-stent wire tracking, particularly with stiff, penetrative wires, which prevents subsequent passage of balloons and stents even if distal true lumen is reached. As reported in several studies, IS CTOs are longer [1, 2], tissue is often harder, not due to calcifications but to fibrous and compact neo-intimal proliferation. An ostial location has also been found to predict procedural failure [2]. Moreover, presence of prior stents interfere with microcatheters, balloons and new stents. Obviously, stent-fractures, undersized stents, deformed and malapposed stents might increase the difficulty to cross with wires, balloons and stents.

The hybrid strategy has been shown to be effective for increasing success rates with IS CTOs, with technical and procedural success now similar in patients with CTOs due to ISR and de novo CTOs, (technical success 89.4 % vs. 92.5 %, $P=0.43$; procedural success 86.0 % vs. 90.3 %, $P=0.31$). In their multicenter study, Christopoulos et al. showed that the most common crossing approach was antegrade wire escalation (41.1 %), followed by the retrograde approach (31.4 %), and antegrade dissection and re-entry (27.4 %). The CrossBoss catheter was used in 54.4 % of cases (26.7 % of de novo CTO cases) [1].

Antegrade wire escalation has been historically used as a first approach, and is still the preferred technique for crossing in-stent CTOs for most operators, although the CrossBoss is now a very helpful tool to add for improved success (Fig. 10.2). Inability to cross the occlusion with a guidewire is the main mode of technical failure, whereas inability to advance or fully inflate a balloon catheter accounts for a minority of cases. As for de novo CTOs, there is no general rule of treatment, as lesion characteristics are highly variable and hardly predictable before a proper dual injection is performed. Soft tip tapered polymer-jacketed wires (such as the Fielder XT) can be first tried a few minutes to search for any central in-stent micro channel, but our experience with this wire in IS CTOs has been deceiving. These soft wires are less steerable and may also slip outside the stent structure, in the sub-intimal plane. Therefore, escalation goes quickly to stiffer polymer jacketed such the Pilot 200 with a special attention not to track the wire under the stent struts. But the most useful guidewire family in that situation are the high torque and hard tip wires like the Miracle 12 which provide a very acute control and torque of the tip to allow the wire to stay within the stent. Because the wire is non-tapered, it is less likely to exit through a stent strut. Several orthogonal views should be taken in order to visualize the wire track within the stent (Fig. 10.2). Hard and tapered wires can be interesting to puncture the proximal cap or go for a short distance trough very hard tissue. In our experience, the Confianza Pro 12 has very good torque control and should be

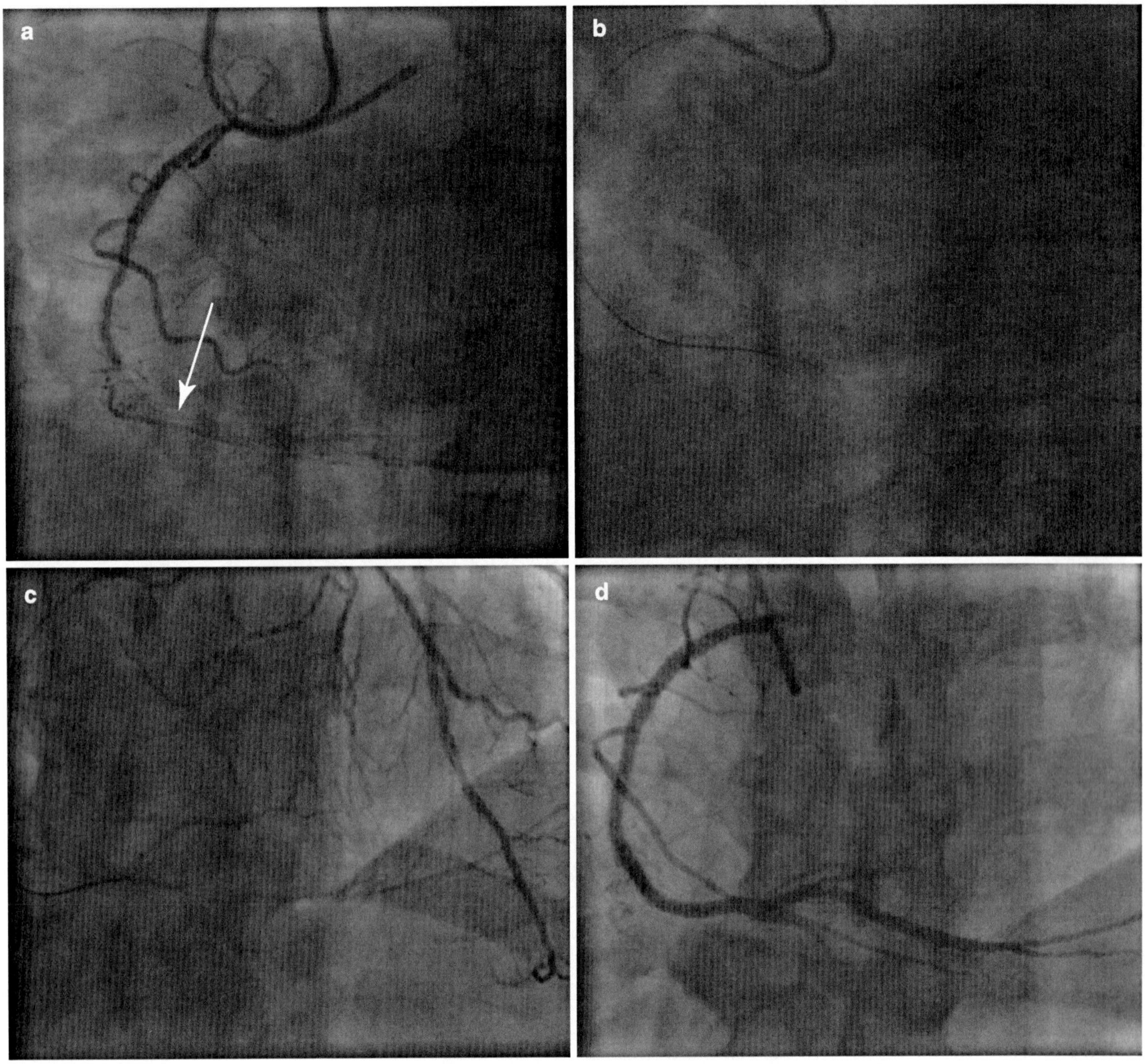

**Fig. 10.2** In-stent restenotic CTO. (**a**) Long in-stent occlusion in the distal RCA ostium, likely due to an in-stent restenosis as highlighted by the presence of an island of patency with contrast at the beginning of the occlusion. (**b**) CrossBoss navigates into the stents and (**c**) is advanced true-to-true into the PDA. (**d**) Final result after deployment of DES

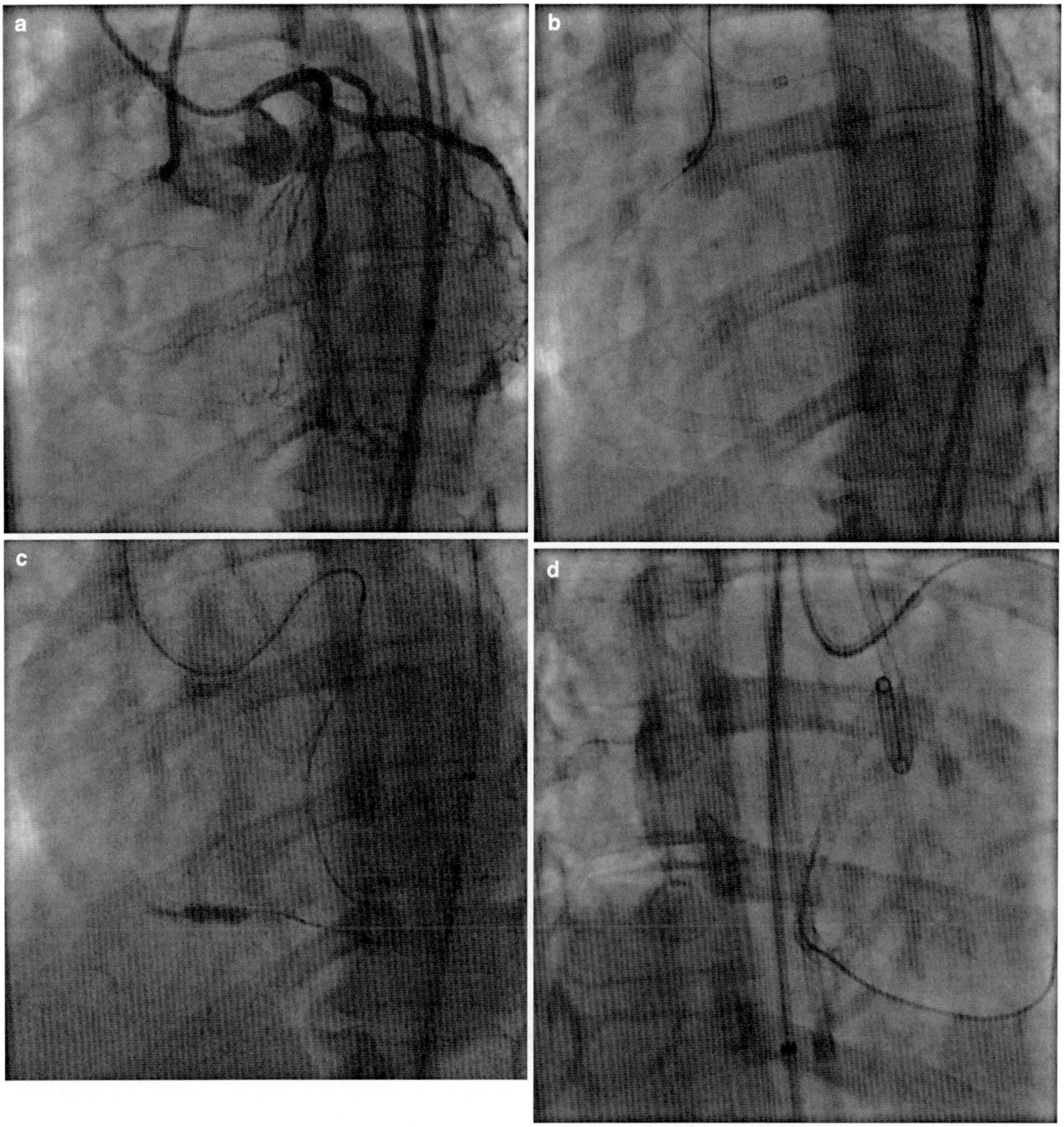


**Fig. 10.3** In-stent CTO from a previous stent thrombosis. (**a**) Very long in-stent occlusion from the RCA ostium to the crux, due to a documented stent thrombosis few years ago. (**b**) This is impossible to progress with the CrossBoss into the occluded stents. (**c**) Antegrade guide changed for an AL0.75. No success with CrossBoss. Retrograde approach and distal contrast injections to modify the plaque. (**d**, **e**) Careful navigation with an alternative use of Pilot 200 and Confianza Pro 12 guidewires to stay within the stents. (**f**) Final result after deployment of DES

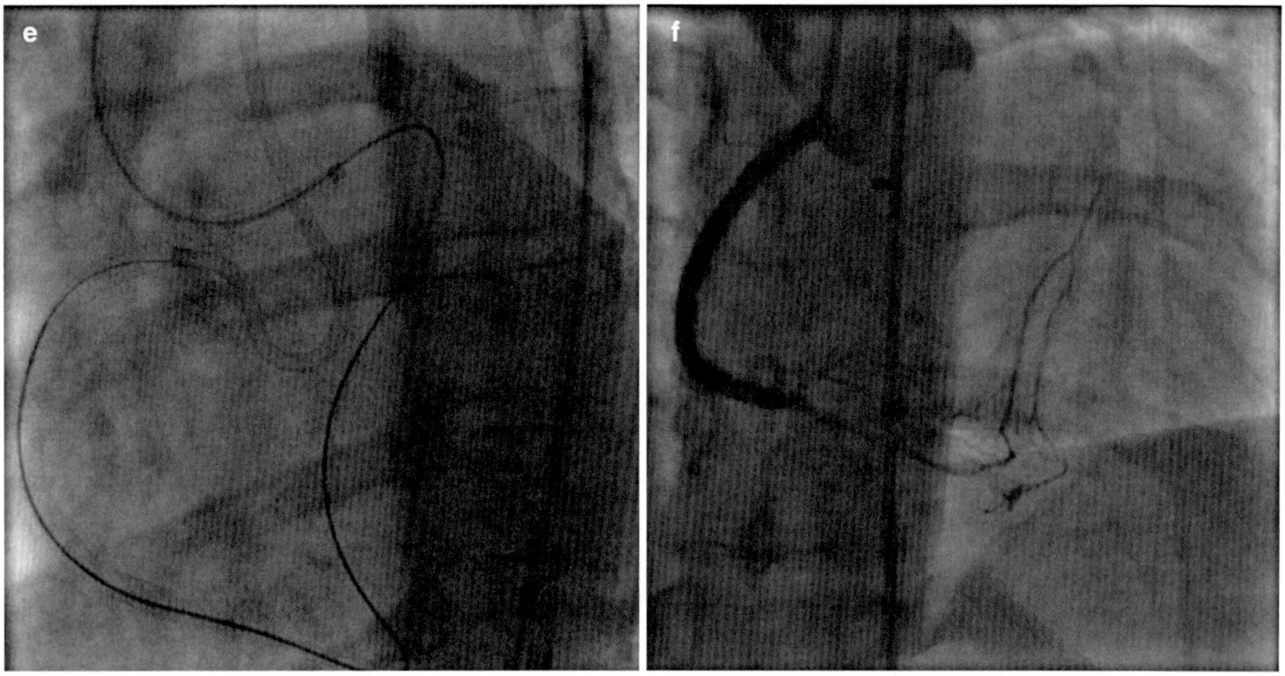


**Fig. 10.3** (continued)

preferred to polymer-jacketed stiff tapered tip like Progress 200 T which can easily slip under the struts. Nevertheless, the latter wire, due to its slippery characteristics, is interesting during cases of very fibrotic and hard restenotic tissue and could facilitate wire progression. Finally, the Gaia family wires have emerged as very efficient wires for in-stent occlusions. Given that the ambiguity of the vessel course is limited with IS CTO, the Gaia wires, especially the less tapered Gaia 3rd version, can be very effective; the wire is pushed up to deflection of its tip. Then, the wire is pulled and redirected away from the resistance. Several orthogonal views should be taken to confirm that the wire stays within the border of the occluded stents.

Although very useful in CTO PCI, knuckled wires should be avoided as a first strategy because of the absence of cleavage space within an IS CTO. Such knuckled wires can track under the stent struts or in the subintimal sub-stent space, resulting in crossing outside the stent structure. Although it has been described [7] with successful stenting in the sub-adventitial layer under the previous occluded stent, extreme caution should be applied for the following reasons: (1) although sub-intimal stenting appears to be safe in the majority of cases, stenting outside a previously deployed stent can lead to substantial overstretching of the adventitia, as a result of non-compressible in-stent tissue leading to potential perforation. (2) Distal re-entry can be laborious and (3) outcomes are unknown with this technique. The key point of a wire-based strategy is to enter the proximal cap in the "true lumen" and avoid to track underneath the stent struts. If the cap is blunt and hard, inflating an OTW balloon (adapted to the size of the proximal vessel) a few millimeter upstream to the in-stent CTO segment can help, as with the performance of an anchoring balloon technique. The back-up support for wire puncture is therefore stronger. Moreover, this technique allows a very good coaxial alignment of the wire in order to puncture the center of the proximal cap instead of the sub-stent space. The Venture catheter is a steerable and orientable micro-catheter that sometimes can be used successfully used with or without Stingray guidewire in that kind of situation [8]. Again, orthogonal angiographic views should be taken most of the time without contrast injection in order to confirm that the wire tracks within the stent borders. If the wire crosses into the distal true lumen but no microcatheter or balloon can cross the occlusion, several solutions could be sought. The first is the CrossBoss catheter that could cross as described later, even over the wire [9]. But in cases of very fibrous and hard tissues we recommend the use of the Tornus or the Corsair microcatheters that can be screwed into the lesion using counter-clockwise motion [10]. After crossing with the microcatheter, the crossing wire can be exchanged for a high support soft tip wire to complete the procedure. However, if the wire crossed outside the stent structure and re-entered more distally, it is wise not to pursue with Tornus or Corsair, as both can get entrapped within the stents struts. In such cases, sequential balloon dilation starting with a very small balloon is the preferred approach, leading to strut enlargement and ability to deliver subsequent new stents in the segment.

The utility of the CrossBoss catheter for refractory CTOs has been established in the FAST-CTO trial [11]; however, ISR cases were excluded from this trial. First description was done in a multicentre European study reporting CrossBoss and Stingray devices for refractory CTOs [12]. The only case of ISR CTO within this study was successfully completed with CrossBoss catheter alone.

Other small series now support the use of CrossBoss catheter for IS CTOs. Indeed, the success rate of crossing with the CrossBoss alone is between 83 % as reported by Papayannis et al. [9] (5 of 6 patients) and 90 % (28 of 31) as reported by Wilson et al. [4]. In that latter study, use of the CrossBoss catheter was the primary strategy in 60 % of IS CTOs cases (31 of 52). Christopoulos et al. reported a use of the CrossBoss for IS CTOs of 54.4 % with a final technical success of 89.4 % [1]. Direct lumen-to-lumen crossing of the catheter was achieved in 88 % of cases in the Wilson et al. series [4], avoiding thus the need for re-entry as long as the distal cap of the CTO is either within or at the very end of the stent struts. Of course, larger series are needed to collect more data.

Efficacy of CrossBoss catheter is based on the fact that stent struts tend to prevent device exit into the subintimal space and ease the passage of the catheter's blunt tip to the distal true lumen. Use of the CrossBoss can lead to a reduction in procedural time. Indeed, the UK ISR-CTO registry reported a median crossing time of the occluded stents of 8 min [4]. Wilson et al. didn't find any differences in baseline characteristics between successful or failed CrossBoss cases. Nevertheless, a few mechanism of failure with the CrossBoss have been reported [4, 9] such as underdeployed stent struts especially with small size stents, tortuosity (defined as a bend more than 45°) within the stented segment which can lead to the CrossBoss tip catching on the stent struts. Although tortuosity proximal to the occlusion does not appear predictive of failure, an occlusion that sits proximal to the stent may be difficult to engage with the device, and may therefore require stiff wires to puncture within the stented segment. Ostial location is a frequent cause of failure probably because of the need for tremendous backup to engage the proximal cap with the CrossBoss catheter. The retrograde approach should be considered if possible in this situation. CTO length and vessel diameter don't seem to predict CrossBoss failure [4]. In the early experience of CB for ISR CTOs [12] and some other series [9], presence of a side branch at proximal cap has been reported as a predictor of failure, but was not found in the UK experience series [4] nor in five high-volume CTO PCI US centers [1]. Although this is poorly documented, it is our belief that stents that occluded as a result of a prior thrombosis offer more resistance to wire and CrossBoss compared to stents that present islands of patency (Fig. 10.3).

In the case of antegrade wire-based or CrossBoss-based failure, a retrograde approach should be considered especially in case of ostial IS CTO [7, 13] (Fig. 10.3). As for de novo CTOs, distal cap is less exposed to systemic blood pressure and tends to be softer allowing wires to penetrate and progress. Of course, antegrade and retrograde techniques should be combined to complete the case. The general principles of the retrograde approach apply here as well, with the exception of the crossing strategy. Although long de novo CTOs will be crossed with retrograde dissection re-entry using knuckled wires, such a technique should be also avoided from the retrograde side, as they will also track underneath the stent. Efforts to stay within the stented segment should be made. The use of the retrograde, in addition to the antegrade approach, can facilitate progression of wires from either sides, serving as targets to one another. The same kind of wires described above for the antegrade escalation strategy should be use to keep maximum steerability and control while traveling retrograde within the stent.

## Problem-Solving Strategies

### Sub-stent Wiring

Especially when hitting stent fractures or malapposed struts, the wire could be at some part tracking under the struts or leaning against struts and thus blocking passage of devices. In these particular situations, Rotablator can be used [14]. After exchanging the 0.014′ wire for a RotaWire, cautious advancement of a small burr (1.25 mm most of the time) can be done. Very slow motion and also slow rotational speed should be used in order to avoid burr stalling and trap beyond the struts or the fibrous lesion. This technique will lead to an ablation of the malapposed struts and will allow advancement of balloons and stents.

In the same way, excimer coronary laser atherectomy can be used. The advantage is that the 0.014′ wire used to cross the in-stent CTO is ready to support the laser device and doesn't need to be exchanged [15]. Moreover, the laser has the ability to ablate tissue that extend beyond the stent borders, increasing the chances of better subsequent apposition. However, laser will not ablate metal struts.

### Sub-stent Subintimal Strategy

If the CrossBoss fails to connect to the true lumen, if antegrade or retrograde wiring fail, subintimal tracking can be used in selected cases. As described by Lee et al. [16], this maneuver is challenging but safe and leads to good midterm outcome, especially if performed in patients who underwent prior cardiac surgery. Re-entry should be performed at distance to the occluded stent using tapered stiff guidewires, the Stingray balloon or from the retrograde side with the reverse-CART technique. In such situation, a new subintimal lumen is created and the occluded stent and its proliferative tissue crushed by balloons and new stents, as mentioned earlier. Sub-stent passage of devices is usually possible as for other subintimal strategy techniques. Nevertheless, crushing occluded stents is difficult and needs cautious sequential dilatation followed with placement of a new stent with high radial strength. Extreme care should be applied not to overstretch the vessel with the new stents; it is safer to accept some under sizing of the newly implanted stents to avoid vessel perforation due to adventitial over dilation.

**Conclusions**

IS CTOs are identified entities that carry their own predictors of success and mechanisms of failure that differ from de novo CTOs. PCI of IS CTO has traditionally been associated with lower success mainly due to wire crossing difficulties. The hybrid strategy, especially including the CrossBoss catheter, seems to be associated with similarly high procedural success and low major complication rates as for patients with de novo CTOs.

## References


1. Christopoulos G, Karmpaliotis D, Alaswad K, et al. The efficacy of "hybrid" percutaneous coronary intervention in chronic total occlusions caused by in-stent restenosis: insights from a US multicenter registry. Catheter Cardiovasc Interv. 2014;84:646–51.
2. Abbas AE, Brewington SD, Dixon SR, Boura J, Grines CL, O'Neill WW. Success, safety, and mechanisms of failure of percutaneous coronary intervention for occlusive non-drug-eluting in-stent restenosis versus native artery total occlusion. Am J Cardiol. 2005;95:1462–6.
3. Werner GS, Moehlis H, Tischer K. Management of total restenotic occlusions. EuroIntervention. 2009;5 Suppl D:D79–83.
4. Wilson WM, Walsh S, Hanratty C, et al. A novel approach to the management of occlusive in-stent restenosis (ISR). EuroIntervention. 2014;9:1285–93.
5. Shah PB, Cutlip DE, Popma JJ, Kuntz RE, Ho KK. Incidence and predictors of late total occlusion following coronary stenting. Catheter Cardiovasc Interv. 2003;60:344–51.
6. Srivatsa SS, Edwards WD, Boos CM, et al. Histologic correlates of angiographic chronic total coronary artery occlusions: influence of occlusion duration on neovascular channel patterns and intimal plaque composition. J Am Coll Cardiol. 1997;29:955–63.
7. Ohya H, Kyo E, Katoh O. Successful bypass restenting across the struts of an occluded subintimal stent in chronic total occlusion using a retrograde approach. Catheter Cardiovasc Interv. 2013;82:E678–83.
8. Brilakis ES, Lombardi WB, Banerjee S. Use of the Stingray guidewire and the Venture catheter for crossing flush coronary chronic total occlusions due to in-stent restenosis. Catheter Cardiovasc Interv. 2010;76:391–4.
9. Papayannis A, Banerjee S, Brilakis ES. Use of the Crossboss catheter in coronary chronic total occlusion due to in-stent restenosis. Catheter Cardiovasc Interv. 2012;80:E30–6.
10. Pagnotta P, Briguori C, Ferrante G, et al. Tornus catheter and rotational atherectomy in resistant chronic total occlusions. Int J Cardiol. 2013;167:2653–6.
11. Whitlow PL, Burke MN, Lombardi WL, et al. Use of a novel crossing and re-entry system in coronary chronic total occlusions that have failed standard crossing techniques: results of the FAST-CTOs (Facilitated Antegrade Steering Technique in Chronic Total Occlusions) trial. JACC Cardiovasc Interv. 2012;5:393–401.
12. Werner GS, Schofer J, Sievert H, Kugler C, Reifart NJ. Multicentre experience with the BridgePoint devices to facilitate recanalisation of chronic total coronary occlusions through controlled subintimal re-entry. EuroIntervention. 2011;7:192–200.
13. Ng R, Hui PY, Beyer A, Ren X, Ochiai M. Successful retrograde recanalization of a left anterior descending artery chronic total occlusion through a previously placed left anterior descending-to-diagonal artery stent. J Invasive Cardiol. 2010;22:E16–8.
14. Ho PC, Leung C, Chan S. Blunt microdissection and rotational atherectomy: an effective combination for the resistant chronic total occlusion. J Invasive Cardiol. 2006;18:E246–9.
15. Fernandez JP, Hobson AR, McKenzie D, et al. Beyond the balloon: excimer coronary laser atherectomy used alone or in combination with rotational atherectomy in the treatment of chronic total occlusions, non-crossable and non-expansible coronary lesions. EuroIntervention. 2013;9:243–50.
16. Lee NH, Cho YH, Seo HS. Successful recanalization of in-stent coronary chronic total occlusion by subintimal tracking. J Invasive Cardiol. 2008;20:E129–32.

# 11 How to Fix Common Problems Encountered in CTO PCI: The Expanded Hybrid Approach

James Sapontis, Steven P. Marso, William L. Lombardi, and J. Aaron Grantham

**Abstract**

There remains a pressing need in the interventional cardiology community to narrow the existing gap in the success rates, safety, and efficiency of chronic total occlusion percutaneous coronary intervention (CTO-PCI) relative to non CTO-PCI. Success rates for non CTO-PCI are high (>98 %). The success rates of CTO-PCI at experienced CTO-PCI centers are catching up (>90 %) but are likely much lower (50–70 %) at the vast majority of other PCI centers. Complication rates appear to be equal between CTO and non-CTO procedures at experienced CTO centers but may not be at others. CTO-PCI is associated with higher procedural time, contrast use, radiation exposure and supply cost than non CTO PCI even at experienced CTO-PCI centers. Thus, a wide variability in the CTO-PCI cases being attempted persists in large part due to these gaps. This chapter provides an overview of the new expanded hybrid approach, commonly employed by successful CTO operators.

**Keywords**

Hybrid approach to CTO-PCI • Dissection reentry (DR) • Antegrade dissection reentry (ADR) • CTO cap • Guidewire escalation • Retrograde cap • Subintimal TRAnscatheter Withdrawal (STRAW) technique

There remains a pressing need in the interventional cardiology community to narrow the existing gap in the success rates, safety, and efficiency of chronic total occlusion percutaneous coronary intervention (CTO-PCI) relative to non CTO-PCI. Success rates for non CTO-PCI are high (>98 %). The success rates of CTO-PCI at experienced CTO-PCI centers are catching up (>90 %) [1–3] but are likely much lower (50–70 %) at the vast majority of other PCI centers [4]. Complication rates appear to be equal between CTO and non-CTO procedures at experienced CTO centers but may not be at others [5]. CTO-PCI is associated with higher procedural time, contrast use, radiation exposure and supply cost than non CTO PCI even at experienced CTO-PCI centers [6]. Thus, a wide variability in the CTO-PCI cases being attempted persists in large part due to these gaps [7].

In April of 2012 the Hybrid Approach to CTO-PCI was described and is now a common construct for approaching CTOs by many operators [8]. Based on this algorithm, four

**Electronic supplementary material** The online version of this chapter (doi:10.1007/978-3-319-21563-1_11) contains supplementary material, which is available to authorized users.

J. Sapontis, BSc, MBBCh, FRACP
Department of Medicine, Monash Heart, Cardiology, Monash Medical Center, Melbourne, VIC, Australia

S.P. Marso, MD
Department of Internal Medicine, University of Texas Southwestern Medical Center, Dallas, TX, USA

W.L. Lombardi, MD
Department of Cardiology, University of Washington Medical Center, Bellingham, WA, USA

J.A. Grantham, MD, FACC (✉)
Department of Cardiology, University of Missouri Kansas City, Kansas City, MO, USA

Department of Cardiology, Saint Luke's Health System's Mid America Heart Institute, Kansas City, MO, USA
e-mail: jgrantham@saint-lukes.org


S. Rinfret (ed.), *Percutaneous Intervention for Coronary Chronic Total Occlusion: The Hybrid Approach*, DOI 10.1007/978-3-319-21563-1_11

**Table 11.1** Four key questions to ask when analyzing a CTO from a hybrid approach

| |
|---|
| 1. Is the proximal cap ambiguous in its location? |
| 2. Is the target distal vessel diseased, or is there a bifurcation at the distal cap? |
| 3. Is the lesion length longer than 20 mm? |
| 4. Is there a collateral or a graft (patent or occluded) that can be used as a conduit to deliver some retrograde gear ('interventional collateral')? |

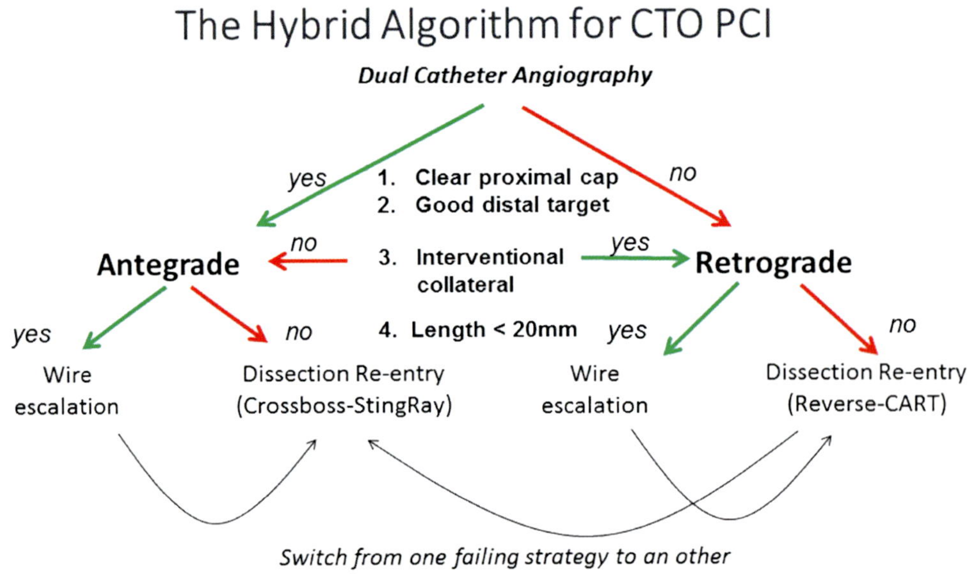


**Fig. 11.1** The original hybrid algorithm

factors are recognized as central in the decision to proceed with an antegrade-first approach, a retrograde-first approach, and with or without dissection re-entry (DR). The four key factors are listed in Table 11.1, and can be remembered as we go from the proximal end to the distal end of the occlusion. Firstly, the proximal coronary vessel anatomy needs to be assessed to clearly determine the location of the proximal cap. Blunt proximal caps are recognized as more difficult targets for an initial antegrade wire escalation strategy, and can increase procedure time and the chances of failure [9]. However, blunt proximal caps are not all ambiguous in location so an alternative description has been proposed by hybrid operators; more simply, if the operator would be uncomfortable to stick the proximal cap with a stiff guidewire, it can be considered ambiguous. The second factor is the lesion length. When a CTO is longer than 20 mm, sub-intimal tracking is likely [10]. Therefore, it is advocated in the algorithm to commit to a dissection and re-entry in such situation. The distal end of the CTO is the third factor, considering significant branches that could be occluded, or disease in the patent segment. Finally, the presence of interventional collaterals is the last factor. This is a collateral or retrograde pathway (like an occluded graft) leading to the distal cap which can be traversed safely by the operator considering his experience level (Chap. 9).

The algorithm is depicted in Fig. 11.1. The philosophy of hybrid is to maximize the likelihood of success while limiting the amount of contrast, radiation and time. This is done by selecting the most appropriate strategy to start with, and then rapidly switching from a failing to alternative approaches allowing testing of multiple strategies during the procedure. A retrograde approach should be adopted first when the proximal cap is unclear (because of either proximal cap bluntness, significant side-branches or poor visualization of the true distal vessel), the distal vessel is diseased, or when the distal cap is at a bifurcation. However, this is conditional to the presence of an interventional collateral. If the proximal cap is clear and the distal vessel is not severely diseased, without major side branches at the distal cap, the first approach should be antegrade. After selecting the direction (antegrade or retrograde), the crossing strategy will depend on occlusion length. When coming retrograde, and facing a short occlusion (<20 mm), a true-to-true (TTT) crossing attempt with sequential wires should be attempted first. However, if the lesion length is >20 mm, a retrograde DR with reverse-Controlled Antegrade and Retrograde Technique (R-CART) should be performed. When coming antegrade, with short lesions (<20 mm), a TTT crossing should also be attempted first. However, for lesions longer than 20 mm, antegrade dissection re-entry (ADR) with CrossBoss and Stingray is the preferred approach. Failing with the first strategy is not uncommon with the approach; nevertheless, success rates with the hybrid approach can reach over 90 %, because of the use of multiple strategies in the case of failing ones.

The hybrid approach adoption has been associated with improved procedural success, adequate procedural safety, and improved efficiency, but among these three barriers to CTO-PCI adoption, procedure time and resource utilization remain well above non CTO-PCI [11]. Since these

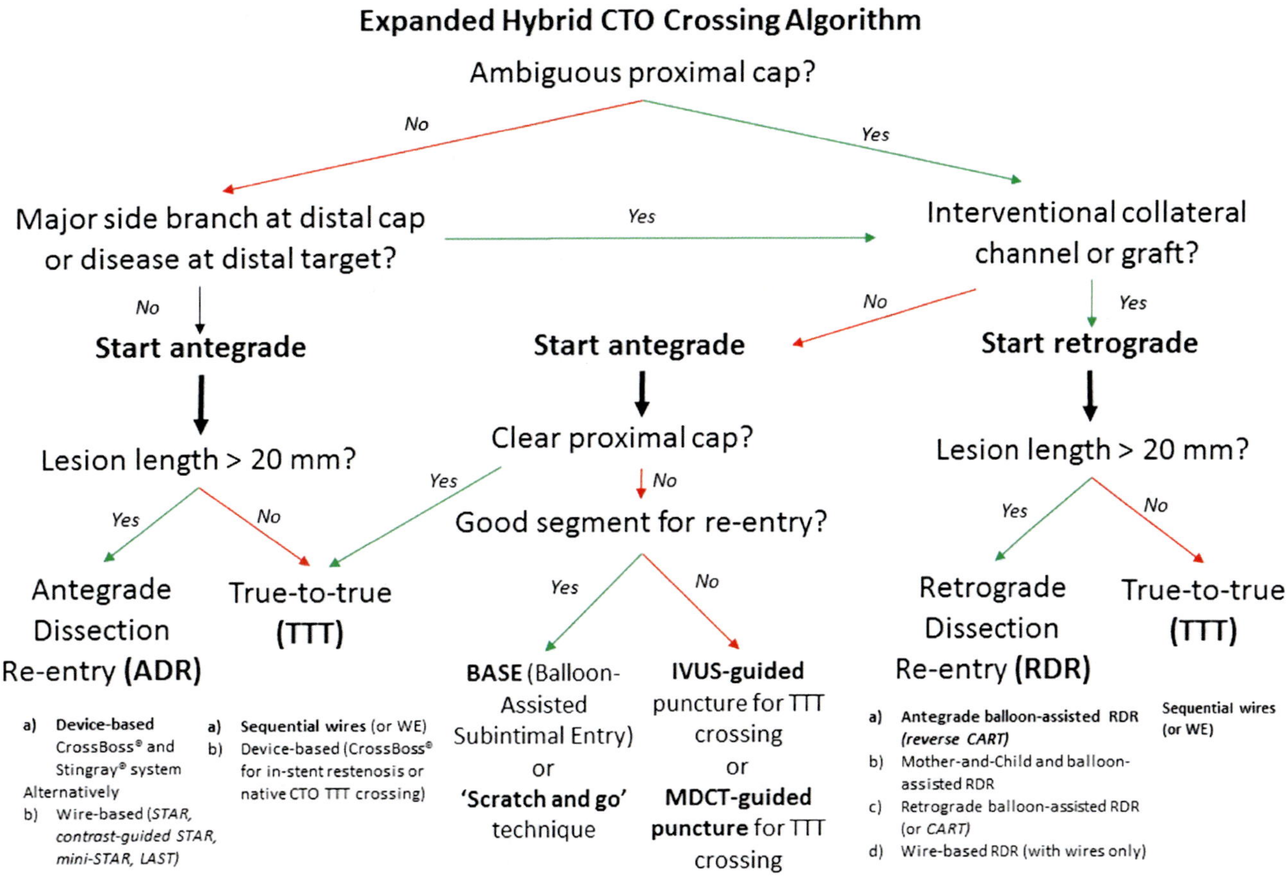


**Fig. 11.2** Enhanced hybrid CTO PCI algorithm. *Acronyms*: *ADR* antegrade dissection and re-entry, *CART* controlled antegrade and retrograde sub-intimal tracking, *CTO* chronic total occlusion, *IVUS* intra-vascular ultrasound, *LAST* limited antegrade subintimal tracking, *MDCT* multi-detector cardiac tomography, *STAR* sub-intimal tracking and re-entry, *TTT* true-to-true, *RDR* retrograde dissection and re-entry, *WE* wire escalation

publications there have been significant advances in the approach to common obstacles encountered during hybrid CTO-PCI procedures, many of which have been published as stand-alone techniques. The purpose of this chapter is to describe ten common obstacles to successful and efficient CTO revascularization and to provide pragmatic procedural solutions in a logical sequence to overcome these barriers, leading to an expanded hybrid CTO PCI algorithm as shown in Fig. 11.2. A structured approach to these CTO-PCI obstacles should facilitate the systematic evaluation and further refinement of the Hybrid approach that ultimately improves operator efficiency and success of CTO PCI.

## Common Problems and Solutions

### Problem 1: Failure to Penetrate a CTO Cap (Antegrade or Retrograde) Using Standard Guidewire Escalation Techniques

#### Definition

Despite optimal guide catheter support, standard wires and catheters are insufficient to penetrate the proximal or distal CTO cap using the previously described hybrid CTO-PCI wire escalation strategy [8] (see Chaps. 4 and 12).

#### Suggested Approach

End around, break the cap, then bailout to the alternate approach.

**End Around** Like the trick American football play "End around", the Hybrid operator with a mastery of re-entry techniques can functionally move around the resistant cap in the subintimal space. The subintimal space should be accessed proximally in the antegrade approach and distally in the retrograde approach. The end around should be avoided if possible when major left ventricular side branches arise near the cap as these branches are at risk for occlusion with dissection techniques. There are two ways to perform an end around:

1. Balloon assisted subintimal entry (BASE) is a technique where the intention is to cause an intimal disruption in the vessel thereby expediting safe wire and catheter access to the subintimal space (Figs. 11.3 and 11.4) [12]. This technique can be used to get around and avoid resistant CTO caps. It is particularly useful in the antegrade approach

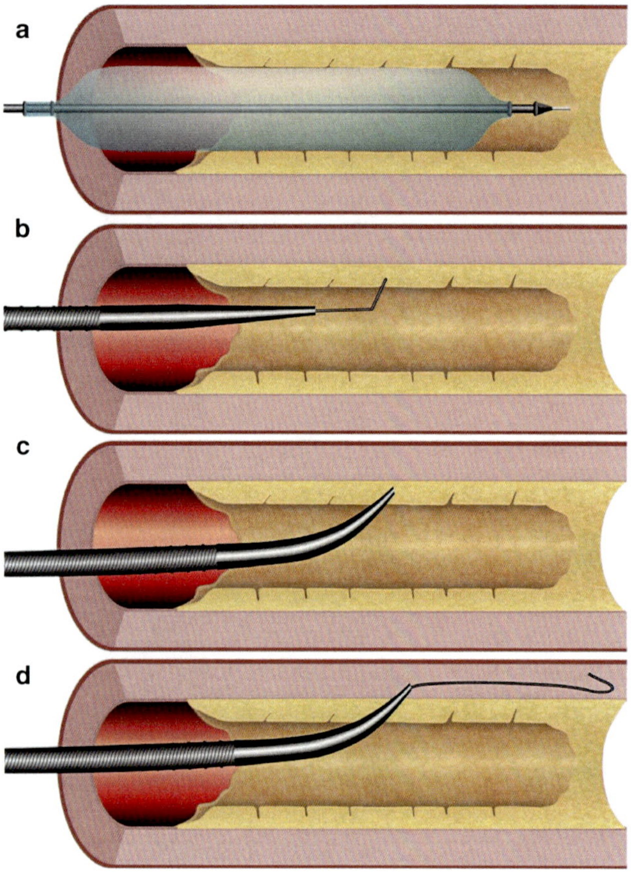


**Fig. 11.3** Balloon-Assisted Sub-intimal Rentry (BASE) technique. (**a**) A balloon is used to dilate and create dissection planes proximal to the ambiguous proximal cap. (**b**) A wire is used to puncture towards the artery wall. (**c**) A microcatheter is advanced, its tip engaging under the plaque. (**d**) A wire is knuckled in the sub-intimal space to gain control of the artery

when there is an adequate stump or segment of vessel in which to place a balloon, and is most effective when there is disease within the segment. Using standard techniques, a balloon sized at a ratio of 1:1 with the artery is inflated above nominal pressure in the vessel proximal to the impenetrable cap. Once the balloon is deflated and removed, a Corsair (Asahi-Intecc, Japan) catheter is advanced to the dilation site. A jacketed wire (e.g. Fielder XT (Asahi-Intecc, Japan) or Pilot 200 (Abbott Vascular, USA)) is advanced toward the vessel wall and manipulated into the subintimal space where it is knuckled over and advanced forward. For very proximal disease, it is not uncommon to notice that the guide catheter moves towards a dissection plane created by the balloon inflation. A very gentle contrast injection (less than 1 cc) is sometimes enough to confirm that the dissection maneuver was effective, and the operator can follow with the knuckled wire as described (Fig. 11.4, Videos 11.1, 11.2, 11.3, 11.4, 11.5, 11.6, 11.7, 11.8, 11.9, 11.10, and 11.11). After confirming the knuckled wire is within the wall of the artery (the wire is moving in concert with the vessel) an antegrade or retrograde dissection and re-entry strategy may be employed depending on the direction chosen for the approach to the CTO. The knuckled wire should be stopped at least 10 mm before the target and the dissection finished with the Crossboss Catheter (Boston Scientific, USA) when employing this technique antegrade (see Chap. 6 and 7). When performing this procedure retrograde, re-entry is made with R-CART described elsewhere [13] and in Chap. 9.

2. The "scratch and go" technique can be employed if BASE is not possible or difficult (i.e. short stump or potential side branch compromise) (Fig. 11.5). In this maneuver a stiff tapered guidewire e.g. Confianza Pro 12 (Asahi-Intecc, Japan) with a 60° 3–4 mm single tip bend, is loaded into a Corsair catheter and used to "scratch" or penetrate the intima proximal to the cap, thereby allowing access to the subintimal space. Once the subintimal space is entered, the Corsair catheter is inserted 1–2 mm into the subintimal space without letting the wire move forward or backward. This requires meticulous control of the wire while rotating and controlling forward advancement of the Corsair. After confirming the catheter is within the wall of the artery (the catheter is moving in concert with the vessel), the stiff wire is exchanged for a polymer jacketed wire which is then intentionally knuckled and pushed in the subintimal space past the cap. At this juncture, an antegrade or retrograde dissection and re-entry strategy may be employed depending on the direction chosen for the approach to the CTO.

**Break the Cap** The second option is to break up the cap with a "hydraulic dissection" or excimer laser (antegrade cap only).

1. Breaking the cap by hydraulic disruption can be performed either antegrade or retrograde using a Corsair catheter driven into the cap often only a millimeter or two (Fig. 11.6). Through this catheter, 0.5–1 ml of contrast is briskly injected under fluoroscopic visualization. If contrast is tracking in the wrong direction the injection should be terminated. This has been called the "modified Carlino technique" [14], and the reader should refer to Chap. 8 for more details. In addition similar to dissecting the vessel with a microcatheter, the same can be accomplished by injection of a small amount (2–3 ml) of contrast through a wedged antegrade guide or guide extension catheter, as described earlier for the BASE technique. While intentionally dissecting a vessel was considered anathema to mainstream interventionalists, the development and use of reliable and safe re-entry techniques [15] by hybrid operators makes these tasks preferable to the use of stiff tapered guidewires which can more easily cause perforations.

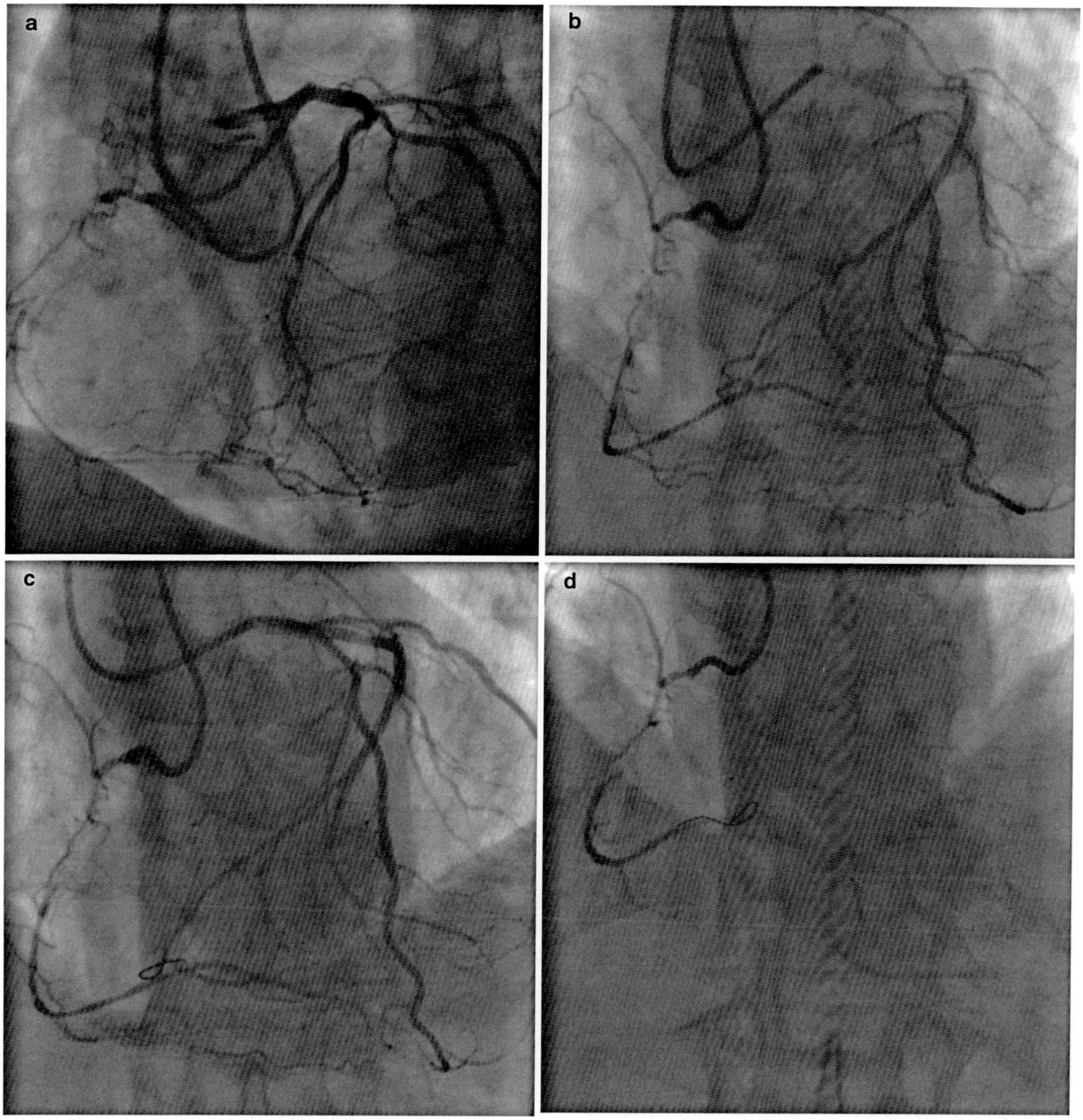


**Fig. 11.4** (Videos 11.1, 11.2, 11.3, 11.4, 11.5, 11.6, 11.7, 11.8, 11.9, 11.10, and 11.11). Balloon-assisted sub-intimal entry (BASE) and blind stick techniques. (**a**, **b**) A more than 20 mm RCA CTO with a very ambiguous proximal cap, largely because of the presence of several ipsilateral bridge collaterals (Videos 11.1 and 11.2). (**c**) Retrograde approach with a Sion through the large epicardial CC from the LCX to the PLV (Video 11.3). (**d**) Failure to connect into the distal RCA, with sub-intimal tracking in the last few mm (Video 11.4). (**e**) Antegrade bailout with BASE (Balloon-Assisted Sub-intimal Entry). After dilating the proximal RCA segment with a 3.0 mm balloon, a very tiny injection was performed with 1 cc of contrast, showing a dissection plane (Video 11.5). (**f**) A Fielder XT is knuckled into the dissection plane, with the support of a CrossBoss (Video 11.6). (**g**) The CrossBoss is advanced to the distal RCA for re-entry (Video 11.7). (**h**) A Stingray ballon is in place (*Circle*), but an antegrade hematoma is compressing the true lumen. Suction of blood from the Stingray ports did not improve visualization (Video 11.8). (**i**) A first stick is performed through the port pointing upward, as the common position of a Stingray following a CrossBoss is following the greater curvature of the artery (Video 11.9). (**j**) Successful swap with a Pilot 200 shaped as the Stingray wire (Video 11.10). (**k**) Final result after DES deployment (Video 11.11)

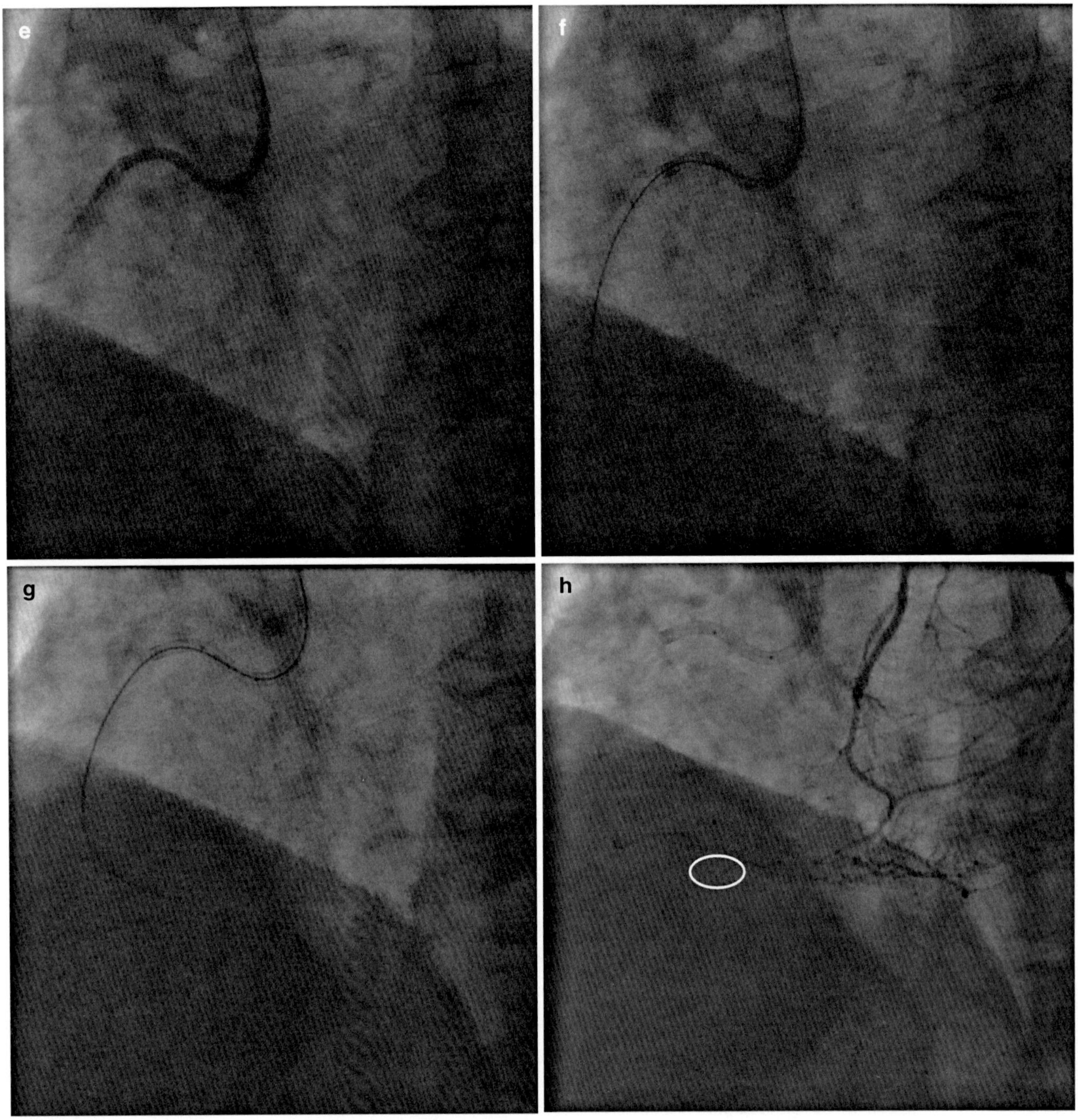


**Fig. 11.4** (continued)

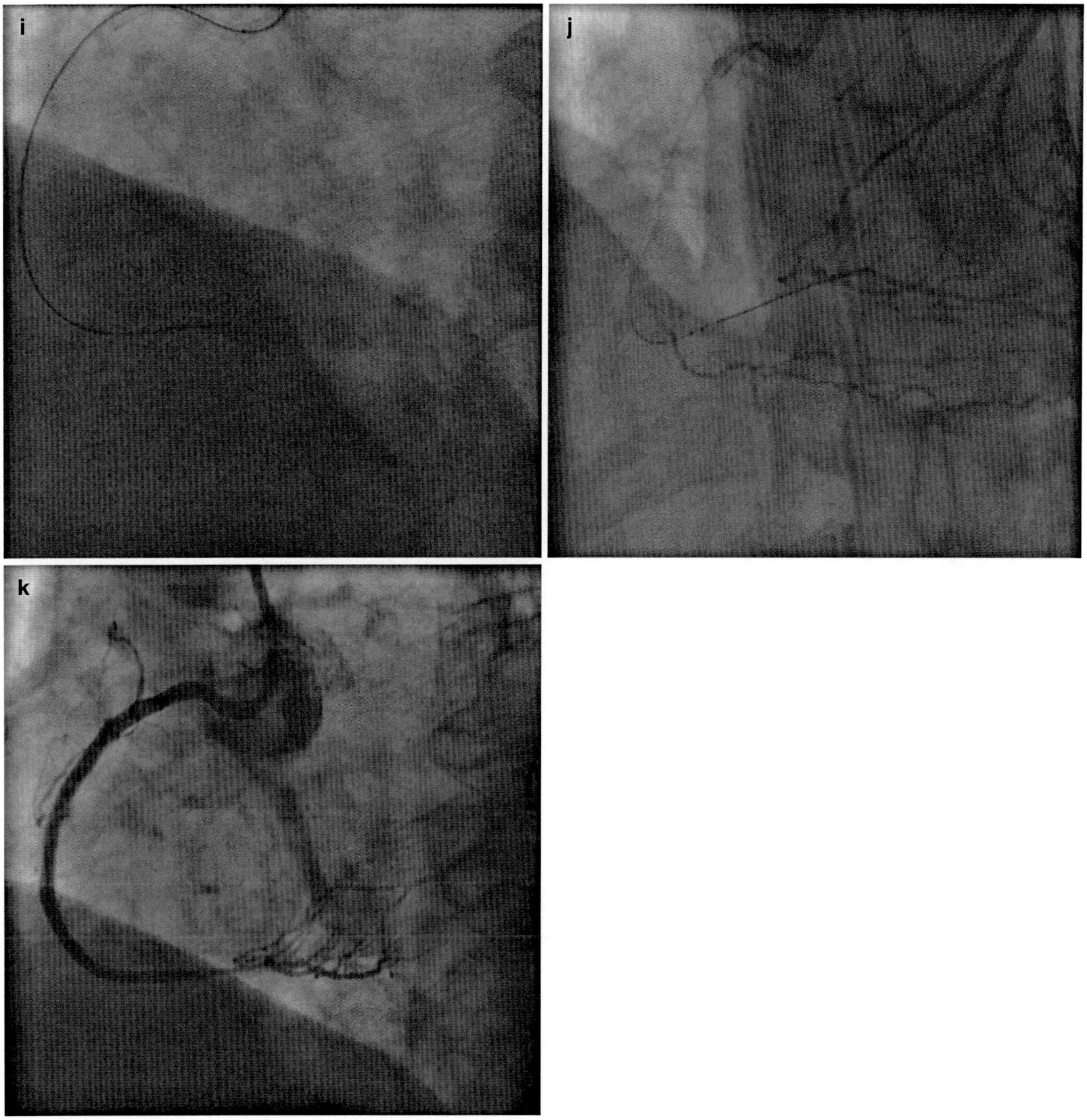


**Fig. 11.4** (continued)

2. In situations where the antegrade proximal cap is defined and tapered, breaking the cap can be performed with the excimer laser (Spectranetics, Inc., USA). This can be achieved with either the coronary or peripheral 0.9 mm excimer laser (ELCA and Turbo elite, Spectranetics, Inc., USA) delivered to the proximal cap. Laser photoablation is then performed for 30 s to 1 min, in order to soften the proximal cap and facilitate either penetration by a wire or Crossboss catheter. It should be emphasized that the proximal cap morphology should funnel the laser toward the occlusion and not the sidewall of the vessel to avoid perforation. Thus the laser is not suited for eccentric or ambiguous proximal caps.

**Bailout** If all of the above fail, the third option is to reverse directions (antegrade to retrograde or retrograde to antegrade). When working antegrade, if suitable collaterals exist, or when working retrograde if proximal cap ambiguity can be solved, a knuckled wire can be pushed to the resistant cap from the opposite direction. The knuckled guidewire will create a space

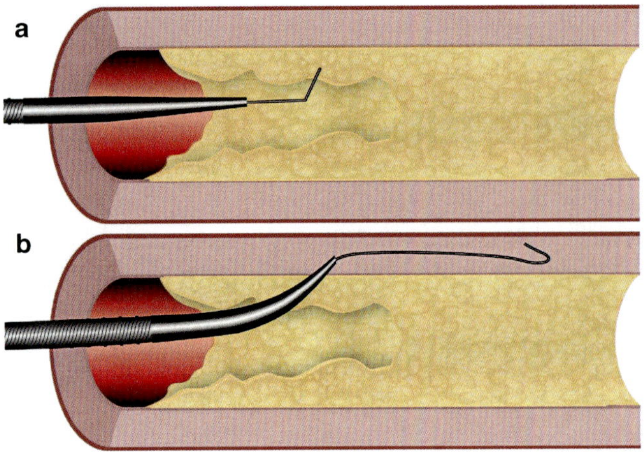


**Fig. 11.5** Scratch and go technique. (**a**) A sharp wire is directed towards the sub-adventitial space. (**b**) Following advancement of the microcatheter, a polymer-jacketed guidewire is knuckled in the space

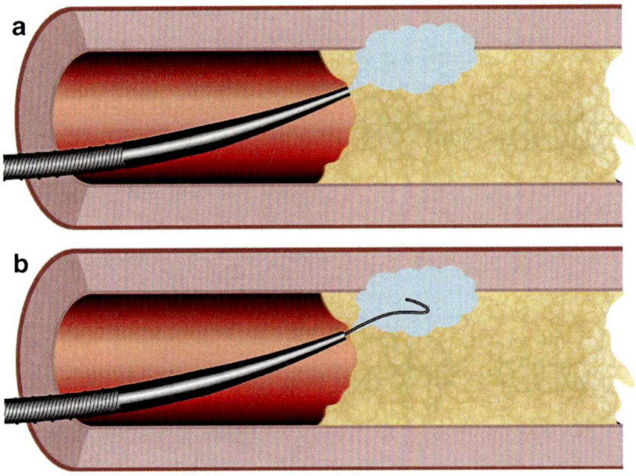


**Fig. 11.6** Contrast-induced hydraulic micro-dissection. (**a**) A small amount of contrast is injected from the tip of the microcatheter, modifying the proximal cap compliance. (**b**) A wire is advanced into the dissection planes

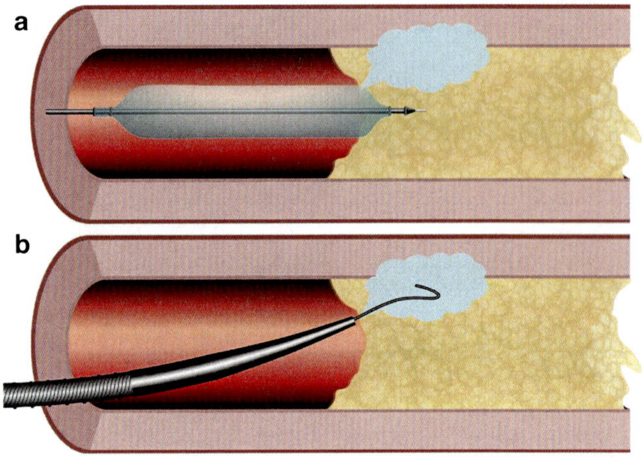


**Fig. 11.7** Balloon-Assisted Microdissection (BAM). (**a**) A small balloon is inflated above its rate-burst pressure, modifying the proximal cap compliance. (**b**) A wire is advanced into the dissection planes

in the vessel wall beside the cap and serve as a target for a stiff tapered guidewire from the opposite direction.

All of these techniques require the operator to be experienced with subintimal crossing and both antegrade and retrograde re-entry techniques. Further, they should be employed in sequence with rapid switching in order to avoid getting stuck in a failure mode.

## Problem 2: The Device-Uncrossable Antegrade or Retrograde Cap

### Definition

A wire has successfully crossed the CTO into the true lumen but no catheter or balloon can cross the lesion. In this instance it is assumed the guide support has been maximized with either a guide extension or anchor balloon.

### Suggested Approaches

The options available include balloon-assisted microdissection (BAM), Laser, Tornus, rotational atherectomy (RA), external crush, and end around techniques. The choice is somewhat dictated by the approach (antegrade vs retrograde).

1. To perform the BAM technique for a 'device resistant' CTO lesion, advance a 1.2–1.5 mm balloon (at least 20 mm because it has a longer length before getting to the marker which is the widest profile on the balloon) and attempt to wedge the balloon into the lesion. Then inflate the balloon up to rated burst pressure and deflate, noting whether the balloon can move forward. If it moves forward, continue to dilate from proximal to distal. If the balloon cannot be advanced further antegrade then inflate the balloon until it ruptures, causing a hydraulic dissection of the proximal cap. The key to limiting the dissection with this strategy is careful attention to the insufflator pressure, as soon as the pressure falls (due to balloon rupture), aspiration is performed and the balloon removed. Afterwards, the operator should retry crossing with a small balloon or microcatheter (Fig. 11.7).
2. If still unsuccessful, or alternatively, a 2.1 or 2.6 Fr Tornus (Asahi-Intecc, Japan) catheter can be utilized to dotter the resistant portion of the lesion and can be especially useful for highly calcified proximal disease [16].
3. Next, if available, a 0.9 mm rapid exchange laser catheter can be used to photoablate the resistant portion of the lesion. The laser catheter is advanced to the point of resistance and activated at a fluency of 60–80 and frequency of 60–80 pulse/s. This technique is preferred when the resistant tissue is fibrous and non-calcified [17].
4. If the wire is in the true lumen and the above techniques do not work or cannot be utilized then the external crush technique can be performed. Here, a second wire is inserted into the subintimal space next to luminal wire. Then a balloon (sized 1:1 to the artery) is inflated to crush

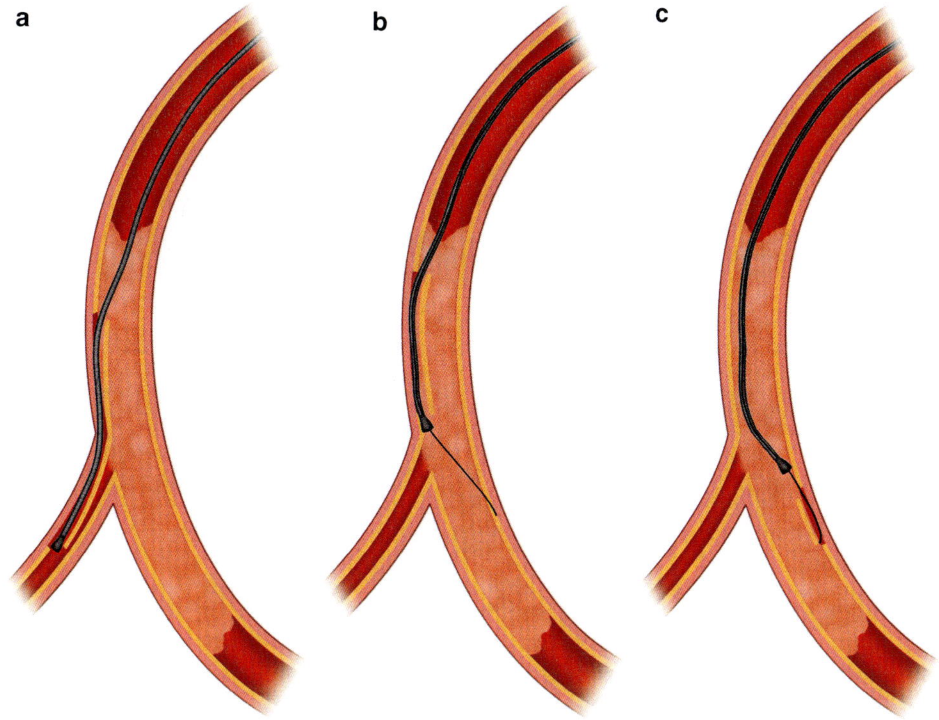


**Fig. 11.8** Wire redirect

the plaque from the subintimal space and enable gear to then move over initial true lumen wire [18].

5. If the above fail, the operator should advance a Finecross (Terumo, Japan), a Valet (Volcano, USA), a Turnpike (Vascular Solutions, USA) or a Corsair (Asahi Intecc, Japan) microcatheter as far distally as possible through the lesion, attempt rewiring the lesion with a RotaWire and performing rotational atherectomy (RA) (Rotablator, Boston Scientific, USA). The tip of the RotaWire should be shaped with a very short 1 mm bend, as for CTO wires, and drilling of the wire should be applied to re-cross through the channel created with the previous wire. The distal end of the RotaWire can hinder effective wiring, if so, one can cut the last 2 cm of the tip off of a rota-floppy wire and position the RotaWire such that the radiopaque transition is more than 5 mm beyond the resistant portion of the lesion. RA is then performed with a 1.25 mm burr, at 180,000 revolutions per minute.
6. If these techniques fail, then entering the subintimal space partially through the lesion with a knuckled wire or the Crossboss catheter and re-entry performed with the Stingray balloon and Stingray wire (Boston Scientific, USA) can also be attempted. Otherwise proceed to the "end around" algorithm or "bailout to another approach" as outlined above.

Tackling device resistant lesions when working via a retrograde approach, primarily involves placement of retrograde wire into the antegrade guide. The operator should bring an Rx balloon into the antegrade guide and inflate at high pressure to trap the tip of the retrograde guidewire in the antegrade guide. This maneuver provides a stronger wire platform with greater pushability for the retrograde microcatheter. Then, we should retry crossing the lesion with the retrograde Corsair followed by a Finecross microcatheter. Next, the operator should consider retrograde balloon dilation of the spot where the Corsair won't cross with 1.2–1.5× 20 mm balloon and progress on to BAM if necessary. If all else fails follow the "end around" algorithm to go around the resistant portion of the lesion in a new tissue plane and repeat retrograde dissection re entry at new more proximal location.

## Problem 3: Antegrade Subintimal Catheter Follows a Side Branch

### Definition

The Crossboss catheter or a knuckled wire tracks along a side branch or graft, rather than the vessel of interest. This problem is identified by discordant motion of the catheter and the vessel as visualized by calcification within the vessel or retrograde filling. The operator can notice that the wire and the vessel 'don't dance together'.

### Suggested Approach

Redirect the system using a straight wire, then a knuckled wire, followed by "end around" techniques to establish a new tissue plane, preferably on the opposite side of the vessel from the first.

1. The Pilot 200 redirect technique is performed by placing Pilot 200 wire with a 3 mm-long 60° tip bend in the CrossBoss catheter (Fig. 11.8). The wire is manipulated until directed away from the branch. Typically resistance

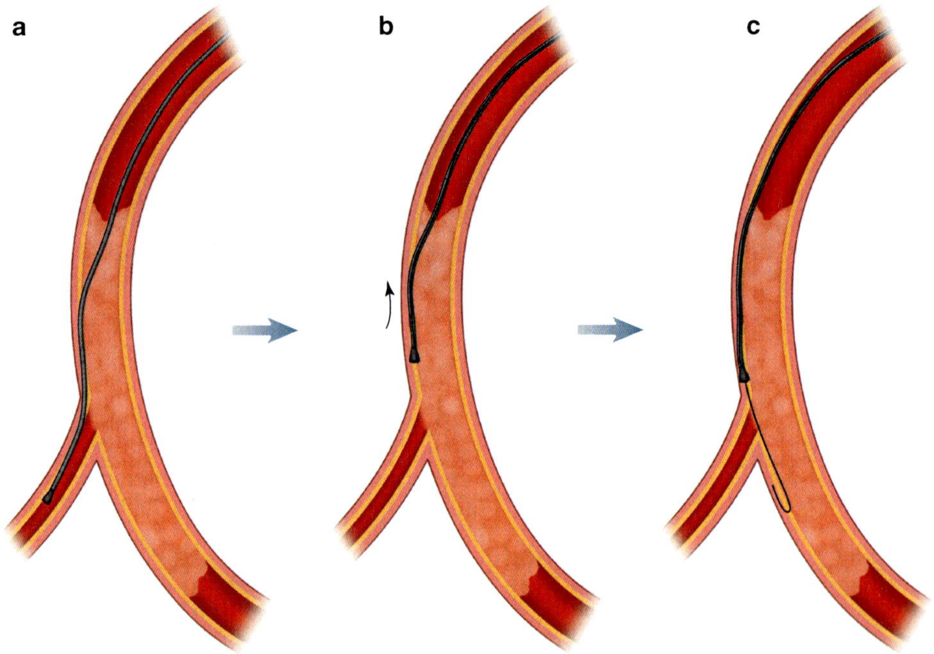


**Fig. 11.9** Knuckle-Boss technique

to the wire is encountered when obtaining the new subintimal location past the branch. The wire is advanced 4–5 mm beyond the sidebranch and the CrossBoss is then advanced over the wire until it is past the branch. Once past the branch the wire is pulled back into the crossboss and it is advanced to the reentry site.

2. If that fails then a "knuckle redirect" or "knuckle-Boss technique" can be employed using a Pilot 200 wire. The Pilot 200 is preferred since it makes a larger loop that is more likely to track alongside the larger branch (i.e. away from the sidebranch). Once the knuckle is past the side branch, the CrossBoss is brought beyond the branch, the wire is pulled back and the CrossBoss is advanced distally into the final re-entry zone (Figs. 11.9 and 11.11).
3. If these both fail, replace the CrossBoss with a Corsair catheter and perform wire redirect with stiff guidewire, usually a Confianza Pro 12 and follow the wire closely with Corsair catheter to a point 3–5 mm past the branch. Remove the stiff Confianza pro 12 and use a softer tipped polymer jacketed wire (Fielder XT or Pilot 200) to create a knuckle to ensure you are in the vessel architecture (wire moving concordantly or dancing with the vessel visualized by calcification or retrograde filling with contrast). Once it is clear that the wire is within the architecture, the CrossBoss is brought back and advanced to the re-entry zone. We discourage the use of the Confianza Pro 12 guidewire into the CrossBoss, as the sudden forward advancement of the CrossBoss can push the sharp wire outside the vessel architecture.
4. If this fails, the operator should try to find a new dissection plane as far proximal to the branch as possible, often with large Pilot 200 knuckle or with a stiff wire redirection with a Confianza Pro 12 with 3–4 mm 60° single tip bend (see "end around").
5. The next option is to use the modified Carlino technique or use of IVUS to identify the side branch origin and steer around it with a stiff wire.
6. Finally if all these techniques fail and it is feasible, bail-out to the alternative approach, place a knuckle wire just beyond the side branch and use it to direct the antegrade wire, or simply complete the case with reverse CART.

## Problem 4: Hematoma Compression of the Re-entry Site Antegrade

### Definition

When performing ADR, retrograde visualization of the target vessel can be lost. This is most often caused by a compressive subintimal hematoma. This causes difficulty performing successful re-entry with the Stingray balloon and Stingray wire.

### Suggested Approach

To minimize the likelihood of hematoma formation in the future reentry zone, the operator must carefully manage the subintimal space. Presence of subintimal hematomas can be tackled with the use of the Subintimal TRAnscatheter Withdrawal (STRAW) technique [19] (Fig. 11.10) or a 'blind stick and swap' (Fig. 11.11, Videos 11.12, 11.13, 11.14, 11.15, 11.16, 11.17, 11.18, 11.19, 11.20, and 11.21).

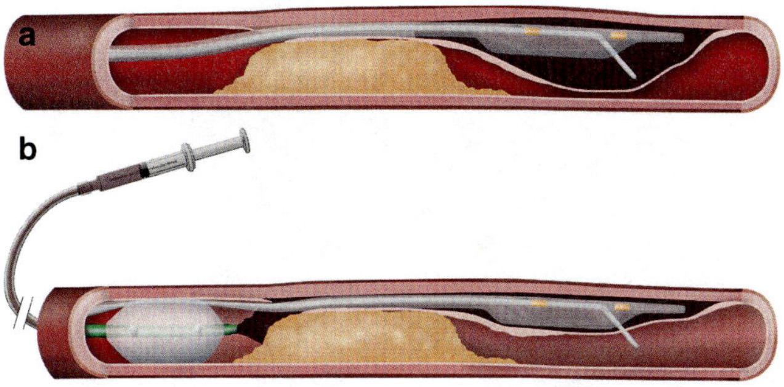


**Fig. 11.10** Subintimal TRAnscatheter Withdrawal (STRAW) technique. (**a**) If subintimal hematoma forms at the target. The Stingray balloon is floating in the hematoma, failing to properly enter in contact with the vessel wall, and the distal true lumen is compressed. (**b**) An over-the-wire low profile balloon is advanced over a second wire into the subintimal entry site alongside the Stingray balloon then inflated to nominal pressure to prevent inflow. The wire is removed and a 10 cc syringe attached to the wire port followed by aspiration for 2–3 min. Repeat retrograde angiography to determine if reconstitution of the target has occurred making re entry easier and more predictable (From Smith et al. [24], with permission)

Subintimal hematoma formation is avoided by refraining from antegrade injection or guide catheter flushing, controlling the size of the knuckle (smaller is better) and always finishing the dissection phase of the procedure with the CrossBoss catheter (i.e. the last 5–10 mm of the antegrade dissection to the reentry zone should be completed with the CrossBoss rather than the knuckled wire). Managing the subintimal space involves optimal deployment of the Stingray balloon. Optimal deployment is accomplished by leaving a wire and the CrossBoss (or the other microcatheter used such as the Corsair) in place during balloon prep. Leaving a microcatheter in place will prevent the sub-intimal space to be filled with antegrade blood flow during the time of Stingray prepping. Leaving the wire in the CrossBoss (and not only the CrossBoss alone) minimizes the time when contrast or blood can also seep into a leak point in the Crossboss catheter and then into the subintimal space. After the Stingray balloon is prepped, the Crossboss should be removed as efficiently as possible and exchanged for the Stingray balloon minimizing the time that the channel into the re entry zone is unplugged, thus minimizing the chance of hematoma formation. Such a technique is best performed with the trapping balloon technique, as described in Chap. 4. Finally, as the operator advances the Stingray wire into the Stingray balloon, if you see contrast staining and accumulation in the re entry zone is visualized, removing the wire and aspirating from the Stingray balloon end hole should solve the problem.

If subintimal hematoma nevertheless forms at the target, re-entry is more difficult because the Stingray balloon is floating in the hematoma, failing to properly enter in contact with the vessel wall, and the distal true lumen is compressed (Figs. 11.4h, 11.10a and 11.11e). The hematoma can be removed by STRAW techniques [19] (Fig. 11.10) or the operator can perform a blind stick and swap technique.

1. STRAW techniques are most effective when one can accomplish occlusion of inflow to the re entry site and aspiration of the hematoma. Figure 11.10 illustrates the optimal STRAW where an over-the-wire low profile balloon (Ryujin, 2.5 mm, Terumo Inc., Japan or Emerge 2.5 mm Boston Scientific, USA) is advanced over a second wire into the subintimal entry site alongside the Stingray balloon then inflated to nominal pressure to prevent inflow. The wire is removed and a 10 cc syringe attached to the wire port followed by aspiration for 2–3 min. Repeat retrograde angiography to determine if reconstitution of the target has occurred making re entry easier and more predictable.

   If these balloons are not available STRAW technique without occlusion of inflow can be attempted by several techniques. Aspiration through the OTW port of the Stingray balloon is the simplest. Remove the wire from the Stingray balloon and attach a 10 cc syringe to the wire port. Pull negative on the syringe and maintain negative pressure. While negative pressure is being applied inflate the balloon to 4 atm then remove the 10 cc syringe and perform re-entry with the guidewire as usual. If this is unsuccessful, position a second guide wire in the dissection plane alongside the balloon shaft. Place a Corsair or Finecross catheter over the second wire just proximal to the balloon and remove the wire. Aspirate through the Corsair wire port while performing re-entry through the balloon. One can also perform aspiration of the hematoma by advancing a guide extension (Guideliner, Vascular Solutions, USA) catheter into the coronary as far distally as possible until it is wedged (as confirmed with a sudden drop in blood pressure) and aspirating through the sidearm of the Copilot (Abbott Vascular, USA) hemostatic valve.
2. The blind stick and swap technique is a modification of stick and swap described in detail in the next section and in Chaps. 5 and 7. Blind implies that the re-entry target is no longer visualized due to compressive hematoma that cannot be removed by the above STRAW techniques. If that hematoma cannot be evacuated then try sticking the Stingray wire 5–7 mm out both ports (because you cannot see the direction needed) then swap that wire for a Pilot 200 and carefully attempt to direct it into one of the fenestrations created by the Stingray wire that communicates with the true lumen. Such a technique can be accomplished sequentially (one side Stick and Swap at the time) (Fig. 11.4, Videos 11.1, 11.2, 11.3, 11.4, 11.5, 11.6, 11.7, 11.8, 11.9, 11.10, and 11.11) or simultaneously (with the two sticks performed, and then swap towards the path of least resistance) (Fig. 11.10).

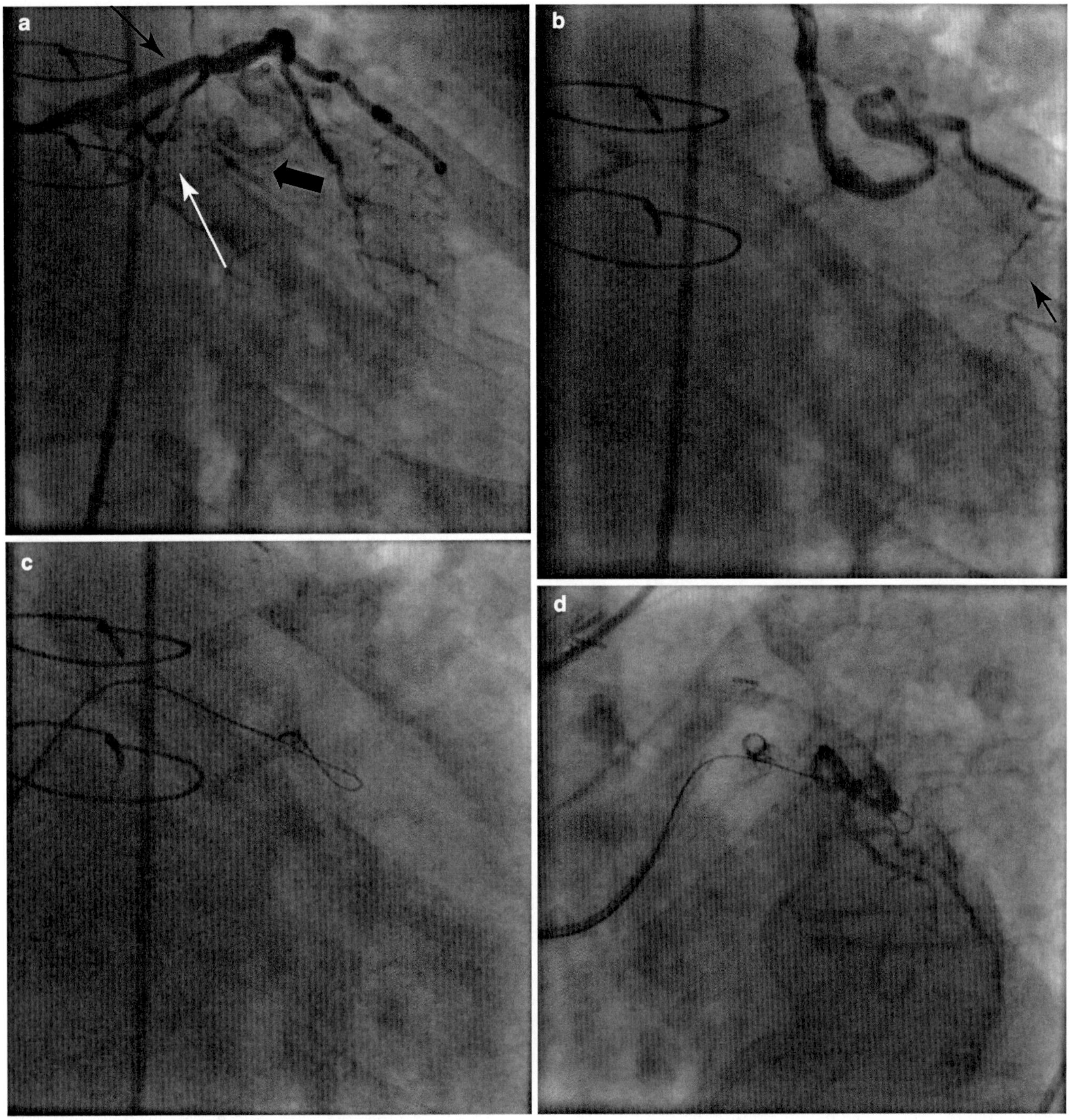


**Fig. 11.11** (Videos 11.12, 11.13, 11.14, 11.15, 11.16, 11.17, 11.18, 11.19, 11.20, and 11.21). Knuckle-Boss and Blind Stick and Swap technique using the CrossBoss and Stingray Antegrade dissection re-entry system. (**a**) Angulated but short CTO of the OM (*white arrow*), that used to be grafted by a sequential SVG to OM and diagonal, which was stented in the past, with occlusion of the first latero-lateral anastomosis (*bold black arrow*) (Video 11.12). (**b**) CrossBoss at the proximal cap; failure to start the dissection. The distal OM is irrigated by a distal epicardial collateral channel from the diagonal branch (*black arrow*) (Video 11.13). (**c**) Knuckled Pilot 200 to start the dissection (Video 11.14). (**d**) The knuckled wire is in the vessel structure, and the CrossBoss is advanced to create a dryer dissection plane (Video 11.15). (**e**) Poor retrograde filling of the OM branch, likely from an hematoma caused by the knuckled wire; the Stingray is visualized from a wrong view (Right Anterior Oblique) (Video 11.16). (**f**) Both wings of the Stingray balloon are overlapped in the Left Anterior Oblique view. Because of poor distal vessel filling, the direction of the stick is ambiguous (Video 11.17). (**g**) A blind stick technique is performed; first, the port pointing upward is punctured; a strong resistance is encountered (Video 11.18). (**h**) Then, the port pointing downward is punctured; a 'pop and release' sensation is felt (Video 11.18). (**i**) A Pilot 200 (swap technique) is used to track the second hole created by the Stingray; it advances without resistance (Video 11.19). (**j**) Retrograde injection that confirms that the Pilot 200 is in the true lumen (Video 11.20). (**k**) Final result post dilation and stenting (Video 11.21)

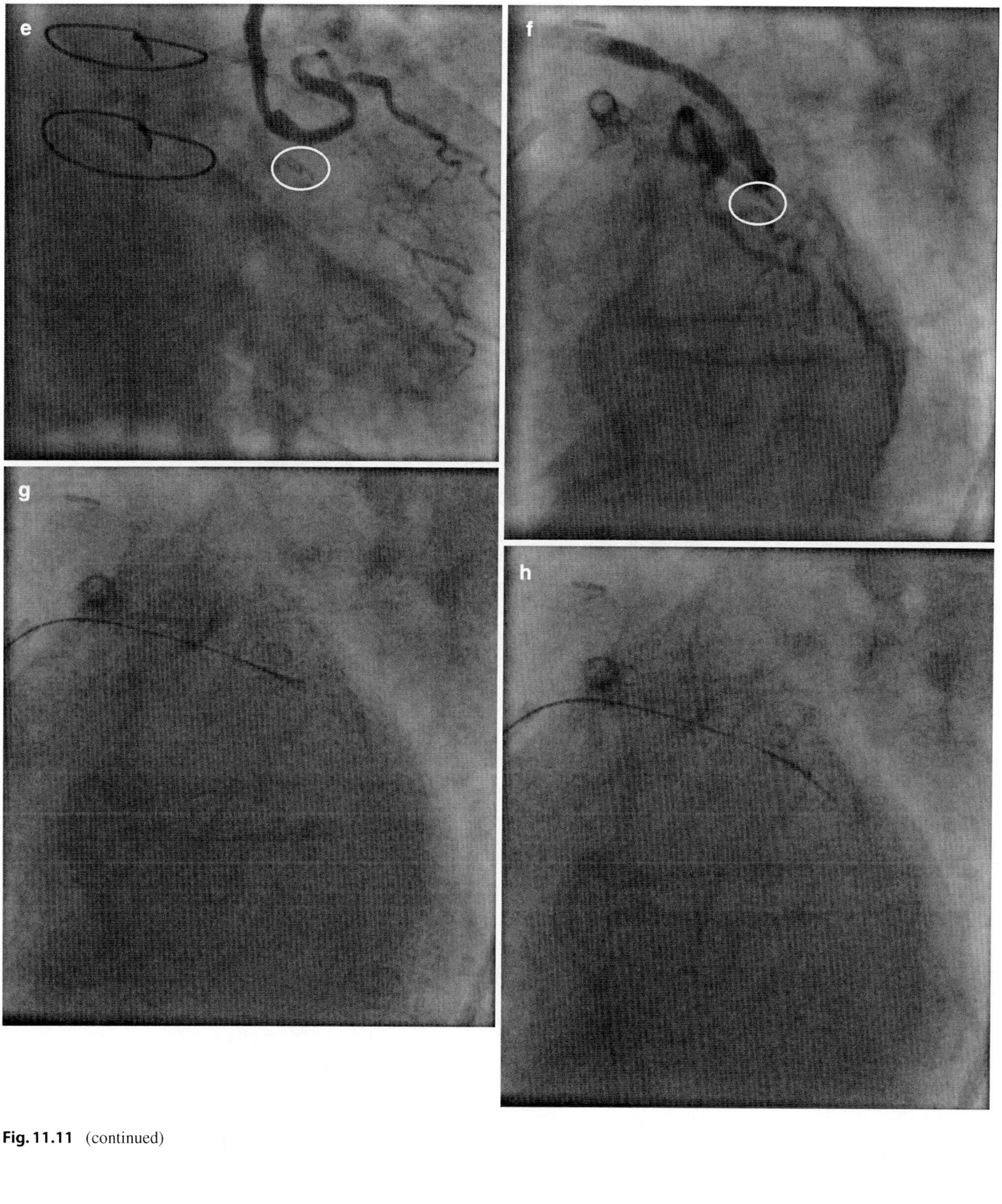


**Fig. 11.11** (continued)

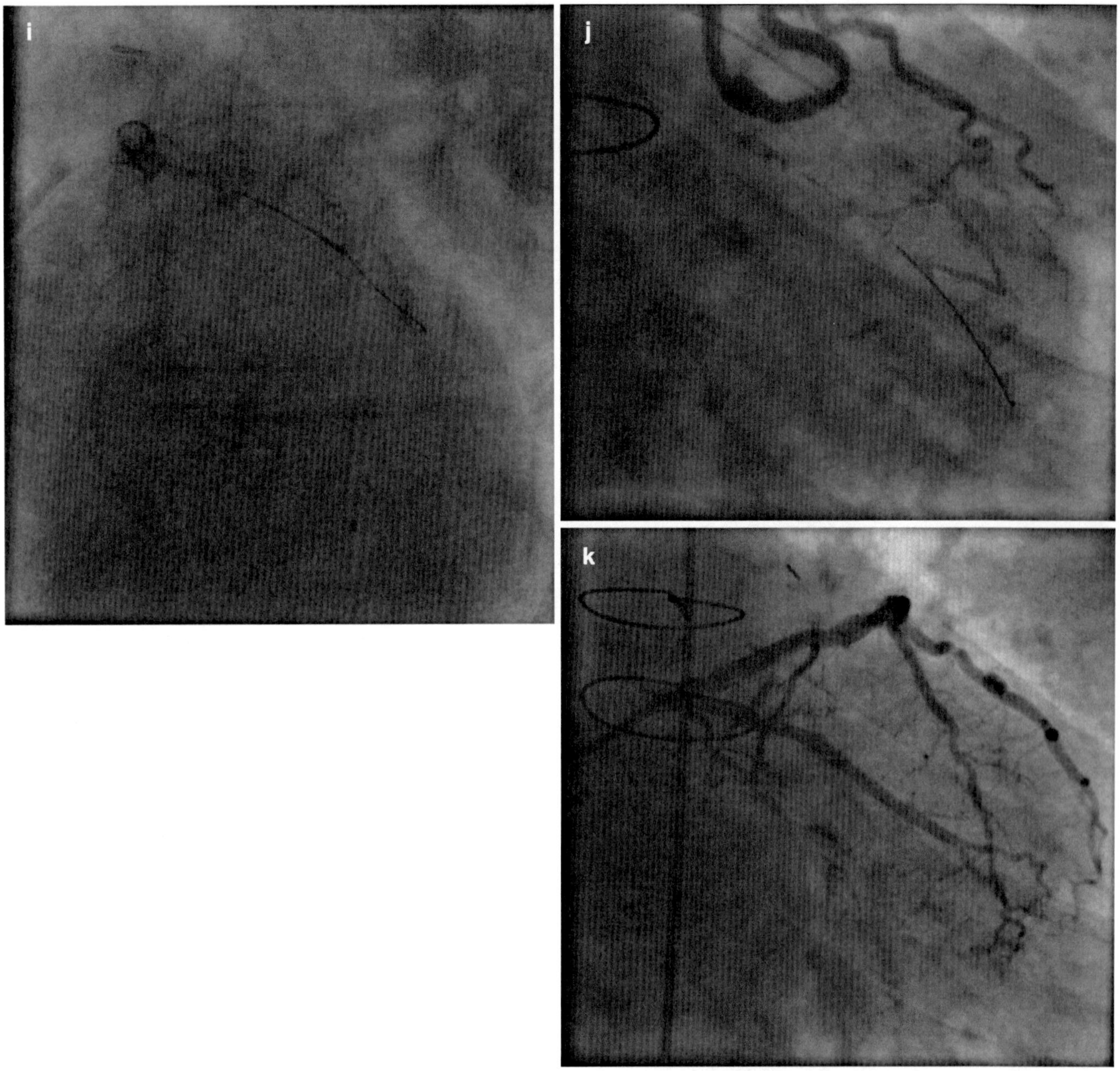


**Fig. 11.11** (continued)

## Problem 5: Inability to Re-enter the Distal Lumen Through Stingray Balloon Antegrade

### Definition

After good placement and successful deployment of the Stingray balloon, 3–4 re entry attempts with the stingray wire are unsuccessful at accessing the distal true lumen.

### Suggested Approach

This is commonly caused by passing the Stingray wire to the opposite back wall of the target vessel. In this situation the first option is the "stick and swap technique" followed by the bobsled maneuver.

1. Stick and swap should be attempted after 3–4 unsuccessful passes of the Stingray wire. The wire should be removed and exchanged for a Pilot 200 with a 1 mm 70–80° tip bend. The wire should be advanced out of the appropriate re-entry port of the stingray balloon to the back wall of the vessel (signified by slight buckling of the wire). The Pilot 200 is then pulled back 1–2 mm, rotated 180° and advanced in an attempt to slide though the Stingray wire channel into the distal true lumen. Given the effectiveness of this technique, some operators prefer to use it as the default reentry technique when using the Stingray system (Chap. 6, Fig. 6.5).
2. If 3–4 attempts of stick and swap are not successful then the operator should move the re-entry site forward using a

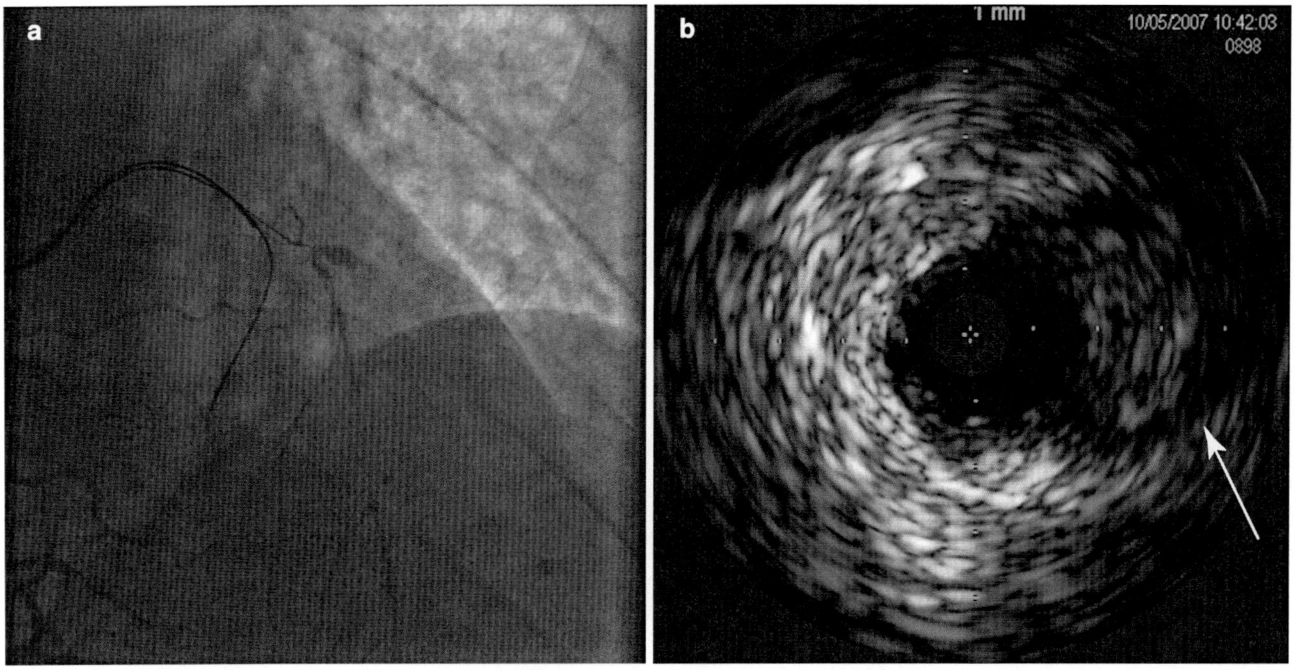


**Fig. 11.12** IVUS-guided proximal cap puncture. (**a**) IVUS guided antegrade puncture is possible when a side branch is close to the presumed cap. (**b**) Careful IVUS examination may clarify the occluded target vessel location. Using IVUS, the operator should be looking for a typical appearance (*arrow*) of the take-off of the occluded cap from the side branch

"bob-sled" technique. With the guidewire inside the balloon and while the balloon is deflated the balloon is gently pushed forward in the dissection plane. The balloon is re inflated and re-entry is re-attempted. The balloon can also be brought more proximal especially if the re-entry zone is larger or the balloon appears to be closer to the lumen at that location. Attempt re entry again after increasing the angle on the Stingray wire from its pre-configured 28.5° to a more acute angle between 45° and 60° and consider using a Confianza Pro 12 to make the re-entry from the balloon, especially if the re entry zone is heavily calcified, or there is a greater amount of tissue between the Stingray balloon and the true lumen, as the Stingray guidewire distal probe can actually be damaged and bended if pushed against calcium.

## Problem 6: Proximal Cap Ambiguity and No Retrograde Option

### Definition

In the setting of proximal cap ambiguity without usable interventional collaterals the original Hybrid Algorithm fails by yielding no solutions.

### Suggested Approach

Since the original publication of the algorithm [8] several techniques to solve this dilemma have been developed. Intravascular ultra sound (IVUS) guided antegrade puncture, non-invasive coronary angiography using multi-detector cardiac tomography (MDCT) and end around techniques can be employed (Fig. 11.2).

1. IVUS guided antegrade puncture is possible when a side branch is close to the presumed cap. Careful IVUS examination may clarify the occluded target vessel location. Using IVUS, the operator should be looking for a typical appearance of the take-off of the occluded cap from the side branch (Fig. 11.12).
2. MDCT can be extremely helpful in those cases as it can reduce proximal cap ambiguity. 3-D reconstruction of the MDCT image, with moving of the angulation to typical coronary angiography incidence can help the operator to figure out where the cap is (Fig. 11.13).
3. If IVUS or MDCT guidance are unsuccessful, or not possible due to absence of side branches or other reasons then go to the "end around" algorithm. Once in the architecture of the vessel proceed with antegrade dissection and re-entry as previously outlined.

## Problem 7: Corsair Will Not Cross the Collateral Channel Retrograde

### Definition

Despite optimal guide catheter support by anchoring or guide extension deployment the Corsair catheter cannot be advanced over the wire through the collateral.

### Suggested Approach

Solutions to this problem depend on whether the channel crossed is septal or epicardial, and involve septal balloon dilation, exchanging out for a new microcatheter or more supportive guidewire. Those solutions can be found in Chap. 9.

1. For septal collaterals, the first choice is to take a 1.25–1.5 mm Rx balloon to dilate the septal. The Corsair catheter is removed using trapping technique if the crossing wire was short. The balloon is passed over the wire with gentle steady pressure until it either crosses completely or goes as far as possible. If it crosses completely, then dilate

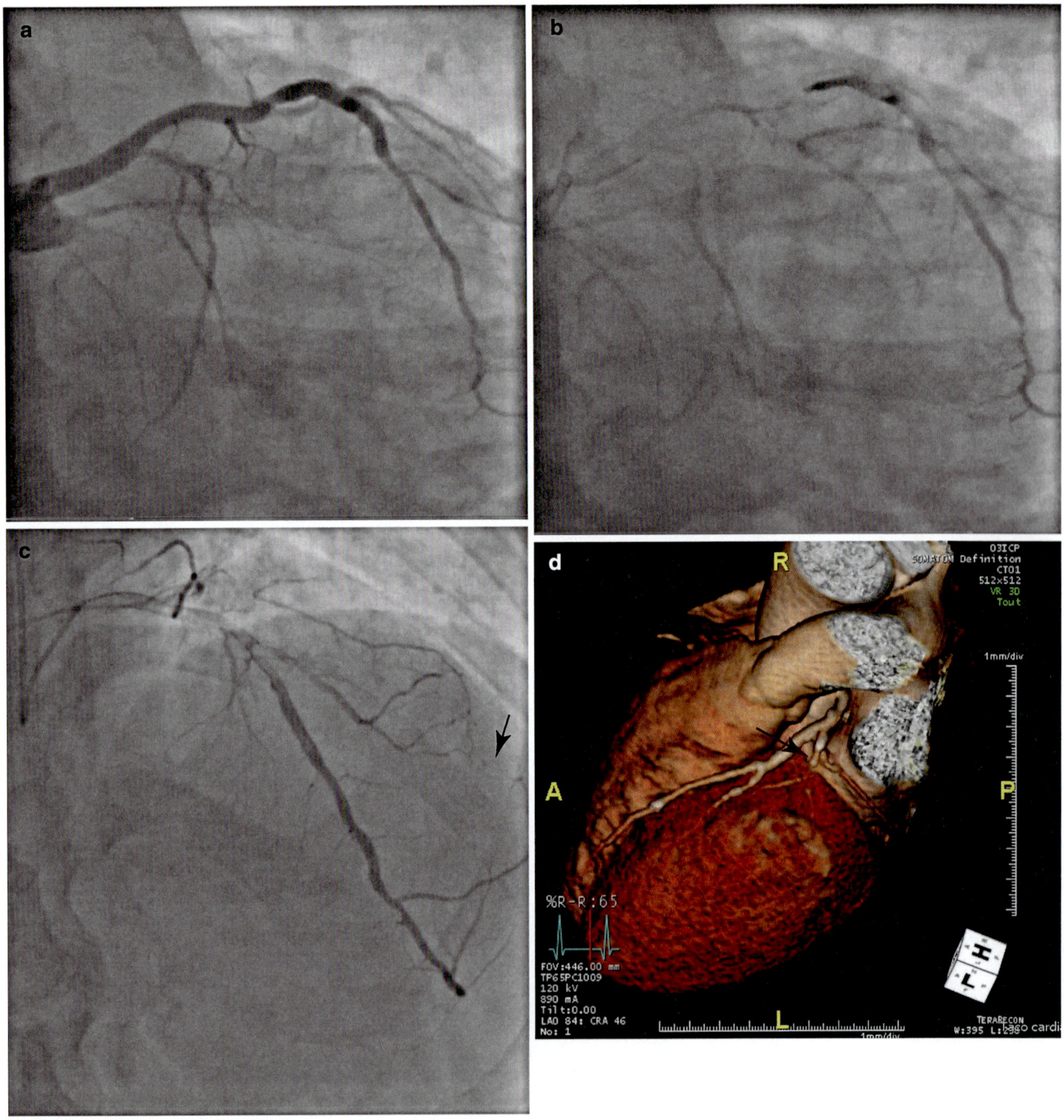


**Fig. 11.13** Ambiguous CTO with no retrograde option. (**a**) Small LCx artery with "missing" vessel on the lateral wall. (**b**) The distal bifurcation of the occluded vessel. (**c**) Only a small tortuous epicardial collateral originating from a distal diagonal branch was visualized in RAO cranial view (shown with *arrows*). (**d**) MDCT shows severely calcified occluded obtuse marginal branch (*black arrow*). (**e**) Final result after wire-based CTO PCI

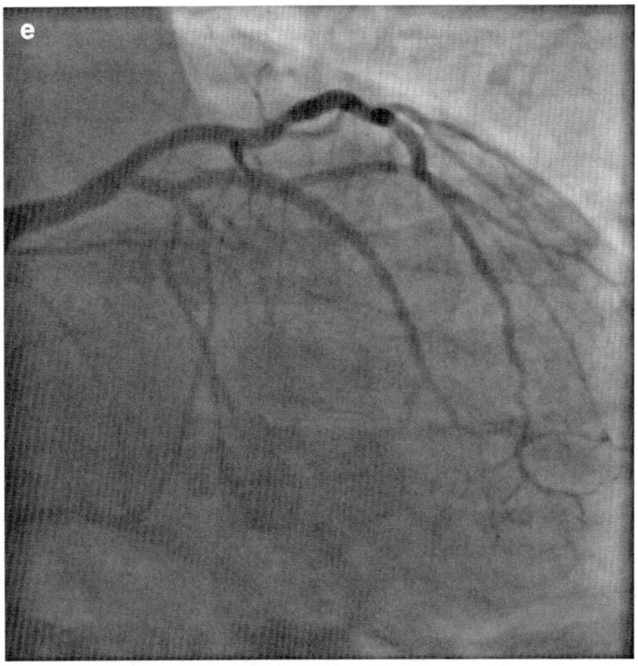


**Fig. 11.13** (continued)

the septal from distal to proximal at low pressure 2–3 atm, unless using a Sprinter legend 1.25 mm (Medtronic Inc., USA) in which case inflation pressures of 6–8 atm are preferred. If the balloon has not completely crossed, then dilate in the most distal position, employing pressures as noted above, and notice if after dilation the balloon moves forward. If it does, continue to dilate the entire septal. If unable to move forward, dilate proximally and then re-try the Corsair, making sure to rewet its outer hydrophilic coating.

2. If the Corsair still will not cross despite balloon dilation then use a new Corsair as these devices can lose their effectiveness with excessive turning. If neither a Corsair nor a balloon will cross, use a Finecross (Terumo, Japan) or a Turpike (Vascular Solutions, USA) catheter. Ensure that 150 cm lengths are used.
3. If these maneuvers are unsuccessful and if the wire used to cross was a Sion (Asahi-Intecc, Japan), place the Corsair as far distally as possible through the collateral channel and exchange the wire with a Fielder FC or Sion Blue (Asahi-Intecc, Japan) which have stiffer bodies, improving support.
4. Consider using a small mother-and-child catheter such as the 6F or 5.5F Guideliner, which could be delivered deeply into the donor vessel and increase the puschability of the Corsair through the collateral (Chap. 9, Fig. 9.15).
5. If these approaches all fail, wire a different collateral or leave the guidewire in place as a target wire and bail out to the antegrade approach and kissing wire technique.

For epicardial collateral channels, after guide support is maximized, consider using a new Corsair, and if this still will not cross, try a Finecross or Turnpike catheter. If neither of these makes further progress, take the Corsair as far as it will go and try to recross the epicardial channel with Fielder FC wire to gain better guidewire support for device passage. It is imperative not to push too hard with micro catheters in epicardial collaterals as they do not have as much structural support and this may result in collateral damage and perforation.

## Problem 8: Failure to Complete a Reverse CART Re-entry

### Definition

Inability to connect the distal true lumen to the proximal true lumen through the dissection path using a retrograde wire (reverse CART).

### Suggested Approach

Increase balloon size, exchanging to a stiffer wire with a longer distal tip bend and addition of an antegrade guide catheter extension help greatly. Finally moving the re-entry site proximally or distally to a more favorable position or changing to a CART approach.

1. The first option is to use a larger antegrade balloon. IVUS can be used to inform the operator of size of the vessel and the site within the occlusion where the antegrade and retrograde wires are in closest proximity. One practical alternative is to use a balloon of the size of the width of the knuckled wire. A balloon at least as large as the vessel should be used. After maximizing balloon size, use a stiffer guidewire with longer 2–4 mm 45° bend retrograde.
2. As mentioned in Chap. 9, mother-and-child catheter facilitated reverse-CART can be performed. It is preferable to deploy an 8 french Guideliner to the antegrade dissection [20], but smaller versions are easier to deliver more distally. To deliver the guide extension to the reentry zone, the reverse-CART balloon can be inflated in the occlusion segment and act as an anchor to help to track the guide extension down at the base of operation. The guide extension facilitates reentry by acting as a target to successfully direct a retrograde stiff wire (Chap. 9, Figs. 9.17 and 9.19).
3. Next, move the re-entry point either distally or proximally, usually to the place where the two systems lie closest together. This is easier when using a mother-and-child extension.
4. Finally, consider bringing in a balloon retrograde and try to pass an antegrade wire into the distal lumen thus converting to a traditional CART technique [21].

## Problem 9: The Wire Cannot Be Externalized Retrograde

### Definition

There are rare times when the retrograde Corsair is in the antegrade guide but externalization can't be completed or the patient is intolerant of the gear in the septum thus requiring conversion to antegrade approach. This situation is more common where the RG 3 wire (Asahi-Intecc, Japan) is not available and occurs in the setting of severe tortuosity or angulation of the collateral channel and donor vessel (e.g. when using grafts as retrograde conduits) or fatigue of the Corsair.

### Suggested Approach

In this situation it may be necessary to perform a "Tip in" or rendezvous technique in the guide described elsewhere [22, 23]. Alternatively, if the externalization has been completed but there is an urgent need to remove the retrograde gear, the use of a Twin-Pass (Vascular Solutions, US) catheter over the externalized wire to quickly deliver an antegrade wire followed by removal of the retrograde system is advocated.

## Problem 10: Retrograde Anatomic Ambiguity

### Definition

Retrograde anatomic ambiguity occurs often when the vessel has been previously bypassed and the retrograde wire keeps entering the bypass graft.

### Suggested Approach

In this situation distal injection through the Corsair into the true vessel lumen can help to highlight the true path of the vessel or the relationship of the vein graft to native artery. If unable to determine the vessel course, use of an antegrade wire or knuckled guidewire and attempting to bring this as close as possible to the retrograde guidewire to sort out the ambiguity and provide a target for a Confianza Pro 12 wire used retrograde through the Corsair can solve the problem (Chap. 9, Fig. 9.19).

## Summary

Narrowing the existing gap in the success rates, safety, and efficiency of chronic total occlusion percutaneous coronary intervention (CTO-PCI) relative to non CTO-PCI may be facilitated by a structured approach to common obstacles encountered even while employing the original Hybrid Approach. The new enhanced hybrid approach and its solutions to common problems is likely to further increase success rate while maintaining safety.

## References


1. Thompson CA, Jayne JE, Robb JF, Friedman BJ, Kaplan AV, Hettleman BD, et al. Retrograde techniques and the impact of operator volume on percutaneous intervention for coronary chronic total occlusions an early U.S. experience. JACC Cardiovasc Interv. 2009;2(9):834–42.
2. Morino Y, Kimura T, Hayashi Y, Muramatsu T, Ochiai M, Noguchi Y, et al. In-hospital outcomes of contemporary percutaneous coronary intervention in patients with chronic total occlusion insights from the J-CTO Registry (Multicenter CTO Registry in Japan). JACC Cardiovasc Interv. 2010;3(2):143–51.
3. Michael TT, Mogabgab O, Fuh E, Patel VG, El Sabbagh A, Alomar ME, et al. Application of the "hybrid approach" to chronic total occlusion interventions: a detailed procedural analysis. J Interv Cardiol. 2014;27(1):36–43.
4. Grantham JA, Marso SP, Spertus J, House J, Holmes Jr DR, Rutherford BD. Chronic total occlusion angioplasty in the United States. JACC Cardiovasc Interv. 2009;2(6):479–86.
5. Patel VG, Brayton KM, Tamayo A, Mogabgab O, Michael TT, Lo N, et al. Angiographic success and procedural complications in patients undergoing percutaneous coronary chronic total occlusion interventions: a weighted meta-analysis of 18,061 patients from 65 studies. JACC Cardiovasc Interv. 2013;6(2):128–36.
6. Karmpaliotis D, Lembo N, Kalynych A, Carlson H, Lombardi WL, Anderson CN, et al. Development of a high-volume, multiple-operator program for percutaneous chronic total coronary occlusion revascularization: procedural, clinical, and cost-utilization outcomes. Catheter Cardiovasc Interv. 2013;82(1):1–8.
7. Fefer P, Knudtson ML, Cheema AN, Galbraith PD, Osherov AB, Yalonetsky S, et al. Current perspectives on coronary chronic total occlusions: the Canadian Multicenter Chronic Total Occlusions Registry. J Am Coll Cardiol. 2012;59(11):991–7.
8. Brilakis ES, Grantham JA, Rinfret S, Wyman RM, Burke MN, Karmpaliotis D, et al. A percutaneous treatment algorithm for crossing coronary chronic total occlusions. JACC Cardiovasc Interv. 2012;5(4):367–79.
9. Morino Y, Abe M, Morimoto T, Kimura T, Hayashi Y, Muramatsu T, et al. Predicting successful guidewire crossing through chronic total occlusion of native coronary lesions within 30 minutes. JACC Cardiovasc Interv. 2011;4(2):213–21.
10. Muhammad KI, Lombardi WL, Christofferson R, Whitlow PL. Subintimal guidewire tracking during successful percutaneous therapy for chronic coronary total occlusions: Insights from an intravascular ultrasound analysis. Catheter Cardiovasc Interv. 2011;79(1):43–8.
11. Pershad A, Eddin M, Girotra S, Cotugno R, Daniels D, Lombardi W. Validation and incremental value of the hybrid algorithm for CTO PCI. Catheter Cardiovasc Interv. 2014;84(4):654–9.
12. Brilakis E, editor. Manual of coronary chronic total occlusion interventions: a step-by-step approach. 1st ed. Amsterdam/Boston: Academic Press; 2013.
13. Rathore S, Katoh O, Tuschikane E, Oida A, Suzuki T, Takase S. A novel modification of the retrograde approach for the recanalization of chronic total occlusion of the coronary arteries intravascular ultrasound-guided reverse controlled antegrade and retrograde tracking. JACC Cardiovasc Interv. 2010;3(2):155–64.
14. Carlino M, Latib A, Godino C, Cosgrave J, Colombo A. CTO recanalization by intraocclusion injection of contrast: the microchannel technique. Catheter Cardiovasc Interv. 2008;71(1):20–6.
15. Whitlow PL, Burke MN, Lombardi WL, Wyman RM, Moses JW, Brilakis ES, et al. Use of a novel crossing and re-entry system in coronary chronic total occlusions that have failed standard crossing techniques: results of the FAST-CTOs (Facilitated Antegrade Steering Technique in Chronic Total Occlusions) trial. JACC Cardiovasc Interv. 2012;5(4):393–401.

16. Brilakis ES, Banerjee S. Crossing the "balloon uncrossable" chronic total occlusion: Tornus to the rescue. Catheter Cardiovasc Interv. 2011;78(3):363–5.
17. Badr S, Ben-Dor I, Dvir D, Barbash IM, Kitabata H, Minha S, et al. The state of the excimer laser for coronary intervention in the drug-eluting stent era. Cardiovasc Revasc Med. 2013;14(2):93–8.
18. Vo M, Ravandi A, Grantham JA. Subintimal space plaque modification for "balloon uncrossable" chronic total occlusions. J Invasive Cardiol. 2014;26(10):E133–6.
19. Lindsay A. Subintimal TRAnscatheter Withdrawal (STRAW) of hematomas compressing the distal true lumen: a novel technique to facilitate distal re-entry during recanalization of chronic total occlusions. J Invasive Cardiol. 2015;27(1):E1–4.
20. Vo M, Brilakis ES. Faster, easier, safer: "guideliner reverse CART" for retrograde chronic total occlusion interventions. Catheter Cardiovasc Interv. 2014;83(6):933–5.
21. Surmely JF, Tsuchikane E, Katoh O, Nishida Y, Nakayama M, Nakamura S, et al. New concept for CTO recanalization using controlled antegrade and retrograde subintimal tracking: the CART technique. J Invasive Cardiol. 2006;18(7):334–8.
22. Kim MH, Yu LH, Mitsudo K. A new retrograde wiring technique for chronic total occlusion. Catheter Cardiovasc Interv. 2010; 75(1):117–9.
23. Funatsu A, Kobayashi T, Nakamura S. Use of the kissing microcatheter technique to exchange a retrograde wire for an antegrade wire in the retrograde approach to intervention in chronic total occlusion. J Invasive Cardiol. 2010;22(5):E74–7.
24. Smith EJ, De Mario C, Spratt JC, et al. Subintimal TRAnscatheter Withdrawal (STRAW) of hematomas compressing the distal true lumen: a novel technique to facilitate distal reentry during recanalization of chronic total occlusion (CTO). J Invasive Cardiol. 2015;27(1):E1–4.

# How to Improve Catheter Support During CTO PCI

**12**

Mohamad Lazkani and Ashish Pershad

**Abstract**

Catheter support during CTO PCI begins with careful selection of the appropriate guide catheter. Careful selection ensures coaxial alignment, allowing for delivery of equipment to the lesion, adequate opacification of the coronary arteries and support during PCI. The guide catheter selected is based on the vascular access used, coronary and aortic anatomy and specific lesion characteristics. Catheter support during CTO PCI relies not only on selecting the appropriate guide catheter, but also on guide catheter size, shape (passive support), sheath length, intubation depth of catheter into the vessel (active support), geometry and surface characteristics of the catheter support point and physical characterizes of the catheter materials. In this chapter nuances of enhancing guide support for CTO PCI will be discussed.

**Keywords**

PCI • CTO • Guide-catheter size • Guide-support • Anchoring • Sheath-length • Trap-balloon • Backup force • Catheter-stiffness

## Introduction

Backup support is defined as "the ability of the guiding catheter to remain in a stable position while PCI hardware is advanced over a guide wire without backing out" [1]. Guiding catheter support is fundamental for procedural success in CTO. Many CTO PCIs fail because of the inability to successfully cross the lesion with a wire, largely due to inadequate guiding catheter support. Selection of a guiding catheter in CTO PCI is different from non CTO PCI. Optimum guide catheter support is paramount for success and inappropriate guide-catheter selection will not only hinder success, but pose increased risk of procedural complications, such as coronary and aortic root dissections. It is imperative to select a guiding catheter that not only provides adequate support and allows for coaxial alignment but also has an adequate inner lumen for accommodating gear needed to successfully perform CTO PCI. The five major factors impacting guiding catheter support include guide catheter size, shape, extensions, anchoring techniques and sheath length.

M. Lazkani, MD
Department of Interventional Cardiology, Banner University Medical Center - Phoenix, Phoenix, AZ, USA

A. Pershad, MD, FACC, FSCAI (✉)
Division of Interventional Cardiology, Banner University Medical Center - Phoenix, Phoenix, AZ, USA
e-mail: ashish.pershad@bannerhealth.com

## Guide Catheter Size

Selecting the appropriately sized guide catheter is an important principle in improving catheter support during CTO PCI. Guide catheter size is determined by the size of the outer diameter. Catheter size is expressed using French (Fr)


S. Rinfret (ed.), *Percutaneous Intervention for Coronary Chronic Total Occlusion: The Hybrid Approach*, DOI 10.1007/978-3-319-21563-1_12

size, by multiplying the diameter of the catheter (in millimeters) by 3 in order to convert it from the metric system to the French scale. Guide catheters have become three times smaller over the last four decades. This is primarily from alteration in catheter design allowing for a larger internal diameter without increasing the external diameter, thus allowing larger devices to be accommodated within the lumen.

A tendency to move to smaller-sized guide catheters makes intuitive sense to reduce access site complications. A major study examining 103,070 consecutive patients that underwent PCI found significant relationship between the guide catheter size and overall PCI complications [2]. Compared with 6 Fr guides, PCIs performed with larger guides (7- and 8-Fr), were associated with more contrast use, more associated nephropathy, more bleeding, more vascular access site complications and greater need for post-procedure transfusions. Even in-hospital MACE and mortality was higher in the group in which larger size guide catheters were used [2]. However, with complex PCI such as with CTO lesions, larger sized catheters maintain their utility, providing better support and improved visualization of the coronary arteries, especially the collaterals. Larger sized guide catheters confer the ability to deliver gear-needed to perform CTO PCI. For example, removing or exchanging equipment through the "trapping balloon" technique is a popular strategy with CTO PCI (see Chap. 4). Seven Fr catheters allow for use of the Corsair (Asahi Intecc, Japan) or CrossBoss (Boston Scientific, US) with a "trapping balloon". Also, 8 Fr catheters allow real time IVUS guidance in conjunction with the Corsair (Asahi Intecc, Japan) or Stingray (Boston Scientific, US) balloon and a "trapping balloon".

Uncomplicated and straightforward PCI can certainly enjoy the perks of smaller guide catheters but with complex CTO PCI, the need for greater catheter support and use of multiple devices necessitates larger guide catheter size. The vascular complications associated with the use of larger guiding catheters can be mitigated by ultrasound-guided access; use of micro puncture technique and careful attention to access site within the common femoral artery [3]. Finally, given that CTO PCI is performed under heparin with close ACT monitoring, most series so far have reported very low rates of femoral complications, even when using bilateral femoral access with 8 F guides. Alternatively, experienced transradial operators can successfully perform CTO PCI using larger-bore (7 or 8 F) guides delivered without a sheath (see Chap. 13).

The guide catheter shafts not only have variable diameters but also have differences in their length and stiffness. The perfect guide catheter maintains the optimal balance between rigidity and flexibility. Guide catheter shaft stiffness is a function of the type of polymer used in its construction and is related to the thickness of its outer layer. Generally, the stiffer the guide catheter, the more support it provides and allows for better navigation through tortuous vessels. Furthermore, stiffer guide catheters have better curve retention. However, there is the potential for dissection and increased traumatic injury with stiff catheters. It is therefore important for even the most experienced operators to exercise caution in CTO PCI with the use of these large bore stiff guide catheters. Shortened guiding catheters (90 cm) such as those needed for retrograde CTO PCI have not been shown to impact catheter support in comparison to other factors such as catheter shape, size, material, configuration, and manipulation technique.

The route of vascular access also limits guide catheter size. CTO PCI can be accomplished from either the femoral approach or the radial approach but requires the operator to be familiar with the advantages and limitations of guide catheter support from each approach. Transradial approach for CTO PCI is not main stream but has been well established as being technically feasible [4]. The wide spread adoption of radial approach for CTO PCI has been limited due to the steep learning curve associated with managing multiple devices through a 6 or 7 Fr guiding catheter and difficult angles making support challenging. The key for successful CTO PCI via transradial approach is appropriate case selection and good non-CTO PCI experience. Sheathless guide catheters are a newer technology developed to address these limitations of transradial CTO PCI but how that impacts guide catheter support and device delivery has not been systematically studied (see Chap. 13).

## Guiding Catheter Shape

The choice of guide catheter shape used for intervention depends on the anatomy of the coronary artery, the location of the ostium (high, low, anterior, posterior, or anomalous) and size of the aortic root. Guide catheter shape can determine procedural outcomes since poor guide support can lead to CTO PCI failure. Prior to their insertion into the coronaries, guide catheters can generally be classified into two major types, those that are "over-bent" (Voda; Judkins; EBU and Q) and those that are "under-bent" (Amplatz and Multipurpose). Both types of catheters can retain "memory" or the ability to return to their default configuration after manipulation. The main difference between over-bent and under-bent guide catheters is the degree of manipulation required. Manipulation of "under-bent" catheters is harder and can lead to aortic root and coronary dissections. Manipulation is usually easier with "over-bent" catheters. Manipulation is vital to catheter alignment, allowing for an ideal coaxial position within the coronary ostium and adequate support along with aortic wall. The importance of coaxial alignment is that it permits transmission of forces

**Table 12.1** Active vs passive support with coronary guide catheters

| | Active support | Passive support |
|---|---|---|
| **Guide catheter tip** | Soft tips | Long tipped |
| **Guide catheter shape** | Can be altered to accommodate aortic root | Rests on aortic valve or opposite wall of the aorta |
| **Guide catheter size** | Active support decreases with larger guide catheter size | Passive support increases with larger guide catheter size |
| **Curves** | More flexible primary curves | Stiffer primary curves |
| **Risk of aortic or ostial coronary dissection** | Low | High |

needed to advance devices safely. This is accomplished by aligning the guide catheter tip along the long axis of the artery. The choice of catheter curve required for coaxial engagement depends on factors that include size of the aortic root, degree of support needed for device delivery and vessel characteristics [1].

For the right coronary artery (RCA), the catheter curves that provide the optimal alignment are the Amplatz, IMA, or Hockey Stick curves. Judkins right catheters may be beneficial if there is a proximal occlusion of the RCA and if retrograde approach is the primary strategy for the RCA CTO PCI and antegrade support is not vital. Inferior take-offs are best intubated with a multipurpose, Judkins, or an Amplatz catheter. With a wide aortic root, RCA cannulation is best accomplished with an Amplatz or multipurpose catheter [5].

For the left coronary system, the extra-back-up (EBU), XB, or Voda left, geometric left, or JCL and left Amplatz guiding catheters are commonly chosen. These catheters have larger primary curves and stiffer tips allowing the catheter to achieve better coaxial engagement and more passive support. XB and EBU catheters are usually preferred for LAD CTO PCI and CTO PCI of the left circumflex system is best managed with AL curves when the radial approach is used.

Guide catheter support has traditionally been divided into passive support and active support (Table 12.1). Active support is seen when the catheter is manipulated into a configuration that conforms to the aortic root. Passive support primarily relies on the stiffness of the guide catheter at the primary curve. An example of passive support is placing the guide catheter back up against the opposite wall for support. Current trends with using guiding catheters for CTO PCI is to maximize both active and passive guide support. With left coronary artery engagement, there are three major factors associated with backup force of guiding catheters: catheter size, angle (theta) of the catheter on the reverse side of the aorta and contact area. The angle (theta) determines the vertical vector that can dislodge the guiding catheter and therefore a lower position is preferable as the point of contact on the reverse side of the aorta because the angle approaches 90° [6]. Larger contact area provides more support due to increased friction. With right coronary artery engagement, the primary attachment site has the greatest impact on backup force, but varies with different catheters. This primary site is the supporting point for generating the required force to pass a device through a tight lesion [7].

Side holed catheters are sometimes essential when there is proximal disease of the coronary and if the pressure wave form dampens on engaging the coronary. The major advantage with the use of guide catheters that have side holes is the ability to monitor arterial pressure although anterograde flow into the vessel may not be adequate and patients may still get ischemic even with an adequate wave form and a side holed catheter. Theoretically, the risk of a hydraulic coronary dissection is also reduced with side holes. The disadvantage of side holed catheters is the additional contrast use and the kinking of the catheter that can occur at the site of the side holes. It is not recommended to use side holed catheters in the left coronaries unless there is ostial left main disease that prevents safe engagement of the guide.

## Guide Catheter Extensions

Guide extensions provide additional guide catheter support by deep intubation of the coronary vessels. Examples include the HeartRail (Terumo, Japan), Guideliner (Vascular Solutions, US) or Guidezilla (Boston Scientific, US) devices which are designed for deep seating in coronary arteries, thereby contributing to increased back-up support. They have also been shown to boost success rates in CTO PCI [8]. Guide catheter extensions are particularly useful when the takeoff of the coronary ostium prevents coaxial engagement of the guiding catheter. The deep-intubation of the target coronary vessel by the softer, flexible extension catheter ensures coaxial alignment, alleviating this problem. For example, the GuideLiner catheter consists of a flexible 20 cm straight guide extension connected to a stainless-steel push shaft, allowing for additional support within the coronary vessel (see Chap. 3). It allows deep engagement into the coronary vessel, providing backup support when device delivery is attempted through challenging anatomy. The Guidezilla guide extension catheter has a 1×1 braid that provides improved back-up guide support without over-straightening the vessel. The HeartRail coronary guiding catheter extension is a coaxial system with a flexible shaft that provides track ability even in tortuous vessels. Its increased lumen size enables lower device friction for delivery of devices to and beyond the lesion. When using the HeartRail or other extension catheters, successful stent delivery is contingent upon the intubation depth, showing markedly improved success rates with depth >2 cm [8]. With all the guide catheter extensions, the support provided is exponentially related to the length seated within the coronary artery. Caution needs to be exercised with their use because of reports of stent shearing and entanglement; proximal vessel dissection and even loss of the distal tip of the catheter in the vessel [9]. These catheter extensions also have niche roles in retrograde CTO PCI [10].

## Anchoring Support

Sometimes modifying the guiding catheter shape is not enough to provide the necessary support needed to complete CTO PCI.

In such instances anchoring techniques are required.

(a) Side branch Anchor Technique:
A workhorse guidewire is advanced into a sidebranch (usually a conus or acute marginal in the setting of the RCA and a diagonal for the LAD) followed by advancing a small diameter balloon like a 1.5 mm or 2 mm balloon. The balloon is inflated at 6–8 atmospheres anchoring the guide in the vessel (Fig. 12.1a). This then facilitates advancement of balloons and micro catheters. Side branch anchor technique offers the advantage of contrast injection and unobstructed access to the CTO [11].

(b) Proximal vessel anchor technique:
Sometimes there are no suitable side branches into which a balloon can be safely inflated. In such situations, inflation of a semi-compliant balloon at nominal inflation pressures in the proximal vessel over a buddy wire can also be done to enhance support within the system.

(c) Power Anchor Modification of the Proximal vessel anchor technique:
When a balloon is inflated adjacent to a microcatheter like a Corsair or Finecross within the proximal vessel to pin the micro catheter against the wall of the artery, the maneuver is called 'power anchor modification' of the proximal anchor technique.

(d) Distal anchor technique – Intimal or subintimal:
In difficult non CTO lesion subsets, it may be possible to advance a buddy wire into the distal vessel and inflate a low profile balloon to facilitate delivery of a stent. Obviously this is not something that can be done in a total occlusion. However a modification of this approach has been described wherein a wire is advanced in the subintimal plane beyond where the microcatheter is stuck and a balloon is inflated distally in the subintimal plane intentionally to anchor the true lumen guide wire enabling the antegrade advancement of the microcatheter past the point it was stuck into the true lumen in the distal vessel (Fig. 12.1b) [12].

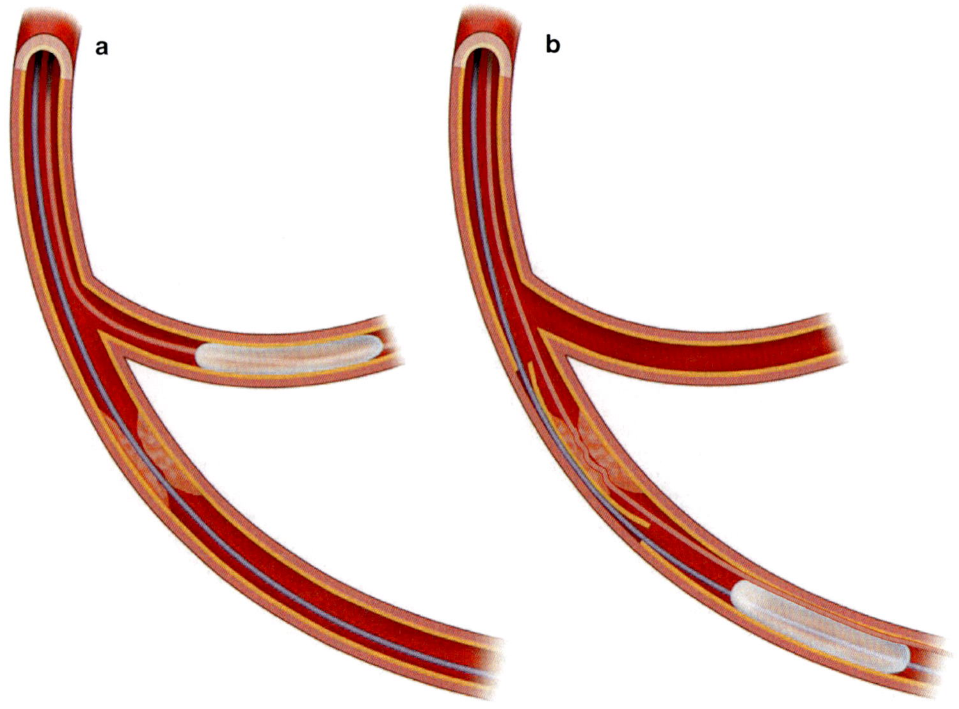


**Fig. 12.1** Different anchoring modalities for guide catheter stabilization. (**a**) Anchoring of a balloon in the side branch proximal to the lesion. (**b**) Subintimal distal anchoring of a balloon in the PDA distal to the lesion-using the subintimal space

Anchoring techniques are not without their risks and limitations. The side branch anchor technique is very safe unless the balloon is oversized or over aggressively dilated. The major problem with anchoring is that with the advancement of gear, the entire system may flail and disengage from the coronary artery. In bench models, the guide extension catheters have been shown to provide greater support than anchoring techniques. Nonetheless the techniques described above are extremely helpful in day to day practice of CTO PCI.

## Newer Support Catheters

The Prodigy (Radius Medical, Boston, MA) support catheter is one such newer support catheter that has the ability to enhance support. It is a 5Fr catheter with an elastomeric balloon inflated to 1 atm that is designed to be used for vessels between 2 and 6 mm diameter. Once inflated it "locks" in place allowing for advancement of wires through the resistant lesion or proximal cap of the CTO without the catheter backing out (Fig. 12.2a). The balloon has a release valve mechanism so as to not allow inadvertent overinflation of the balloon thereby preventing vessel injury or balloon slippage. The clinical experience with this catheter is still limited.

Another set of new catheters, CenterCross (Fig. 12.2b) and MultiCross (Fig. 12.2c) (Roxwood Medical, US) help boost antegrade guide support. They have a unique design to enable centering within the vessel architecture with the ability to even advance a microcatheter like a Corsair through one of the multichannels present within the lumen of the microcatheter thereby greatly enhancing support for antegrade CTO PCI. Again, the experience with such novel catheters is limited and their effectiveness in current practice needs to be established.

## Sheath Length

The length of the sheath inserted into the arterial system is another underappreciated yet important factor in providing maximal support for the guide catheter. Long, reinforced sheaths help improve passive support to the guiding catheters as well as improve ability to torque catheters in patients that have peripheral vascular disease and tortuosity. Because the use of long sheaths increases passive support with minimal additional risks, the adage that longer is better applies to sheaths for CTO PCI. Standard sheath lengths range from 6 to 23 cm, the majority of sheaths being 10 cm in length. In traditional PCI, compared to CTO PCI, shorter sheaths are typically recommended to minimize amount of material in the vascular space. However, in CTO PCI, guiding catheter support and manipulation is paramount and therefore routine use of long sheaths is advocated, even up to 45 cm in length, usually reaching the level of the diaphragm. To give perspective, the standard length of a guide catheter is 100 cm, therefore long sheaths provide up to 45 % coverage of a standard guide catheter.

The most common configuration of sheaths for CTO PCI is bi-femoral. In this approach, 8 Fr long sheaths are used because they eliminate the potential issues with iliac and aortic tortuosity that may impede the ability to torque devices within the coronary artery. Longer sheaths straighten tortuosity in the iliac arteries and therefore allow for enhanced guide catheter manipulation and one-to-one torque transmission.

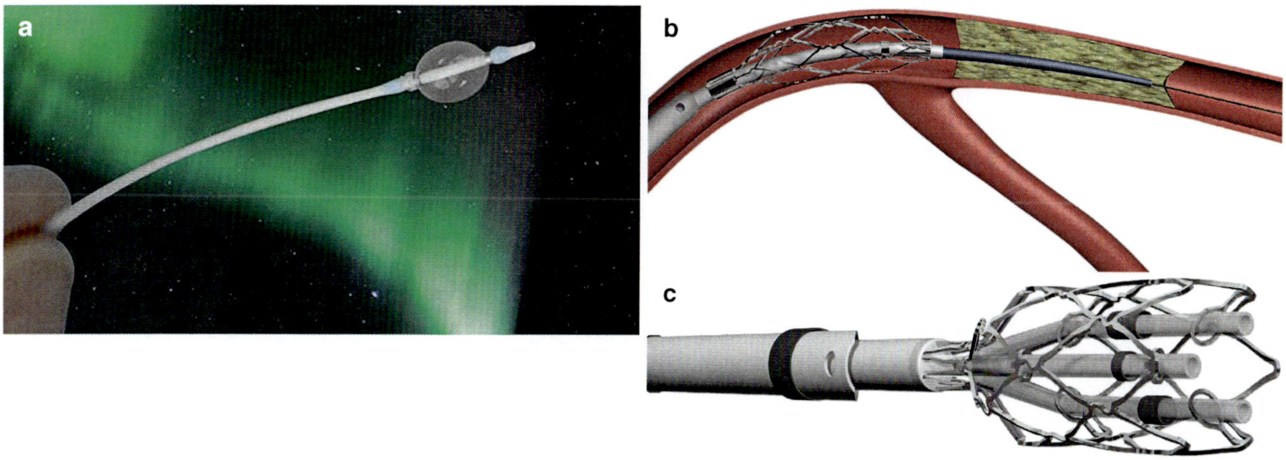


**Fig. 12.2** (a) Prodigy support catheter. (b) CenterCross support catheter. (c) Multicross support catheter (a: Courtesy of Radius Medical; b and c: Courtesy of Roxwood Medical)

There is a small potential for increased thrombotic risk with the use of long sheaths, but in CTO PCI, careful attention is paid to adequate anticoagulation to mitigate this concern.

**Conclusions**

In summary, enhancing guide catheter support for successful CTO PCI is one of the most important components of the procedure. Multiple techniques for enhancing guide support have been described in this comprehensive review. These techniques are not mutually exclusive and often have to be used together. These techniques are not only useful in CTO PCI but also in other complex PCI procedures.

## References


1. Prashant PU. Current and emerging catheter technologies for percutaneous transluminal coronary angioplasty. Re Rep Clin Cardiol. 2014;2014(5):213–26.
2. Grossman PM, Gurm HS, McNamara R, Lalonde T, Changezi H, Share D, Smith DE, Chetcuti SJ, Moscucci M, Blue Cross Blue Shield of Michigan Cardiovascular Consortium (BMC2). Percutaneous coronary intervention complications and guide catheter size: bigger is not better. JACC Cardiovasc Interv. 2009;2(7):636–44.
3. Lee MS, Applegate B, Rao SV, Kirtane AJ, Seto A, Stone GW. Minimizing femoral artery access complications during percutaneous coronary intervention: a comprehensive review. Catheter Cardiovasc Interv. 2014;84(1):62–9.
4. Rinfret S, Joyal D, Nguyen CM, Bagur R, Hui W, Leung R, Larose E, Love MP, Mansour S. Retrograde recanalization of chronic total occlusions from the transradial approach; early Canadian experience. Catheter Cardiovasc Interv. 2011;78(3):366–74.
5. Ge JB. Current status of percutaneous coronary intervention of chronic total occlusion. J Zhejiang Univ Sci B. 2012;13(8):589–602.
6. Ikari Y, Nagaoka M, Kim JY, Morino Y, Tanabe T. The physics of guiding catheters for the left coronary artery in transfemoral and transradial interventions. J Invasive Cardiol. 2005;17(12):636–41.
7. Ikari Y, Masuda N, Matsukage T, Ogata N, Nakazawa G, Tanabe T, Morino Y. Backup force of guiding catheters for the right coronary artery in transfemoral and transradial interventions. J Invasive Cardiol. 2009;21(11):570–4.
8. Mamas MA, Eichhofer J, Hendry C, El-Omar M, Clarke B, Neyses L, Fath-Ordoubadi F, Fraser D. Use of the Heartrail II catheter as a distal stent delivery device; an extended case series. EuroIntervention. 2009;5(2):265–71.
9. Brilakis ES, Grantham JA, Banerjee S. "Ping-pong" guide catheter technique for retrograde intervention of a chronic total occlusion through an ipsilateral collateral. Catheter Cardiovasc Interv. 2011;78(3):395–9.
10. Chang YC, Fang HY, Chen TH, Wu CJ. Left main coronary artery bidirectional dissection caused by injection of guideliner catheter from the guiding catheter. Catheter Cardiovasc Interv. 2013;82(3):E215–20.
11. Shah SB, Heuser RR. CTO: Current Technique Overview: a look at today's strategies used to treat coronary chronic total occlusions. Cardiac Interv Today. 2009;109(2):58–63.
12. Michael TT, Banerjee S, Brilakis ES. Subintimal distal anchor technique for "balloon uncrossable" chronic total occlusions. J Invasive Cardiol. 2013;25(10):552–4.

# When and How to Perform a Transradial Approach for CTO PCI

# 13

Khaldoon Alaswad and Stéphane Rinfret

**Abstract**

The radial artery (RA) access has been used to perform chronic total occlusion percutaneous coronary intervention (CTO PCI) with similar success and safety to CTO PCI using the common femoral artery (CFA) access. The success of a complex CTO PCI depends at the beginning on the use of two supportive guiding catheters with large enough lumen to accommodate multiple devices simultaneously. Two arterial accesses are needed in most CTO PCIs. Bilateral CFA accesses are frequently used to accommodate large bore supportive guiding catheters. Few CTO PCI operators combine one CFA access with one RA access to decrease potential bleeding complications from bilateral CFA accesses. However, operators from Canada and the United States have shown that CTO PCI using bilateral RA accesses have similar success rates and safety to CTO PCI from CFA accesses. They adapted all the current CTO PCI techniques to the 6 Fr guiding catheters from the RA access. They routinely perform antegrade dissection and re-entry (ADR) and retrograde techniques including controlled antegrade and retrograde tracking and reentry (CART) and reverse CART, using 6 Fr guiding catheters from bilateral RA accesses. More recently, techniques have been developed to use 7 or 8 Fr guiding catheters from the radial artery. This chapter describes the procedure of CTO PCI from bilateral RA accesses, and some of the difficulties encountered and their troubleshooting during these complex procedures.

**Keywords**

Radial artery access in CTO PCI • Patient positioning for radial artery access • Access to radial artery • Guiding catheter • Guiding catheter and radial artery • Hybrid algorithm and transradial approach

## Rationale for Radial Artery Access in CTO PCI

The radial artery (RA) access has been used to perform chronic total occlusion percutaneous coronary intervention (CTO PCI) with similar success and safety to CTO PCI using the common femoral artery (CFA) access [1–4]. The success of a complex CTO PCI depends at the beginning on the use of two supportive guiding catheters with large enough lumen to accommodate multiple devices simultaneously. Two arterial accesses are needed in most CTO PCIs [3, 5, 6]. Bilateral CFA accesses are frequently used to accommodate large bore supportive guiding catheters. Few CTO PCI operators

K. Alaswad, MD
Section of Cardiology, Department of Medicine, Henry Ford Hospital, Detroit, MI, USA

S. Rinfret, MD, SM (✉)
CTO Recanalization Program, Interventional Cardiology, Multidisciplinary Department of Cardiology, Quebec Heart and Lung Institute, Laval University, Quebec City, QC, Canada
e-mail: Stephane.Rinfret@criucpq.ulaval.ca


S. Rinfret (ed.), *Percutaneous Intervention for Coronary Chronic Total Occlusion: The Hybrid Approach*, DOI 10.1007/978-3-319-21563-1_13

combine one CFA access with one RA access to decrease potential bleeding complications from bilateral CFA accesses [2]. However, operators from Canada and the United States have shown that CTO PCI using bilateral RA accesses have similar success rates and safety to CTO PCI from CFA accesses [1, 7]. They adapted all the current CTO PCI techniques to the 6 Fr guiding catheters from the RA access. They routinely perform antegrade dissection and re-entry (ADR) and retrograde techniques including controlled antegrade and retrograde tracking and reentry (CART) and reverse CART, using 6 Fr guiding catheters from bilateral RA accesses. More recently, techniques have been developed to use 7 or 8 Fr guiding catheters from the radial artery.

Because CTO PCI requires two arterial accesses, the bleeding risk reduction with bilateral RA accesses as compared to bilateral CFA accesses is more pronounced during CTO PCI than non-CTO PCI, which mostly requires only one arterial puncture site. In addition to reduction in access site bleeding complications, bilateral RA access during CTO PCI decreases non-bleeding access site complications and facilitate early ambulation and discharge [8]. CTO PCI from bilateral RA access as compared to bilateral CFA access can decrease the cost of the procedure; nursing care of patients post CTO PCI with bilateral RA access is likely less demanding than patient care after bilateral femoral artery access; in addition, currently available closure devices for radial artery access are significantly cheaper than closure devices for the common femoral artery access. More importantly, quality of life parameters and patient's satisfaction are significantly better after transradial artery CTO PCI when compared to procedures performed via CFA access [9–11].

Operators trying to learn CTO PCI from radial artery accesses should be proficient in complex non-CTO PCI from the RA access. Meanwhile they should continue to use their default arterial access for CTO PCI during the learning processes [12]. This chapter describes the procedure of CTO PCI from bilateral RA accesses, and some of the difficulties encountered and their troubleshooting during these complex procedures.

## When to Choose the Radial Artery Access for CTO PCI

Bilateral RA accesses can be the default access during CTO PCI by operators who are proficient with the RA access. Several studies have shown that transradial CTO PCI is associated with similar success rates to CTO PCI from bilateral CFA access [1, 3, 7, 13]. However transradial CTO PCI was associated with increased radiation and procedure time [1].

CTO PCI operators who routinely use the CFA access should also develop the skills required to perform transradial CTO PCI, because certain conditions require the use of at least one radial artery access site to ensure success and to improve safety (Table 13.1). Radial artery access is necessary when the CTO PCI procedure requires more than two arterial access sites; for example, in patients with previous coronary artery bypass grafting (CABG), a third arterial access during the CTO PCI might be needed if a graft provides flow to additional collaterals, especially if the visualization is lost while trying to cross another collateral channel. A third guiding catheter from a third arterial access in patients with previous CABG will save time, radiation and contrast by avoiding guiding catheter exchanges to engage different collaterals from different donor arteries. Also, at least one radial artery access is necessary in patients who need hemodynamic support device placement from a common femoral artery access during the CTO PCI procedure that precludes the use of one common femoral artery for the second guiding catheter. Finally, the radial artery might be the last available access site in patients with occlusion in the common femoral or iliac arteries, and will be certainly safer than a brachial access. Patients at high risk for groin complications are better treated from radial artery access [8, 14].

Few conditions make radial artery access either difficult or contraindicated (Table 13.1). The common femoral artery is the preferred access if the radial artery is absent surgically, occluded, cannot be crossed with the wire, or cannot accommodate a 6 Fr introducer sheath. CFA access is preferred in

**Table 13.1** Conditions where the radial or the femoral access should be preferred during CTO PCI

| Radial artery access is critically important for the success of the CTO PCI | Common femoral artery access is preferred during CTO PCI |
|---|---|
| Post CABG patients when CTO PCI requires more than 2 arterial accesses | Anatomically absent radial artery |
| The need of hemodynamic support device via common femoral artery access | Radial artery that cannot accommodate a 6 Fr introducer |
| Peripheral artery disease with occlusion of the aorta, iliac or common femoral arteries | Anatomic variation that prevent radial artery crossing with the wire or the guiding catheter |
| Patients at high risk for femoral access site complications | Significant subclavian or brachiocephalic tortuosity |
| | Patients who may need permanent hemodialysis access |
| | Ostial or very proximal chronic total occlusion |

cases of severe subclavian or brachiocephalic tortuosity that makes the manipulation of the guiding catheter very difficult. The radial artery should not be used in patients with end stage renal disease that might need future permanent hemodialysis access in the upper extremities [10]. At the current level of technology development, a 5 Fr guiding catheter should never be used to perform CTO PCI. Therefore, if a 6 Fr guiding catheter cannot be advanced through the radial artery, a CFA access should be used instead. Finally, CFA access with a large bore catheter might be needed for technical reasons during CTO PCI if the lesion is ostial or very proximal in the coronary artery, because guiding catheter support enhancement techniques like deep guide catheter engagement or mother-and-child techniques are not possible. At the same time, with the lack of a proper landing zone for the tip of the guide catheter, it may become extremely difficult to keep the guiding catheter engaged in the coronary ostium during deep inspiration; the guiding catheter from the radial access does not move in the same direction as the diaphragm and the heart and might disengage from the coronary artery ostium during the respiratory cycle. On the other hand, a guiding catheter inserted from a CFA access tends to move in sync with the diaphragm and the heart during the respiratory cycle and stays engaged in the coronary artery ostium during deep inspiration.

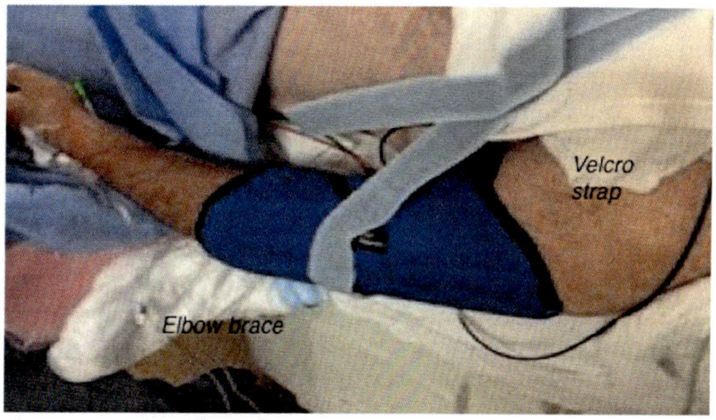


**Fig. 13.1** Velcro that help pull the patient's left arm to the right side of the table closer to the operator. Please notice the elbow immobilizer that keeps the arm straight to facilitate catheter and wire manipulations

## Patient Positioning and Gaining Access

Radial artery access should be obtained per common practices. The wrist should be retroflexed during access with a micro-puncture kit or an angiocath and a 0.035″ straight tip guide wire. The preferred right arm position for CTO PCI from the right radial artery is next to the patient because the operator needs to stay close to the patient to reach the other access in the left radial artery. The left radial artery access poses ergonomic difficulties, because most operators stand on the right side of the patient and have to reach over the patient; otherwise, the patient's left arm should be pulled to the right side close to the operator. Currently, there are no good available systems to keep the left arm in position close to the operator on the right side of the patient. The left arm tends to fall away from the operator standing on the right side of the patient causing discomfort to the patient, and/or the operator. One solution to the left arm positioning problem is to pull the arm to the right side of the patient using an arm restraint that is tied to the right side of the cath lab table (Fig. 13.1). The patient sometimes tends to bend the left elbow, which will pull the guiding catheter away from the operator and decrease equipment-control; left elbow orthopedic immobilizer will keep the left elbow straight and facilitate the manipulation of the left arm guiding catheter and the interventional gear from the same side. Placing a pillow to prop the left arm up might keep the arm close to the operator standing on the right side of the catheterization table. Until we find better techniques to keep the left arm of the patient pulled close to the right side toward the operator, it is easier to position both arms next to the patient after obtaining access (Fig. 13.2). However, reaching over the patient to the left wrist might be difficult in obese patients with large abdomens. The patient's hands should be placed in a natural position after obtaining access to avoid discomfort to the patient during lengthy CTO PCI procedures.

## Introducer Sheath Selection for Radial Artery Access for CTO PCI

Because the CTO PCI frequently requires the use of multiple devices simultaneously in one guiding catheter [6], it is important to use the largest sheath that can fit in the radial artery when obtaining radial artery access for CTO PCI for the antegrade side. While most patients tolerate a 6 Fr sheath, 7 or 8 Fr sheaths can sometimes be used for CTO PCI from the RA access. Studies showed that hydrophilic sheaths are easier to insert in the radial artery with less risk of entrapment [15]. However, the outer diameter of commercially available sheaths is considerably larger than the outer diameter of the corresponding size guiding catheter. If the patient cannot tolerate a large sheath, a thin wall sheath, or ad hoc or dedicated sheathless guiding catheters can be used. Thin wall sheaths are now commercially available, with smaller outer diameter than the same French size conventional sheath; the outer diameter of a 6 Fr thin wall sheath is similar to the outer diameter of a conventional 5 Fr sheath (Fig. 13.3). Patients might have better tolerance if the sheath outer diameter is smaller or the guiding catheter is introduced without an introducer sheath. Moreover, it may prevent subsequent radial artery occlusion, a benign

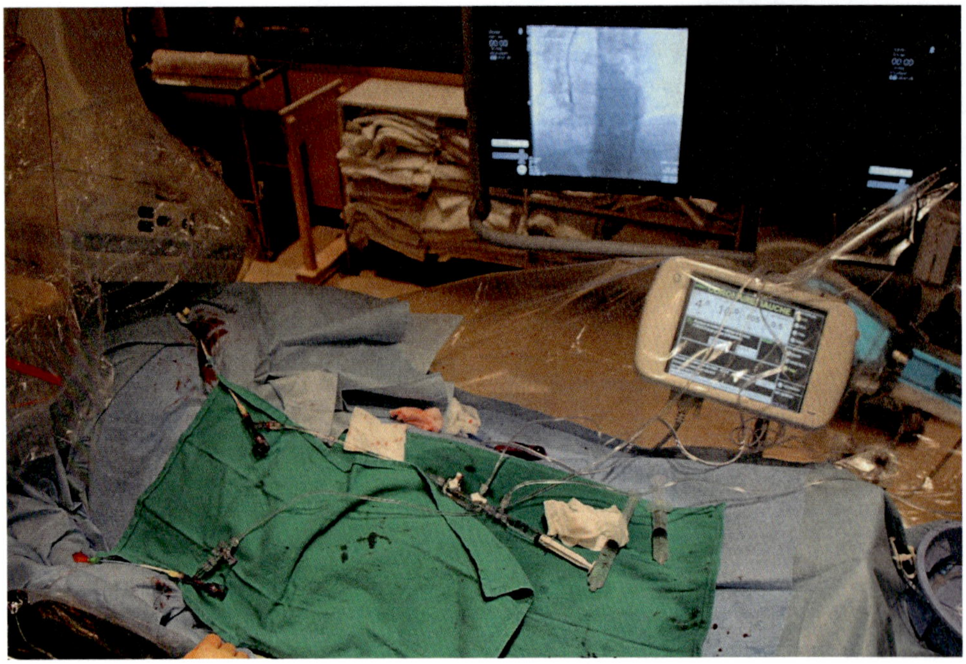

**Fig. 13.2** Dual radial set up at the table

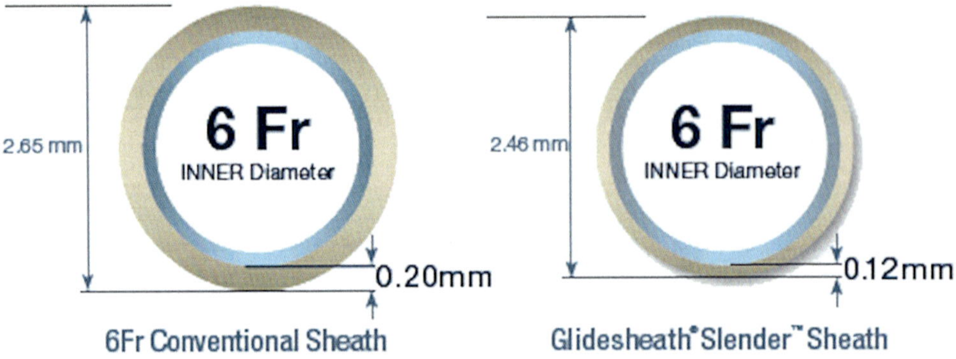


**Fig. 13.3** Thin wall sheath outer diameter and wall thickness are smaller than conventional sheath (Glidesheath Slender ® Introducer Sheath image provided courtesy of Terumo Medical Corporation)

complication, yet precluding future access from the occluded site.

Unlike in femoral artery access, longer sheaths do not provide incremental support from the radial artery access and might increase patients' discomfort and the risk of sheath entrapment at the end of the procedure. Therefore, the preferred sheath length for radial artery access is 13 cm or shorter. The sheath should not be forced in the radial artery if it encounters significant resistance; in this case, the sheath could be used despite being partly advanced in the radial artery, or the operator could use an ad hoc or predesigned sheathless guide catheter system, described later in this chapter.

The left hand tends to pronate during the procedure, which will hide the sheath from the operator. The left radial artery sheath might slip out of the artery unnoticed during the guiding catheter manipulation; thus the left radial artery sheath can be sutured to the skin or secured in place with adhesive material to prevent the sheath from slipping out of the radial artery.

## Guiding Catheter Selection During CTO PCI from the Radial Artery

Large guiding catheters with supportive configuration are needed to facilitate the use of multiple wires, balloons, and specialized devices simultaneously in one guiding catheter. The most important limitation during CTO PCI from a bilateral radial artery access is the need to use smaller guiding catheter size (6 Fr versus 7 or 8 Fr); otherwise, there should be few technical differences related to guiding catheter manipulation and patient positioning between CTO PCI from bilateral CFA accesses and bilat-

**Table 13.2** Compatibility of different CTO PCI techniques with different guiding catheters

| Guiding catheters | 5 Fr sheath + GC | 6 Fr sheath + GC | 6.5 Fr sheathless | 7 Fr sheath + GC | 7.5 Fr sheathless | 8 Fr sheath + GC |
|---|---|---|---|---|---|---|
| Internal diameter (inches) | 0.56–0.58 | 0.70–0.71 | 0.7 | 0.78–0.81 | 0.81 | 0.88–0.90 |
| External diameter at the arterial access site (mm) | 2.3 | 2.52–2.60 | 2.16 | 2.85–3.10 | 2.49 | 3.20–3.50 |
| Parallel wire technique (antegrade CTO PCI technique) | | | | | | |
| Wire + 1 microcatheter | Yes | Yes | Yes | Yes | Yes | Yes |
| 2 microcatheters | No | Yes | Yes | Yes | Yes | Yes |
| 1 microcatheter + 1 OTW balloon | No | No | No | Yes | Yes | Yes |
| 2 OTW balloons | No | No | No | No | No | Yes |
| Side-branch anchoring balloon and balloon trapping (useful for both antegrade and retrograde CTO PCI techniques) | | | | | | |
| 1 monorail balloon + 1 microcatheter | No | Yes[a] | Yes[a] | Yes | Yes | Yes |
| 1 monorail balloon + 1 OTW balloon | No | Yes[b] | Yes[b] | Yes | Yes | Yes |
| CTO PCI: IVUS-guidance (useful for both antegrade and retrograde CTO PCI techniques) | | | | | | |
| With simultaneous wire inside | Yes | Yes | Yes | Yes | Yes | Yes |
| With simultaneous microcatheter inside | No | No | No | Yes | Yes | Yes |
| Adjunctive devices (useful for both antegrade and retrograde CTO PCI techniques) | | | | | | |
| Rotablator 1.25–1.75 mm burr | No | Yes[c] | Yes | Yes | Yes | Yes |
| Rotablator 2.0–2.25 mm burr | No | No | No | Yes | Yes | Yes |
| Laser 0.9–1.4 mm | Yes | Yes | Yes | Yes | Yes | Yes |
| Laser 1.7–2.2 mm | No | No | No | Yes | Yes | Yes |
| Tornus 2.1 F | No | Yes | Yes | Yes | Yes | Yes |
| Tornus 2.6 F | No | Yes | Yes | Yes | Yes | Yes |
| Corsair | No | Yes | Yes | Yes | Yes | Yes |
| CrossBoss catheter | No | Yes | Yes | Yes | Yes | Yes |
| Stingray CTO re entry device | No | Yes | Yes | Yes | Yes | Yes |

From Burzotta et al. [3] with permission
Data from bench testing with the following materials:
Guiding Catheters (GC): 5, 6, 7, and 8 Fr Vista Brite Tip (Cordis) and Sherpa NX Active and Launcher (Medtronic), Eaucath Sheathless 6.5 and 7.5 Fr (Asahi)
Microcatheters: Finecross (Terumo); Quickcross (Spectranetis); over-the-wire (OTW)
Monorail Balloons: Sprinter Legend 1.25 mm (Medtronic); Mini Trek 1.20 mm (Abbott), Ryujin 1.25 mm (Terumo), Emerge 1.25 mm (Boston Scientific)
IVUS: Atlantis Pro (Boston Scientific)
[a]Feasible with Finecross, Quickcross, Tornus 2.1 Fr microcatheters but not with Corsair and CrossBoss and Stingray device
[b]Feasible but not advisable (too much friction)
[c]Feasible with a 1.75 mm burr but not advisable (too much friction) GC, guiding catheter

eral RA accesses. Several CTO PCI techniques require simultaneous introduction of two or more devices in the same guiding catheter. Most commercially available devices fit simultaneously with other device in an 8 Fr guiding catheter. However, 7 Fr and 6 Fr guiding catheters are most commonly used during RA access CTO PCI. The choice of devices that can fit simultaneously inside 7 or 6 Fr guiding catheter is more complex, as listed in Table 13.2 [3].

The inner diameter of same size guiding catheters varies according to the manufacturers. Operators should choose a catheter that provides the largest inner diameter, as the guiding catheter inner diameter choice becomes more important when using a 6 Fr guiding catheter. However, a larger inner diameter will turn the catheter to be more prone to kinking; therefore, careful manipulation of such guides is required.

Similar to those used in CTO PCI from bilateral CFA accesses, guiding catheters shapes for CTO PCI from bilateral RA accesses should provide optimal passive support. Larger guiding catheter curves should be used during CTO PCI procedures when possible from the antegrade side [16]. However, a 6 F guide catheter provides enough space and support on the retrograde side for the majority of cases, while preventing to some extent donor artery trauma.

## Advancing and Manipulating the Guiding Catheter from the Radial Artery

The guiding catheter can be advanced most of the time through an introducer sheath over a 0.035″ guide wire. Occasionally, other maneuvers have to be used to facilitate advancing the guiding catheter through a small radial artery:

1. Balloon-assisted tracking of the guiding catheter through the radial artery, where the guiding catheter is advanced with a 3 mm coronary balloon inflated at the tip of the guiding catheter over a 0.014 coronary wire [17].
2. Advancing the guiding catheter sheathless with either a 110 cm long 5 or 6 Fr sheath dilator or a 0.035 un-inflated peripheral vascular balloon.

Some operators will flush the radial artery with lubricant like Rotaglide (Boston Scientific, US) or ViperSlide (CSI, US) to facilitate the guiding catheter advancement, especially when using a sheathless technique. After the guiding catheter is advanced to the aortic root, it is frequently necessary to keep a 0.035″ or larger guide wire inside the guiding catheter to facilitate the manipulation of the guiding catheters from the radial artery accesses. If a guide wire larger than 0.035″ is not available, two 0.035″ guide wires might facilitate the guiding catheter manipulation in patients with extreme tortuosity in the brachiocephalic artery. Extra stiff guidewire can also help with the manipulations in these circumstances.

Because engaging the guiding catheter in the RCA requires more manipulation than engaging in the left main, it is technically easier to engage the RCA first then the LCA. Manipulating the RCA guiding catheter is more difficult if the LCA guiding catheter is already engaged and it could move the LCA guiding catheter out of its position.

## Enhancing Guiding Catheter Support from the Radial Artery Access Site

It is important to use the largest diameter possible and the most supportive shapes during CTO PCI, especially for the antegrade guide. An 8 Fr guiding catheter provides considerably more support than a 6 Fr guiding catheter [18]. Passively supportive guiding catheters that sit against the opposite aortic wall while extending deep in the coronary artery ostia provide better support than actively supportive guiding catheters, which need dynamic deep engagement to provide additional guiding catheter support. A choice of supportive guiding catheter from the beginning will save time, radiation and contrast by decreasing the need for guiding catheter support enhancing techniques.

The orientation of the guiding catheter from the subclavian artery to the coronary artery ostia is crucial for support enhancement; the left radial artery access provides better guiding catheter engagement and support in the RCA, while the right radial artery access provides better engagement and support in the LCA.

Other techniques to enhance the support of guiding catheters are frequently necessary during CTO PCI regardless of the arterial access; these methods are well explained in another chapter in this book (Chap. 12), and include buddy wire, balloon anchoring, and or mother-and-child extension catheters.

A 6 Fr guiding catheter has less space to accommodate a microcatheter, and anchoring wire or anchoring balloon (Table 13.3). It is important to remember that the internal effective lumen of the guiding catheter becomes a 5 Fr when using a mother-and-child extension to enhance the guiding catheter support in a 6 Fr guiding catheter; a 5 Fr guiding catheter lumen is not large enough to accommodate multiple devices simultaneously. The commercially available 6 Fr guiding catheters are associated with additional limitations during CTO PCI beside potential lack of support; the effective lumen does not allow the trapping of the coronary guide wire during exchanges of bulky devices like the CrossBoss

**Table 13.3** Lists the maneuvers that can or cannot be performed in a 6 Fr guiding catheter

| | Yes | No |
|---|---|---|
| IVUS-guided prox cap puncture with a microcatheter | | ✓ |
| Trapping balloon + Tornus 2.6 Fr/CrossBoss/Stingray Balloon | | ✓ |
| Deliver Jomed RX covered stent (graft master) | ✓ | |
| Trapping balloon + Tornus 2.1 Fr | ✓ | |
| Trapping balloon + Corsair | ✓ | |
| Deep seating | ✓ | |

Corsair, and Tornus 2.1 and 2.6 Fr are made by Assahi Intecc, Japan; Stingray balloon, Crossboss are made by Boston Scientific, US. Jomed Rx Graftmaster made by Abbott, US

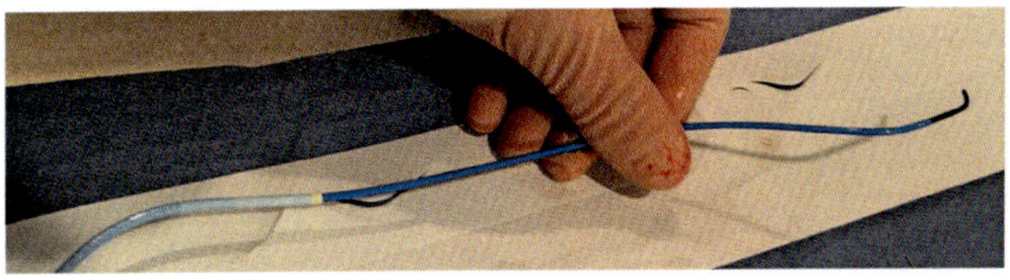

**Fig. 13.4** Sheathless delivery of regular 8 F Cordis Vista Bright tip guiding catheter using a 125 cm 6 F Shuttle Select Slip-Cath inside. The tip of the Shuttle catheter enters very smoothly into the radial over an 0.035′ guidewire, after removal of the 6 F sheath

and the Stingray Balloon (Boston Scientific, US). However, trapping the wire during exchanges of most other devices and anchoring maneuvers can be performed in a 6 Fr guiding catheter (Table 13.3).

## Introducing Guiding Catheters Without an Introducer Sheath

If the patient cannot tolerate a large diameter sheath, the guiding catheter should be introduced without an introducer sheath to improve the patient's tolerance of a larger size guiding catheter and avoid the entrapment of the introducer sheath in the radial artery. The guiding catheter introduction through the skin and the arterial puncture is facilitated by cutting the skin with a size 11 blade. The guiding catheter is then advanced over a long sheath dilator (Flexor Shuttle Sheath, Cook, US) that is 2 Fr smaller than the size of the guiding catheter (6 Fr sheath dilator in an 8 Fr guiding catheter) or over a 3–4 mm peripheral undilated angioplasty balloon. Alternatively, a 125 cm 6 Fr Shuttle Select Slip-Cath (Cook, US), usually used for carotid selective angiography, can be used into an 8 Fr guide. Moreover, the 125 cm 5 Fr Shuttle Select Slip-Cath will perfectly fit into a 7 Fr guide (Figs. 13.4 and 13.5).

## Commercially Available Sheathless Guiding Catheters

Sheathless guiding catheters with dilators are commercially available [19, 20]. The outer diameter of the SheathLess EauCath guiding catheters (Asahi Intecc, Japan) is similar to the outer diameter of a significantly smaller introducer sheath, while inner diameter is significantly larger (Fig. 13.6). However, a 7.5 sheathless guide only provides an inner diameter similar to a 7 Fr guide. Moreover, these catheters only provide limited support for complex PCI, and tend to slip out of the coronary ostium. Their tip is also relatively sharp, increasing the risk of guide-induced trauma. For these reasons, we think they have limited value for transradial CTO PCI in their current version.

## The Hybrid Algorithm and the Transradial Approach for CTO PCI

If the patient cannot tolerate a 7 Fr or larger introducer in the radial artery, a 6 Fr guiding catheter can be used. A CFA or brachial artery access should be considered for patients who cannot tolerate 6 Fr guiding catheters from the radial.

The most important disadvantages of using 6 Fr guiding catheters in CTO PCI is inability to accommodate multiple devices simultaneously, and to a lesser extent the decreased guiding catheter support. However, most CTO PCI maneuvers can be performed with 6 Fr guiding catheters, such as CTO PCI antegrade wire escalation. Wire trapping in 6 Fr guiding catheters can be achieved with a 2.0 or 2.5 mm semi-compliant monorail balloon. With few exceptions most microcatheters can fit with a monorail trapping balloon in a 6 Fr guiding catheter. However, the CrossBoss, the Stingray Balloon (Boston Scientific, US) or the 2.6 Fr Tornus (Asahi Intecc, Japan) cannot fit with a monorail trapping balloon simultaneously in a 6 Fr guiding catheter. As a result, committing to a smaller antegrade guide can limit treatment options.

Antegrade dissection and re-entry strategy using the CrossBoss catheter and the Stingray balloon (Boston Scientific, US) requires the use of long 300 cm coronary guide wires if performed with 6 Fr guides, because there are no commercially available trapping balloons that can fit simultaneously with these devices in a 6 Fr guiding catheter.

Crossing the collaterals and advancing retrograde gear during retrograde strategies can easily be performed though 6 Fr catheters. Guiding catheter support enhancement techniques are sometimes needed to deliver retrograde microcatheter (Fig. 13.5). Wire or balloon anchoring techniques can be used; however, the mother-and-child technique is used more frequently to enhance the support of 6 Fr guiding catheters during CTO PCI from the radial artery. We especially like the 5.5 Fr version of the GuideLiner (Vascular Solutions, US), that can accommodate the Corsair microcatheter (Asahi Intecc, Japan) while reducing the risk of donor artery trauma because of its smaller outer diameter. Once a mother-and-child technique is used in a 6 Fr guiding catheter, it becomes impossible to use a balloon anchoring technique, because the daughter guiding catheters effective lumen is 5 Fr or less, which precludes the introduction of the anchoring balloon simultaneously with the retrograde microcatheter.

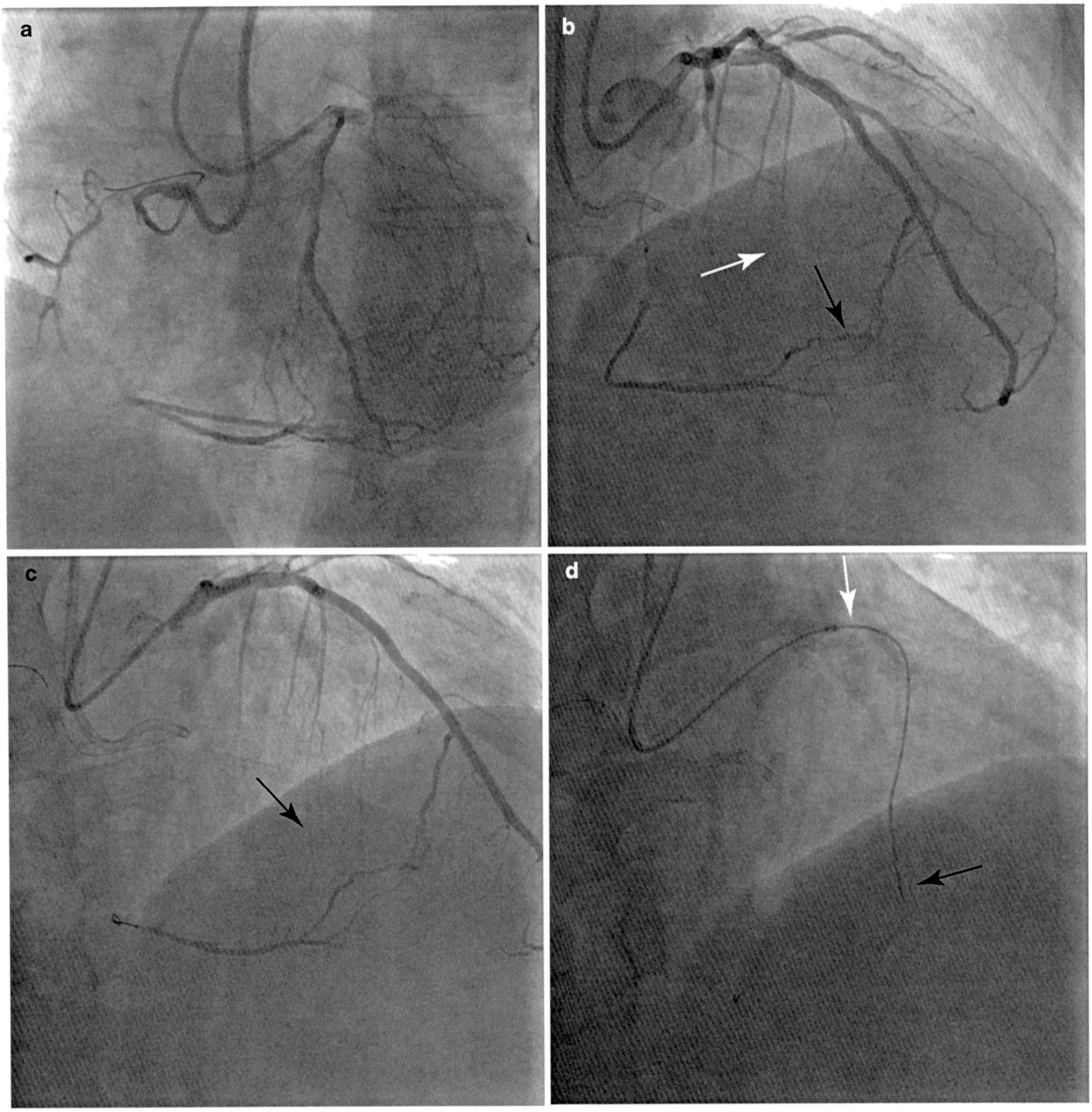


**Fig. 13.5** Dual radial approach for complex retrograde CTO PCI. (**a**) Long RCA CTO with an island of patent RCA in the mid segment, with an ambiguous proximal cap, and a distal cap at the crux bifurcation, mandating a retrograde approach. An 8 Fr catheter, delivered without a sheath, is used antegrade from the left radial, and a 6 Fr is used on the retrograde side. A guidewire is placed in the auricular branch to stabilize the antegrade guide. (**b**) Very large but tortuous CC2 septal CCs are visualized from the LAD to the PDA (*black arrow*). There are other septal branches that give CC0 collateral channels (*white arrow*). (**c**) After 5 min of surfing one of the most proximal septals with a Sion through a Finecross, a connection to the PDA was achieved. The *arrow* indicate the trajectory of the wire. (**d**) The Finecross is exchanged for a Corsair (*black arrow*), which is advanced through the septal CC with the support of a 5.5 Fr Guideliner MAC catheter (*white arrow*). (**e**) A Pilot 200 is used to create a retrograde dissection up to the proximal cap. The *arrow* indicate the tip of the knuckled wire. (**f**) An anchoring balloon technique (using a 2.0 mm balloon) is used to stabilise the antegrade guide, and to improve support (*black arrow*). A Pilot 200 is advanced targeting the knuckled wire and subsequently knuckled beside the retrograde system. Both the antegrade and the retrograde wires are in the sub-intimal space. A 3.0 mm balloon in used to connect both system together (reverse CART). (**g**) The balloon is moved more proximally (reverse CART). There is a very close contact of the antegrade balloon with the retrograde Corsair. (**h**) A straight Pilot 200 is used to navigate through the dissection plane, up to the aorta. (**i**) After advancing the Corsair to the RCA ostium, a soft workhorse wire is redirected into the antegrade guide. (Alternatively, snaring could have been performed). (**j**) After pulling out the retrograde system, we cannot even see where the Corsair navigated through the septum. (**k**) Final result, showing preserved distal branches, but also some few side branches of the RCA in the mid segment, despite a dissection-reentry technique used. Please note that there remain a small channel above the stent from previous retrograde re-entry attempt. It will close within days after the CTO PCI

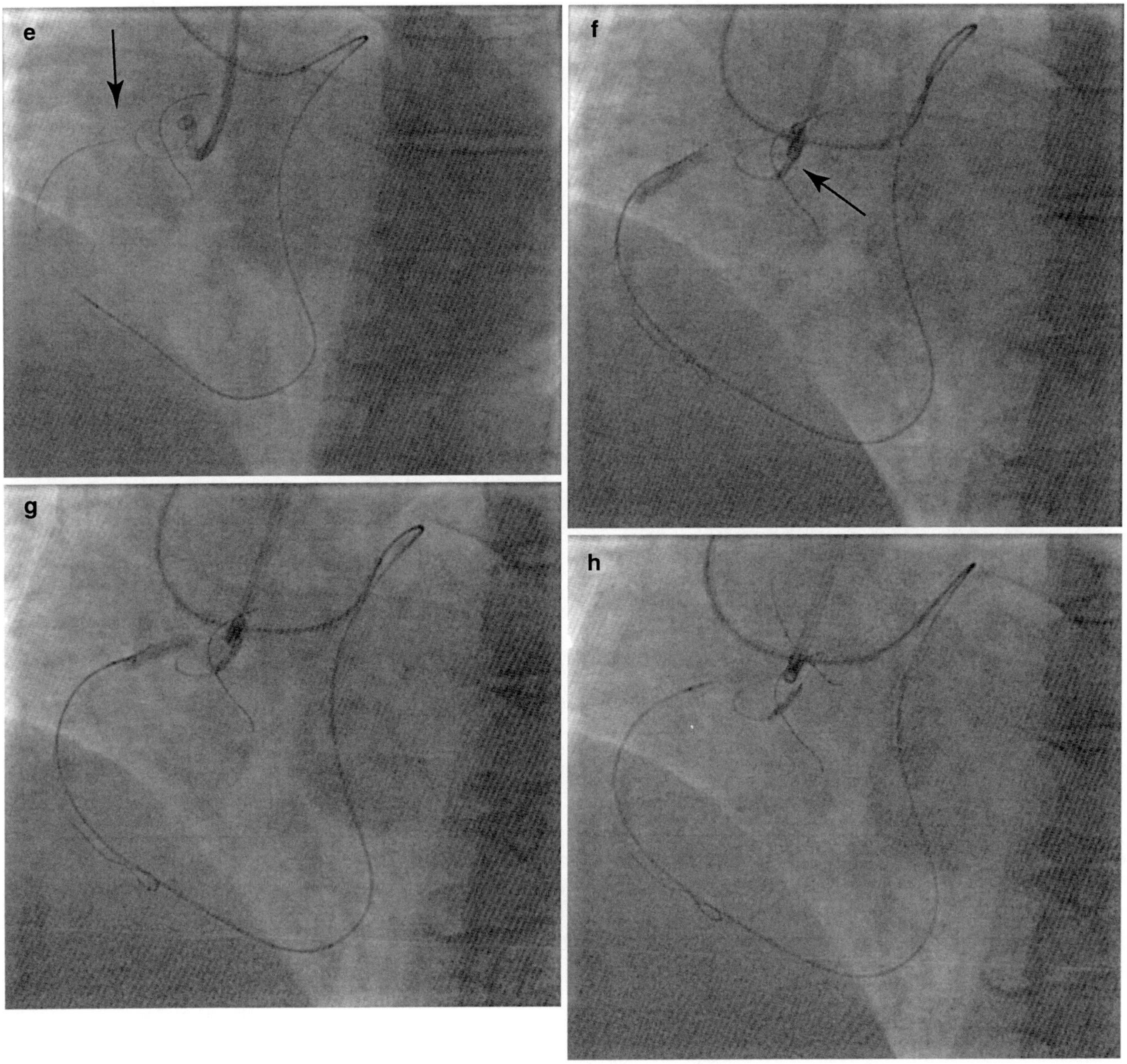


**Fig. 13.5** (continued)

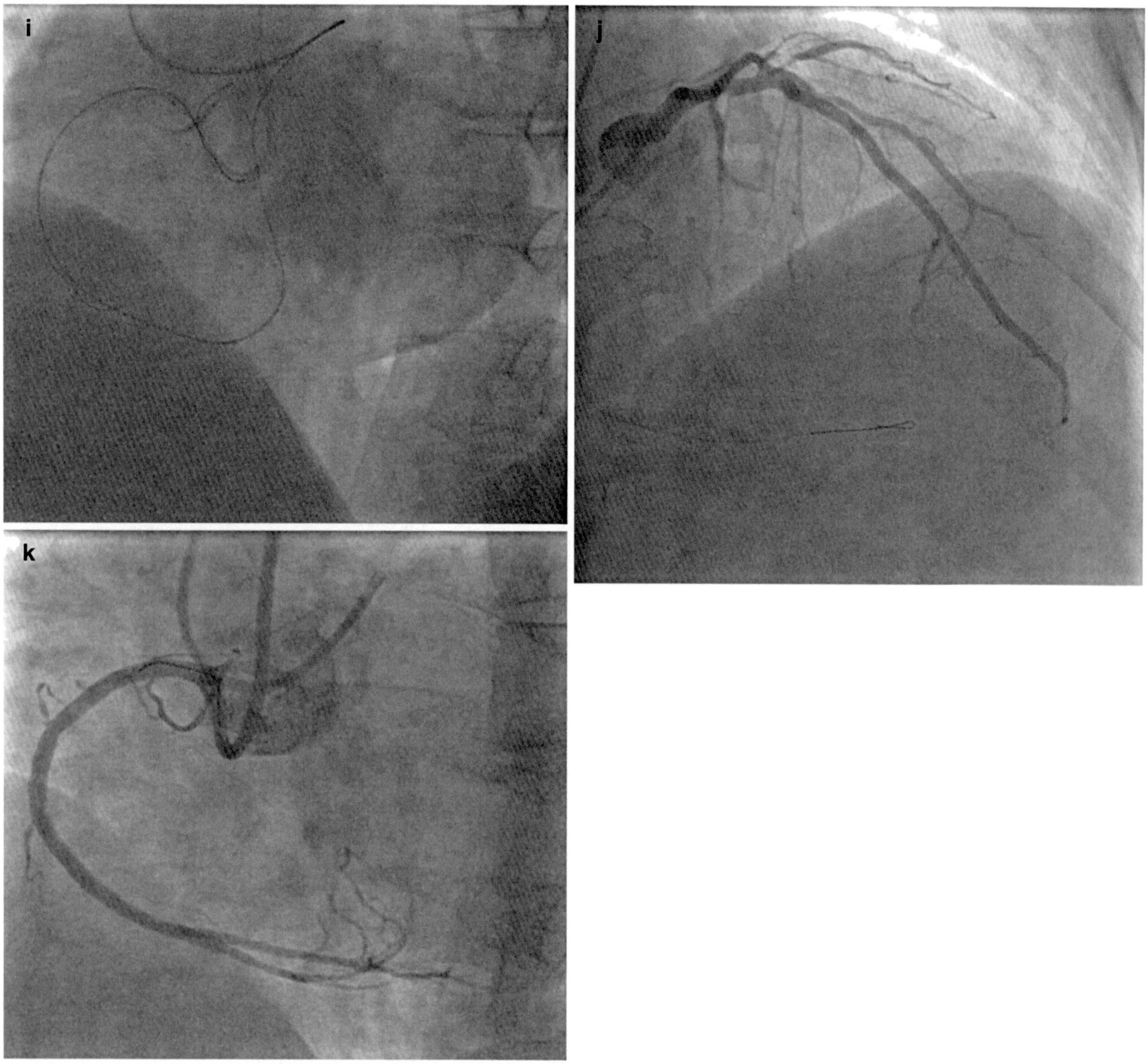


**Fig. 13.5** (continued)

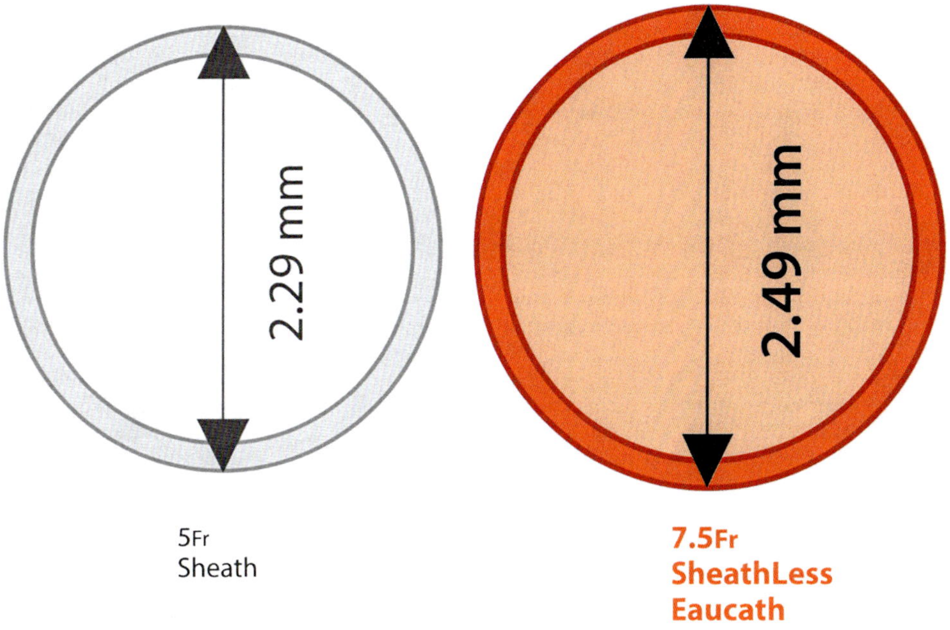


**Fig. 13.6** The Outer Diameter (OD) of the 7.5 Fr SheathLess Eaucath is 2.49 mm, similar to the OD of the 5 Fr sheath at 2.29 mm (From Asahi Intecc. with permission)

**Conclusion**

The transradial approach can be the default access strategy for CTO PCI with similar success rates and possibly better safety than CTO PCI performed from the common femoral artery accesses. Most radial arteries will be large enough to tolerate 6 Fr guiding catheters, however, 7 and 8 Fr guiding catheters are increasingly being used during CTO PCI from radial artery accesses, especially when delivered without a sheath. The hybrid algorithm for CTO PCI can be applied from using one or 2 radial artery accesses with minimal iterations. The choice of the arterial access site should be dictated by safety and clinical considerations. All interventional cardiologists should master the skills necessary to perform PCI the from radial artery access. Advances in guiding catheters and device technology will provide solutions to most of the limitations of radial artery access during CTO PCI.

## References


1. Alaswad K, Menon RV, Christopoulos G, Lombardi WL, Karmpaliotis D, Grantham JA, Marso SP, Wyman MR, Pokala NR, Patel SM, Kotsia AP, Rangan BV, Lembo N, Kandzari D, Lee J, Kalynych A, Carlson H, Garcia SA, Thompson CA, Banerjee S, Brilakis ES. Transradial approach for coronary chronic total occlusion interventions: insights from a contemporary multicenter registry. Catheter Cardiovasc Interv. 2015. doi:10.1002/ccd.25827.
2. Rathore S, Hakeem A, Pauriah M, Roberts E, Beaumont A, Morris JL. A comparison of the transradial and the transfemoral approach in chronic total occlusion percutaneous coronary intervention. Catheter Cardiovasc Interv. 2009;73(7):883–7. Wiley Subscription Services, Inc., A Wiley Company.
3. Burzotta F, De Vita M, Lefevre T, Tommasino A, Louvard Y, Trani C. Radial approach for percutaneous coronary interventions on chronic total occlusions: technical issues and data review. Catheter Cardiovasc Interv. 2014;83(1):47–57.
4. Kim PH, Gwon HC, Kim YH, Ahn SJ, Rhee I, You CW, et al. Safety and feasibility in trans-radial coronary interventions for chronic total occlusion. Korean Circ J. 2004;34(8):767–74.
5. Christopoulos G, Menon RV, Karmpaliotis D, Alaswad K, Lombardi W, Grantham JA, et al. Application of the "hybrid approach" to chronic total occlusions in patients with previous coronary artery bypass graft surgery (from a Contemporary Multicenter US registry). Am J Cardiol. 2014;113(12):1990–4.
6. Brilakis ES, Grantham JA, Rinfret S, Wyman RM, Burke MN, Karmpaliotis D, et al. A percutaneous treatment algorithm for crossing coronary chronic total occlusions. J Am Coll Cardiol Intv. 2012;5(4):367–79.
7. Bagur R, Rinfret S. Transradial approach for chronic total occlusion percutaneous coronary intervention. Int Cardiol Clin. 2012;1(3):355–63.
8. Nathan S, Rao SV. Radial versus femoral access for percutaneous coronary intervention: implications for vascular complications and bleeding. Curr Cardiol Rep. 2012;14(4):502–9. Current Science Inc.
9. Rao SV, Tremmel JA, Gilchrist IC, Shah PB, Gulati R, Shroff AR, et al. Best practices for transradial angiography and intervention: a consensus statement from the society for cardiovascular angiography and intervention's transradial working group. Catheter Cardiovasc Interv. 2014;83(2):228–36.
10. Caputo RP, Tremmel JA, Rao S, Gilchrist IC, Pyne C, Pancholy S, et al. Transradial arterial access for coronary and peripheral procedures: executive summary by the transradial committee of the SCAI. Catheter Cardiovasc Interv. 2011;78(6):823–39. Wiley Subscription Services, Inc., A Wiley Company.
11. Cooper CJ, El-Shiekh RA, Cohen DJ, Blaesing L, Burket MW, Basu A, et al. Effect of transradial access on quality of life and cost of cardiac catheterization: a randomized comparison. Am Heart J. 1999;138(3 Pt 1):430–6. Elsevier.

12. Sciahbasi A, Romagnoli E, Trani C, Burzotta F, Pendenza G, Tommasino A, et al. Evaluation of the "learning curve" for left and right radial approach during percutaneous coronary procedures. Am J Cardiol. 2012;108(2):185–8. Elsevier.
13. Rinfret S, Joyal D, Nguyen CM, Bagur R, Hui W, Leung R, et al. Retrograde recanalization of chronic total occlusions from the transradial approach; early Canadian experience. Catheter Cardiovasc Interv. 2011;78(3):366–74. Wiley Subscription Services, Inc., A Wiley Company.
14. Jolly SS, Amlani S, Hamon M, Yusuf S, Mehta SR. Radial versus femoral access for coronary angiography or intervention and the impact on major bleeding and ischemic events: a systematic review and meta-analysis of randomized trials. Am Heart J. 2009;157(1): 132–40. Elsevier.
15. Rathore S, Stables RH, Pauriah M, et al. Impact of length and hydrophilic coating of the introducer sheath on radial artery spasm during transradial coronary intervention: a randomized study. J Am Coll Cardiol Intv. 2010;3(5):475–83.
16. Alaswad K. Toolbox and inventory requirements for chronic total occlusion percutaneous coronary interventions. Int Cardiol Clin. 2012;1(3):281–97.
17. Patel T, Shah S, Pancholy S. Balloon-assisted tracking of a guide catheter through difficult radial anatomy: a technical report. Catheter Cardiovasc Interv. 2013;81(5):E215–8.
18. Di Mario C, Ramasami N. Techniques to enhance guide catheter support. Catheter Cardiovasc Interv. 2008;72(4):505–12. Wiley Subscription Services, Inc., A Wiley Company.
19. Mamas MA, Fath Ordoubadi F, Fraser DG. Atraumatic complex transradial intervention using large bore sheathless guide catheter. Catheter Cardiovasc Interv. 2008;72(3):357–64. Wiley Subscription Services, Inc., A Wiley Company.
20. Mamas M, D'Souza S, Hendry C, Ali R, Iles Smith H, Palmer K, et al. Use of the sheathless guide catheter during routine transradial percutaneous coronary intervention: a feasibility study. Catheter Cardiovasc Interv. 2010;75(4):596–602. Wiley Subscription Services, Inc., A Wiley Company.

# 14 How to Manage Radiation and Contrast During Chronic Total Occlusion Percutaneous Coronary Intervention

Antonis N. Pavlidis and Elliot J. Smith

**Abstract**

Although successful CTO recanalization is associated with significant clinical benefits, including improvement of angina, quality of life, reduced need for surgical revascularization, and improvement of left ventricular function, CTO procedures may require prolonged x-ray exposure and use of larger volumes of contrast compared to non CTO procedures. Careful selection of cases, assessment of patient related risks and application of specific measures to prevent complications from contrast and radiation is of crucial importance.

**Keywords**

Coronary artery disease • Chronic total occlusions • Coronary intervention • Radiation • Contrast • Acute kidney injury • Renal failure • Diuresis • Skin burn

## Contrast-Induced Acute Kidney Injury in CTO Percutaneous Coronary Interventions

Contrast-induced acute kidney injury (CI-AKI) is defined as the decline of renal function that occurs in a narrow time window after administration of iodinated contrast agents and represents a major cause of morbidity and mortality in patients undergoing percutaneous coronary intervention (PCI). CI-AKI is more prevalent in patients with pre-existing chronic kidney disease (CKD) and has been associated with high mortality rates, prolonged hospital stay and increased healthcare costs [1]. Contrast media volume has been shown to be an independent predictor for CI-AKI [2], therefore patients undergoing CTO PCI represent a high risk group due to large contrast doses used and frequent need for repeat attempts.

## Definitions of Contrast-Induced Acute Kidney Injury

CI-AKI is broadly defined as a rise in serum creatinine or a decline of the estimated glomerular filtration rate (eGFR) within 24–72 h after contrast administration. In a recent meta-analysis the definition of CI-AKI ranged from 0.3 to 0.5 mg/dL for an absolute increase and from 25 to 50 % for a relative increase in serum creatinine levels [3]. The most commonly used definitions of CI-AKI are summarised in Table 14.1.

A widely used simplified definition of CI-AKI is the rise of serum creatinine by ≥0.5 mg/dL within 24–72 h after exposure to contrast media [4, 7]. Barrett et al. [5] proposed that CI-AKI can be diagnosed in the presence of an absolute increase in serum creatinine by ≥0.5 mg/dL or a relative

**Table 14.1** Most common definitions of contrast-induced acute kidney injury (CI-AKI)

| |
|---|
| Serum creatinine increase ≥0.5 mg/dl or ≥25 % from baseline within 72 h [4, 5] |
| Serum creatinine rise by ≥ 0.3 mg/dl within 48 h ***or***<br>Serum creatinine rise ≥150 % from baseline value within 1 week ***or***<br>Urine output <0.5 ml/kg/h for >6 consecutive hours [6] |

A.N. Pavlidis, MD, PhD, FACC (✉)
Department of Cardiology, Barts Health NHS Trust, London, UK
e-mail: antonispav@yahoo.com

E.J. Smith, MD, MRCP
Department of Cardiology, London Chest Hospital, Barts Health NHS Trust, London, UK


S. Rinfret (ed.), *Percutaneous Intervention for Coronary Chronic Total Occlusion: The Hybrid Approach*,
DOI 10.1007/978-3-319-21563-1_14

**Table 14.2** RIFLE and AKIN criteria for staging of contrast-induced acute kidney injury (CI-AKI)

| AKIN | | Serum creatinine | Urine output |
|---|---|---|---|
| | *Stage 1* | ≥0.3 mg/dl ***or*** ≥150 to 200 % | <0.5 ml/kg/h for >6 h |
| | *Stage 2* | >200 to 300 % | <0.5 ml/kg/h for >12 h |
| | *Stage 3* | >300 % ***or*** ≥4.0 mg/dl with an acute increase of at least 0.5 mg/dl ***or*** on RRT | <0.3 ml/kg/h for 24 h ***or*** anuria for 12 h |
| **RIFLE** | | **Serum creatinine or GFR** | **Urine output** |
| | *Risk* | Increase in serum creatinine × 1.5 ***or*** decrease in GFR >25 % | <0.5 ml/kg/h for >6 h |
| | *Injury* | Increase in serum creatinine × 2.0 ***or*** decrease in GFR >50 % | <0.5 ml/kg/h for >12 h |
| | *Failure* | Increase in serum creatinine × 3.0 ***or*** serum creatinine >4.0 mg/dl with an acute increase of at least 0.5 mg/dl ***or*** decrease in GFR >75 % | <0.3 ml/kg/h for 24 h ***or*** anuria for 12 h |
| | *Loss* | Persistent acute renal failure = complete loss of kidney function >4 weeks | |
| | *ESRD* | ESRD > 3 months | |

Data from KDIGO Clinical Practice Guideline for Acute Kidney Injury [6]
For both AKIN stage and RIFLE criteria, only one criterion needs to be fulfilled. For AKIN, the increase in creatinine must occur in <48 h. For RIFLE, AKI should be both abrupt (within 1–7 days) and sustained (more than 24 h). For RIFLE, when baseline creatinine is elevated, an abrupt rise of at least 0.5 mg/dl to >4 mg/dl is sufficient
*AKIN* Acute Kidney Injury Network, *RIFLE* risk injury failure loss and end stage, *RRT* renal replacement therapy, *GFR* glomerular filtration rate, *ESRD* end-stage renal disease

increase in serum creatinine by ≥25 % from baseline within 72 h after contrast administration. The most recently published Kidney Disease: Improving Global Outcomes (KDIGO) definition of CI-AKI has been widely adopted by the majority of the national cardiovascular intervention societies and is based on the fulfilment of at least one of the following criteria: (a) an absolute increase in serum creatinine by ≥0.3 mg/dL from baseline within 48 h, (b) a relative increase in serum creatinine by ≥1.5 fold from the baseline value, which is known or presumed to have occurred within 1 week from administration of contrast agent, or (c) a decline in urine output by ≤0.5 mL/kg/h for a period of at least 6 h [6].

The Acute Dialysis Quality Initiative (ADQI) RIFLE and Acute Kidney Injury Network (AKIN) staging systems have demonstrated that the risk of mortality is higher when the stage of AKI is higher [8, 9]. Patients with CI-AKI should be staged according to the criteria (serum creatinine or urine output) that give them the highest stage. The staging criteria are summarized in Table 14.2.

## Incidence of Contrast-Induced Acute Kidney in CTO Procedures

The incidence of CI-AKI in patients undergoing CTO intervention varies in different registries according to the used diagnostic criteria. In a recently published large scale meta-analysis including almost 19,000 CTO cases the pooled estimated rate of CI-AKI was 3.8 %, although only 20 % of the studies reported data on contrast nephropathy [10]. In another meta-analysis including 3493 CTOs a lower incidence of CI-AKI at 1.8 % was found [11]. The incidence of CI-AKI in the most recently published registries and studies varies between 0.9 and 5.4 % (Table 14.3). No significant differences with regards to contrast volume have been shown between different subsets such as femoral vs radial access [22], in-stent restenosis vs de novo lesions [23] and patients with vs without previous coronary artery bypass grafting (CABG) [13]. The recent development of the "hybrid approach" to CTO crossing has resulted in a significant reduction in total fluoroscopy time and contrast utilization along with an improved technical success rate [24].

## Risk Factors for Contrast-Induced Acute Kidney in CTO Procedures

The risk of CI-AKI in patients undergoing a coronary procedure may be estimated using a range of validated scores. The most commonly used scoring system, the Mehran score, includes variables of age, gender, eGFR or serum creatinine, haematocrit, diabetes mellitus (DM), presence of congestive heart failure, contrast volume, hypotension and haemodynamic support with intra-aortic balloon pump (IABP) [2].

The presence of established renal impairment is the single most important risk factor for development of CI-AKI following a CTO procedure. The incidence of CI-AKI in patients with pre-existing chronic kidney disease (CKD) undergoing standard PCI procedures has been reported as high as 55 %, despite adequate pre-procedure hydration [25].

**Table 14.3** Prevalence of contrast-induced acute kidney injury (CI-AKI) and contrast volume use in most recent CTO registries and meta-analyses

| | Study type | Characteristics | Year | CTO lesions (n) | CI-AKI (%) | Contrast (ml) |
|---|---|---|---|---|---|---|
| Lin et al. [12] | Retrospective study | | 2014 | 516 | 5.4 | 296 ± 225[a] 277 ± 121[b] |
| El Sabbagh et al. [11] | Metanalysis | Retrograde only | 2014 | 3493 | 1.8 | 350 ± 71 |
| Christopoulos et al. [13] | Registry | | 2014 | 496 | NR | 250 (180–360)[c] |
| Karmpaliotis et al. [14] | Registry | Retrograde only | 2012 | 462 | NR | 345 ± 177 |
| Michael et al. [15] | Registry | | 2013 | 1361 | NR | 294 ± 158 |
| Tsuchikane et al. [16] | Registry | Retrograde only | 2013 | 801 | NR | 307 ± 137 |
| Patel et al. [17] | Metanalysis | | 2013 | 18,941 | 3.8 | NR |
| Danzi et al. [18] | Registry | Multiple CTOs | 2013 | 249 | NR | 400 (300–500)[c] |
| Galassi et al. [19] | Registry | | 2011 | 1983 | 0.9 | 313 ± 184 |
| Morino et al. [20] | Registry | | 2010 | 528 | 1.2 | 293 (53–1097)[c] |
| Aguiar-Souto et al. [21] | Retrospective study | | 2010 | 227 | 0.88–6.16[d] | 260 (200–350)[c] |

*CTO* total chronic occlusion, *NR* not reported, *CI-AKI* contrast induced acute kidney injury
[a]CI-AKI group
[b]Non CI-AKI group
[c]Median (range)
[d]Depending on criteria used for diagnosis of CI-AKI

The correlation of contrast media volume during CTO PCI and the development of CI-AKI has been well documented in several studies [26, 27]. During CTO PCI patients receiving ≥400 ml of contrast have an almost twofold higher incidence of CI-AKI compared to those receiving <400 ml of contrast [21]. However, in the absence of coexistent CKD and DM the incidence of CI-AKI remains low, even after high volumes of contrast media [28]. Although the existing data is limited, no significant correlations between the CTO lesion characteristics and the development of CI-AKI have been shown. Lin et al. [12] showed that severe tortuosity of CTO lesions was an independent predictor of CI-AKI, however none of the other established J-CTO criteria for lesion complexity (calcification, length, ambiguous cap) reached statistical significance. In the same study, a Mehran score >11 was clearly correlated to the development of CI-AKI after CTO PCI. On the contrary, Aguiar-Souto et al. [21] showed that clinical parameters, procedural characteristics, target vessels and Mehran scoring were not predictors for CI-AKI in CTO intervention. The risk factors for CI-AKI in CTO procedures are summarized in Table 14.4.

**Table 14.4** Risk factors for development of contrast-induced acute kidney injury (CI-AKI) in patients undergoing CTO interventions

| Patient-related | Procedure-related |
|---|---|
| Chronic kidney disease (eGFR <60 ml/min/1.73 m$^2$) | High contrast media volume |
| Renal transplant | Multiple procedures |
| Older age (>75 years old) | Lesion complexity (e.g. tortuosity of CTO segment) |
| Female sex | IABP |
| Congestive heart failure | Hemodynamic instability |
| LV impairment | |
| Volume depletion | |
| Nephrotoxic medication (diuretics, NSAIDs) | |
| Anemia | |
| Low serum albumin (<35 g/L) | |

*eGFR* estimated glomerular filtration rate, *NSAIDs* non-steroidal anti-inflammatory drugs, *LV* left ventricle, *CTO* chronic total occlusion, *IABP* intra-aortic balloon pump

## Prognostic Impact of Contrast-Induced Acute Kidney

The occurrence of CI-AKI has been associated with poor short and longterm outcomes, including increased cardiovascular mortality [29]. Patients with CI-AKI have up to fivefold higher risk of death [30, 31], while CI-AKI has been shown to be an independent predictor of 1-year mortality [32, 33]. In the majority of cases CI-AKI is transient and complete or near-complete recovery of renal function occurs within a period of 3 months [33]. However, all patients who develop AKI following coronary interventions are at increased risk for progressive longterm renal impairment [34].

In the Alberta registry [34], which included a large number of patients who underwent coronary angiography, CI-AKI was independently associated with a twofold increase in the risk of death, fourfold increase in the risk of end-stage renal disease, 1.5-fold increase in the risk of

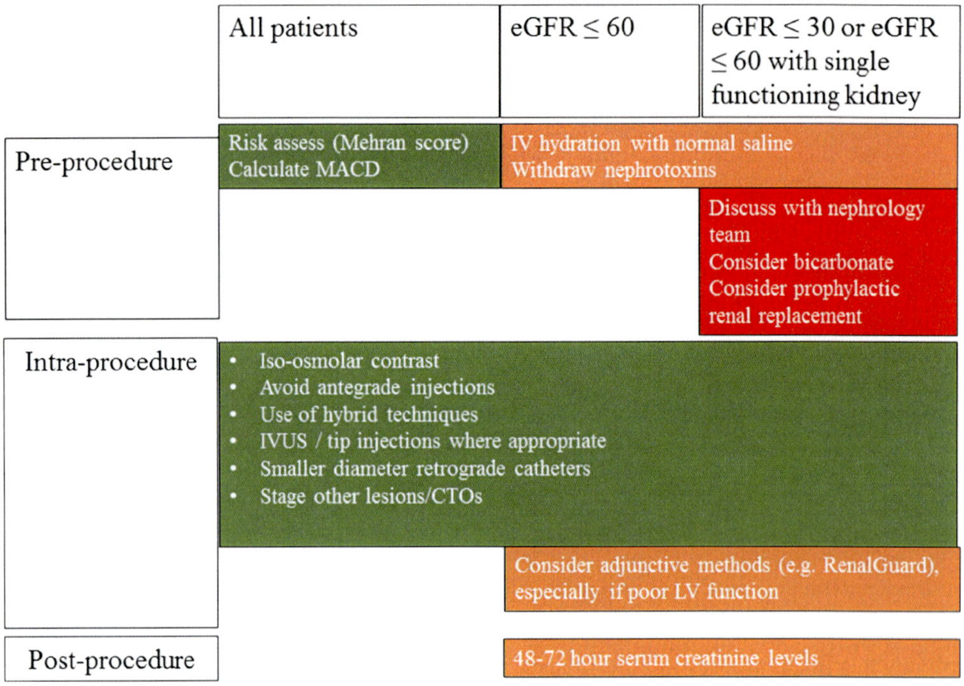


**Fig. 14.1** Proposed algorithm for prevention of contrast-induced acute kidney injury in CTO interventions. *CTO* chronic total occlusion, *eGFR* estimated glomerular filtration rate (ml/min/1.73 m$^2$), *MACD* maximal acceptable contrast dose, *IVUS* intravascular ultrasound, *LV* left ventricle

hospitalization for heart failure, and twofold increase in the risk of hospitalization with acute renal failure. This can only partially be explained by the co-existence of several comorbidities in these patients including hypertension, DM, impaired left ventricular function or heart failure. Patient with CI-AKI have been shown to be more susceptible to persistent microvascular renal dysfunction after an acute episode of ischemic tubular injury, while recurrent CI-AKIs due to frequent exposures to contrast or recurrent acute clinical events can also contribute to the chronic deterioration of renal function towards end-stage disease [32].

## Prevention of Contrast-Induced Acute Kidney in CTO Procedures

Several preventive methods have been described in the literature, however the data remain controversial for the majority of them. So far, no strategies have been shown to be effective in preventing CI-AKI beyond thorough patient selection, minimizing the amount of contrast media and meticulous hydration of the patient. Preventive modalities can be distinguished in pre-procedural and intra-procedural methods and follow up. A proposed algorithm for prevention of CI-AKI in CTO interventions is shown in Fig. 14.1.

### Pre-procedural Strategies

#### Patient Selection

The first step in prevention of CI-AKI in CTO procedures is the identification of patients at high risk. A thorough assessment of the risk factors and calculation of validated scores, such as the Mehran score, should be performed routinely for all patients in the CTO pre-assessment clinic. Nephrology consultation should be obtained prior to procedure for all patients at very high risk (eGFR <30 ml/min/1.73 m$^2$).

#### Hydration

Patients at high risk of CI-AKI should have a thorough assessment of their volume status and receive appropriate volume expansion prior to the procedure. Intravenous 0.9 % sodium chloride has been shown to be more effective than 0.45 % sodium chloride or oral hydration in prevention of CI-AKI [35, 36]. Although most of the trials have not directly addressed the ideal protocol, the most widely used approach is the administration of intravenous 0.9 % sodium chloride at a rate of 1 mL/kg/h for 24, beginning 12 h before administration of the contrast medium, in order to achieve a urine output of >150 ml/h. This approach seems to be superior to either bolus volume expansion during the procedure [37] or removal of restrictions on oral fluid intake [36]. Patients with moderate to severe left ventricular dysfunction should receive cautious hydration with isotonic 0.45 % saline and close monitoring of urine output aiming to maintain a euvolemic state [38].

#### Calculation of Maximum Allowable Contrast Dose

In 1989 Cigarroa et al. [39] reported an empiric formula for calculating the maximal acceptable contrast dose (MACD):

MACD = 5 ml × weight (kg)/baseline serum creatinine (mg/dl)

The use of contrast beyond the MACD was later correlated to an increased risk of CI-AKI [40]. A ratio of less than

3.7 for the volume of contrast media to creatinine clearance has also been proposed as a stricter limit [41].

#### N-Acetylcysteine

N-acetylcysteine (NAC) has been shown to reduce the nephrotoxic effects of contrast media via antioxidant and vasodilatory mechanisms. The initial enthusiasm following publication of the study by Tepel et al. in 2000 [42], which showed the beneficial effects of NAC in preventing CI-AKI, has now subsided following numerous heterogeneous studies and meta-analyses [43–45]. More recently, a large randomized trial demonstrated that NAC does not reduce the risk of CI-AKI or affect any relevant outcomes in high risk patients undergoing percutaneous coronary procedures [46]. There is currently no compelling evidence for the routine use of N-acetylcysteine to prevent CI-AKI [47].

#### Sodium Bicarbonate

Sodium bicarbonate prevents CI-AKI by inhibiting the production of free radicals. Several recent trials [48–50], including a large meta-analysis [51], suggest that volume expansion with intravenous bicarbonate is more effective compared to normal saline. Nevertheless, other studies have failed to show a clear benefit for bicarbonate volume expansion in preventing contrast-induced AKI [52, 53]. Whilst more convincing data are awaited, intravenous bicarbonate can be a useful alternative in patients with impaired LV function or heart failure undergoing prolonged CTO interventions.

#### Hemodialysis and Hemofiltration

Studies have shown that 2–3 h of hemodialysis can eliminate up to 90 % of the contrast [54]. Hemofiltration reduces oliguria and volume overload and maintains electrolyte balance. However, only limited data on the efficacy of hemofiltration in preventing CI-AKI in high risk patients undergoing PCI exist [55] and until the results of large randomized trials are available, it cannot be recommended as standard prophylaxis in patients undergoing CTO procedures.

#### Statins

Statins are known to exert several pleiotropic effects including decreased systemic inflammation and improvement of endothelial function. They can therefore demonstrate beneficial effects in CI-AKI prevention by decreasing the inflammatory response induced by contrast media and improving the renal tubular endothelial function. Indeed, several studies have demonstrated reduced CI-AKI rates in patients with renal impairment undergoing PCI following treatment with statins [56, 57], although these results have not been consistent [58, 59]. In a meta-analysis of 8 trials, Giacoppo et al. [60] showed that pre-treatment with statins was associated with significant reduction in CI-AKI, both in patient with and without baseline renal impairment. Despite the above findings the use of statins prior to PCI in order to prevent CI-AKI is not yet routine practice.

#### CTO Road Mapping with Computed Tomography

Computed tomography coronary angiography (CTCA) is rapidly emerging as an important component to CTO planning. It provides important information regarding the length of the occlusion, the presence of tortuosity in the occluded segment and the amount of calcification. More importantly, it is extremely useful in identifying an ambiguous proximal cap and assessing the presence of potential interventional collaterals. Several prospective studies have correlated the lesion length and the presence of calcification, measured with pre-procedure CTCA, to the procedural success [61]. Disadvantages of CT angiography include the lack of soft tissue contrast which can impair localization of the luminal borders of the CTO, a relatively high degree of radiation exposure and the use of contrast, although in the majority of cases adequate information can be achieved by a single venous injection of only 100 ml of contrast [62]. Therefore, CTCA is an extremely useful tool for CTO planning which can be translated in significant peri-procedural contrast reduction.

### Intra-Procedural Strategies

#### General Measures

General principles for preventing CI-AKI during CTO recanalization include the administration of the lowest possible dose of contrast medium, use of iso-osmolar contrast agents, such as Iodixanol, and maintenance of haemodynamic stability throughout the procedure in order to ensure adequate renal perfusion. Further interventions to bystander coronary disease or other CTOs should be performed as staged procedures in patients with pre-existing renal impairment.

#### Procedural Techniques

CTO operators should be trained in all key skillsets of antegrade wiring, antegrade dissection-re-entry and retrograde CTO PCI. Adoption of the hybrid approach with early switch from a failing strategy maximizes the chance of procedural success, reduces procedure time and minimises radiation and contrast use [63]. Although there are no specific time limits for each of the algorithm steps, operators should stop pursuing a technique that has not resulted in any significant progress during a reasonable period of time [63]. In particular, antegrade contrast injections are avoided in order to prevent hydraulic expansion of the sub-intimal space. Meanwhile the use of knuckle wire techniques and specific catheters such as the CrossBoss (Boston Scientific, USA) may allow the operator to cross long vessel segments where there is anatomical ambiguity without the need for the use of contrast.

The benefits of intravascular ultrasound (IVUS) in CTO recanalization have been very well validated [64]. IVUS use during CTO interventions can reduce radiation exposure, contrast volume and procedure time. It is an excellent tool for identification of the proximal cap in stumpless occlusions, guidance of re-entry from sub-intimal tracks, assessment of appropriate stent coverage of the diseased segment and confirmation of satisfactory stent expansion and apposition. During reverse Controlled Antegrade and Retrograde Tracking (reverse CART) it can be utilised to assess the position of the retrograde wire in the subintimal space and the size of the subintimal space for optimal balloon dilatation. Moreover, tracking of the antegrade (CART) or the retrograde wire (reverse CART) towards the true lumen can be performed using direct IVUS visualization, thereby avoiding contrast.

The use of smaller size 5 Fr diagnostic catheters for retrograde opacification and tip injections via the retrograde microcatheter in order to assess the appropriateness of retrograde interventional collaterals can reduce the amount of contrast volume and should be considered in high risk patients. Uehara et al. [65] reported a case of reverse CART CTO recanalization of a right coronary artery in a high risk patient where only 10 ml of contrast media was used. The procedure was successfully performed with tip injections via the retrograde Corsair microcatheter and utilization of IVUS to guide balloon dilatation, stent sizing and post-deployment optimisation.

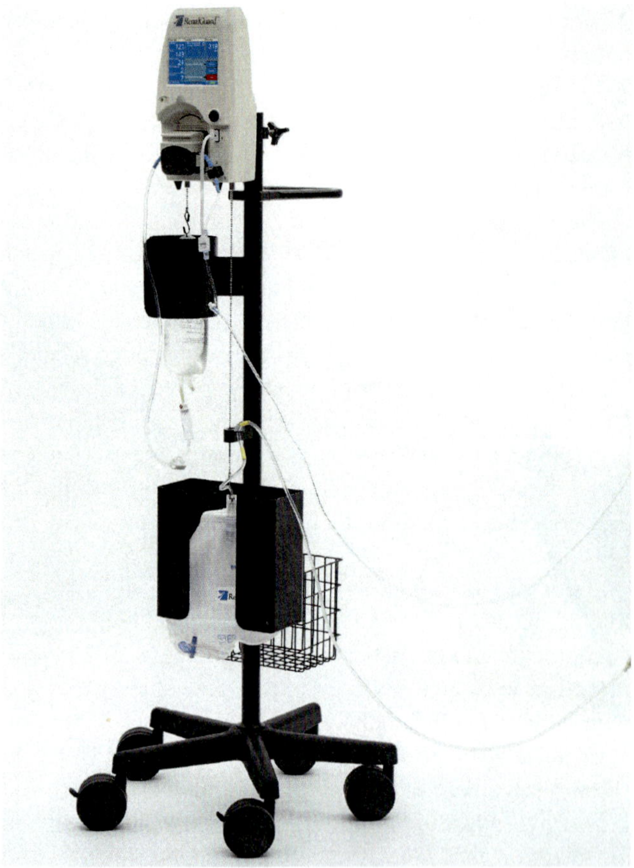

**Fig. 14.2** The RenalGuard system (Reproduced with permission from PLC Medical Systems)

### Forced Diuresis (RenalGuard System)

The RenalGuard system (PLC Medical Systems, Milford, Massachusetts) represents a novel approach to prevention of CI-AKI in high risk patients undergoing PCI. It is designed to reduce the toxic effects of contrast media on the kidneys by achievement of high urine output rates while maintaining euvolemia. The physiological benefits include a more rapid transit of contrast through the kidneys and reduced oxygen consumption in the medulla of the kidney [66].

The RenalGuard system is comprised of a urinary collection bag, which connects to the patient's Foley catheter, and a high volume infusion set which connects to a standard intravenous catheter (Fig. 14.2). A console measures the volume of urine in the collection set and continuously adjusts the infusion rate to an equal volume to match the patient's urine output. An initial bolus of ~3 ml/kg is initially infused over 30 min (*pre-procedural phase*). In the presence of impaired LV function (ejection fraction ≤30 %) the bolus is reduced to ≤150 ml. Following the initial bolus, diuresis is initiated with a small dose of furosemide (0.25 mg/kg). Once an optimal urine flow of ≥300 mL/h has been achieved the patient is transferred to the catheterization laboratory and the procedure begins. Controlled hydration by the RenalGuard system continues throughout the procedure (*procedure phase*) and for 4 h after the procedure (*post-procedural phase*). Additional furosemide doses should be administered when there is a decrease in urine flow below the target value. A schematic representation of the RenalGuard protocol is depicted in Fig. 14.3.

The first trial was conducted in 2012 [67] and randomized 170 patients with eGFR <30 ml/min/1.73 m$^2$ undergoing coronary procedures to standard intravenous isotonic saline hydration versus forced diuresis with the RenalGuard system. A percentage of 4.6 % of the patients in the RenalGuard group developed CI-AKI versus 18 % in the saline group (p=0.005). The threefold reduction in CI-AKI was also associated with a lower incidence of post-procedural major adverse clinical events, although the study was not powered to detect differences in clinical outcomes. In this study PCI was performed in 59 % of the patients.

The REMEDIAL II trial [68] was a randomized, open-label controlled trial which assigned 292 patients with baseline eGFR ≤30 ml/min/1.73 m$^2$ or a Mehran risk score of ≥11 to either RenalGuard and NAC or intravenous sodium bicarbonate and NAC. PCI was performed in 55 % of the patients. CI-AKI occurred in 11 % in the RenalGuard group and 20.5 % in the control group (p=0.025). Major adverse cardiac events (MACE) were similar in the two groups after

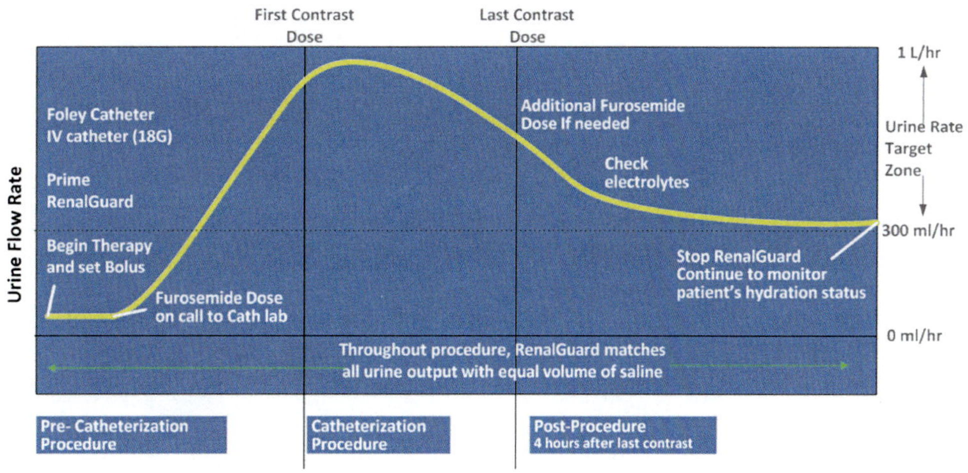


**Fig. 14.3** Treatment protocol for the RenalGuard system (Reproduced with permission from PLC Medical Systems)

1 month of follow up, while 3 patients in the RenalGuard group and 1 patient in the control group developed congestive heart failure post-procedure.

The CIN-RG trial is a pivotal trial which is currently in progress and aims to compare RenalGuard and NAC against intravenous saline plus NAC in high risk patients scheduled to receive at least 75 ml of contrast during angiography [69]. Although the use of the RenalGuard system in high risk CTO patients has not yet been standardised, it appears to be an attractive solution for preventing CI-AKI.

### Coronary Sinus Contrast Media Extraction (CINCOR System)

Another promising strategy to reduce contrast volume in CTO procedures is the coronary sinus contrast media extraction system (CINCOR Contrast Removal System, Osprey Medical, St. Paul, Minnesota). The CINCOR system comprises of an 11 Fr coronary sinus aspiration catheter which is inserted via the jugular vein. Upon activation it exerts a vacuum effect and removes contrast from the coronary sinus. Duffy et al. [70] reported no change in renal function from baseline in 26 patients with eGFR <60 ml/min/1.73 $m^2$ undergoing coronary angiography and PCI with the use of the device. The safety and capacity of the CINCOR system to reduce the risk of CI-AKI are currently being evaluated in a large-scale randomized trial (PRESERV: Prospective Randomized Evaluation to Study the Effects of Reduced Contrast Media on the Vitality of the Kidney) [71].

### Follow Up

Repeat contrast administration within a short period of time should be avoided in patients that have undergone complex CTO recanalization procedures. Renal function should be routinely assessed 48–72 h following the procedure to ensure stable renal function.

Key measures for prevention of CI-AKI during CTO are listed in Table 14.5.

**Table 14.5** Methods for prevention of contrast-induced acute kidney injury (CI-AKI) in CTO interventions

| Pre-procedure | Intra-procedure |
|---|---|
| Patient selection and risk assessment | Limitation of contrast volume |
| Calculation of MACD | Iso-osmolar contrast (Iodixanol) |
| Intravenous hydration | Maintain haemodynamic stability |
| NAC | Hybrid CTO strategy |
| Sodium bicarbonate | Stage procedures for other lesions or multiple CTOs |
| Hemodialysis or hemofiltration | IVUS |
| Statins | Tip injections |
| Antioxidants | Reverse CART |
| Theophylline | Small size retrograde catheters |
| Withdrawal of nephrotoxic agents | Forced diuresis (RenalGuard) |
| CTCA | Coronary sinus contrast media extraction |

*CTO* chronic total occlusion, *MCAD* maximum allowable contrast dose, *NAC* *N*-acetylcysteine, *ACE* angiotensin enzyme, *NSAIDs* non-steroidal anti-inflammatory drugs, *CTCA* computed tomography coronary angiography, *IVUS* intravascular ultrasound, *R-CART* reverse controlled antegrade and retrograde tracking

## Radiation Exposure Complications in CTO Interventions

Radiation exposure is higher during CTO PCI compared to non-CTO interventions because of the prolonged fluoroscopic time and repeated cine angiography [72]. Although radiation skin injury is rare, the risks of radiation-related complications are greater in CTO procedures. Moreover, operator and lab staff exposure can result in longterm adverse outcomes, such as cataract and malignancies, therefore reducing radiation exposure is a key factor in CTO interventions.

## Radiation Doses in CTO Procedures

There are three different values that are currently measured by modern interventional fluoroscopic equipment: (a) the *entrance surface air kerma* (*ESAK*), measured in Gray (Gy), which represents the radiation energy released at the point where the X-ray beam enters the patient's skin surface and includes both the incident air kerma and radiation backscattered from the tissue, (b) the *dose area product* (*DAP*), measured in Gy.cm$^2$, which represents the product of the dose in air within the X-ray beam and the beam area, and is therefore a measure of all the radiation that enters the patient and (c) *Fluoroscopic time* (*FT*), measured in minutes, which is the time during a procedure that fluoroscopy is used. FT does not include cine acquisition imaging and is therefore inadequate to assess patient radiation. The ESAK is used to measure the deterministic risk to the patient such as skin injury, while the DAP is used to measure the stochastic risk of the patient, which involves the likelihood of developing malignancies or genetic defects in the future.

A plain chest x-ray produces a DAP of 0.08 Gy.cm$^2$ and a background equivalent of 3 days, while the equivalents for a non-CTO PCI with one stent are 36 Gy.cm$^2$ and 3.7 years [73]. According to a study by Suzuki et al. [72] the median ESAK for CTOs PCI was 4.6 Gy, compared to 2.4, 1.5 and 1.2 Gy for multivessel, single-vessel multiple stenosis and single stenosis PCIs respectively. Several lesion- and patient-related risk factors have been shown to affect radiation dose during percutaneous interventions. In a study of 1933 PCI procedures Fetterly et al. [74] found that lesion complexity, PCI of left circumflex artery, previous CABG, body mass index (BMI) and the number of treated lesions correlated to an increased ESAK. Similar results were found in a larger study by Delewi et al. [75] which included 9850 PCI procedures. They demonstrated that high BMI, previous history of CABG, the number of treated lesions and CTO interventions were associated with the highest patient radiation exposure.

## Deterministic Effects

Radiation-induced skin injury is an infrequent complication during PCI, but appears more often in CTO interventions as a result of prolonged fluoroscopy times. Radiation toxicity is rare with <5 Gy but patients with higher doses should be followed up 2–3 weeks after the procedure and assessed for development of new skin changes. At Grade I radiation-induced skin injury a faint erythema can be seen at the first 48 h after exposure. Following a latent phase that can last up to 5 weeks, moderate to brisk erythema with oedema can be observed. Larger doses of radiation can result in Grade IV injury with skin necrosis or ulceration within 2 weeks after exposure (Table 14.6) [76].

**Table 14.6** Staging of radiation skin injury

| Grade | Skin appearance | Radiation dose | Time after radiation exposure |
|---|---|---|---|
| 1 | Faint erythema or desquamation | >2 Gy | First 48 h |
| 2 | Moderate to brisk erythema or moist desquamation. Moderate swelling. | >15 Gy | 2–5 weeks |
| 3 | Confluent, moist desquamation >1.5 cm diameter, which is not confined to the skin folds. Pitting oedema | >40 Gy | 6–7 weeks |
| 4 | Skin necrosis or ulceration of full thickness dermis | >550 Gy | 2 weeks |

Data from Bernier et al. [96]

Radiation-induced skin injury appears to be the least frequently reported complication following CTO intervention. In a meta-analysis of 65 studies Patel et al. [10] showed an incidence of <0.01 % with only 3 reported cases among 2857 patients. However, radiation skin injury was the least frequently reported CTO complication, with only 11 % of the studies reporting on its occurrence. In another metanalysis of retrograde CTO interventions, El Sabbagh et al. [11] reported an incidence of 0.5 %, although only 2 out of the 26 studies (0.08 %) reported this complication. Morino et al. [20] published the outcomes for 498 patients and 528 CTO lesions included in J-CTO registry (Multicenter CTO Registry of Japan) and no incidents of radiation-induce skin injuries were reported. The reported incidence of radiation skin in the most recent CTO registries and meta-analyses is summarised in Table 14.7.

## Stochastic Effects

Radiation dose exposure has been related to an additional risk of developing solid tumours [77]. The Biological Effects of Ionizing Radiation (BEIR) VIII risk model suggests that the risk of cancer increases proportionally to the dose of the radiation, with no low-dose threshold [78]. At such low doses of exposure, the risk of developing cancer is naturally low, but not zero. Minimal data on the risk of cancer related to radiation exposure during PCI are available. Godino et al. [79] estimated

**Table 14.7** Radiation doses in recent CTO registries and meta-analyses

| | Study type | Characteristics | Year | CTO lesions (n) | Radiation skin injury (%) | Fluoroscopy time |
|---|---|---|---|---|---|---|
| Lin et al. [12] | Retrospective study | | 2014 | 516 | NR | 43 ± 27[a]<br>42 ± 24[b] |
| El Sabbagh et al. [11] | Metanalysis | Retrograde only | 2014 | 3493 | 0.5 % | 82 ± 34 |
| Christopoulos et al. [13] | Registry | | 2014 | 496 | NR | 41 (26–65)[c] |
| Michael et al. [15] | Registry | | 2013 | 1361 | NR | 42 ± 29 |
| Karmpaliotis et al. [14] | Registry | Retrograde only | 2012 | 462 | NR | 61 ± 40 |
| Tsuchikane et al. [16] | Registry | Retrograde only | 2013 | 801 | NR | 95 ± 52 |
| Patel et al. [17] | Metanalysis | | 2013 | 18,941 | <0.01 | NR |
| Galassi et al [19] | Registry | | 2011 | 1983 | NR | 42 ± 47 |
| Morino et al. [20] | Registry | | 2010 | 528 | 0 | 45 (1–301)[c] |
| Aguiar-Souto et al. [21] | Retrospective study | | 2010 | 227 | NR | 32 (19–47)[c] |

*CI-AKI* contrast induced acute kidney injury
[a]CI-AKI group
[b]Non CI-AKI group
[c]Median (range)

the cancer risk due to radiation exposure in patients undergoing PCI for acute ST-elevation myocardial infarction (STEMI) and patients undergoing CTO PCI by incorporating the effective radiation dose into the Biological Effects of Ionizing Radiation (BEIR) VII model [80]. They found that the number of estimated additional lung and bone marrow cancer cases was on average two times higher in patients treated for CTOs compared to STEMI patients. Nevertheless, the above observations have not yet been confirmed in epidemiological studies and there is therefore insufficient evidence to defer a CTO intervention based on concerns for radiation exposure [81].

## Radiation Exposure Effects to Operators

Chronic exposure to low doses of ionising radiation has shown to cause DNA damage in interventional cardiologists which seems to correlate with the number of years of catheterization laboratory experience [82]. Venneri et al. [83] used the BEIR VII model to show that interventionalists had an increased cancer risk caused by professional radiation exposure. Recently published case clusters of interventional cardiologists with left sided brain neoplasms have raised the existing concerns, since radiation exposure to the left side is higher during PCI [84–86]. Despite the above, the risks related to radiation exposure in operators remains uncertain and further studies are required.

Radiation-induced cataract represents another occupational hazard to interventional cardiologists. The RELID (Retrospective evaluation study of lens injuries and dose) study showed that they have a threefold higher rate of posterior subcapsular lens opacities compared to unexposed individuals. Although the risk of developing cataract appears is dose-dependent [87], it appears to be lower for regular users of protective lead glasses [88]. The International Commission on Radiological Protection (ICRP) have suggested a threshold dose to the lens of 20 mSv per year, averaged over 5 consecutive years, with a maximum of 50 mSv in a single year [89].

## Methods for Reducing Radiation during CTO Interventions

### Pre-procedural Strategies

Careful **selection of patients** and early **assessment of the risk factors** that are associated with high risk for radiation injury is of primary importance. Patients with recent radiation exposure are at particularly high risk of radiation skin injury [90]. Every patient should be **consented** on the risks of radiation-related complications and careful examination of the skin should be performed prior to starting a CTO procedure. Moreover, the 'CTO team', including physicians, nurses and technicians, should always **review the films** prior to the procedure in order to understand the anatomy and plan the interventional strategy. Specific radiographic views that are most likely to be useful should be identified early in order to avoid unnecessary radiation exposure. As mentioned earlier **CTCA** is a useful tool for CTO pre-procedural planning. Although the contribution of multislice CT (MSCT) is approximately 19 mSv [61] the total radiation dose can be decreased significantly with successful CTO road mapping, based on the additional information on lesion characteristics. Incorporation of ECG-pulsed modulation of the tube current [91] and the use of new generation MSCT equipment can lower the effective radiation dose significantly [73]. Finally, each cardiac lab should have an established **radiation safety program** and operators should undergo **compulsory training** on radiation dose management and safety. Studies have shown that radiation doses can be reduced up to 34 % if operators have recently attended an informative conference on appropriate use of radiation and changes in x-ray delivery settings [92].

### Intra-Procedural Strategies

General Measures. Staff radiation dose should be closely monitored with **personal dose monitors** and dosimeter records should be provided to operators regularly. The ICRP recommends the use of two dosimeters [89]: one under the protective garment, usually at waist height, and a second outside the thyroid collar. If unusually high doses are recorded a review of staff practice patterns and adoption of further safety measures should be applied.

Protective 0.5 mm **lead aprons**, **thyroid shielding**, **shin leg covers and radiation-specific glasses** can stop up to 95 % of the scattered radiation and should be worn by all CTO operators [8]. Apart from the commonly used **radiation shielding**, additional protection could be achieved during CTO interventions with below table mounted shielding and the recently developed Trinity Radiation Protection system [93]. The latter consists of a combination of fixed shields, radiation drapes and interconnecting flexible radiation resistant materials that create a complete radiation protection environment for the operators. All CTO operators should be familiar with and apply the **ALARA** (As Low As Reasonably Achievable) principle, which means using all relevant methods and strategies in order to minimize radiation dose. Radiation exposure should be monitored closely at any time during the procedure. The **operator should be alerted** by the cardiac lab team when radiation levels exceed certain limits in order to balance the risks and benefits of discontinuing the procedure. A dose of 10 Gy ESAK has been suggested as a threshold at which a CTO operator should discontinue the procedure provided it is safe to do so, unless lesion crossing has occurred and the procedure is expected to be completed within a short period of time [63].

Increasing the distance between the patient and the X-ray tube by **positioning the table at a higher level** can result in significant reduction of radiation dose, although this should never affect the operator's comfort [94]. Higher **magnification** (zoom) increases patient's dose and should only be utilized in special circumstances. Moreover, all CTO operators should be familiar with operating at **lower framing rates per second** (fps) (6.0–7.5 fps instead of 15 fps) and using pulsed **fluoroscopy mode** rather than the digital cine mode storage. The number of acquisition runs should be held for optimising the strategy and assessing possible complications. **Altering the beam angulation** during the procedure by rotating the x-ray tube more than 40° can reduce the patient's skin dose at a given point [95]. Steep angles result in higher radiation doses due to penetration through more layers of tissue and should therefore be avoided [94]. **Collimation** decreases scatter radiation and the overall dose received by the patient. The use of additional copper filters reduces primary beam exposure and can enhance focused visualization.

**Table 14.8** Methods for reducing radiation during CTO interventions

| Pre-procedure | Intra-procedure | Post-procedure |
|---|---|---|
| Patient selection and risk assessment<br>Consent<br>Review films<br>CTCA<br>Radiation safety program<br>Compulsory training on radiation safety and management | Dosimeters<br>Protection clothing<br>Shielding<br>ALARA principle<br>Alert operator when radiation exceeds limits<br>Table position at higher level<br>Lower magnification<br>Lower frame rates<br>Changing beam angulation<br>Collimation<br>Procedure techniques | Dose documentation<br>Follow up |

*CTO* chronic total occlusion, *CTCA* computed tomography coronary angiography, *ALARA* as low as reasonably achievable

### CTO Specific Techniques

The use of CTO specific techniques can result in significant reduction of total radiation exposure:

- The **trapping technique** for equipment exchange (balloon inflation inside the guiding catheter to fix the wire).
- During dual injections, the **donor vessel is injected first** to allow time to fill the distal vessel. Fluoroscopy or cine acquisition begins 1–2 s later and it is followed by injection of the occluded vessel.
- The use of **IVUS** for proximal cap identification, re-entry guidance, assessment of retrograde wire position in reverse CART and stent optimisation.
- **Marking the length of the wire** that can be advanced safely without exiting the microcatheter during wire exchanges or when modifying the wire's tip bend. A pre-attached torquer at the end of the inserted wire or a stable marker on the table can be used.

The methods for reducing radiation during CTO interventions are summarised in Table 14.8. Adoption of these measures should avoid excessive doses, such that a target of <5 Gy should be achievable for the vast majority of cases, and many operators now use an absolute stopping point of 8 Gy ESAK.

## Post-Procedural Strategies and Follow Up

Post-procedure dose analysis is important in order to determine further management and follow up, especially if a repeat procedure is planned and the initial procedure resulted in high radiation exposure. The CTO procedure report should include all available radiation dose parameters, such as the fluoroscopy time, ESAK and DAP.

Post-procedure follow up should be guided by the Air Kerma Dose that the patient received during the CTO intervention [90]:

- **>5 Gy**: patients should be educated regarding potential skin changes on their back. A thorough examination of the skin should be performed 1 month following the procedure and if there is evidence of radiation-induced skin injury an appropriate specialist referral should be considered.
- **>10 Gy**: patients should be educated accordingly and followed up after 2–4 weeks. A qualified physicist should promptly be asked to calculate peak skin dose.
- **>15 Gy**: dosed above this level are identified by the Joint Commission as a sentinel event, therefore hospital risk management and regulatory authorities need to be contacted within 24 h after the procedure. No interventional procedure should reach this level unless there is a life threatening complication that necessitates obligatory percutaneous fluoroscopic reversal.

### Conclusions

The field of CTO-PCI has evolved significantly in recent years and the hybrid approach to CTO offers the opportunity to treat more complex anatomy successfully and therefore meet the needs of a wider patient population. Prevention of complications related to use of contrast and radiation represents a major component of a successful CTO intervention. Operator awareness and use of all the required precautions improve patient, staff and physician safety.

## References


1. McCullough PA. Contrast-induced acute kidney injury. J Am Coll Cardiol. 2008;51:1419–28.
2. Mehran R, Aymong ED, Nikolsky E, Lasic Z, Iakovou I, Fahy M, Mintz GS, Lansky AJ, Moses JW, Stone GW, Leon MB, Dangas G. A simple risk score for prediction of contrast-induced nephropathy after percutaneous coronary intervention: development and initial validation. J Am Coll Cardiol. 2004;44:1393–9.
3. McDonald JS, McDonald RJ, Comin J, Williamson EE, Katzberg RW, Murad MH, Kallmes DF. Frequency of acute kidney injury following intravenous contrast medium administration: a systematic review and meta-analysis. Radiology. 2013;267:119–28.
4. Meinel FG, De Cecco CN, Schoepf UJ, Katzberg R. Contrast-induced acute kidney injury: definition, epidemiology, and outcome. Biomed Res Int. 2014;2014:859328.
5. Barrett BJ, Parfrey PS. Prevention of nephrotoxicity induced by radiocontrast agents. N Engl J Med. 1994;331:1449–50.
6. KDIGO clinical practice guideline for acute kidney injury. Kidney Int Suppl. 2012;2:8–12.
7. McDonald RJ, McDonald JS, Bida JP, Carter RE, Fleming CJ, Misra S, Williamson EE, Kallmes DF. Intravenous contrast material-induced nephropathy: causal or coincident phenomenon? Radiology. 2013;267:106–18.
8. Hoste EA, Clermont G, Kersten A, Venkataraman R, Angus DC, De Bacquer D, Kellum JA. RIFLE criteria for acute kidney injury are associated with hospital mortality in critically ill patients: a cohort analysis. Crit Care. 2006;10:R73.
9. Thakar CV, Christianson A, Freyberg R, Almenoff P, Render ML. Incidence and outcomes of acute kidney injury in intensive care units: a Veterans Administration study. Crit Care Med. 2009;37:2552–8.
10. Patel VG, Michael TT, Mogabgab O, Fuh E, Banerjee A, Brayton KM, Cipher DJ, Abdullah SM, Brilakis ES. Clinical, angiographic, and procedural predictors of periprocedural complications during chronic total occlusion percutaneous coronary intervention. J Invasive Cardiol. 2014;26:100–5.
11. El Sabbagh A, Patel VG, Jeroudi OM, Michael TT, Alomar ME, Mogabgab O, Fuh E, Roesle M, Rangan BV, Abdullah S, Hastings JL, Grodin J, Kumbhani DJ, Alexopoulos D, Fasseas P, Banerjee S, Brilakis ES. Angiographic success and procedural complications in patients undergoing retrograde percutaneous coronary chronic total occlusion interventions: a weighted meta-analysis of 3,482 patients from 26 studies. Int J Cardiol. 2014;174:243–8.
12. Lin YS, Fang HY, Hussein H, Fang CY, Chen YL, Hsueh SK, Cheng CI, Yang CH, Chen CJ, Hang CL, Yip HK, Wu CJ. Predictors of contrast-induced nephropathy in chronic total occlusion percutaneous coronary intervention. EuroIntervention. 2014;9:1173–80.
13. Christopoulos G, Karmpaliotis D, Alaswad K, Lombardi WL, Grantham JA, Rangan BV, Kotsia AP, Lembo N, Kandzari DE, Lee J, Kalynych A, Carlson H, Garcia S, Banerjee S, Thompson CA, Brilakis ES. The efficacy of "hybrid" percutaneous coronary intervention in chronic total occlusions caused by in-stent restenosis: Insights from a US multicenter registry. Catheter Cardiovasc Interv. 2014;84(4):646–51.
14. Karmpaliotis D, Michael TT, Brilakis ES, Papayannis AC, Tran DL, Kirkland BL, Lembo N, Kalynych A, Carlson H, Banerjee S, Lombardi W, Kandzari DE. Retrograde coronary chronic total occlusion revascularization: procedural and in-hospital outcomes from a multicenter registry in the United States. JACC Cardiovasc Interv. 2012;5:1273–9.
15. Michael TT, Karmpaliotis D, Brilakis ES, Fuh E, Patel VG, Mogabgab O, Alomar M, Kirkland BL, Lembo N, Kalynych A, Carlson H, Banerjee S, Lombardi W, Kandzari DE. Procedural outcomes of revascularization of chronic total occlusion of native coronary arteries (from a multicenter United States registry). Am J Cardiol. 2013;112:488–92.
16. Tsuchikane E, Yamane M, Mutoh M, Matsubara T, Fujita T, Nakamura S, Muramatsu T, Okamura A, Igarashi Y, Oida A, Retrograde Summit Investigators. Japanese multicenter registry evaluating the retrograde approach for chronic coronary total occlusion. Catheter Cardiovasc Interv. 2013;82:E654–61.
17. Patel VG, Brayton KM, Tamayo A, Mogabgab O, Michael TT, Lo N, Alomar M, Shorrock D, Cipher D, Abdullah S, Banerjee S, Brilakis ES. Angiographic success and procedural complications in patients undergoing percutaneous coronary chronic total occlusion interventions: a weighted meta-analysis of 18,061 patients from 65 studies. JACC Cardiovasc Interv. 2013;6:128–36.
18. Danzi GB, Valenti R, Migliorini A, Parodi G, Vergara R, Antoniucci D. Percutaneous coronary intervention for multiple chronic total occlusions. Am J Cardiol. 2013;112:1849–53.

19. Galassi AR, Tomasello SD, Reifart N, Werner GS, Sianos G, Bonnier H, Sievert H, Ehladad S, Bufe A, Shofer J, Gershlick A, Hildick-Smith D, Escaned J, Erglis A, Sheiban I, Thuesen L, Serra A, Christiansen E, Buettner A, Costanzo L, Barrano G, Di Mario C. In-hospital outcomes of percutaneous coronary intervention in patients with chronic total occlusion: insights from the ERCTO (European Registry of Chronic Total Occlusion) registry. EuroIntervention. 2011;7:472–9.
20. Morino Y, Kimura T, Hayashi Y, Muramatsu T, Ochiai M, Noguchi Y, Kato K, Shibata Y, Hiasa Y, Doi O, Yamashita T, Morimoto T, Abe M, Hinohara T, Mitsudo K, J-CTO Registry Investigators. In-hospital outcomes of contemporary percutaneous coronary intervention in patients with chronic total occlusion insights from the J-CTO Registry (Multicenter CTO Registry in Japan). JACC Cardiovasc Interv. 2010;3:143–51.
21. Aguiar-Souto P, Ferrante G, Del Furia F, Barlis P, Khurana R, Di Mario C. Frequency and predictors of contrast-induced nephropathy after angioplasty for chronic total occlusions. Int J Cardiol. 2010;139:68–74.
22. Rathore S, Hakeem A, Pauriah M, Roberts E, Beaumont A, Morris JL. A comparison of the transradial and the transfemoral approach in chronic total occlusion percutaneous coronary intervention. Catheter Cardiovasc Interv. 2009;73:883–7.
23. Christopoulos G, Menon RV, Karmpaliotis D, Alaswad K, Lombardi W, Grantham JA, Michael TT, Patel VG, Rangan BV, Kotsia AP, Lembo N, Kandzari DE, Lee J, Kalynych A, Carlson H, Garcia S, Banerjee S, Thompson CA, Brilakis ES. Application of the "hybrid approach" to chronic total occlusions in patients with previous coronary artery bypass graft surgery (from a Contemporary Multicenter US registry). Am J Cardiol. 2014;113:1990–4.
24. Michael TT, Karmpaliotis D, Brilakis ES, Alomar M, Abdullah SM, Kirkland BL, Mishoe KL, Lembo N, Kalynych A, Carlson H, Banerjee S, Luna M, Lombardi W, Kandzari DE. Temporal trends of fluoroscopy time and contrast utilization in coronary chronic total occlusion revascularization: insights from a multicenter United States registry. Catheter Cardiovasc Interv. 2015;85(3):393–9.
25. Rihal CS, Textor SC, Grill DE, Berger PB, Ting HH, Best PJ, Singh M, Bell MR, Barsness GW, Mathew V, Garratt KN, Holmes Jr DR. Incidence and prognostic importance of acute renal failure after percutaneous coronary intervention. Circulation. 2002;105:2259–64.
26. Betge S, Krack A, Figulla HR, Werner GS. Analysis of location and pattern of target vessel failure in chronic total occlusions after stent implantation and its potential for the efficient use of drug-eluting stents. J Interv Cardiol. 2006;19:226–31.
27. Ivanhoe RJ, Weintraub WS, Douglas Jr JS, Lembo NJ, Furman M, Gershony G, Cohen CL, King 3rd SB. Percutaneous transluminal coronary angioplasty of chronic total occlusions. Primary success, restenosis, and long-term clinical follow-up. Circulation. 1992;85:106–15.
28. Kahn JK, Rutherford BD, McConahay DR, Johnson WL, Giorgi LV, Shimshak TM, Hartzler GO. High-dose contrast agent administration during complex coronary angioplasty. Am Heart J. 1990;120:533–6.
29. Brown J, Malenka DJ, DeVries JT, Robb JF, Jayne JE, Friedman BJ, Hettleman BD, Niles NW, Kaplan AV, Schoolwerth AC, Thompson CA. Transient and persistent renal dysfunction are predictors of survival after percutaneous coronary intervention: insights from the Dartmouth Dynamic Registry. Catheter Cardiovasc Interv. 2008;72: 347–54.
30. Levy EM, Viscoli CM, Horwitz RI. The effect of acute renal failure on mortality: a cohort analysis. JAMA. 1996;275:1489–94.
31. Gruberg L, Mintz GS, Mehran R, Gangas G, Lansky AJ, Kent KM, Pichard AD, Satler LF, Leon MB. The prognostic implications of further renal function deterioration within 48 h of interventional coronary procedures in patients with pre-existent chronic renal insufficiency. J Am Coll Cardiol. 2000;36:1542–8.
32. Maioli M, Toso A, Leoncini M, Gallopin M, Musilli N, Bellandi F. Persistent renal damage after contrast-induced acute kidney injury: incidence, evolution, risk factors, and prognosis. Circulation. 2012; 125:3099–107.
33. James MT, Ghali WA, Tonelli M, Faris P, Knudtson ML, Pannu N, Klarenbach SW, Manns BJ, Hemmelgarn BR. Acute kidney injury following coronary angiography is associated with a long-term decline in kidney function. Kidney Int. 2010;78:803–19.
34. James MT, Ghali WA, Knudtson ML, Ravani P, Tonelli M, Faris P, Pannu N, Manns BJ, Klarenbach SW, Hemmelgarn BR, Alberta Provincial Project for Outcome Assessment in Coronary Heart Disease (APPROACH) Investigators. Associations between acute kidney injury and cardiovascular and renal outcomes after coronary angiography. Circulation. 2011;123:409–16.
35. Mueller C, Buerkle G, Buettner HJ, Petersen J, Perruchoud AP, Eriksson U, Marsch S, Roskamm H. Prevention of contrast media-associated nephropathy: randomized comparison of 2 hydration regimens in 1620 patients undergoing coronary angioplasty. Arch Intern Med. 2002;162:329–36.
36. Trivedi HS, Moore H, Nasr S, Aggarwal K, Agrawal A, Goel P, Hewett J. A randomized prospective trial to assess the role of saline hydration on the development of contrast nephrotoxicity. Nephron Clin Pract. 2003;93:C29–34.
37. Bader BD, Berger ED, Heede MB, Silberbaur I, Duda S, Risler T, Erley CM. What is the best hydration regimen to prevent contrast media-induced nephrotoxicity? Clin Nephrol. 2004;62:1–7.
38. Caixeta A, Nikolsky E, Mehran R. Prevention and treatment of contrast-associated nephropathy in interventional cardiology. Curr Cardiol Rep. 2009;11:377–83.
39. Cigarroa RG, Lange RA, Williams RH, Hillis LD. Dosing of contrast material to prevent contrast nephropathy in patients with renal disease. Am J Med. 1989;86:649–52.
40. Brown JR, Robb JF, Block CA, Schoolwerth AC, Kaplan AV, O'Connor GT, Solomon RJ, Malenka DJ. Does safe dosing of iodinated contrast prevent contrast-induced acute kidney injury? Circ Cardiovasc Interv. 2010;3:346–50.
41. Laskey WK, Jenkins C, Selzer F, Marroquin OC, Wilensky RL, Glaser R, Cohen HA, Holmes Jr DR, NHLBI Dynamic Registry Investigators. Volume-to-creatinine clearance ratio: a pharmacokinetically based risk factor for prediction of early creatinine increase after percutaneous coronary intervention. J Am Coll Cardiol. 2007;50:584–90.
42. Tepel M, van der Giet M, Schwarzfeld C, Laufer U, Liermann D, Zidek W. Prevention of radiographic-contrast-agent-induced reductions in renal function by acetylcysteine. N Engl J Med. 2000;343:180–4.
43. Briguori C, Manganelli F, Scarpato P, Elia PP, Golia B, Riviezzo G, Lepore S, Librera M, Villari B, Colombo A, Ricciardelli B. Acetylcysteine and contrast agent-associated nephrotoxicity. J Am Coll Cardiol. 2002;40:298–303.
44. Kshirsagar AV, Poole C, Mottl A, Shoham D, Franceschini N, Tudor G, Agrawal M, Denu-Ciocca C, Magnus Ohman E, Finn WF. N-acetylcysteine for the prevention of radiocontrast induced nephropathy: a meta-analysis of prospective controlled trials. J Am Soc Nephrol. 2004;15:761–9.
45. Nallamothu BK, Shojania KG, Saint S, Hofer TP, Humes HD, Moscucci M, Bates ER. Is acetylcysteine effective in preventing contrast-related nephropathy? A meta-analysis. Am J Med. 2004;117:938–47.
46. Investigators ACT. Acetylcysteine for prevention of renal outcomes in patients undergoing coronary and peripheral vascular angiography: main results from the randomized Acetylcysteine for Contrast-induced nephropathy Trial (ACT). Circulation. 2011;124:1250–9.
47. Lewington A, MacTier R, Hoefield R, Sutton A, Smith D, Downes M, The Renal Association, British Cardiovascular Intervention Society, Royal College of Radiologists. Prevention contrast induced acute kidney injury (CI-AKI) in adult patients, 2013. Available at: http://www.renal.org/Clinical/OtherGuidelines.aspx.

48. Merten GJ, Burgess WP, Gray LV, Holleman JH, Roush TS, Kowalchuk GJ, Bersin RM, Van Moore A, Simonton 3rd CA, Rittase RA, Norton HJ, Kennedy TP. Prevention of contrast-induced nephropathy with sodium bicarbonate: a randomized controlled trial. JAMA. 2004;291:2328–34.
49. Recio-Mayoral A, Chaparro M, Prado B, Cózar R, Méndez I, Banerjee D, Kaski JC, Cubero J, Cruz JM. The reno-protective effect of hydration with sodium bicarbonate plus N-acetylcysteine in patients undergoing emergency percutaneous coronary intervention: the RENO Study. J Am Coll Cardiol. 2007;49:1283–8.
50. Ozcan EE, Guneri S, Akdeniz B, Akyildiz IZ, Senaslan O, Baris N, Aslan O, Badak O. Sodium bicarbonate, N-acetylcysteine, and saline for prevention of radiocontrast-induced nephropathy. A comparison of 3 regimens for protecting contrast-induced nephropathy in patients undergoing coronary procedures. A single-center prospective controlled trial. Am Heart J. 2007;154:539–44.
51. Hogan SE, L'Allier P, Chetcuti S, Grossman PM, Nallamothu BK, Duvernoy C, Bates E, Moscucci M, Gurm HS. Current role of sodium bicarbonate-based preprocedural hydration for the prevention of contrast-induced acute kidney injury: a meta-analysis. Am Heart J. 2008;156:414–21.
52. Maioli M, Toso A, Leoncini M, Gallopin M, Tedeschi D, Micheletti C, Bellandi F. Sodium bicarbonate versus saline for the prevention of contrast-induced nephropathy in patients with renal dysfunction undergoing coronary angiography or intervention. J Am Coll Cardiol. 2008;52:599–604.
53. From AM, Bartholmai BJ, Williams AW, Cha SS, Pflueger A, McDonald FS. Sodium bicarbonate is associated with an increased incidence of contrast nephropathy: a retrospective cohort study of 7977 patients at mayo clinic. Clin J Am Soc Nephrol. 2008;3:10–8.
54. Sterner G, Frennby B, Kurkus J, Nyman U. Does post-angiographic hemodialysis reduce the risk of contrast-medium nephropathy? Scand J Urol Nephrol. 2000;34:323–6.
55. Marenzi G, Marana I, Lauri G, Assanelli E, Grazi M, Campodonico J, Trabattoni D, Fabbiocchi F, Montorsi P, Bartorelli AL. The prevention of radiocontrast-agent-induced nephropathy by hemofiltration. N Engl J Med. 2003;349:1333–40.
56. Ozhan H, Erden I, Ordu S, Aydin M, Caglar O, Basar C, Yalcin S, Alemdar R. Efficacy of short-term high-dose atorvastatin for prevention of contrast-induced nephropathy in patients undergoing coronary angiography. Angiology. 2010;61:711–4.
57. Patti G, Ricottini E, Nusca A, Colonna G, Pasceri V, D'Ambrosio A, Montinaro A, Di Sciascio G. Short-term, high-dose Atorvastatin pretreatment to prevent contrast-induced nephropathy in patients with acute coronary syndromes undergoing percutaneous coronary intervention (from the ARMYDA-CIN [atorvastatin for reduction of myocardial damage during angioplasty–contrast-induced nephropathy] trial. Am J Cardiol. 2011;108:1–7.
58. Jo SH, Koo BK, Park JS, Kang HJ, Cho YS, Kim YJ, Youn TJ, Chung WY, Chae IH, Choi DJ, Sohn DW, Oh BH, Park YB, Choi YS, Kim HS. Prevention of radiocontrast medium-induced nephropathy using short-term high-dose simvastatin in patients with renal insufficiency undergoing coronary angiography (PROMISS) trial–a randomized controlled study. Am Heart J. 2008;155:499.e1–8.
59. Toso A, Maioli M, Leoncini M, Gallopin M, Tedeschi D, Micheletti C, Manzone C, Amato M, Bellandi F. Usefulness of atorvastatin (80 mg) in prevention of contrast-induced nephropathy in patients with chronic renal disease. Am J Cardiol. 2010;105:288–92.
60. Giacoppo D, Capodanno D, Capranzano P, Aruta P, Tamburino C. Meta-analysis of randomized controlled trials of preprocedural statin administration for reducing contrast-induced acute kidney injury in patients undergoing coronary catheterization. Am J Cardiol. 2014;114:541–8.
61. García-García HM, van Mieghem CA, Gonzalo N, Meijboom WB, Weustink AC, Onuma Y, Mollet NR, Schultz CJ, Meliga E, van der Ent M, Sianos G, Goedhart D, den Boer A, de Feyter P, Serruys PW. Computed tomography in total coronary occlusions (CTTO registry): radiation exposure and predictors of successful percutaneous intervention. EuroIntervention. 2009;4:607–16.
62. Courtney BK, Munce NR, Anderson KJ, Thind AS, Leung G, Radau PE, Foster FS, Vitkin IA, Schwartz RS, Dick AJ, Wright GA, Strauss BH. Innovations in imaging for chronic total occlusions: a glimpse into the future of angiography's blind-spot. Eur Heart J. 2008;29:583–93.
63. Brilakis ES, Grantham JA, Rinfret S, Wyman RM, Burke MN, Karmpaliotis D, Lembo N, Pershad A, Kandzari DE, Buller CE, DeMartini T, Lombardi WL, Thompson CA. A percutaneous treatment algorithm for crossing coronary chronic total occlusions. JACC Cardiovasc Interv. 2012;5:367–79.
64. Dai J, Katoh O, Kyo E, Tsuji T, Watanabe S, Ohya H. Approach for chronic total occlusion with intravascular ultrasound-guided reverse controlled antegrade and retrograde tracking technique: single center experience. J Interv Cardiol. 2013;26:434–43.
65. Uehara Y, Shimizu M, Yoshimura M. A case of CTO treated with minimum use of contrast media. Catheter Cardiovasc Interv. 2013;82:E884–7.
66. Stevens MA, McCullough PA, Tobin KJ, Speck JP, Westveer DC, Guido-Allen DA, Timmis GC, O'Neill WW. A prospective randomized trial of prevention measures in patients at high risk for contrast nephropathy: results of the P.R.I.N.C.E. Study. Prevention of radiocontrast induced nephropathy clinical evaluation. J Am Coll Cardiol. 1999;33:403–11.
67. Marenzi G, Ferrari C, Marana I, Assanelli E, De Metrio M, Teruzzi G, Veglia F, Fabbiocchi F, Montorsi P, Bartorelli AL. Prevention of contrast nephropathy by furosemide with matched hydration: the MYTHOS (Induced Diuresis With Matched Hydration Compared to Standard Hydration for Contrast Induced Nephropathy Prevention) trial. JACC Cardiovasc Interv. 2012;5:90–7.
68. Briguori C, Visconti G, Focaccio A, Airoldi F, Valgimigli M, Sangiorgi GM, Golia B, Ricciardelli B, Condorelli G, REMEDIAL II Investigators. Renal Insufficiency After Contrast Media Administration Trial II (REMEDIAL II): RenalGuard System in high-risk patients for contrast-induced acute kidney injury. Circulation. 2011;124:1260–9.
69. Evaluation of RenalGuard System to Reduce the Incidence of Contrast Induced Nephropathy in At-Risk Patients (CIN-RG). ClinicalTrials.gov NCT01456013.
70. Duffy SJ, Ruygrok P, Juergens CP, Sievert H, Richards M, Blake J, Whitbourn R, Farouque HO, Pertile T, Kaye DM. Removal of contrast media from the coronary sinus attenuates renal injury after coronary angiography and intervention. J Am Coll Cardiol. 2010;56:525–6.
71. Contrast Media Reduction and Removal in Patients With CKD (PRESERV). ClinicalTrials.gov NCT01168024.
72. Suzuki S, Furui S, Kohtake H, Yokoyama N, Kozuma K, Yamamoto Y, Isshiki T. Radiation exposure to patient's skin during percutaneous coronary intervention for various lesions, including chronic total occlusion. Circ J. 2006;70:44–8.
73. Sianos G, Werner GS, Galassi AR, Papafaklis MI, Escaned J, Hildick-Smith D, Christiansen EH, Gershlick A, Carlino M, Karlas A, Konstantinidis NV, Tomasello SD, Di Mario C, Reifart N, EuroCTO Club. Recanalisation of chronic total coronary occlusions: 2012 consensus document from the EuroCTO club. EuroIntervention. 2012;8:139–45.
74. Fetterly KA, Lennon RJ, Bell MR, Holmes Jr DR, Rihal CS. Clinical determinants of radiation dose in percutaneous coronary interventional procedures: influence of patient size, procedure complexity, and performing physician. JACC Cardiovasc Interv. 2011;4:336–43.
75. Delewi R, Hoebers LP, Råmunddal T, Henriques JP, Angerås O, Stewart J, Robertsson L, Wahlin M, Petursson P, Piek JJ, Albertsson P, Matejka G, Omerovic E. Clinical and procedural characteristics associated with higher radiation exposure during percutaneous coronary interventions and coronary angiography. Circ Cardiovasc Interv. 2013;6:501–6.

76. Slovut DP. Cutaneous radiation injury after complex coronary intervention. JACC Cardiovasc Interv. 2009;2:701–2.
77. Wrixon AD. New ICRP recommendations. J Radiol Prot. 2008;28:161–8.
78. Einstein AJ, Henzlova MJ, Rajagopalan S. Estimating risk of cancer associated with radiation exposure from 64-slice computed tomography coronary angiography. JAMA. 2007;298:317–23.
79. Godino C, Maccagni D, Pavon AG, Viani G, Cappelletti A, Margonato A, Colombo A. Estimating incidence of organ cancer related to PCI radiation exposure in patients treated for acute and chronic total occlusions. J Invasive Cardiol. 2013;25:441–5.
80. Committee to Assess Health Risks from Exposure to Low Level of Ionizing Radiation. Health risks from exposure to low levels of ionizing radiation: BEIR VII phase 2. Washington, DC: National Academies; National Research Council.
81. Shah N, Deshmukh A, Sachdeva R. Radiation exposure after percutaneous coronary intervention: is the cancer risk real? J Invasive Cardiol. 2013;25:447–8.
82. Andreassi MG, Cioppa A, Botto N, Joksic G, Manfredi S, Federici C, Ostojic M, Rubino P, Picano E. Somatic DNA damage in interventional cardiologists: a case-control study. FASEB J. 2005;19: 998–9.
83. Venneri L, Rossi F, Botto N, Andreassi MG, Salcone N, Emad A, Lazzeri M, Gori C, Vano E, Picano E. Cancer risk from professional exposure in staff working in cardiac catheterization laboratory: insights from the National Research Council's Biological Effects of Ionizing Radiation VII Report. Am Heart J. 2009;157:118–24.
84. Roguin A, Goldstein J, Bar O. Brain tumours among interventional cardiologists: a cause for alarm? Report of four new cases from two cities and a review of the literature. EuroIntervention. 2012;7:1081–6.
85. Roguin A, Goldstein J, Bar O. Brain malignancies and ionising radiation: more cases reported. EuroIntervention. 2012;8:169–70.
86. Roguin A, Goldstein J, Bar O, Goldstein JA. Brain and neck tumours among physicians performing interventional procedures. Am J Cardiol. 2013;111:1368–72.
87. Ciraj-Bjelac O, Rehani MM, Sim KH, Liew HB, Vano E, Kleiman NJ. Risk for radiation-induced cataract for staff in interventional cardiology: is there reason for concern? Catheter Cardiovasc Interv. 2010;76:826–34.
88. Jacob S, Boveda S, Bar O, Brézin A, Maccia C, Laurier D, Bernier MO. Interventional cardiologists and risk of radiation-induced cataract: results of a French multicenter observational study. Int J Cardiol. 2013;167:1843–7.
89. International Commission on Radiological Protection. Avoidance of radiation injuries from medical interventional procedures. Ann ICRP. 2000:25–43.
90. Chambers CE, Fetterly KA, Holzer R, Lin PJ, Blankenship JC, Balter S, Laskey WK. Radiation safety program for the cardiac catheterization laboratory. Catheter Cardiovasc Interv. 2011;77: 546–56.
91. Abada HT, Larchez C, Daoud B, Sigal-Cinqualbre A, Paul JF. MDCT of the coronary arteries: feasibility of low-dose CT with ECG-pulsed tube current modulation to reduce radiation dose. AJR Am J Roentgenol. 2006;186:S387–90.
92. Azpiri-López JR, Assad-Morell JL, González-González JG, Elizondo-Riojas G, Dávila-Bortoni A, García-Martínez R, Treviño-Frutos R. Effect of physician training on the X-ray dose delivered during coronary angioplasty. J Invasive Cardiol. 2013;25:109–13.
93. Fattal P, Goldstein JA. A novel complete radiation protection system eliminates physician radiation exposure and leaded aprons. Catheter Cardiovasc Interv. 2013;82:11–6.
94. Brilakis ES, editor. Manual of coronary chronic total occlusion interventions. A step-by-step approach. Waltham: Elsevier; 2013.
95. Abdelaal E, Plourde G, MacHaalany J, Arsenault J, Rimac G, Déry JP, Barbeau G, Larose E, De Larochellière R, Nguyen CM, Allende R, Ribeiro H, Costerousse O, Mongrain R, Bertrand OF, Interventional Cardiologists at Quebec Heart-Lung Institute. Effectiveness of low rate fluoroscopy at reducing operator and patient radiation dose during transradial coronary angiography and interventions. JACC Cardiovasc Interv. 2014;7:567–74.
96. Bernier J, Bonner J, Vermorken JB, Bensadoun RJ, Dummer R, Giralt J, Kornek G, Hartley A, Mesia R, Robert C, Segaert S, Ang KK. Consensus guidelines for the management of radiation dermatitis and coexisting acne-like rash in patients receiving radiotherapy plus EGFR inhibitors for the treatment of squamous cell carcinoma of the head and neck. Ann Oncol. 2008;19:142–9.

# Complications of Chronic Total Occlusion Percutaneous Coronary Intervention

# 15

Rolf Graning and Tony DeMartini

**Abstract**

Percutaneous coronary intervention of chronic total occlusions has gained attention over the past 10 years. This is due to advances in technology, techniques and the hybrid algorithm. A systematic approach to these complex procedures may reduce the risk of complications. Complications are inevitable but awareness of the etiology and treatment of the complications is imperative. An algorithmic approach to complication management will allow the operator to more skillfully diagnose and manage the situation.

**Keywords**

Chronic total occlusion • Percutaneous coronary intervention • Complication(s) • Perforation • Dissection • Entrapment • Contrast induced nephropathy • Radiation injury

## Introduction

Chronic total occlusions (CTO) are one of the most challenging and complex types of percutaneous coronary interventions (PCI), namely due to the marked anatomic and lesion variability that hallmark CTOs and the variety of techniques and devices required for recanalization. The rate of successful recanalization of CTOs continues to improve and is currently ≥80 % in contemporary practice at centers with higher CTO PCI volumes [1, 2]. Further, advances in techniques and devices have also reduced the rate of major complications (death, emergent coronary artery bypass graft, and stroke) to as low as 0.5 % [2]. However, as many of the devices used in CTO revascularization are unique to the procedure, the complication rates differ compared with those from a routine PCI (Table 15.1). Because of this, it is important for the CTO operator to be aware of the complications that are unique to CTOs in order to identify them and treat them accordingly. CTO complications can be categorized according to timing (acute *versus* chronic) and location (cardiac *versus* non-cardiac) (Fig. 15.1). Chronic complications predominantly relate to in-stent restenosis and thrombosis and will not be reviewed in this chapter. We will discuss the complications and causes of CTO revascularization and strategies for prevention and treatment.

**Electronic supplementary material** The online version of this chapter (doi:10.1007/978-3-319-21563-1_15) contains supplementary material, which is available to authorized users.

R. Graning, MD (✉)
Department of Cardiology, William Beaumont Hospital, Royal Oak, MI, USA
e-mail: graningr@gmail.com

T. DeMartini, MD
Department of Cardiology, Advocate Heart Institute, Downers Grove, IL, USA

## Acute Cardiac Complications

### Coronary Perforation

Coronary perforations represent one of the most dreaded complications of any interventional operator. Because of the potential sub-intimal position of wires and equipment with CTOs, routine use of stiff and polymer-jacketed guidewires, and frequent uncertainty regarding the vessel course there is an increased risk of perforation compared with non-CTO


S. Rinfret (ed.), *Percutaneous Intervention for Coronary Chronic Total Occlusion: The Hybrid Approach*, DOI 10.1007/978-3-319-21563-1_15

**Table 15.1** Frequency of complications in the largest reported series of CTO interventions

| Author | Year | Patients | Success (%) | Retrograde (%) | MI (%) | Tamponade (%) | In-hospital mortality (%) | Emergent CABG (%) |
|---|---|---|---|---|---|---|---|---|
| Suero et al. [3] | 2001 | 2007 | 69.9 | 0 | 2.4 | 0.5 | 1.3 | 0.7 |
| Prasad et al. (Mayo clinic) [4] | 2007 | 634 ('97-'05) | 72 | 0 | 7.2 | 0.9 | 0.3 | 0.7 |
| Rathore et al. (Toyohashi) [5] | 2009 | 806 | 87.5 | 17.1 | 3.0 | 1.5 | 0.5 | 0.2 |
| Morino et al. (J-CTO) [6] | 2010 | 498 | 87.7 | 25.7 | 2.3 | 0.4 | 0.4 | 0 |
| Galassi et al. (ERCTO) [7] | 2011 | 1914 | 82.9 | 11.8 | 1.3 | 0.5 | 0.3 | 0.1 |
| Christopoulos et al. [8] | 2014 | 497 | 91.5 | 32 | 1.0 | 0.4 | 0.4 | NR |

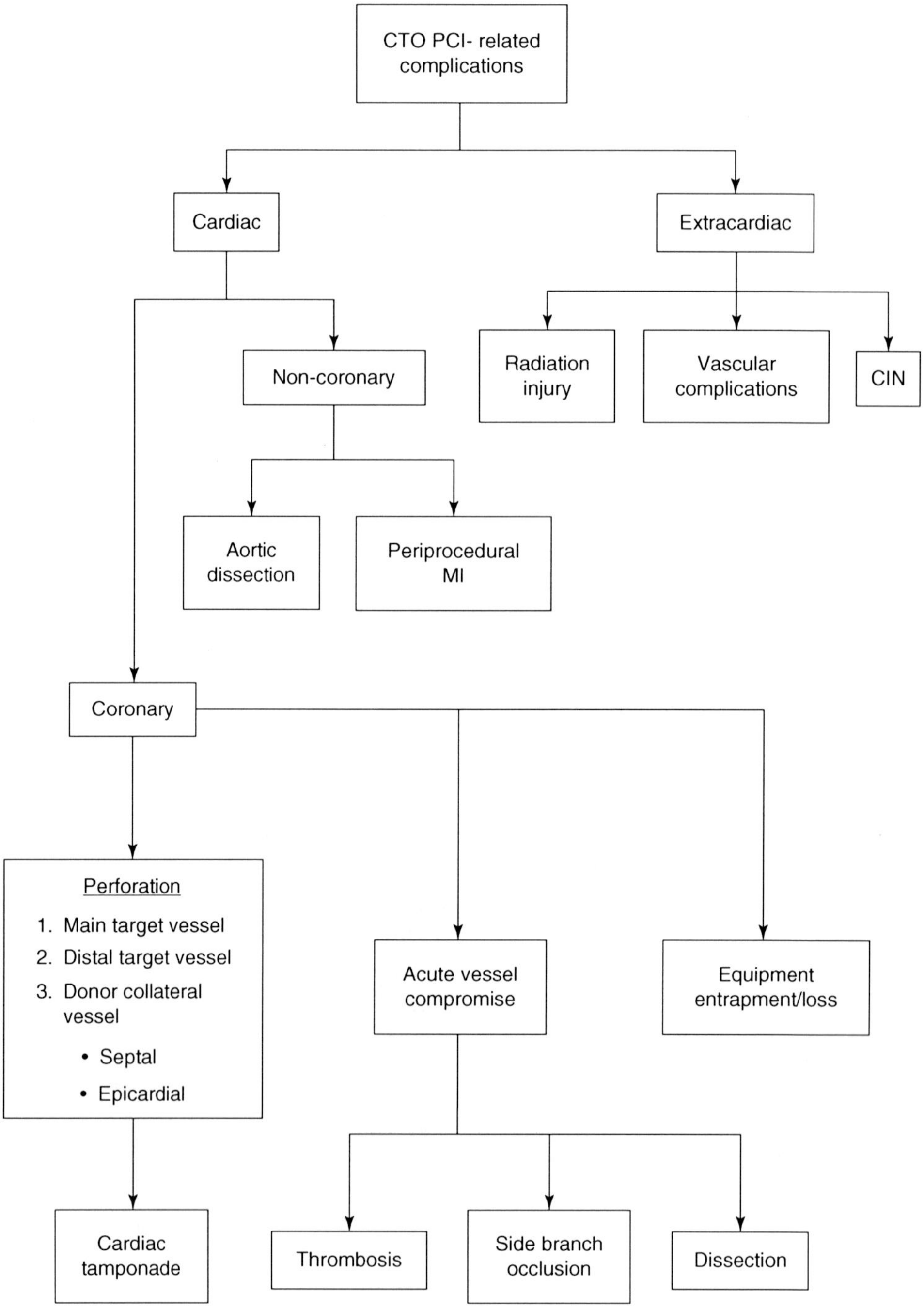


**Fig. 15.1** Complications of percutaneous coronary intervention of chronic total occlusions. *CIN* contrast induced nephropathy, *CTO* chronic total occlusion, *MI* myocardial infarction, *PCI* percutaneous coronary intervention

**Table 15.2** Ellis classification of coronary perforations

| Perforation type | Description |
|---|---|
| Type I | Extraluminal crater without myocardial blush, extravasation, or evidence of dissection |
| Type II | Myocardial or pericardial blush without extravasation |
| Type III | Extravasation through a ≥1 mm perforation |
| Type III: cavity spilling | Perforation and extravasation into an anatomic cavity chamber |

PCI where the incidence is approximately 0.2 % [9]. The estimated incidence of coronary perforation for CTO PCI is 2.9 % (95 % confidence interval [CI] 2.3–3.6 %), however observed rates are as high as 11.9 % in the literature [2]. The most feared complication of perforation is tamponade requiring emergent pericardiocentesis or cardiac surgery. In a large meta-analysis of over 18,000 patients who had undergone CTO PCI, approximately 10 % of patient with coronary perforations developed tamponade (pooled incidence rate = 0.3 %, 95 % CI 0.2–0.5 %) [2]. Therefore, while the incidence of perforation is higher than in non-CTO PCI, the majority of perforations are self-limited and can be managed without progression to tamponade.

Not surprisingly, the rate of coronary perforation and tamponade is higher in unsuccessful PCI attempts compared with successful recanalization (perforation = 10.7 % vs. 2.1 %, $p<0.0001$; tamponade = 1.7 % vs. 0 %, $p<0.0001$) [2]. Further, the risk of coronary perforation is higher using a retrograde approach compared with antegrade (4.7 % vs. 2.1 %, $p=0.04$) however the rates of tamponade are similar [7].

Perforations are classified according to the Ellis Criteria (Table 15.2). While this is a simplistic view of perforations in general, it helps to stratify patients according to risk for development of complications such as tamponade and provides a rough framework in order to guide further intervention. Further, perforations can be classified according to vessel location. This is important as the mechanisms and subsequent management greatly differs and range from conservative therapy for septal perforations to percutaneous intervention with coils or covered stents and even emergent surgery for epicardial or main vessel perforations. In general, the three main coronary vessel locations for perforations are: (1) main target vessel (i.e. at or near the CTO); (2) distal target vessel; and (3) donor collateral vessel, either epicardial or septal.

Main target vessel coronary perforation can occur with either antegrade or retrograde percutaneous approaches. Guidewire perforations alone via wire escalation or dissection and reentry techniques are typically self-limited and rarely lead to a hemorrhagic pericardial effusion and/or cardiac tamponade. However, if a balloon or device (e.g. stent or microcatheter) is advanced outside of the coronary architecture after guidewire perforation then the risk for hemorrhagic pericardial effusion and cardiac tamponade increases due to manual expansion of the coronary perforation. Inadvertent antegrade injection can also lead to hydraulic expansion of the guidewire perforation, leading to an uncontrolled perforation. It is also important to recognize that over-sized balloons or stents can also lead to main target vessel coronary perforation. As many target vessels undergo negative remodeling due to chronic under-filling it can be difficult to adequately size balloons/stents appropriately, in which case use of intravascular ultrasound can be helpful.

Following identification of a main target vessel perforation of any type, the initial step in management is to position an appropriately sized balloon proximal to the area of contrast extravasation in order to occlude the perforation with balloon inflation. This can also be performed with the stent delivery balloon in the case of a post stent perforation. Prolonged balloon inflations may be required to achieve hemostasis. If bleeding persists despite balloon occlusion, then a covered stent (e.g. JOSTENT Graftmaster, Abbott Vascular, Santa Clara, CA; Symbiort stent, Boston Scientific Corp., Natick, MA; Over and Under stent, IGTI Medical, Or Akiva, Israel) should be placed [10]. Type III (Table 15.2) coronary perforations usually result in cardiac tamponade and a covered stent should be implanted for this type of perforation [11]. The most efficient method to minimize bleeding in patients requiring a covered stent is to use a dual-catheter, or "ping pong" guide technique [12]. With this technique, a second guide catheter is advanced near the coronary ostium next to the first guide catheter that is currently engaged with the balloon occluding the perforation. While maintaining balloon occlusion the first guide catheter is pulled back into the aorta while the second guide catheter is engaged. The vessel is then wired from the second guide with the balloon rapidly deflated and re-inflated in order to allow wire passage distally. The covered stent is positioned proximal to the occluding balloon which is then rapidly deflated and withdrawn proximally while the covered stent is advanced and deployed to fully cover the perforated site [12]. In the case of covered stent delivery failure, a balloon can be inflated more proximally while maintaining hemostasis from the first guide catheter with the balloon inflated at the perforation site. Reattempt to deliver the covered stent will usually be successful. Prior to removing any equipment, adequate sealing of the coronary perforation should be verified.

Distal target vessel perforation typically occurs after crossing the CTO using an antegrade approach. After crossing a CTO either through wire escalation or dissection and reentry, advancement of the guidewire distally can lead to coronary vessel perforation. This scenario occurs more often when the guidewire is advanced into a smaller branch of the distal target vessel, particularly when using stiff or polymer jacketed wires. One reason dual injection is essential for CTO PCI is the ability to delineate the natural course of the target vessel and identify branches beyond the distal cap of the CTO [1]. Importantly, exchanging the stiffer crossing guidewire for workhorse wires immediately after crossing the CTO lesion and reentering the true lumen can minimize the risk for distal target vessel perforation, ideally using a trapping technique (see Chap. 4). Distal target vessel perforation can be less angiographically apparent than main target vessel perforation, thus it is critical that operators pay careful attention to the distal guidewire position during CTO PCI.

As with main vessel perforation, the initial step with distal target perforation is to use balloon occlusion proximal to the perforation which may itself lead to hemostasis. Other options include advancing a microcatheter into the distal target vessel, typically a small side branch, and aspirating using a 30–60 ml lure lock syringe to collapse the vessel [13]. If bleeding persists despite these techniques then embolization is typically required using coils, vascular plugs, thrombin, subcutaneous fat, or fibrin glue [14–16].

Unique to retrograde CTO PCI is the risk for donor collateral vessel perforation. However, progression to cardiac tamponade following a donor collateral vessel perforation depends on the location of the collateral vessel (i.e. septal versus epicardial). Collateral vessel perforation normally occurs due to advancing the guidewire and/or devices when attempting to reach the distal cap of the CTO. To facilitate passage to the target vessel, some operators may dilate the septal collateral vessels, which can also lead to coronary vessel perforation.

Septal collateral vessel perforation carries a unique set of downstream consequences however cardiac tamponade rarely occurs [17]. Guidewire perforation of a septal collateral results in bleeding into the interventricular septum (i.e. septal wall hematoma) and not the pericardial space. It is also possible to perforate a septal collateral coronary vessel into any cardiac chamber, including the coronary sinus, yet this rarely leads to any adverse clinical consequence [18]. Rarely, septal hematomas can result in chest discomfort and also heart block depending on its size and location [19, 20]. (Fig. 15.2) Exceptionally, a septal wall hematoma can progress to a septal wall rupture requiring percutaneous or surgical treatment [21].

Epicardial coronary vessel perforation carries a higher risk of hemorrhagic pericardial effusion and cardiac tamponade compared with septal collaterals. Bleeding from an epicardial vessel perforation can be difficult to control due to the limited options available for management. Thus, only experienced retrograde CTO operators, able and ready to treat a perforation, should attempt recanalization through an epicardial collateral vessel. If an epicardial vessel perforation is noticed, one initial measure is to balloon occlude either the perforated epicardial collateral or its donor vessel. Then, the perforation should be approached both antegrade (if the CTO has been successfully reanalyzed, which is not always the case) and retrograde, with an attempt to achieve hemostasis using microcatheters with suction to collapse the perforated vessel and/or embolization (e.g. coils) (Fig. 15.3). Unfortunately, this approach presupposes that the CTO has been recanalized and the perforated vessel can be approached from both sides. If bleeding continues despite these measures, cardiac surgery may be required.

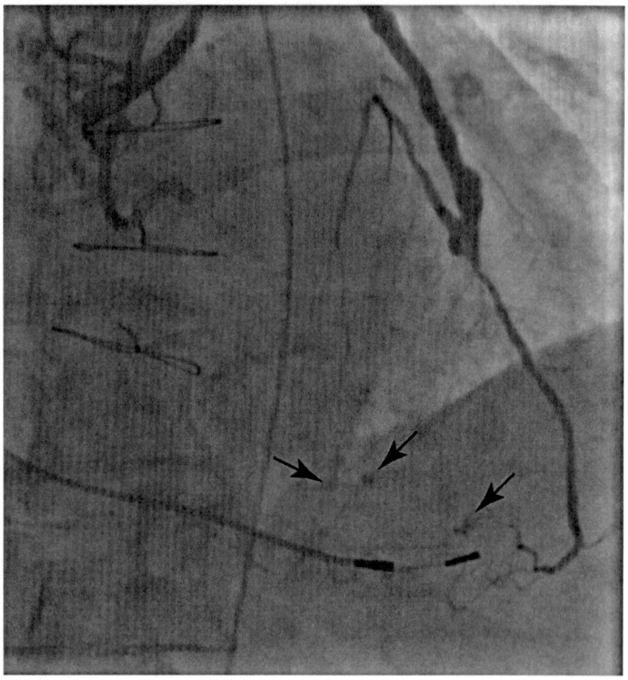

**Fig. 15.2** Failed attempt to connect retrograde from the LAD with some benign septal stains of contrast (*arrows*)

In general, operators should be aware of the natural history of coronary perforation in CTO PCI. Complications resulting from a perforation may not manifest for hours to days after PCI. Thus, the threshold for prompt evaluation of any cardiac or atypical symptoms is essential following CTO PCI. Anticoagulation with unfractionated heparin may be considered over bivalirudin given the opportunity to reverse the anticoagulant effects of heparin with protamine [1]. Routine use of glycoprotein IIb/IIIa inhibitors is also not advised during CTO PCI and should only be administered if clinically indicated to minimize the risk of bleeding with any coronary perforation.

It is critical that all catheterization centers performing CTO PCI have emergency equipment immediately available to treat a perforated coronary vessel which includes a pericardiocentesis kit, varying sizes of covered stents, embolization equipment and a two-dimensional echocardiography machine. Intravenous fluids and or vasoactive agents should be administered rapidly for hypotension and

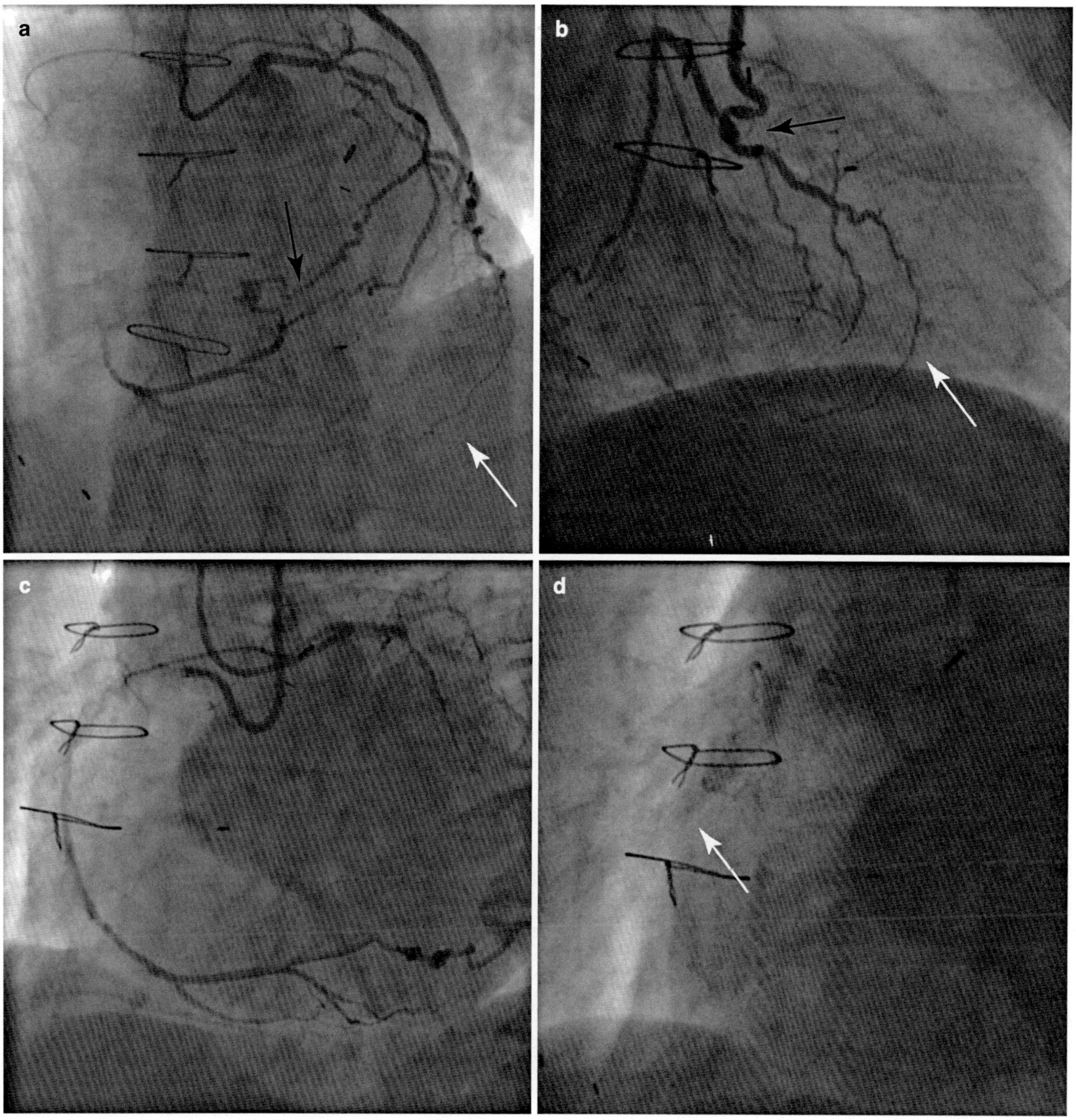


**Fig. 15.3** Post CABG RCA CTO; Retrograde CTO PCI complicated by a type 2 coronary perforation, myocardial ischemia, and epicardial collateral perforation requiring coils. (**a**) Dual retrograde injection (left main and LIMA to OM) reveals a very large but tortuous epicardial collateral (*black arrow*) from the native distal LCX to the PLV and also a straighter interventional epicardial CC from the OM branch (grafted with a LIMA) to the PDA (*white arrow*). (**b**) Nice epicardial collateral from the distal OM (*white arrow*) but very tortuous anastomosis of the LIMA (*black arrow*) (**c**). Nice distal target for antegrade dissection re-entry. (**d**) Failed antegrade knuckling with type 2 perforation (*arrow*). (**e**, **f**). Retrograde attempt from the LIMA that had to be aborted because of cessation of flow by the Corsair through the anastomosis. (**g**) Retrograde attempt with a Finecross and a Sion wire, complicated by a brisk perforation at the level of severe tortuority (not on image). (**h**) 0.018" Cook Tornado coils delivered through a Progreat (Terumo, Japan) delivery catheter, with successful hemostasis from the left circumflex. (**i**) LIMA injection revealing persistent leaking from the distal extremity of the collateral (*arrow*). (**j**) Reattempt from the LIMA with the Finecross instead of the Corsair, that did not result in flow cessation. (**k**) Reverse CART. (**l**) After stenting, antegrade injection reveals persistent perforation from the other extremity of the collateral. (**m**) Antegrade delivery of the same coils. (**n**) Final result

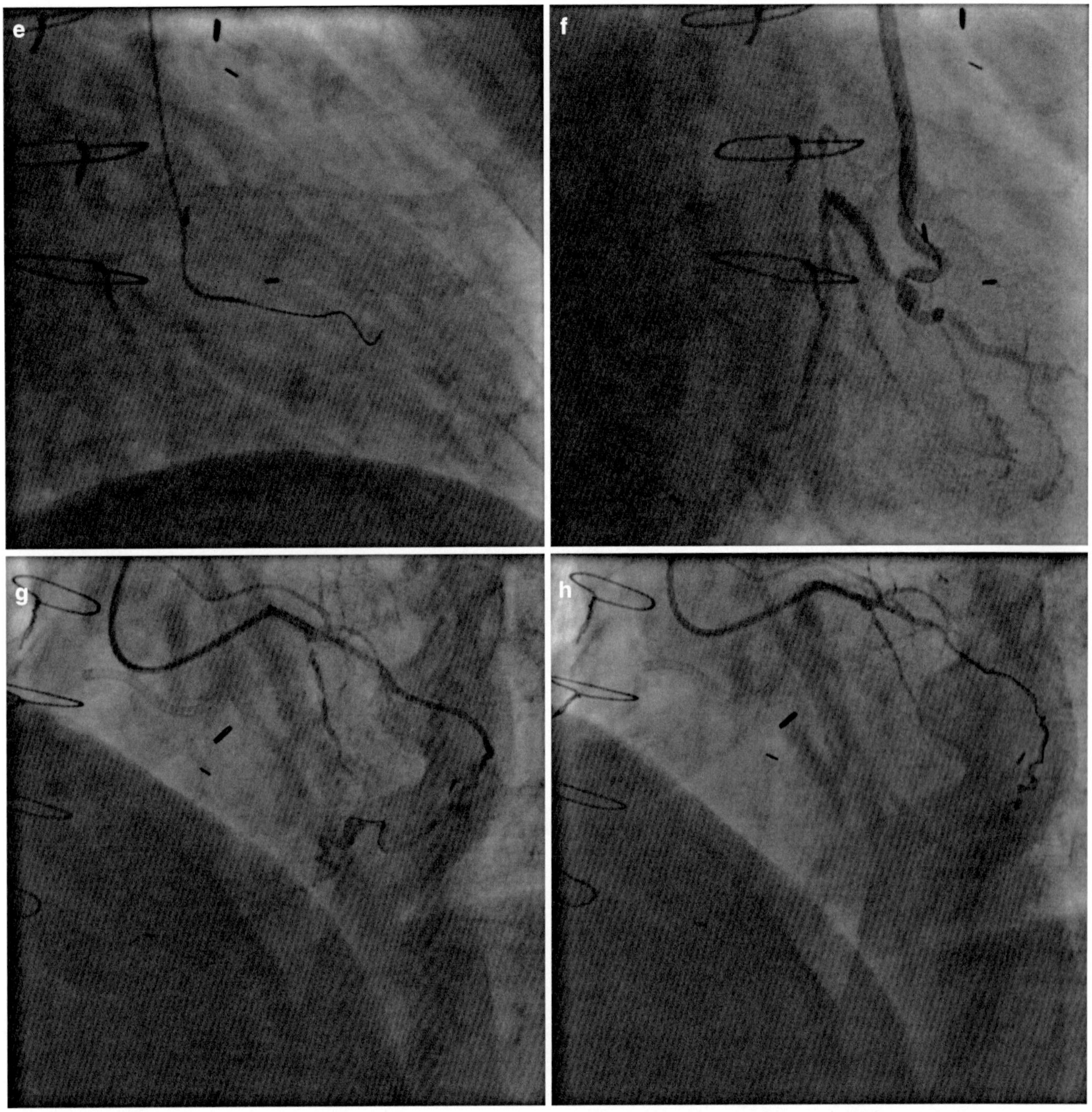


**Fig. 15.3** (continued)

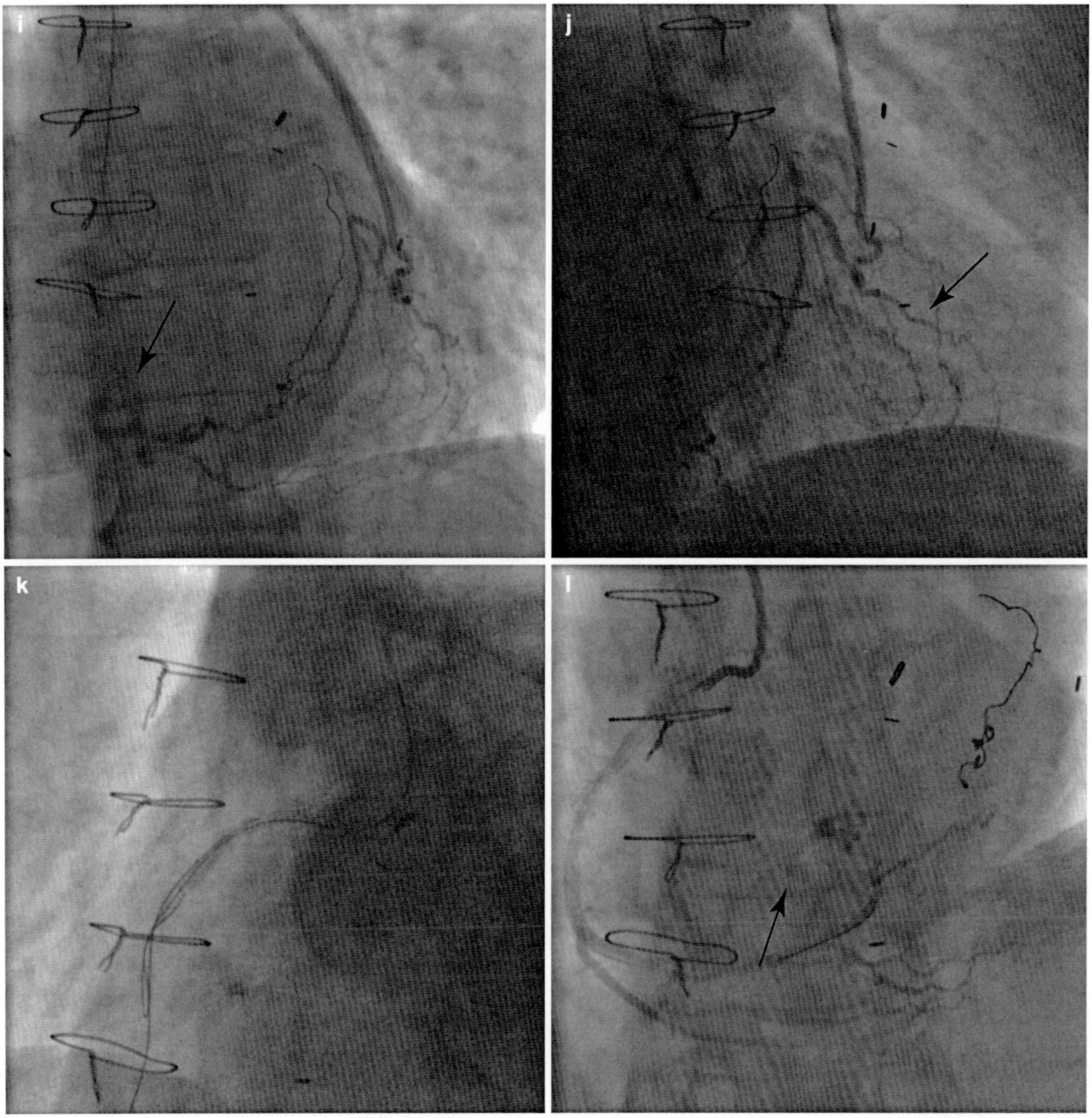


**Fig. 15.3** (continued)

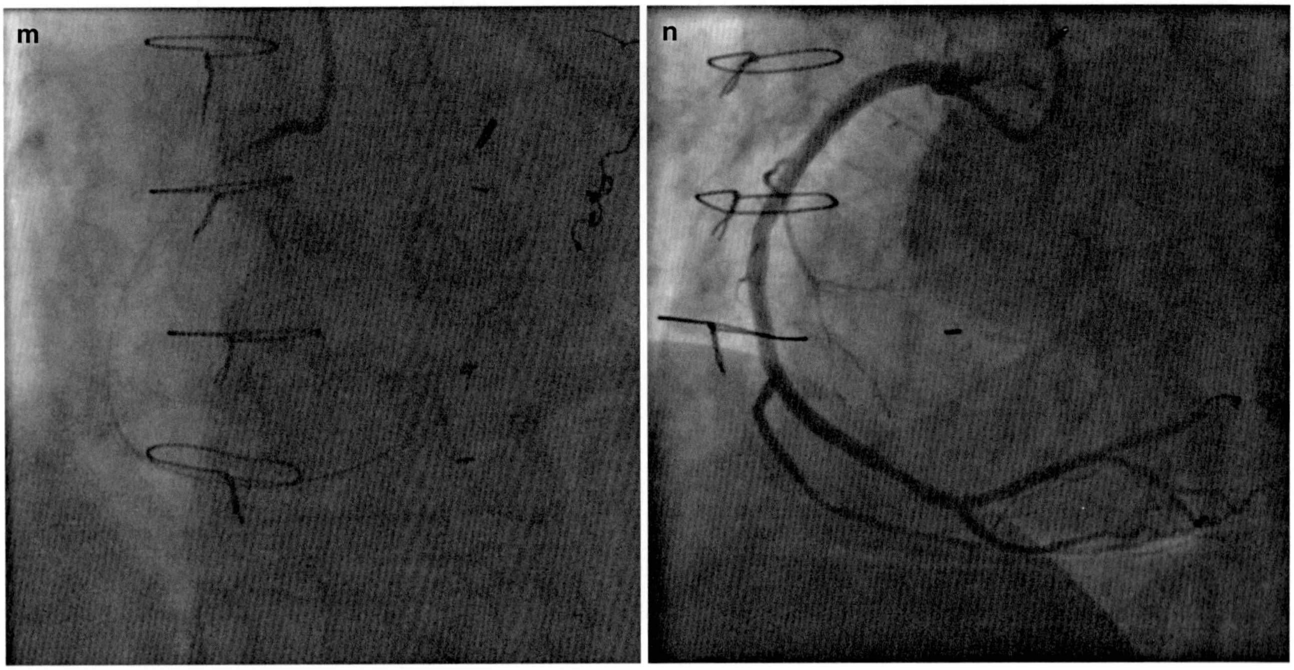


**Fig. 15.3** (continued)

suspected coronary perforation. In this setting, the patient should also undergo immediate evaluation for pericardial effusion and meticulous review of the coronary angiogram. The decision to perform emergent pericardiocentesis should be dictated based on the patient's hemodynamics. In certain patients, a hemorrhagic effusion may be focal (e.g. prior CABG) and can potentially self-tamponade the perforation. Despite the history of CABG, the risk remains for isolated atrial tamponade if the perforation is within the AV groove or over the atrium. The steps described previously to ensure hemostasis are essential to the management of coronary perforation.

## Donor Vessel Injury

During retrograde CTO PCI, non-target donor vessel injury with or without acute closure can occur as attempts are made to advance guidewires and devices to the distal cap of the CTO. In addition, the aggressive guide catheters that are required to support retrograde CTO PCI can dissect the proximal donor vessel, particularly as equipment or wires are externalized and withdrawn which can cause deep seating of the guide catheter. The incidence of coronary dissection during retrograde PCI ranges from 0.5 to 10 % and is significantly higher in unsuccessful versus successful attempts (10 versus 3.1 %) [5, 22–24]. The consequences of coronary dissection largely rest on the amount of myocardium supplied and the severity of the dissection (Fig. 15.4, Videos 15.1, 15.2, 15.3, 15.4, 15.5, 15.6, 15.7, 15.8, 15.9 and 15.10). It is also important to note that acute vessel closure of the donor vessel may occur without dissection due to thrombosis. While rare, the risk of vessel thrombosis may be higher compared with non-CTO PCI due to the prolonged guidewire times, large guiding catheters, and burden of equipment required for CTO recanalization. For this reason, activated clotting times should be closely monitored and maintained above 350 s to minimize the risk.

## Target Vessel Injury

In any attempt to recanalize a CTO, there is a risk of target vessel injury both proximal and distal to the CTO lesion. Side branches at or near the CTO are common and observed in 16–79 % of CTO lesions [5, 6, 22]. In one study, side branch compromise occurred in 22 % of patients, and the rate of side branch occlusion was significantly higher in successful CTO procedures compared with unsuccessful attempts (4.4 % vs. 0.88 %, $p=0.008$) [5]. Side branch occlusion is particularly common during dissection and reentry techniques, but also may occur during stent deployment after successfully crossing the CTO. Given the risk for periprocedural myocardial infarction (MI) with side branch compromise, it is critical that attempts are made to reduce its occurrence. Dual injection of the target and contralateral

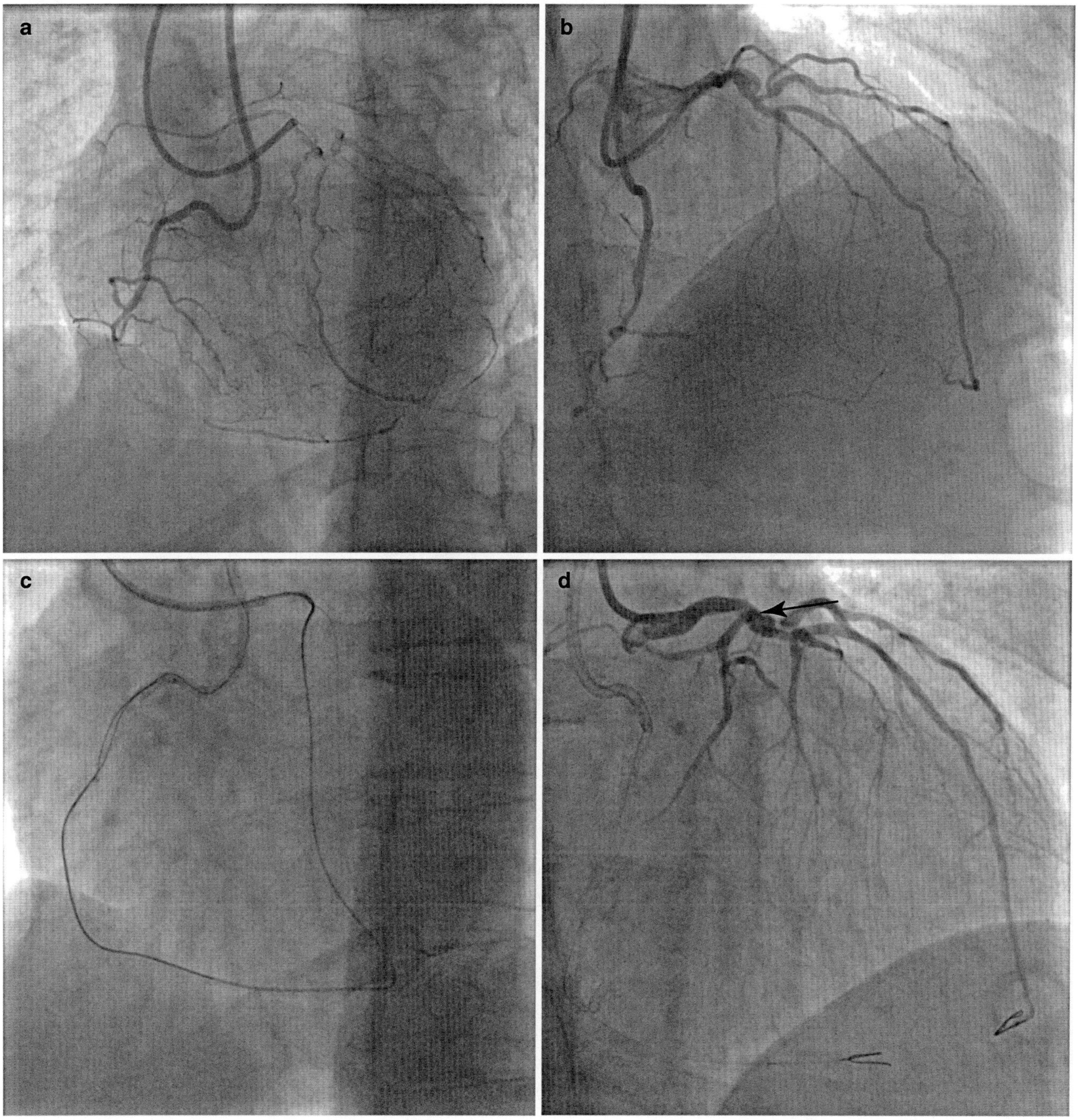


**Fig. 15.4** Donor artery dissection that manifested a few hours after the CTO PCI. (**a**, **b**) Dual transradial injection using an AL 1 in the RCA and a 7 F XB 3.5 in the LM both delivered without a sheath (Video 15.1 and 15.2). (**c**) Retrograde approach and GuideLiner Reverse CART (Video 15.3). (**d**) Suspicion of a small intimal tear in the mid segment of the left main (Video 15.4). (**e–g**) IVUS in the distal (**e**), mid (**f**) and proximal (**g**) segments of the left main that did not reveal any tear or flap (Video 15.5). (**h**) Final RCA result (Video 15.6). (**i**) Final angiography on the left; the suspected image in the left main had disappeared (Video 15.7). (**j**) 3 h later, patient presented sudden chest pain associated with high-blood pressure (180/95), followed by hypotension and sweating. Urgent catheterization revealed a clear dissection of the left main, with reduced flow (Video 15.8). (**k**) Following complex trifurcation stenting of the left main (Video 15.9). (**l**) Control angiography on the right showed patent stents and significant remodelling of the PDA. The patient was sent home 2 days later. In retrospective, a stent should have been placed as soon as a doubt was raised about a potential intimal tear (Video 15.10)

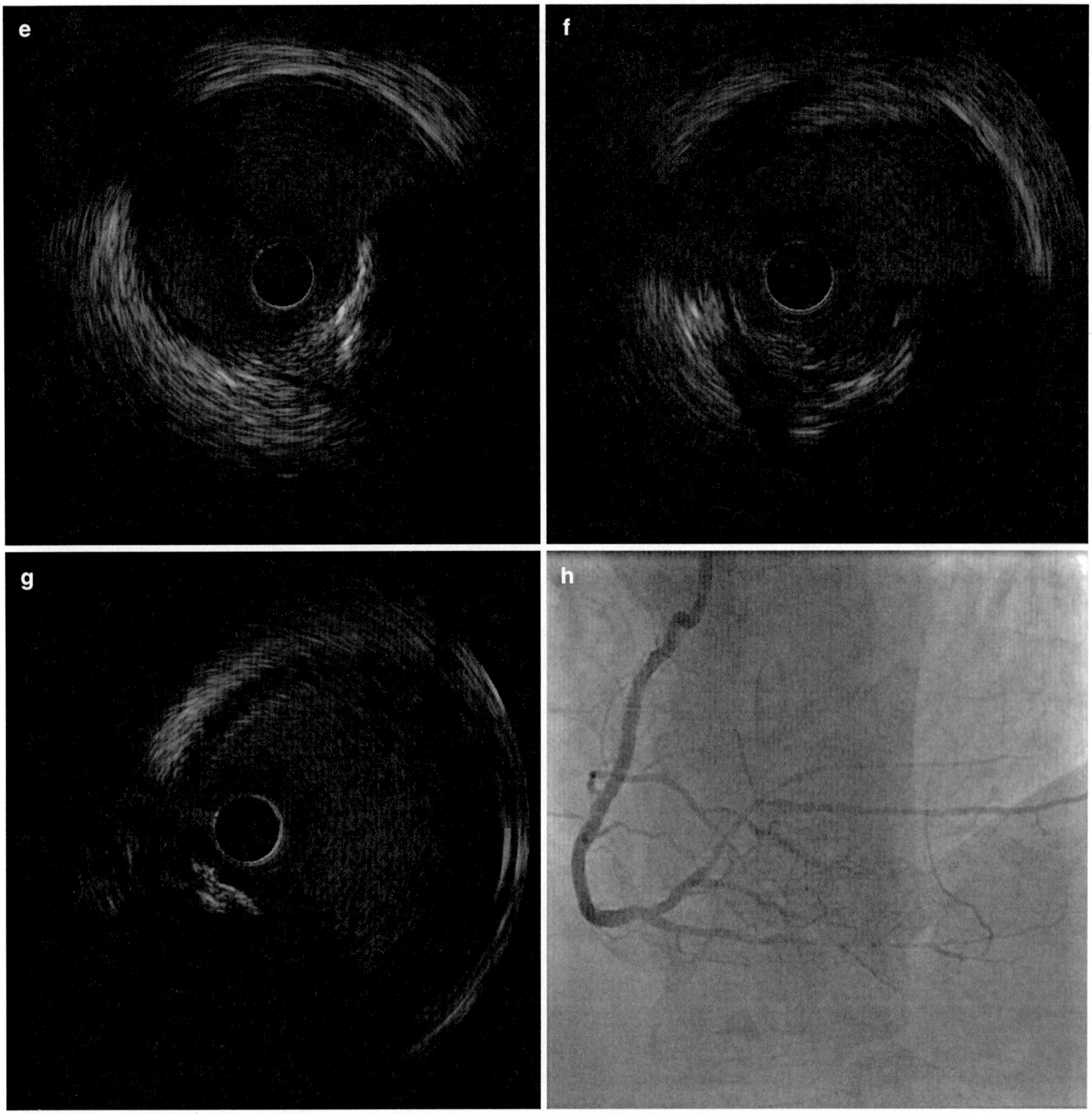


**Fig. 15.4** (continued)

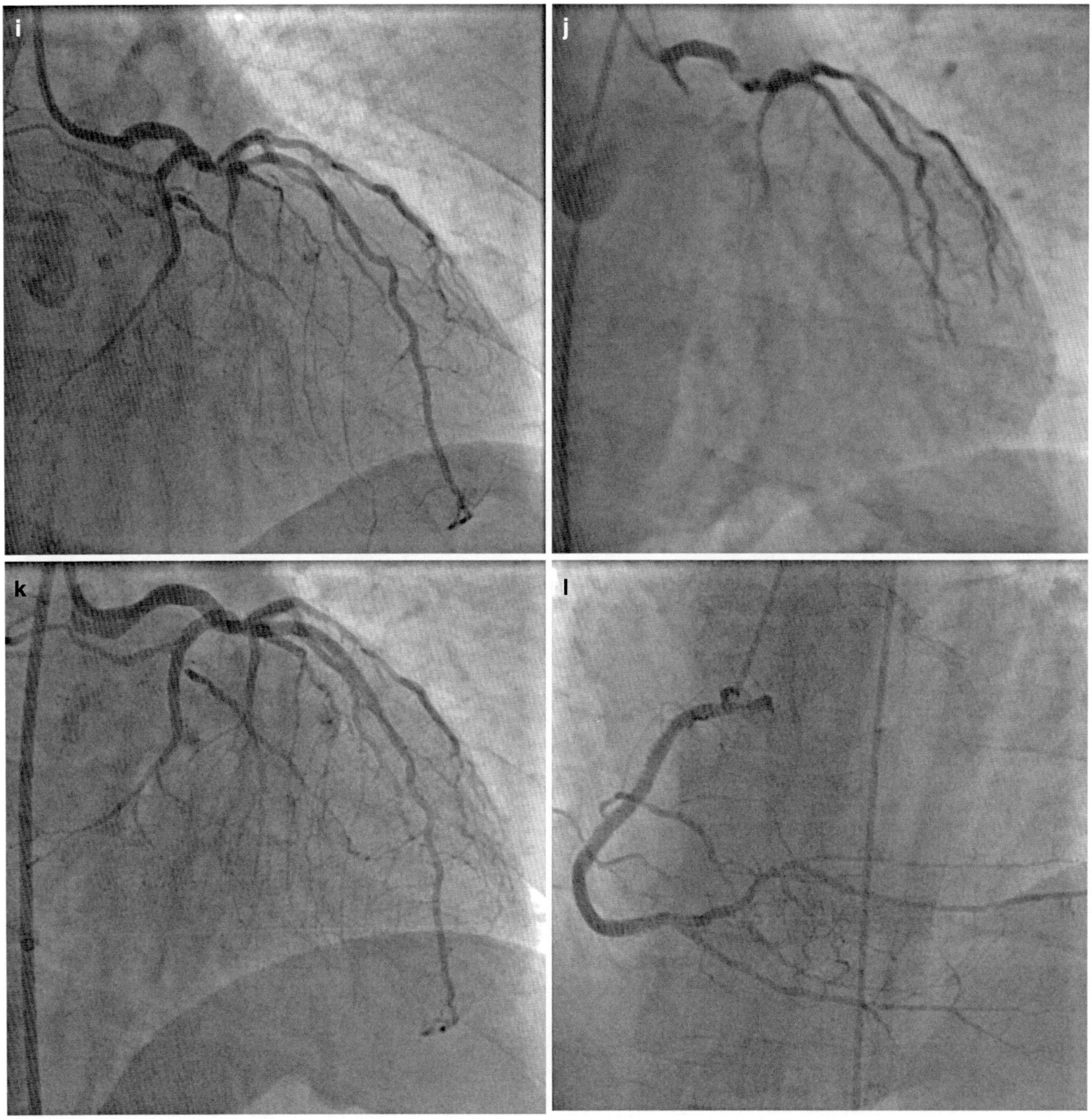


**Fig. 15.4** (continued)

donor vessels is mandatory in all CTO PCIs to allow for visualization of any side branches associated with the CTO lesion [1].

With any dissection and re-entry technique, the subintimal dissection length should be minimized by reentering the true lumen as soon as possible after successfully crossing the lesion. Distal target vessel dissection can arise from long subintimal dissection planes, where wire position is unknown or proximal reentry was unsuccessful. Specialized techniques such as crossing/reentry devices (CrossBoss catheter and Stingray balloon/guidewire system, Boston Scientific, Boston, Massachusetts) should be utilized to facilitate successful crossing and lessen the risk for side branch occlusion. Intravascular imaging with IVUS may also facilitate CTO PCI and minimize target vessel complications by enhanced subintimal wire tracking [25].

## Equipment Loss or Entrapment

Entrapment or loss of any equipment required for CTO recanalization including stents, guidewires, and other devices is considered a very rare complication [26, 27]. The risk for entrapment or device loss increases in CTO PCI due to the lesion complexity, extent of calcification, vessel tortuosity, and techniques required for recanalization. This complication can lead to vessel injury and/or acute vessel closure and retrieval should be pursued in all cases of equipment loss. Any equipment that is embolized and not retrievable should be crushed against the coronary vessel well via a series of balloon inflations and stent deployment [26, 27]. Intravascular imaging with intravascular ultrasound (IVUS) or optical coherence tomography (OCT) should be used to ensure that the crushed equipment is not exposed anywhere in the coronary vessel [27].

## Aortic Dissection

While possible with any PCI, aortic dissection is more common with CTO PCI and typically occurs in the right coronary artery. The incidence of aortic dissection in CTO PCI is low (<1 %) [5]. As the guide catheters used in CTO PCI are typically large, stiff and aggressively shaped to facilitate back-up it is usually caused by guide catheter trauma however can also be caused by forceful contrast injection, subintimal wire passage, or balloon rupture. Use of guide catheters with side holes for the right coronary artery and avoiding injections with dampened waveforms may help with prevention.

Historically, iatrogenic aortic dissection is associated with high mortality rates (~35 %) and myocardial infarction (15 %) [28]. However, the clinical presentation of iatrogenic aortic dissection can be insidious. Patients will not present with the "classical" symptoms associated with spontaneous aortic dissection. Instead, atypical symptoms or the absence (25 %) of chest discomfort is common, and hemodynamic compromise occurs in approximately one-fourth of patients [28]. It is important to consider aortic dissection in any patient with sudden hemodynamic collapse and/or ischemia during CTO PCI.

If an aortic dissection occurs, further antegrade injections should be avoided as they can expand the dissection plane. The ostium of the coronary artery should then be stented to seal the dissection and protect from further compromise of the coronary circulation [29]. The dissection should then be followed with non-invasive imaging such as computed tomography or transesophageal echocardiography. Early consultation with cardiac surgery is also critical for the management of iatrogenic aortic dissection.

One minor variation of aortic dissection is when it occurs limited to the coronary sinus, as a result of guide trauma, sub-intimal tracking to the aorta, or other circumstances. In most instances, such an event is benign and associated with very favorable outcomes, after successful stenting of the coronary ostium.

## Periprocedural Myocardial Infarction

Any of the acute complications discussed previously can result in periprocedural MI. It is one of the most common procedural complications occurring in approximately 2.5 % of cases (95 % CI 1.9–3.0) however its incidence may be underdiagnosed due to variability in post-procedure biomarker measurement. The vast majority of periprocedural MI's are non-Q wave, with only 0.2 % of patient's experiencing a Q wave MI (95 % CI 0.1–0.3 %) [2]. The rates of periprocedural MI are similar between antegrade and retrograde approaches as well as in successful versus unsuccessful PCI attempts.

# Acute Non-cardiac Complications

## Contrast Induced Nephropathy

Contrast induced nephropathy (CIN) is a major cause of morbidity and mortality. In CTO PCI, rates of CIN range from 2.4 to 18.1 % with a pooled estimate of 3.8 % (95 % CI 2.4–5.3 %) [2]. However, CIN is only reported in 20 % of studies published on CTO PCI complications, thus the pooled estimate is likely underestimated [2]. One concern with CTO PCI is the risk for CIN with the administration of higher volumes of contrast compared with non-CTO PCI. Renal function should be assessed in all patients undergoing CTO PCI by measuring the estimated glomerular filtration rate (GFR) and appropriate measures taken to reduce CIN, in particular with contrast volume minimization as appropriate and pre- and post-procedure hydration.

## Radiation Injury

CTO PCI requires longer fluoroscopy times compared with non-CTO PCI [30]. In a meta-analysis of 18,061 patients radiation injury was reported in only three cases out of 2857 patients; however it was infrequently reported in studies thus underestimating its incidence [2]. The risk of radiation injury is dose-dependent, and there is a wide variability in the radiation dose ranges with different operators and institutions [30, 31]. In all cases of CTO PCI, careful attention to the fluoroscopy time and radiation dose is necessary. Any patient with an exposure dose >5-Gy can present radiation skin injury, while doses >10-Gy may cause significant injury [1].

**Table 15.3** Steps to minimize radiation dose during percutaneous treatment of chronic total occlusions

| |
|---|
| **Minimize exposure to patient and operator** |
| Utilize radiation only when necessary |
| Minimize use of cine |
| Minimize use of steep angles |
| Minimize use of magnification modes |
| Minimize frame rate of fluoroscopy and cine (<15 frames/s) |
| Keep the image receptor close to the patient |
| Utilize collimation |
| Monitor radiation dose real time |
| **Minimize exposure to operator** |
| Use appropriate protective garments |
| Maximize distance from X-ray source |
| Keep shields in optimal position at all times |
| Keep all body parts out of the field of view at all times |
| **Minimize exposure to patient** |
| Keep table height as high as possible |
| Vary the beam angle to reduce repeated skin exposure of one area |
| Keep all extremities out of the radiation beam |

Patients who do receive more than 5-Gy should be evaluated in 2–4 weeks for radiation skin injury and followed for a minimum of 1-year. Steps to minimize radiation exposure during CTO PCI are shown in Table 15.3.

## References


1. Brilakis ES, Grantham JA, Rinfret S, Wyman RM, Burke MN, Karmpaliotis D, et al. A percutaneous treatment algorithm for crossing coronary chronic total occlusions. JACC Cardiovasc Interv. 2012;5(4):367–79.
2. Patel VG, Brayton KM, Tamayo A, Mogabgab O, Michael TT, Lo N, et al. Angiographic success and procedural complications in patients undergoing percutaneous coronary chronic total occlusion interventions: a weighted meta-analysis of 18,061 patients from 65 studies. JACC Cardiovasc Interv. 2013;6(2):128–36.
3. Suero JA, Marso SP, Jones PG, Laster SB, Huber KC, Giorgi LV, Johnson WL, Rutherford BD. Procedural outcomes and long-term survival among patients undergoing percutaneous coronary intervention of a chronic total occlusion in native coronary arteries: a 20-year experience. J Am Coll Cardiol. 2001;38(2):409–14.
4. Prasad A, Rihal CS, Lennon RJ, Wiste HJ, Singh M, Homes Jr DR. Trends in outcomes after percutaneous coronary intervention for chronic total occlusions: a 25-year experience from the mayo clinic. J Am Coll Cardiol. 2007;49(15):1611–8.
5. Rathore S, Matsuo H, Terashima M, Kinoshita Y, Kimura M, Tsuchikane E, et al. Procedural and in-hospital outcomes after percutaneous coronary intervention for chronic total occlusions of coronary arteries 2002 to 2008: impact of novel guidewire techniques. JACC Cardiovasc Interv. 2009;2(6):489–97.
6. Morino Y, Kimura T, Hayashi Y, Muramatsu T, Ochiai M, Noguchi Y, et al. In-hospital outcomes of contemporary percutaneous coronary intervention in patients with chronic total occlusion insights from the J-CTO Registry (Multicenter CTO Registry in Japan). JACC Cardiovasc Interv. 2010;3(2):143–51.
7. Galassi AR, Tomasello SD, Reifart N, Werner GS, Sianos G, Bonnier H, et al. In-hospital outcomes of percutaneous coronary intervention in patients with chronic total occlusion: insights from the ERCTO (European Registry of Chronic Total Occlusion) registry. EuroIntervention. 2011;7(4):472–9.
8. Christopoulos G, Menon RV, Karmpaliotis D, Alaswad K, Lombardi W, Grantham A, Patel VG, Rangan BV, Kotsia AP, Lembo N, et al. The efficacy and safety of the "hybrid" approach to coronary chronic total occlusions: Insights from a contemporary multicenter US registry and comparison with prior studies. J Invasive Cardiol. 2014;26(9):427–32.
9. Javaid A, Buch AN, Satler LF, Kent KM, Suddath WO, Lindsay Jr J, et al. Management and outcomes of coronary artery perforation during percutaneous coronary intervention. Am J Cardiol. 2006;98(7):911–4.
10. Romaguera R, Waksman R. Covered stents for coronary perforations: is there enough evidence? Catheter Cardiovasc Interv. 2011;78(2):246–53.
11. Al-Mukhaini M, Panduranga P, Sulaiman K, Riyami AA, Deeb M, Riyami MB. Coronary perforation and covered stents: an update and review. Heart Views. 2011;12(2):63–70.
12. Ben-Gal Y, Weisz G, Collins MB, Genereux P, Dangas GD, Teirstein PS, et al. Dual catheter technique for the treatment of severe coronary artery perforations. Catheter Cardiovasc Interv. 2010;75(5):708–12.
13. Yasuoka Y, Sasaki T. Successful collapse vessel treatment with a syringe for thrombus-aspiration after the guidewire-induced coronary artery perforation. Cardiovasc Revasc Med. 2010;11(4):263.e1–3.
14. Fischell TA, Korban EH, Lauer MA. Successful treatment of distal coronary guidewire-induced perforation with balloon catheter delivery of intracoronary thrombin. Catheter Cardiovasc Interv. 2003;58(3):370–4.
15. Oda H, Oda M, Makiyama Y, Kashimura T, Takahashi K, Miida T, et al. Guidewire-induced coronary artery perforation treated with transcatheter delivery of subcutaneous tissue. Catheter Cardiovasc Interv. 2005;66(3):369–74.
16. Ponnuthurai FA, Ormerod OJ, Forfar C. Microcoil embolization of distal coronary artery perforation without reversal of anticoagulation: a simple, effective approach. J Invasive Cardiol. 2007;19(8):E222–5.
17. Matsumi J, Adachi K, Saito S. A unique complication of the retrograde approach in angioplasty for chronic total occlusion of the coronary artery. Catheter Cardiovasc Interv. 2008;72(3):371–8.
18. Sachdeva R, Hughes B, Uretsky BF. Retrograde approach to a totally occluded right coronary artery via a septal perforator artery: the tale of a long and winding wire. J Invasive Cardiol. 2010;22(4):E65–6.
19. Lin TH, Wu DK, Su HM, Chu CS, Voon WC, Lai WT, et al. Septum hematoma: a complication of retrograde wiring in chronic total occlusion. Int J Cardiol. 2006;113(2):e64–6.
20. Fairley SL, Donnelly PM, Hanratty CG, Walsh SJ. Images in cardiovascular medicine. Interventricular septal hematoma and ventricular septal defect after retrograde intervention for a chronic total occlusion of a left anterior descending coronary artery. Circulation. 2010;122(20):e518–21.
21. Joyal D, Thompson CA, Grantham JA, Buller CE, Rinfret S. The retrograde technique for recanalization of chronic total occlusions: a step-by-step approach. JACC Cardiovasc Interv. 2012;5(1):1–11.
22. Ma JY, Qian JY, Ge L, Fan B, Wang QB, Yan Y, et al. Retrograde approach for the recanalization of coronary chronic total occlusion: collateral selection and collateral related complication. Chin Med J (Engl). 2013;126(6):1086–91.
23. Muramatsu T, Tsukahara R, Ito Y, Ishimori H, Park SJ, de Winter R, et al. Changing strategies of the retrograde approach for chronic total occlusion during the past 7 years. Catheter Cardiovasc Interv. 2013;81(4):E178–85.
24. Karmpaliotis D, Michael TT, Brilakis ES, Papayannis AC, Tran DL, Kirkland BL, et al. Retrograde coronary chronic total occlusion

revascularization: procedural and in-hospital outcomes from a multicenter registry in the United States. JACC Cardiovasc Interv. 2012;5(12):1273–9.
25. Tsujita K, Maehara A, Mintz GS, Kubo T, Doi H, Lansky AJ, et al. Intravascular ultrasound comparison of the retrograde versus antegrade approach to percutaneous intervention for chronic total coronary occlusions. JACC Cardiovasc Interv. 2009;2(9):846–54.
26. Utsunomiya M, Kobayashi T, Nakamura S. Case of dislodged stent lost in septal channel during stent delivery in complex chronic total occlusion of right coronary artery. J Invasive Cardiol. 2009;21(11): E229–33.
27. Sianos G, Papafaklis MI. Septal wire entrapment during recanalisation of a chronic total occlusion with the retrograde approach. Hellenic J Cardiol. 2011;52(1):79–83.
28. Januzzi JL, Sabatine MS, Eagle KA, Evangelista A, Bruckman D, Fattori R, et al. Iatrogenic aortic dissection. Am J Cardiol. 2002; 89(5):623–6.
29. Abdou SM, Wu CJ. Treatment of aortocoronary dissection complicating anomalous origin right coronary artery and chronic total intervention with intravascular ultrasound guided stenting. Catheter Cardiovasc Interv. 2011;78(6):914–9.
30. Grantham JA, Marso SP, Spertus J, House J, Holmes Jr DR, Rutherford BD. Chronic total occlusion angioplasty in the United States. JACC Cardiovasc Interv. 2009;2(6):479–86.
31. Suzuki S, Furui S, Isshiki T, Kozuma K, Endo G, Yamamoto Y, et al. Factors affecting the patient's skin dose during percutaneous coronary intervention for chronic total occlusion. Circ J. 2007; 71(2):229–33.

# How to Prevent Perforation During CTO PCI

16

Parag Doshi

**Abstract**

Coronary perforations remain a dreaded complication during percutaneous coronary intervention (PCI) for coronary chronic total occlusion (CTO). However, with the hybrid algorithm-driven approach, the incidence can be minimized; and if they do occur, the situation can be controlled and PCI completed in most cases.

The incidence of perforation in CTO PCI was found to be 2.9 % in a large meta-analysis of 18,061 patients from 65 studies. Most of these perforations were however self-limited and only 0.3 % resulted in cardiac tamponade. It should be noted that increasing experience and confidence along with more advanced techniques do not necessarily reduce the frequency of perforations due to more complex lesions attempted. However, experience results in better understanding of the situations that can result in improved outcomes related to the perforation.

**Keywords**

Coronary perforation • Prevention of coronary perforation • Coronary perforation and CTO PCI • Predictors of coronary perforation • Classification of coronary perforation

Coronary perforations remain a dreaded complication during percutaneous coronary intervention (PCI) for coronary chronic total occlusion (CTO). However, with the hybrid algorithm-driven approach, the incidence can be minimized; and if they do occur, the situation can be controlled and PCI completed in most cases.

The incidence of perforation in CTO PCI was found to be 2.9 % in a large meta-analysis of 18,061 patients from 65 studies [1]. Most of these perforations were however self-limited and only 0.3 % resulted in cardiac tamponade. It should be noted that increasing experience and confidence along with more advanced techniques do not necessarily reduce the frequency of perforations due to more complex lesions attempted. However, experience results in better understanding of the situations that can result in dramatic outcomes related to the perforation.

P. Doshi, MD, FACC, FSCAI
Department of Cardiology, Chicago Cardiology Institute, Schaumburg, IL, USA
e-mail: pdoshi@chicagocardiology.com

Coronary perforation may result in one of the following potential consequences:

- Tamponade
- Myocardial hematoma, especially with septal branches
- Coronary fistula into a cardiac vein, chamber or great vessels
- Limited pericardial hematoma compressing a valve or chamber.

It should be noted that, many times, wire perforations are self-limited without any clinical consequences, especially in patients with previous surgery and resultant adherent pericardial space.

## Predictors of Coronary Perforation

In a published review [2], Al-Mukhaini et al. evaluated the predictors of perforation. More specific to CTO, the following factors should be considered:



S. Rinfret (ed.), *Percutaneous Intervention for Coronary Chronic Total Occlusion: The Hybrid Approach*, DOI 10.1007/978-3-319-21563-1_16

1. Clinical factors: Advanced age, female sex, renal impairment, non ST-elevation myocardial infarction.
2. Angiographic factors: Calcification, Type C lesions (all of which are CTOs), tortuosity, target lesions in the circumflex and right coronary arteries, long lesions.
3. Technique-associated factors: Use of hydrophilic or stiff guidewires, atherectomy devices, increased balloon-to-artery ratio, high-pressure stent post-dilatation and cutting balloons.

## Classification of Coronary Perforations

In 1994, Ellis et al. created a classification, which is still commonly used today:

- Type I—Extra luminal crater without extravasation
- Type II—Pericardial or myocardial blush without contrast jet extravasion
- Type III—Extravasion through frank (>1 mm) perforation
- Cavity Spilling—Perforation into an anatomic cavity or chamber [3].

It should be noted that Type I is essentially an adventitial hematoma, seen frequently during CTO PCI and should not be necessarily reported as a true perforation. Specifically, this should be considered as adventitial hematoma or dye hang up with poor washout. Also, perforation into the pericardium can either be associated with minor contrast leak or major and brisk contrast washout. Pericardial hematomas and intramyocardial hematoma can result from either type 2 or type 3 perforation. Finally, coronary fistula into an anatomic chamber (pericardium or a cardiac chamber) is a benign form of type 3 perforation.

In general, perforation into pericardium, resulting in either tamponade or pericardial hematomas is associated with serious consequences. Pericardial hematoma may create an inaccessible collection of blood compressing a vital structure such as a ventricle or an atrium. This is especially the case with perforation of a coronary or a collateral that tracks the atrio-ventricular groove in a patient with previous cardiac surgery; a perforation in such patient may result in localized collection of blood behind the atrium as it cannot flow in the mid or apical portion of the adherent pericardium. Similarly, intra-myocardial hematoma may cause varying degrees of subaortic obstruction. Any of those dangerous sequelae may be immediate or occur slowly over several hours. Use of contrast echocardiography can be of great help to ascertain if a given perforation that occurred during the procedure, which is associated with some pericardial effusion but equivocal signs of tamponade, is still leaking blood actively [4].

## Prevention of Coronary Perforation During CTO PCI

With the basic understanding of perforation, we can now develop strategies to minimize the risk, beginning before the procedure all the way to the post-procedure period as described below:

### Pre-procedure

It is important to assess the patient and patient-specific factors, most important being previous cardiac surgery, which provides some protection and ability to manipulate wires with less apprehension. Indeed, it has been well recognized that patients who underwent a previous pericardiotomy have healed with some adherence of the pericardium to the surface of the heart. Other risk factors listed previously should also be carefully considered. If a previous angiogram is available, a careful review will give knowledge of the vessel course before complete occlusion. Side branches and ipsilateral collateral (bridges) should be carefully noted, as tracking of such structure can lead to perforation, especially with 'bridges' can be mistakenly identified as the true lumen of the vessel.

### Adjunctive Medications

Heparin is the anticoagulant of choice. Bivalirudin should be avoided due to the lack of an effective antidote. GPIIbIIIa inhibitors are expressly avoided except in rare situations. It is important to note that non-intentional guidewire exits from the vessel are common during CTO PCI and may not be apparent: use of GPIIbIIIa inhibitors can lead to continuous oozing from these exit points and delayed tamponnade that would not have happened otherwise.

### Angiographic Technique

Guiding catheters are typically large bore in CTO PCI. In an occluded vessel, dampening of the pressure curve from guide catheter engagement is frequent. Forceful injection can easily create a spiral dissection or even perforation. Our approach is to let an assistant inject through the retrograde guide catheter, and have operator to follow with a controlled antegrade injection. If the subintimal space is accessed, antegrade injections should be minimized until after stents have been implanted. To avoid erroneous injections, antegrade manifold may be covered by a towel or the injection syringe removed from the manifold. Even after stenting, all the subintimal space may not be covered and gentle post-stenting injections are still advised.

## Wire Manipulation

Hydrophilic tapered wires maneuvers such as with the Fielder XT do not provide tactile feedback. In addition, typical curve used for CTO is very shallow and thus guide wire can exit the vessel very easily. The Confianza Pro 12 is another wire that can easily create a perforation due to its high tip load concentrated on a 0.009 tip. Even though its tip is hydrophobic for 1 mm, it is immediately followed by hydrophilic coating. Its sharp distal end can therefore easily exit the vessel and tactile feedback is then lost instantly. Even after the guidewire exits the vessel, it may not be immediately apparent in the same single view. To avoid complications, it is important to take following precautions.

1. Avoid short cuts. Use workhorse guide wire to deliver a microcatheter to the proximal cap and then exchange for specialty guide wire
2. Check the wire position in one additional view with contralateral injection
3. Either with contralateral injection or by calcium in the occluded vessel, confirm that the guidewire is moving in synchrony with the vessel, often referred to 'dancing with the vessel'.
4. Once the specialty wire achieves its purpose, it should be switched to a less aggressive guide wire, to avoid distal vessel perforation.
5. The Confianza Pro 12 is a very effective and essential wire to puncture the proximal cap. However, as soon as it has advanced few millimeters, it is wise to follow with the microcatheter (such as Corsair) into the cap and exchange it for a less aggressive guidewire to track the vessel structure. An exception to this rule is when a calcified straight vessel is tracked with a very easily identifiable course.
6. In long CTO lesions, especially if non-calcified, it is far safer to advance a knuckled wire than trying to advance a stiff wire. This is due to the fact that knuckles create blunt force and simply expand adventitia in contrast to sharp wire that can penetrate and exit the adventitial border. There is an adage in the hybrid CTO PCI philosophy that tells operators to "Trust the knuckle"

## Gear Perforation

As noted above, it is not uncommon for guidewires to exit the vessel structure within the occluded segment. Such events are usually self-limited. However, it is critically important to recognize the extraluminal guidewire course as described above and avoid advancing catheters or balloon over it, which will expand the exit point. Another very important cause of gear-induced perforation is the operator forcing a microcatheter in a tiny branch. For example, in CTO PCI of an RCA, guidewires frequently track small side branches the mid vessel portion, on the greater curvature of the coronary, and may not be apparent in the working fluoroscopic projection. However, before advancing CTO catheters such as the Corsair or the CrossBoss, it is crucial to check the position in a perpendicular projection.

## Retrograde-Specific Considerations

When using the retrograde approach, septal collateral channels (CC) are considered safer, but it is important to remember that the guidewire frequently exits the septal channel and enters a ventricle. Excessive motion is the hallmark that confirms the lack of connection to the distal CTO vessel, and gear should not be advanced prior to performing contrast injection or checking from a different projection. Use of epicardial CC is associated with increased perforation risk, and only appropriate for experienced operators, especially with small tortuous collaterals. Even if wire passage is successful, microcatheter or excessive straightening may still result in perforation.

Typically, after successful retrograde crossing, a long guidewire, such as the RG3 or the Viper wire, is externalized. At that point, the stiff shaft portion of the wire is across the collateral. It is extremely important to keep the microcatheter across the collateral and into the distal CTO vessel all the time to avoid the stiff shaft of the wire slicing the tiny collateral. After stenting, microcatheter should be re- advanced to the antegrade guide or into the deployed stents before pulling the externalized guidewire.

Also, it is important to note that epicardial CC perforation may not be apparent until after the microcatheter has been removed. To preserve access to the collateral for delivering therapy such as coils, the operator should leave the floppy portion of the guide wire in the collateral, pull the microcatheter back and perform the angiogram. Only after a careful review of the collateral ruling out a leak, the guidewire can then be pulled. Otherwise, the microcatheter may have to be readvanced to deliver therapy to occlude the perforation.

Management of perforations: techniques can be found in Chap. 15.

## References

1. Patel VG, Brayton KM, Tamayo A, Mogabgab O, Michael TT, Lo N, Alomar M, Shorrock D, Cipher D, Abdullah S, Banerjee S, Brilakis ES. Angiographic success and procedural complications in patients undergoing percutaneous coronary chronic total occlusion

interventions: a weighted meta-analysis of 18,061 patients from 65 studies. JACC Cardiovasc Interv. 2013;6:128–36.
2. Al-Mukhaini M, Panduranga P, Sulaiman K, Riyami AA, Deeb M, Riyami MB. Coronary perforation and covered stents: an update and review. Heart Views. 2011;12:63–70.
3. Ellis SG, Ajluni S, Arnold AZ, Popma JJ, Bittl JA, Eigler NL, Cowley MJ, Raymond RE, Safian RD, Whitlow PL. Increased coronary perforation in the new device era. Incidence, classification, management, and outcome. Circulation. 1994;90:2725–30.
4. Bagur R, Bernier M, Kandzari DE, Karmpaliotis D, Lembo NJ, Rinfret S. A novel application of contrast echocardiography to exclude active coronary perforation bleeding in patients with pericardial effusion. Catheter Cardiovasc Interv. 2013;82:221–9.

# How to Prevent and Manage Ischemic Complications During CTO PCI

17

Minh N. Vo

**Abstract**

Percutaneous coronary interventions (PCIs) of chronic total occlusions (CTOs) are relatively safe, but procedural complications can occur. In addition to the standard complications of non-CTO PCIs, CTO PCIs carry unique complications, especially with retrograde approaches. One common procedural complication is ischemia which can be devastating. Such a complication, if unrecognized and not treated immediately, may result in myocardial infarction, hemodynamic collapse, and death. Ischemic complications during CTO PCIs occur when there is injury to one of three vessels: (1) target CTO vessel, (2) donor vessel, or (3) collateral vessels. In this chapter, we will briefly discuss the causes of and ways to prevent and treat ischemic complications.

**Keywords**

Percutaneous coronary intervention (PCI) • Chronic total occlusion (CTO) • Ischemia • Ischemic complications • Ischemic complications from target CTO vessel injury • Ischemic complications from donor vessel injury • Ischemic complications from collateral vessel injury

## General Overview

Percutaneous coronary interventions (PCIs) of chronic total occlusions (CTOs) are relatively safe, but procedural complications can occur [1]. In addition to the standard complications of non-CTO PCIs, CTO PCIs carry unique complications, especially with retrograde approaches [2]. One common procedural complication is ischemia which can be devastating. Such a complication, if unrecognized and not treated immediately, may result in myocardial infarction, hemodynamic collapse, and death. Ischemic complications during CTO PCIs can can occur when there is injury to one of three vessels (Fig. 17.1): (1) target CTO vessel, (2) donor vessel, or (3) collateral vessels. In this chapter, we will briefly discuss the causes of and ways to prevent and treat ischemic complications.

M.N. Vo, MD
Department of Cardiology, St. Boniface Hospital, Winnipeg, MB, Canada
e-mail: mvo@sbgh.mb.ca

## Ischemic Complications from Target CTO Vessel Injury

Target vessel injury can cause ischemic complications when side branches or dominant ipsilateral collaterals are compromised. For example, if the chronically occluded segment is distal to major side branches and dominant ipsilateral collaterals, injury to the proximal vessel such as dissection will compromise blood flow to these vessels resulting in ischemia. Common causes of proximal vessel injury include coronary and aortocoronary dissection [3]. Coronary dissection can result from aggressive guide catheter engagement, hydraulic dissection from aggressive contrast injection, guidewire manipulation, and advancement of mother-and-child catheters. Prevention of this type of injury is important in order to avoid potentially lethal ischemic complications. Upon engagement, the guide catheter may occlude the vessel and cause hydraulic dissection with aggressive injections. The use of side-hole catheters may prevent ischemia but may also give a false sense of security. It is best to adjust guide



S. Rinfret (ed.), *Percutaneous Intervention for Coronary Chronic Total Occlusion: The Hybrid Approach*,
DOI 10.1007/978-3-319-21563-1_17

**Fig. 17.1** Ischemic complications during CTO PCI

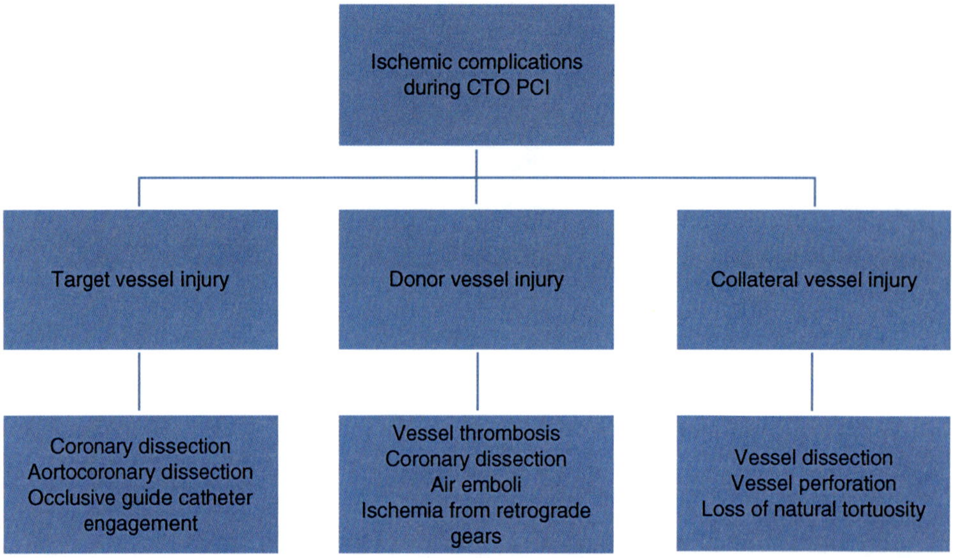


catheter engagement to prevent pressure damping and avoid aggressive injections especially with non-coaxial or occlusive engagement. The use of less aggressive guide catheters can also reduce the risk of catheter-induced dissection.

When wiring a proximal vessel, especially a tortuous proximal vessel, use a low-tip load workhorse guidewire to avoid proximal injury. Once the distal cap of the CTO is reached, an over-the-wire device such as a microcatheter and an over-the-wire (OTW) balloon can then be advanced over the workhorse wire. The workhorse wire is then removed and exchanged for a more aggressive, higher tip load CTO guidewire for proximal cap puncture. If insertion of a mother-and-child catheter is required, preparation may be needed with proximal vessel ballooning and advance it over a balloon to prevent mechanical injury.

Aortocoronary dissection, similar to coronary dissection, may cause ischemia by acutely occluding the proximal target vessel (Fig. 17.2). This type of complication may occur from guide catheter hydraulic dissection, aggressive guide engagement, or balloon rupture. More commonly, this type of dissection occurs from retrograde crossing attempts especially of the right coronary artery (RCA) [3]. Aortocoronary dissections may involve only the coronary sinus or extension into the ascending aorta and more distally. Prevention includes strategies described above for coronary dissection such as meticulous engagement of aggressive guide catheters or use of less aggressive guide catheters, and avoiding high balloon pressure inflation at the aortocoronary ostium. When performing dissection reentry techniques, limit subintimal space wiring and dissection to the occluded segments in order to prevent aortocoronary dissections and proximal vessel injury. This allows sparing of important side branches and dominant ipsilateral collaterals. If there are side branches at the proximal or distal cap, avoid using dissection re-entry techniques and if necessary, limit the dissection as mentioned and if possible, protect the side branch with a wire. Once proximal vessel injury or aortocoronary dissections occur with resultant significant ischemia, treatment includes urgent revascularization, mainly with stenting of the injured segment and ensuring full coverage of the ostium in the case of aortocoronary dissection. Urgent bail-out retrograde techniques may be required to revascularize the target vessel [4].

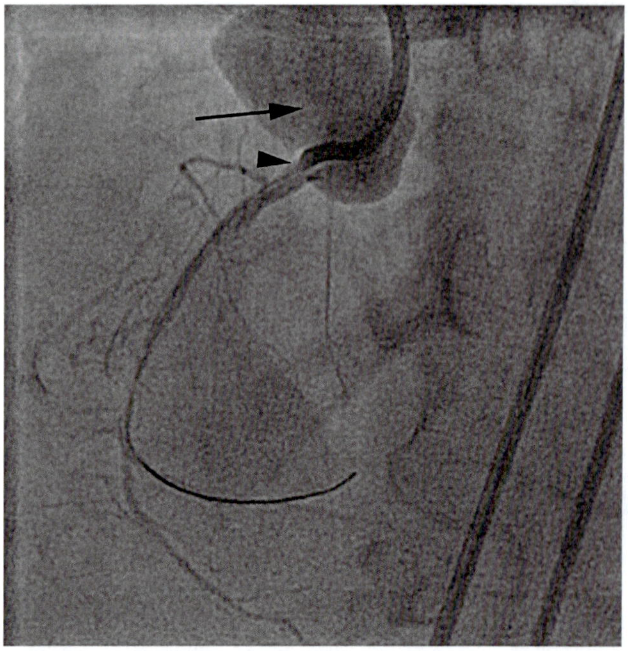

**Fig. 17.2** Aortic dissection (*arrow*) during CTO PCI caused by aggressive guide engagement and forceful contrast injection (*arrow head*)

## Ischemic Complications from Donor Vessel Injury

With retrograde approaches, donor vessel compromise is a serious and potentially lethal complication due to global ischemia [5], especially when the donor vessel is the last

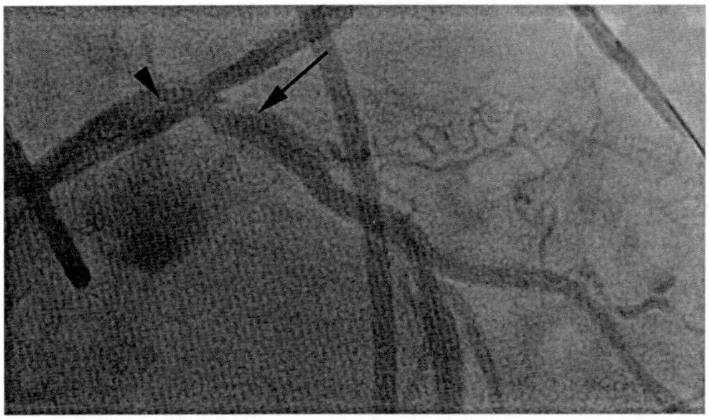

**Fig. 17.3** Donor vessel dissection during retrograde RCA CTO PCI. Dissection of the left main artery (*arrow head*) and the left circumflex artery (*arrow*). This occurred during removal of retrograde equipment which caused unintentional advancement of the LM guide resulting donor vessel dissection

remaining vessel (commonly seen in patients with prior coronary artery bypass surgery). Main causes of donor artery injury include thrombosis, dissection, and ischemia from presence of retrograde devices, especially in a moderate to severe diffusely diseased vessel. Donor artery thrombosis may occur due to prolonged procedure time and with inadequate anticoagulation [5, 6]. Prevention includes keeping procedure time short and meticulous monitoring of activated clotting time (ACT). We recommend keeping ACT above 350 seconds for retrograde approach and to check ACTs every 30 min. Flush catheters routinely to prevent catheter thrombosis. If thrombosis occurs, standard treatments are utilized such as additional heparin bolus to achieve target ACT, additional glycoprotein IIbIIIa inhibitor may be required, thrombus aspiration, and prolonged balloon inflations. Stenting may be necessary if significant amounts of thrombus persist. Retrograde devices in the donor vessel poses a major problem for emergent stenting. Multiple options exist: (1) stenting on the externalized wire if anatomically feasible, (2) withdrawing the retrograde OTW device back into the donor vessel and using it to exchange the externalized wire for a workhorse wire which can be used for stent delivery, or (3) advancing a second wire for stenting which would jail the externalized wire (and therefore, should be done with great caution) [7].

Similar to donor vessel thrombosis, donor vessel dissection, although rare, can be catastrophic [2, 8]. It can be caused by guide catheters, retrograde equipment especially during removal (Fig. 17.3), and guidewire manipulation [6]. Prevention is the key treatment. When wiring the donor vessel to access the appropriate collaterals for retrograde approach, use a soft tip workhorse wire with appropriate bends to prevent injury. Once collaterals have been crossed and the wire has been externalized, the donor vessel along with collaterals should be protected with a microcatheter or an OTW balloon to prevent injury. If snaring is required to achieve externalization, the wire should be pushed from the retrograde limb rather than being pulled from the antegrade limb to prevent tension and sheer stress, which may cause transection of the vessels involved [5]. Pulling on any intracoronary equipment, especially retrograde devices and externalized wires causes unintentional advancement of guide catheters, especially retrograde guides which can cause dissection of donor vessel. Therefore, careful manipulation and being vigilant of guide catheter position at all times is mandatory. For example, during removal of an externalized wire, aggressive pulling will cause the retrograde guide catheter to dive deep into the donor vessel and cause dissection. Therefore, it is recommended that the retrograde guide is disengaged and the externalized wire is pulled with just enough force during diastole to slowly remove the wire. If donor vessel dissection occurs, prompt treatment with stenting is usually needed to prevent global ischemia and hemodynamic collapse [6]. Emergent stenting of the donor vessel can be problematic due to the presence of retrograde equipment but there are multiple options as discussed above.

Donor vessel ischemia can also occur without injury. In diseased donor vessels, insertion of devices for retrograde access may impede blood flow, resulting in clinically significant ischemia (Fig. 17.4). If the patient becomes agitated from ischemic pain, aggressive sedation will be required. Some even advocate the use of general anesthesia to enable completion of the CTO PCI. If hemodynamic compromise becomes evident, then treating the donor vessel may be the only option to allow continuation of the procedure. Prevention of such complications can be accomplished by carefully assessing for donor vessel ischemia with either intracoronary ultrasonography or fractional flow reserve and treat as needed prior to CTO PCI.

Air emboli is another cause of donor vessel ischemia without actual vessel injury. This is caused by injection of air from the retrograde guide catheter. The most common source of air emboli during CTO PCI is from the "trapping" technique which can entrain air. Air emboli can cause significant ischemia resulting in hemodynamic collapse, dysrhythmias, and possibly death [9–11]. Primary treatment is prevention with meticulous attention and avoidance of potential causes especially during "trapping" techniques which always entrain air. Routinely bleed back from guide catheters to remove air after "trapping". Once air emboli occurs, management includes administration of 100 % oxygen, analgesics for pain control, treat clinically significant arrhythmias, and supportive measures such as vasopressors if necessary [10, 11]. Air bubbles may be aspirated or broken up with coronary guidewires [10–13]. In the majority of cases, adverse effects of air emboli only lasts several minutes and therefore, supportive measures as previously mentioned should be employed to avoid catastrophic outcome.

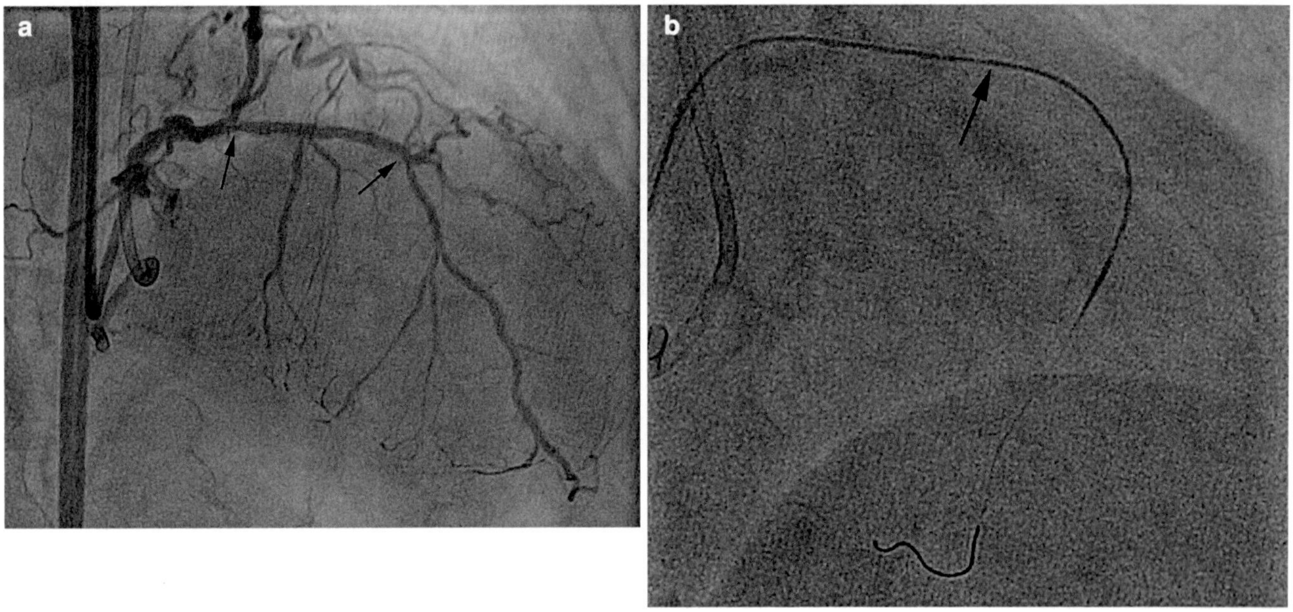


**Fig. 17.4** Moderately diffuse disease in donor vessel (*arrows*, panel **a**) can result in ischemia when retrograde equipment such as Corsair (*arrow*, panel **b**) is inserted. In this particular case, the patient developed cardiac arrest when Corsair was occupying the LAD. Removal of retrograde equipment resolved the hemodynamic compromise

## Ischemic Complications from Collateral Vessel Injury

The retrograde approach requires accessing collateral vessels which can be injured with guidewire and/or device manipulation. Epicardial collaterals are often more tortuous and carry higher risk for complications [5]. Dissection or perforation of a collateral vessel can cause significant ischemia in the recipient vessel if it is the primary or only source of collateral flow (Fig. 17.5). Wiring and delivering OTW devices in tortuous collateral vessels such as tortuous epicardial or LIMA graft collaterals, may result in the loss of natural collateral tortuosity and impedes blood flow causing ischemia [14] (Fig. 17.5). Primary treatment is prevention of collateral vessel injury. Use low-tip force wire to wire collateral vessels and have a heightened awareness especially when working with epicardial collaterals. We suggest using epicardial collaterals as a last resort for reasons just mentioned [14]. If recipient vessel ischemia occurs due to straightening of tortuous collaterals with wires and devices, then withdraw retrograde equipment and change strategy by using a different collateral or switching to the antegrade approach.

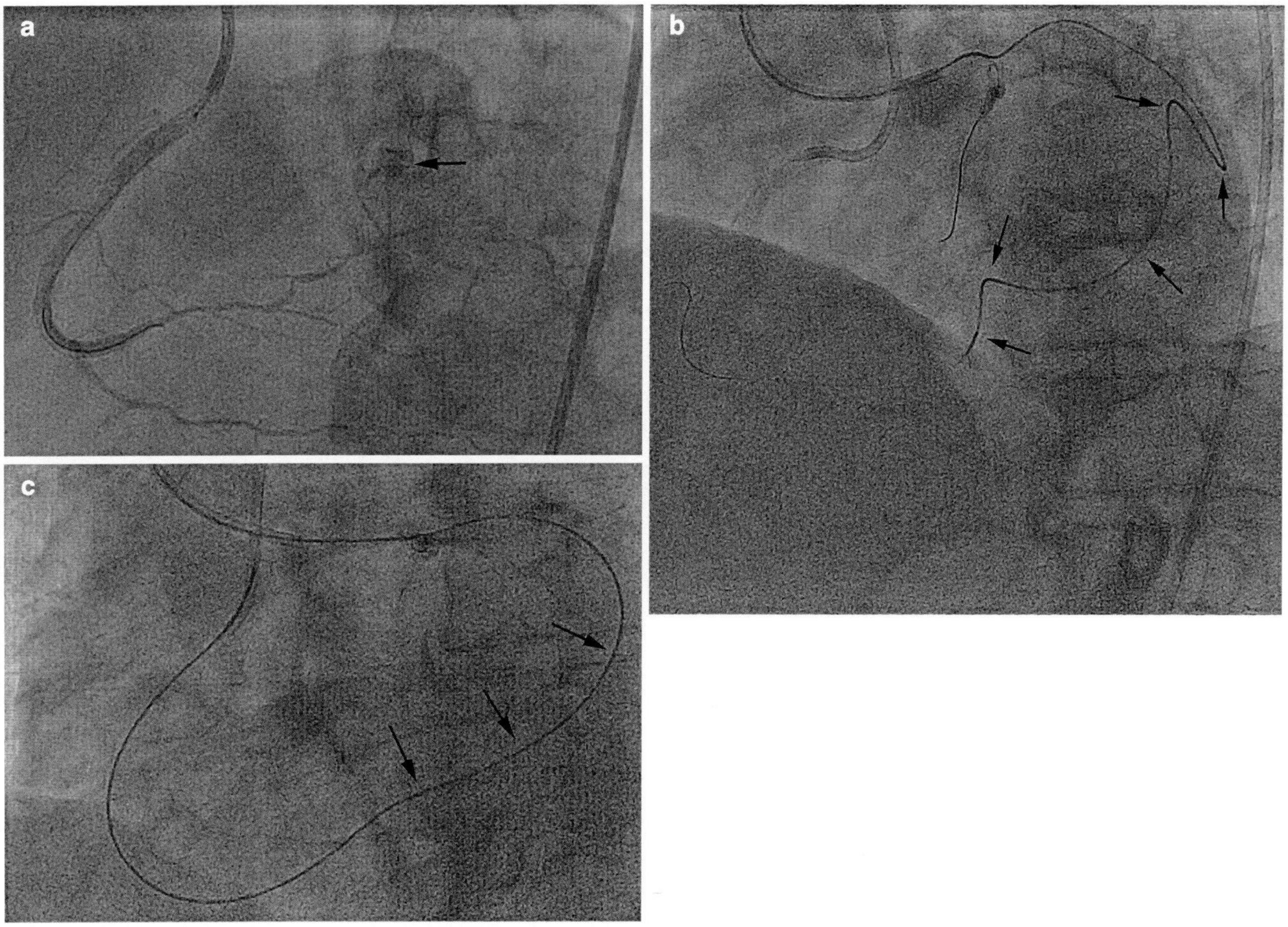


**Fig. 17.5** Common causes of epicardial collateral vessel injury. Perforation (*arrow*, panel **a**) can be catastrophic due to tamponade and/or severe ischemia especially when it is the dominant or sole collateral. Severely tortuous collateral vessel (*arrows*, panel **b**) will lose its natural tortuosity with introduction of devices, Corsair in this case (*arrows*, panel **c**), resulting in blood flow impediment and ischemia

## References


1. Patel VG, et al. Angiographic success and procedural complications in patients undergoing percutaneous coronary chronic total occlusion interventions: a weighted meta-analysis of 18,061 patients from 65 studies. JACC Cardiovasc Interv. 2013;6(2):128–36.
2. Patel VG, et al. Clinical, angiographic, and procedural predictors of periprocedural complications during chronic total occlusion percutaneous coronary intervention. J Invasive Cardiol. 2014;26(3):100–5.
3. Shorrock D, et al. Frequency and outcomes of aortocoronary dissection during percutaneous coronary intervention of chronic total occlusions: a case series and systematic review of the literature. Catheter Cardiovasc Interv. 2014;84(4):670–5.
4. Suh J, Cho YH, Lee NH. Bail-out reverse controlled antegrade and retrograde subintimal tracking accompanied by multiple complications in coronary chronic total occlusion. J Invasive Cardiol. 2008;20(12):E334–7.
5. Brilakis ES, et al. The retrograde approach to coronary artery chronic total occlusions: a practical approach. Catheter Cardiovasc Interv. 2012;79(1):3–19.
6. Lee NH, et al. Recanalization strategy of retrograde angioplasty in patients with coronary chronic total occlusion -analysis of 24 cases, focusing on technical aspects and complications. Int J Cardiol. 2010;144(2):219–29.
7. Brilakis ES. Manual of coronary chronic total occlusion interventions. A step-by step approach. Elsevier, Waltham, MA, USA 2014.
8. Sianos G, et al. European experience with the retrograde approach for the recanalisation of coronary artery chronic total occlusions. A report on behalf of the euroCTO club. EuroIntervention. 2008;4(1):84–92.
9. Bentivoglio LG, Leo LR. Death from coronary air embolism during percutaneous transluminal coronary angioplasty. Cathet Cardiovasc Diagn. 1985;11(6):585–90.
10. Kahn JK, Hartzler GO. The spectrum of symptomatic coronary air embolism during balloon angioplasty: causes, consequences, and management. Am Heart J. 1990;119(6):1374–7.
11. Khan M, et al. Coronary air embolism: incidence, severity, and suggested approaches to treatment. Cathet Cardiovasc Diagn. 1995;36(4):313–8.
12. Patterson MS, Kiemeneij F. Coronary air embolism treated with aspiration catheter. Heart. 2005;91(5), e36.
13. Solodky A, et al. Coronary air embolism treated by bubble aspiration. Catheter Cardiovasc Interv. 2000;49(4):452–4.
14. Joyal D, et al. The retrograde technique for recanalization of chronic total occlusions: a step-by-step approach. JACC Cardiovasc Interv. 2012;5(1):1–11.

# Managing Entrapped Gear During Chronic Total Occlusion Interventions

# 18

Creighton W. Don and William L. Lombardi

**Abstract**

Entrapment of interventional equipment is an infrequent complication of percutaneous coronary interventions, with an incidence of less than 0.3 % in the contemporary era, but when it does occur, it can potentially lead to major complications such as vessel perforation, thrombosis, and early and late myocardial infarctions. Where attempts at percutaneous retrieval fail, emergent surgical extraction or coronary bypass may be required.

Percutaneous interventions on chronic total occlusions (CTO) may have a greater risk for device entrapment and embolization due to the significant calcification and tortuosity of occluded vessels. Furthermore the aggressive wiring and ballooning techniques used in CTO interventions, and retrograde passage of gear through small sharply angulated collateral branches and may predispose to device entrapment.

This chapter will discuss the risk factors and common procedural scenarios associated with device entrapment, and provide a review of the bail-out strategies operators should know when these situations are encountered.

**Keywords**

Entrapment of interventional equipment • Entrapment of interventional devices • Percutaneous coronary interventions (PCI) and device entrapment • Trapped wires and PCI • Trapped stents and PCI • Trapped microcatheters and PCI • Trapped balloons and PCI • Retrograde entrapment and PCI

## Introduction

Entrapment of interventional equipment is an infrequent complication of percutaneous coronary interventions, with an incidence of less than 0.3 % in the contemporary era [1–4], but when it does occur, it can potentially lead to major complications such as vessel perforation, thrombosis, and early and late myocardial infarctions [1–3]. Where attempts at percutaneous retrieval fail, emergent surgical extraction or coronary bypass may be required [1–3].

Percutaneous interventions on chronic total occlusions (CTO) may have a greater risk for device entrapment and embolization due to the significant calcification and tortuosity of occluded vessels [5, 6]. Furthermore the aggressive wiring and ballooning techniques used in CTO interventions, and retrograde passage of gear through small sharply angulated collateral branches and may predispose to device entrapment [7].

This chapter will discuss the risk factors and common procedural scenarios associated with device entrapment, and provide a review of the bail-out strategies operators should know when these situations are encountered (Table 18.1).

C.W. Don, MD
Division of Cardiology, University of Washington Medical Center, Seattle, WA, USA

W.L. Lombardi, MD (✉)
Department of Cardiology,
University of Washington Medical Center,
Seattle, WA, USA
e-mail: mongocto@gmail.com


S. Rinfret (ed.), *Percutaneous Intervention for Coronary Chronic Total Occlusion: The Hybrid Approach*,
DOI 10.1007/978-3-319-21563-1_18

**Table 18.1** Causes for device entrapment and techniques for device retrieval

| Scenario | Causes | Bail-out techniques |
|---|---|---|
| **Trapped equipment** | | |
| Wires | Prolapsed or knuckled wire is trapped in a calcified or tortuous segment<br>Wire used to protect a side branch is trapped behind a newly deployed stent | Advance microcatheter or over-the-wire balloon to provide controlled, local traction at the site of entrapment.<br>Advance the microcathter beyond the highest point of resistance, and the wire can then be removed. |
| Knotted wires | During aggressive wire 'knuckling' or excessive torquing, a knot can be formed | Advance a microcatheter to the point where the wire is knotted and gently pull on the wire to untangle it |
| Balloons, stents and microcatheters | Stent or microcatheter is aggressively advanced or drilled into a calcified and tortuous vessel<br>Balloon is ruptured in calcified, fibrotic lesion, becoming entrapped<br>Device snags on the struts of a newly placed stent | Cut off device hub and advance a guide or telescoping 'mother-in-child' guide to the lesion to provide local coaxial countertraction while attempting to withdraw the device<br>Advance a gooseneck snare over the trapped device shaft to provide traction on the device close to the site of entrapment<br>Advance a parallel wire and perform angioplasty of the culprit region in the lesion or subintimal space |
| Rota-burr | Small Rota burr is advanced too quickly past a lesion and cannot be withdrawn<br>Rota burr is embedded into a calcified lesion or within a previously placed stent | Apply gentle negative pressure while using Dynaglide<br>Use 'mother-in-child' guide or gooseneck snare as above.<br>Advance a parallel wire and perform angioplasty of the culprit region<br>Pull on the RotaWire while pulling on the burr |
| **Retrograde scenarios** | | |
| Wires | Wire trapped in small tortuous collateral | Use a microcatheter to relieve the resistance on the wire, as above |
| Balloons and microcatheters | Collateral is small and tortuous, has a sharply angulated takeoff, or is jailed by a stent | Remove the externalized wire from the microcatheter to allow it to become more pliable and conform to the tortuous vessel, then remove the microcatheter<br>Use 'mother-in-child' guide or gooseneck snare as above. |
| Entanglement of antegrade and retrograde gear | Tips of the antegrade and retrograde microcatheters become coupled | Pull both catheters from their proximal extremities<br>Cut off antegrade device hub and pull back on the retrograde equipment, pulling out all the gear through the collateral and out the retrograde guide |
| **Embolized equipment** | | |
| Wires, stents, and microcatheter tips | Entrapped portion of device fractures during attempt to withdraw device<br>Aggressive or careless wire advancement causes the wire tip to prolapse and fracture<br>Calcified/tortuous lesion causes the delivery balloon to separate from the stent | Micro snare retrieval<br>Entangle the fragment with 2 or 3 wires and remove<br>Advance a small balloon or protection device/basket distal to the fragment and drag back<br>Biopsy forceps can be used for devices in proximal coronaries<br>Stent the fragment into the vessel wall |

## Risk Factors

Device entrapment and embolization is most frequently associated with interventions on tortuous and severely calcified vessels [1] and can occur in the left and right coronary arteries equally [3]. The use of collaterals in CTO interventions can predispose to device entrapment. Tortuous collateral channels and septal branches with sharply angulated takeoffs have been associated with retrograde wire [8], balloon, and stent entrapment [7].

During antegrade interventions, it is imperative that the target vessel is properly prepared and the operator avoids forcing stents and other devices to cross lesions. Now that the vast majority of stents are pre-crimped, stent dislodgment is almost always due to aggressive advancement of stents into improperly prepared lesions or distal to previously deployed stents. It is also advised to prep the stent delivery balloon only when the stent is in place; otherwise, negative suction on the balloon can weaken the stent crimping, and increase the chance of stent dislodgment. The use of debulking devices to modify plaque characteristics and create channels through 'non-crossable' lesions helps reduce this risk. Inflation of balloons to high enough pressures to cause rupture may lead to the balloon becoming embedded into the vessel and entrapped [9], so there should be a low threshold to utilize atherectomy if a lesion appears non-dilatable.

Advancing equipment through recently placed stents also presents a situation with increased risk for device entrapment. The exposed stent struts can shear off parts of the devices crossing through the cells or along the stent edge. Pulling directly on the device without disentangling it from the stent can cause stent deformation, leading to entrapment. This situation has been described by operators who entagled an IVUS catheter within the struts of a newly placed stent [10] or were performing rotational atherectomy with a stent [11].

The risk for device breakage or stripping stents off of delivery balloons can be reduced by making sure coaxial traction is directed as close as possible to the site of resistance. The non-coaxial force applied to stent delivery balloons due to vessel tortuosity or poor guide positioning has been described as a significant risk associated with stent embolization [1]. Additionally, pulling forcefully on trapped wires and devices can cause trauma to the proximal vessel, or to the weaker weld points on the device, while very little of this force is transmitted to the site of resistance.

## Entrapped Equipment

### Wires

Although it happens less commonly with newer flexible wires, with more durable weld points, wire entrapment has been reported with prolapsing and extreme torquing of the end of the wire within tortuous distal vessels, along sharply angulated branches, and within calcified, fibrotic lesions. More commonly, wires can become entangled within fresh stents struts, or inadvertently jailed behind stents deployed to high pressure [4].

Continuously increasing traction without any movement of the trapped segment will lead to wire fracture and embolization, or stripping of the polymer coat, so an attempt should be made to apply controlled coaxial traction as close as possible to the entrapped segment using a guide or microcathter while withdrawing the wire. It may be possible to advance a microcatheter beyond the trapped region, or if the wire has been stented, underneath the stent, at which point the wire can be withdrawn through the microcatheter [12]. A braided catheter such as a Tornus or Corsair (Asahi Intecc, Aichi, Japan) may be required to push through the calcified lesion.

During aggressive wire knuckling, while creating or tracking a subintimal channel, concomitant torquing of the wire can lead to the wire being tied into a knot. If as a result the wire cannot be withdrawn, then a microcatheter should be advanced to the knot to help disentangle the wire. Often the wire and microcatheter can then be withdrawn simultaneously. Suggestions for managing embolized wire fragments is described at the end of the chapter.

**Bail-Out Technique for Trapped Wires**

- Use a microcatheter to disentangle and free entrapped wires to avoid fracturing wires while pulling back on them.

### Microcatheters, Balloons and Stents

In tortuous, highly angulated vessels, or in severely calcified lesions, microcatheters and stents can become entrapped, especially if the operator progressively advances the catheter by torquing the device, thoroughly embedding it into a lesion. Equipment can also become entangled by advancing it through the cells of a freshly deployed stent into a sharply angulated branch [13] or snagging the balloon on a stent edge [14]. Balloons become entrapped when they are ruptured within a lesion or when the irregular balloon fragments prevent withdrawal of the ruptured balloon through a lesion [9].

If the lesion can be modified, the device can sometimes be extricated. If a large enough guide was used, a second wire can be advanced across the lesion and balloon angioplasty of the lesion can be performed. If the lesion cannot be crossed with a wire, it may be reasonable to track the second wire subintimally around the lesion and perform a high-pressure inflation, attempting to modify the calcified plaque by crushing it from the extraluminal space. If the first guide will not accommodate another wire and balloon, a second guide catheter may be required from a second access site to intubate the coronary artery alongside the first guide (ping pong technique).

Another approach is to cut off the hub of the device to allow advancement of a telescoping 'mother-in-child' catheter through the guiding catheter, over the shaft of the trapped device. This second guide catheter can be deep seated and provide coaxial countertraction at the site of entrapment [9].

If a large enough guide was used, it may be possible to loop a gooseneck snare around the shaft of the entrapped device and slide the snare and snare microcatheter as distal as possible along the device and provide additional negative traction on the device. If the guide cannot fit the snare catheter, the hub of the device can be cut and the guide catheter removed. The snare catheter can then be inserted directly through the sheath.

### Bail-Out Techniques for Trapped Stents, Microcatheters, and Balloons

- Use a second wire and balloon to dilate the lesion where the device is entrapped
- Advance a telescoping guide to provide local countertraction at the site of entrapment
- Slide a gooseneck snare and snare microcatheter along the shaft of device as close to the site of entrapment as possible to provide additional negative traction

## Rotablator Burr

The Rotablator burr can be advanced forward too quickly, insufficiently atherectomizing the lesion, and then pushed beyond the lesion. Since the atherectomy surface on the Rotablator is only on the distal tip surface, it is possible that the burr cannot be withdrawn back through the vessel in this situation. It is also possible that the burr becomes embedded in a fibrotic and calcified lesion and the device stalls and will not rotate. Gently withdrawing the burr using Dynaglide, with constant low RPMs, typically will disentangle a stalled device; however this is occasionally insufficient to remove the device.

Expanding the lesion with an angioplasty balloon may reduce the resistance of the lesion and allow the burr to be withdrawn. If an 8 F guide is used, a second wire and 1.5 mm balloon can be passed alongside the rotablation catheter and an attempt can be made to pass a wire alongside the entrapped rotablation burr and angioplasty the resistant lesion. A second guide can be used from a second access site (ping pong technique) or a smaller guide can be upsized by cutting the distal hub off of the Rotablator burr, removing the smaller guide, and advancing a larger guide over the Rotablator shaft. Alternatively, once the distal hub of the Rotablator burr is cut, the outer plastic sheath covering the burr can be removed [15]. This will allow for a second wire and balloon to be passed through a 6 or 7 F guide [11].

As described in the section above, a telescoping 5 F guide to provide countertraction [16] or a gooseneck snare to provide negative traction [17] have been described to successfully remove entrapped Rotablator burrs. The hub of the Rotablator catheter and the outer plastic sheath needs to be removed so a telescoping 'mother-in-child' guide can be advanced over the Rotablator shaft assembly or the snare and snare microcatheter will fit alongside the Rotablator within the guide.

Finally, when exerting traction on the Rotablator burr, it is also useful to apply traction on the RotaWire also, as its 0.014′ extremity cannot be retrieved into the catheter and can serve as a powerful distal anchor to pull the device.

### Bail-Out Techniques for Trapped Rotablator Burr

- Apply gentle traction while using Dynaglide
- Use a second wire and balloon to dilate the lesion where the device is entrapped
- Use a telescoping guide to provide local countertraction or gooseneck snare to provide additional negative traction
- Pull the RotaWire to help retrieve the burr out of the plaque

## Retrograde Scenarios

Removing retrograde equipment can be challenging when the collateral vessel is very small and tortuous, the takeoff of the septal branch is sharply angulated from the main branch, or the retrograde equipment needed to pass through stent struts [7]. In CART procedures (controlled antegrade retrograde tracking) balloons and other devices are advanced retrograde through the collateral branches. The larger profile of used or ruptured balloons may have difficulty being withdrawn through collaterals, particularly septal channels that have not been adequately dilated. Guidewires can also become entrapped in the collateral channels [8], and have been reported in as many as 1.2 % of retrograde CTO cases [5]. Extrication of wires and devices is generally similar to the techniques described previously.

If the cause for microcatheter entrapment is a severely tortuous collateral, it is sometimes helpful to remove the wire within the catheter first. The stiff body of externalized wires can sometimes over-straighten the vessel causing vessel pleating to increase resistance on the device.

In rare situations, when antegrade and retrograde microcatheters or balloons have been used simultaneously, it is possible that the nose of one catheter can telescope within the other catheter, entrapping both catheters. If the catheters cannot be disengaged by pulling both catheters from their proximal extremity, one solution is to cut the hub off of the antegrade catheter and withdraw the retrograde collateral, removing the antegrade catheter by pulling in through the collateral and into the retrograde guide.

### Bail-Out Techniques for Retrograde Entrapment

- Use similar techniques for antegrade entrapment, from the retrograde approach
- Remove the externalized wire from the microcatheter to allow it to become more pliable and conform to the tortuous vessel, then remove the microcatheter
- Cut off antegrade device hub and pull back on the retrograde equipment, pulling out all the gear through the collateral and out the retrograde guide

## Embolized Equipment

Aggressive pulling of entrapped devices can eventually cause fracturing and embolization of distal parts of the devices. Multiple techniques have been described to retrieve embolized stents [1, 3]. The most frequently used method is to remove the stent delivery balloon while maintaining wire control into the stent. Over the wire, a small Goose Neck snare with its microcatheter can be advanced as close as possible to the stent and then attempts are made to snare the stent. If wire control of the stent is lost, a wire should be advanced distal to the stent and snaring attempted. If this is unsuccessful, a balloon can be advanced along this wire and inflated distal to the stent and the stent can be dragged back to another position where it can be snared or trapped in the guide. Other authors have described using a distal protection device deployed beyond the stent to drag the stent back. One novel idea is to hook a wire through a stent and then advance the wire back into the guide where it can be trapped, thereby allowing the operator to pull out the stent [18]. If the stent can be dragged back to the guide it can be trapped in the guide and removed, or a bioptome can grasp the stent in the aorta [19].

Similar snare and trapping techniques can be used for embolized wire and microcatheters fragments. Wire fragments can also be retrieved by entangling 2 or 3 wires around the fragment and quickly spinning the new wires around the embolized one. Very small fragments in small branches may not need to be removed if they are not threatening closure of major territories [19]. Finally, if the fragment cannot be removed and there is a concern that it might affect vessel patency, stenting the fragment into the vessel wall may be considered.

## Bail-Out Techniques for Retrieving Embolized Wires, Microcatheters and Stents

- Micro snare retrieval
- Entangle the fragment with wires and remove
- Advance a small balloon or protection device/basket distal to the fragment and drag back
- Biopsy forceps can be used for devices in proximal coronaries
- Stent the fragment into the vessel wall

## Managing Complications

The major complication of entrapped and embolized gear is related to vessel perforation caused by attempts to forcefully remove the gear, or thrombosis due to retained fragments. The decision to abandon wires and devices must of course weigh the risk for vessel closure against the potential complications of aggressive percutaneous or surgical attempts at retrieval. Small wire fragments in distal branches, or trapped underneath stents are not likely to cause problems, whereas devices occluding a large branch or extending into the aorta clearly need treatment. If the vessel is large and remains obstructed, or the device cannot be removed without causing further risk to the patient, urgent bypass surgery needs to be considered.

Operators need to be prepared to quickly treat acute vessel perforation and respond to the hemodynamic consequences thereof. Prior to attempting a forceful, aggressive retrieval maneuver, occlusion balloons need to be on the ready to be deployed quickly, and coils and covered stents must be also be available, with operators who are familiar with using these devices on the ready. Assessment of vessel competence and the need for urgent pericardiocentesis should also be performed immediately following aggressive device retrieval.

## Management of Major Complications

- Consider urgent coronary bypass for large retained fragments and persistent occlusion caused by entrapped device
- Have pericardiocentesis kits, occlusion balloons, covered stents and coils readily available to treat vessel perforations

### Conclusions

Device entrapment is rare, but remains one of the most dreaded complications, even by experiences CTO PCI operators. The incidence of device entrapment can be reduced by avoiding rapid advancement, excessive force or torquing on devices in small, tortuous calcified lesions. If significant resistance is encountered, operators should consider alternative approaches than those that rely only on applying greater forward force. Vessel preparation is paramount, and the threshold to utilize atherectomy should be low if a lesion appears non-dilatable, in order to modify plaque characteristics that will prevent device passage or removal. Post-entrapment modification of the plaque is helpful, if possible. Likewise, for entrapped devices, careful tension on the device should be directed at the site of resistance, by using microcatheters, snares, or deep seated telescoping guides in order to directly apply focused, coaxial force on the embedded device.

## References

1. Brilakis ES, Best PJ, Elesber AA, Barsness GW, Lennon RJ, Holmes Jr DR, Rihal CS, Garratt KN. Incidence, retrieval methods, and outcomes of stent loss during percutaneous coronary intervention: a large single-center experience. Catheter Cardiovasc Interv. 2005;66:333–40.

2. Iturbe JM, Abdel-Karim AR, Papayannis A, Mahmood A, Rangan BV, Banerjee S, Brilakis ES. Frequency, treatment, and consequences of device loss and entrapment in contemporary percutaneous coronary interventions. J Invasive Cardiol. 2012;24: 215–21.
3. Alomar ME, Michael TT, Patel VG, Altomare CG, Rangan BV, Cipher D, Banerjee S, Brilakis ES. Stent loss and retrieval during percutaneous coronary interventions: a systematic review and meta-analysis. J Invasive Cardiol. 2013;25:637–41.
4. Alomari I, Snider R, Ponce S, Ahmed B. Entrapped devices after pci. Cardiovasc Revasc Med. 2014;15:182–5.
5. El Sabbagh A, Patel VG, Jeroudi OM, Michael TT, Alomar ME, Mogabgab O, Fuh E, Roesle M, Rangan BV, Abdullah S, Hastings JL, Grodin J, Kumbhani DJ, Alexopoulos D, Fasseas P, Banerjee S, Brilakis ES. Angiographic success and procedural complications in patients undergoing retrograde percutaneous coronary chronic total occlusion interventions: a weighted meta-analysis of 3,482 patients from 26 studies. Int J Cardiol. 2014;174: 243–8.
6. Christopoulos G, Menon RV, Karmpaliotis D, Alaswad K, Lombardi W, Grantham A, Patel VG, Rangan BV, Kotsia AP, Lembo N, Kandzari D, Carlson H, Garcia S, Banerjee S, Thompson CA, Brilakis ES. The efficacy and safety of the "hybrid" approach to coronary chronic total occlusions: Insights from a contemporary multicenter us registry and comparison with prior studies. J Invasive Cardiol. 2014;26:427–32.
7. Utsunomiya M, Kobayashi T, Nakamura S. Case of dislodged stent lost in septal channel during stent delivery in complex chronic total occlusion of right coronary artery. J Invasive Cardiol. 2009;21: E229–33.
8. Sianos G, Papafaklis MI. Septal wire entrapment during recanalisation of a chronic total occlusion with the retrograde approach. Hellenic J Cardiol. 2011;52:79–83.
9. Chang W-T, et al., A two-case series of entrapment of a ruptured balloon in the coronary artery: Avoidable complications and nonsurgical management, Journal of the Formosan Medical Association (2013), http://dx.doi.org/10.1016/j.jfma.2013.05.008.
10. Hamamoto M, Futagami D. Successful surgical removal of an entrapped intravascular ultrasonography catheter in the left circumflex coronary artery. Gen Thorac Cardiovasc Surg. 2012;60:830–3.
11. Dahdouh Z, Abdel-Massih T, Roule V, Sarkis A, Grollier G. Rotational atherectomy as endovascular haute couture: A road map of tools and techniques for the interventional management of burr entrapment. J Interv Cardiol. 2013;26:586–95.
12. Cho YH, Park S, Kim JS, Lee SY, Choi D, Jang Y, Cho SY. Rescuing an entrapped guidewire using a tornus catheter. Circ J. 2007;71: 1326–7.
13. Bruschi G, Colombo P, Piccalo G, Trunfio S, Colombo T, Vitali E. Successful emergent surgical revascularization and retrieval of entrapped drug eluting stent. J Cardiovasc Med (Hagerstown). 2008;9:182–3.
14. Pappy R, Gautam A, Abu-Fadel MS. Angiosculpt ptca balloon catheter entrapment and detachment managed with stent jailing. J Invasive Cardiol. 2010;22:E208–10.
15. Sakakura K, Ako J, Momomura S. Successful removal of an entrapped rotablation burr by extracting drive shaft sheath followed by balloon dilatation. Catheter Cardiovasc Interv. 2011;78:567–70.
16. Kimura M, Shiraishi J, Kohno Y. Successful retrieval of an entrapped rotablator burr using 5 fr guiding catheter. Catheter Cardiovasc Interv. 2011;78:558–64.
17. Hyogo M, Inoue N, Nakamura R, Tokura T, Matsuo A, Inoue K, Tanaka T, Fujita H. Usefulness of conquest guidewire for retrieval of an entrapped rotablator burr. Catheter Cardiovasc Interv. 2004; 63:469–72.
18. Brilakis ES, Abdel-Karim AR, Banerjee S. Hairpin-trap: a novel stent retrieval technique. Catheter Cardiovasc Interv. 2011;77:213–6.
19. Hartzler GO, Rutherford BD, McConahay DR. Retained percutaneous transluminal coronary angioplasty equipment components and their management. Am J Cardiol. 1987;60:1260–4.

# How to Start and Build Your CTO Practice and Maintain Referrals in a Competitive Environment

19

M. Nicholas Burke and Stéphane Rinfret

**Abstract**

Starting and building a CTO practice can be one of the most challenging things that an interventional cardiologist may encounter in his or her professional career. Even in the best of situations, the new CTO operator will likely encounter a host of critics including from non-invasive cardiologists, cardiovascular surgeons, other interventional cardiologists, and even from his or her partners. CTO PCI can be long, costly, and present complications that are uncommon even in a busy cath lab. Administrators, cath lab staff, and nursing staff can either be supportive or they can make it even more challenging. The best way to minimize and or avoid such issues is to approach CTO PCI programmatically and deliberately with the goal of providing the most effective and safest care possible.

**Keywords**

CTO practice • CTO operator • CTO interventionalist • CTO PCI • CTO community • CTO program

## Introduction

Starting and building a CTO practice can be one of the most challenging things that an interventional cardiologist may encounter in his or her professional career. Even in the best of situations, the new CTO operator will likely encounter a host of critics including from non-invasive cardiologists, cardiovascular surgeons, other interventional cardiologists, and even from his or her partners. CTO PCI can be long, costly, and present complications that are uncommon even in a busy cath lab. Administrators, cath lab staff, and nursing staff can either be supportive or they can make it even more challenging. The best way to minimize and or avoid such issues is to approach CTO PCI programmatically and deliberately with the goal of providing the most effective and safest care possible.

M.N. Burke, MD (✉)
Department of Medicine, Minneapolis Heart Institute, Minneapolis, MN, USA

S. Rinfret, MD, SM
CTO Recanalization Program, Interventional Cardiology, Multidisciplinary Department of Cardiology, Quebec Heart and Lung Institute, Laval University, Quebec City, QC, Canada

## The New CTO Operator Should Know the Data

Possibly the most important consideration in CTO PCI is "why do it at all?" To understand when and where PCI is appropriate is vital to the success of the CTO program. It is important that any CTO Interventionalist be well versed in the data both supporting and refuting CTO PCI, as discussed in Chap. 1. It is usually not enough to be able to perform the procedure. The new operator should be thoroughly familiar with the current and historic literature regarding medical management, surgery, completeness of revascularization, ischemia-driven therapy, long term outcomes, and current indications for CTO PCI. In this day of increasing scrutiny, there is a strong need to be aware of Appropriate Use Criteria



S. Rinfret (ed.), *Percutaneous Intervention for Coronary Chronic Total Occlusion: The Hybrid Approach*,
DOI 10.1007/978-3-319-21563-1_19

(AUC) and how they apply to the CTO PCI practice. "Because it's there" might have been a good enough reason for George Mallory to attempt to climb Mount Everest, it is not a good enough reason to perform CTO PCI.

## The New CTO Operator Should Know Himself or Herself

CTO PCI is difficult. If it were easy, Interventionalists would have always done it and there never would have been any issues. As a result of its difficulty, there will be many times when the new operator will be unsuccessful and, unfortunately, will encounter complications. As such, any operator contemplating in starting to perform advanced CTO PCI should ask him- or herself several questions: Is this the right time in my career for me to be doing this? Do I have enough experience as an Interventionalist to take this on? Will I have the time, ability, volume, and commitment to do this correctly? Am I doing this for the right reasons? Is this about making patients better, or is this about me? Those questions are of paramount importance.

## The New CTO Operator Should Educate Him or Herself

CTO PCI is not the same as standard PCI. The CTO operator will be approaching lesions in ways that were taught to be avoided. Much of the equipment, terminology, and techniques are unfamiliar to even the most experienced Interventionalists. Even if someone has performed thousands of cases in a career, CTO PCI will still need to be approached with a novice perspective. For this reason, it is imperative that he or she educate him/herself though reading. Textbooks such as this one help explain the concepts. We also encourage the new operator to use the Internet. The CTO community has an educational website, CTOFundamentals.org, which has a series of lectures which cover all of the basics. Once the didactic sessions are completed, the operator is invited to join the online community where cases are discussed, new information is shared, and questions can be asked. Meetings are also a great source of education. All of the large meetings have CTO PCI specific sessions. There are meetings specific to CTO PCI including those put on by SCAI as well as CRF's CTO Summit. Attending a course (or more than one) is strongly advocated. Currently there are several industry sponsored CTO courses throughout the year. These are small, live courses where experienced CTO PCI operators do cases on site and interact directly with the attendees in dynamic discussions illustrating all aspects of CTO PCI.

## The New CTO Operator Should Get a Mentor

This is important. There is nothing like learning through a one-to-one experience with a mentor. Perhaps it could be someone who was a faculty member at an attended course, or someone the operator heard speak. Most established CTO PCI operators have made a commitment to training other interventionists. Probably the best way to develop a mentor/mentee relationship is by having a CTO proctor come do cases at the new CTO operator site. Some of the key equipment currently used in CTO PCI requires a formal proctoring for several cases. These proctors are generally the same experienced CTO operators who serve as faculty at the CTO courses.

## The New CTO Operator Should Start a Program

The new CTO operator should at least have the support of colleagues and institution. If not, it might be best to wait. It is best to approach CTO PCI programmatically. Perhaps the best example of this is the CTO Program at Piedmont Heart Institute in Atlanta, GA where they implemented a formal multi-operator CTO program. Operators were identified who then underwent extensive training. They received on site proctoring. Indications for the procedure were formalized. Procedural criteria such as strategies, contrast and radiation limits were set. Patients were discussed at a weekly CTO meeting, and a database following outcomes was established. They also decided to have two Interventionalists scrubbed on each case which is not a widespread practice. They then published their results and their program is widely regarded as the model for implementation. While a program of this magnitude might not be possible for most institutions, a vetting process for each case with input from more than one cardiologist is best. The Minneapolis Heart Institute program requires 2 Interventionalists to approve each case. We also double scrub our CTOs and have found this to be of value. Same thing in Quebec City. A second pair of eyes and set of hands are particularly helpful in long cases where fatigue can be a factor for errors and complication and to help in making clinical decisions such as when to stop or change course. In addition, you will find it advantageous if you can develop a team of techs/nurses who are interested in CTO PCI. Finally, splitting cath lab priorities with a colleague for CTO PCI increases the available spots for CTO PCI while preserving each other time in the lab to also perform non-CTO PCI work.

## The New CTO Operator Should Go Slowly

Generally speaking, CTOs should not be done *ad hoc*. This applies also to experienced CTO operators, not just novices. There are several reasons for this. CTO PCI does have a somewhat higher complication rate and most often requires 2 catheters. These cases can be long, requiring significant doses of contrast and radiation. It is best to separate the diagnostic and interventional procedures to try to limit the patient's exposure. Patients should be informed of this and consented appropriately. Perhaps most importantly, performing the intervention in a staged fashion allows for the Interventionalist to make certain that the procedure is appropriate and to carefully study the angiogram to determine strategies. Once a few appropriate cases have been identified, having a proctor come to the new CTO PCI institution to help with first CTOs cases is helpful. One should aim at utilizing several strategies with the proctor in a 1–2 days' worth of cases.

## The New CTO Operator Should Learn to Walk Before Running When Starting Alone

Initial case selection is of paramount importance, not just on clinical but also on anatomic grounds. We often say that it takes years to develop a good reputation and just one day to develop a bad one. This means that the new operator should choose cases which appear to have the highest chance of success (J-CTO scores of 0 and 1) with good distal targets and visible septal collaterals or even bypass grafts for possible retrograde routes. Cases with epicardial collaterals and or high J-CTO scores (≥2) should be attempted only after gaining significant experience and success with more straightforward procedures.

## An Ounce of Prevention...

The best way to avoid complications is to be ready for them. The new operator should be familiar with techniques to deal with perforations, pericardial effusions, and retained equipment. A full complement of snares, coils, covered stents should be readily available prior to the cases and the operator should know how to use them in case of an emergency. Proficiency with pericardiocenteses techniques is a must. On site surgical backup is considered an asset, but several institutions have started very successful CTO PCI program without on-site surgery.

## The New CTO Operator Should Get Ready to Fail

CTO PCI is difficult. Nobody becomes an Interventional Cardiologist because they want to fail. But the new operator certainly will, and repeatedly. That is one of the reasons why it is better to be an experienced Interventionalist when starting this sub-specialty, with a track record of success that can be used for support in tough times. Sometimes it is just not going to happen. One need to be able to accept defeat graciously and learn from it rather than to refuse to give up and harming someone. The CTO operator should also have someone to refer failures. If it's worth doing, the operator's ego should not prevent the CTO from being opened by someone else in case of failure.

## The New CTO Operator Should Track Outcomes

To do this correctly, the new CTO operator need to be able to report to partners, referring providers, administrators, and patients procedural outcomes. Information on success rate, techniques used, and complications should be collected. Patients should be aware of what they are signing up for. Furthermore, this will enable the program to identify trends as well as track changes.

## The New CTO Operator Should Grow His or Her Program

The best way to grow a program is to start correctly and to stay focused on it being safe and effective. If done correctly, non-invasive cardiologists generally come on board first and start referring their patients. It is more difficult to get Interventionalists to refer to other Interventionalists. By far the best way to encourage inter-specialty referrals is to be as open and welcoming as possible. If someone else is interested in learning CTO PCI, the best way to get referral if to teach them and help them build new programs. There are way more cases out there than one can handle. Plus, it's the right thing to do. Many of them will not pursue this long term. We have proctored at numerous competing programs in our environment and we try to encourage these Interventionalists to send failed cases. We have developed a very nice network throughout our regions by supporting other Interventionalists at other programs.

It is important to understand the referral pattern with CTOs. Over the years, we think they split into a 2 by 2 factorial table, with attempt and referring as crucial factors, as shown in Table 19.1.

**Table 19.1** Referral pattern with CTOs

| | The CTO was referred for PCI to the CTO PCI program | The CTO was not referred to the CTO PCI program |
|---|---|---|
| **CTO PCI was attempted but failed** | Educate the operator who failed<br>Good message for team work | Disconnection between the original indication for CTO PCI and recommendation of subsequent medical therapy<br>Cases usually will be referred by treating physicians; if an attempt was done, it gives at least the message that the CTO can be revascularized |
| **CTO PCI was not attempted** | Usually cases where the likely techniques to be required are beyond the expertise of the referring operator | This group is only appropriate if a message of potential referral to the CTO PCI program is possible is case of failure of medical therapy<br>Otherwise, such an approach reduces treatment options for patients |

As illustrated, efforts should be made to make sure the partners refer failed cases, but especially that non-attempted, non-referred cases get on mention about the CTO PCI program in case of failure of medical therapy.

## The New CTO Operator Should Keep Learning

CTO PCI is still in its infancy. New techniques and tools are continuing to evolve. Scientific data is slowly accumulating. Keeping up with the literature is key to growing success. Another ways to keep learning are to go to meetings, participate regularly on the CTO Fundamentals website. The learning curve is a long but satisfying one.

**Conclusion**

We became interested in CTO PCI many years ago before we had all of these tools and strategies. We knew we needed to do better and that somehow we could. And we spent years failing and made every mistake possible. We often learned what to do by doing it incorrectly. Now, one of the most satisfying things that we have experienced professionally is to have a patient come back and say that their life has been dramatically changed when they had been told previously that there was nothing more that could be done for them. The new CTO operator has the opportunity to do it right. There are currently only a minority of CTO cases attempted. The quest for quality and safety will invariably lead to sustained referral to CTO PCI programs.

# Index

**A**
Activated clotting time (ACT), 213
Acute cardiac complications
 aortic dissection, 204
 coronary perforation
  collateral vessel perforation, 196
  coronary vessel locations, 195
  distal target vessel perforation, 196
  Ellis classification, 195
  epicardial coronary vessel perforation, 196–200
  hemodynamics, 200
  ping pong guide technique, 195
  septal hematomas, 196
  stent delivery balloon, 195
  stiff and polymer-jacketed guidewires, 193
  tamponade, 195
 donor vessel injury, 200–203
 equipment loss or entrapment, 203
 periprocedural myocardial infarction, 204
 target vessel injury, 200, 203
Acute non-cardiac complications
 contrast induced nephropathy, 204
 radiation injury, 204–205
ADR approach. *See* Antegrade dissection/re-entry (ADR) approach
Air emboli, 213
Ambiguous proximal cap
 balloon-assisted sub-intimal entry, 67–71
 blind stick technique, 67, 69–71
 IVUS-guided proximal cap puncture, 66
 scratch and go technique, 66–67
Ambiguous proximal fibrous cap (PFC), 84
Anchoring support, 164–165
Angiographic technique, 208
Antegrade challenges
 CrossBoss challenges, 73–74
 hybrid algorithm, 65
 reentry challenges, 74–80
 sub-intimal dissection planes and management, 72–73
 unique to antegrade dissection reentry, 72
 WE and ADR
  ambiguous proximal cap, 66–71
  impenetrable cap, 67–68, 72
  uncrossable lesion, 72
Antegrade dissection/re-entry (ADR) approach
 antegrade challenges, 72
 basic principles
  CrossBoss and Stingray Dissection and Reentry System, 55–56
  8 F guiding catheter, 56
  haematoma, 56
  landing zone, 54
  Luer-lock syringe, 58
  Miracle Bros 12, 57
  occluded right coronary artery, 56
  stent deployment, 54
  stick and drive technique, 58, 60–61
  stick and swap technique, 58, 62–63
  Stingray balloon orientation, 58–59
  Stingray based re-entry, 56–57
 CrossBoss catheter, 54–55
 LAST technique, 54
 proximal cap ambiguity, 61
 STAR technique, 54
 target vessel, 61
 vascular access site and guide catheter selection, 59, 61
Antegrade subintimal catheter
 blind stick and swap technique, 150, 152–154
 definition, 149
 Knuckle-Boss technique, 150
 wire redirect, 149
Antegrade wire escalation (AWE)
 advancing equipment
  anchor balloon, 49–50
  guide extension, 50
  higher support microcatheter, 50
  rotational atherectomy, 50
 anatomical subsets
  distal landing zone, 45
  in-CTO tortuosity, 45
  interventional collaterals, 45–46
  lesion length, 44
  presence of intra-CTO calcium, 45
  previous procedural failure, 45
  proximal cap anatomy, 44–45
 basic principles of CTO PCI
  back-up support, 46
  high gram weight wires, 47
  medium weight highly toqueble wires, 47
  medium weight wires, 47
  over-the-wire equipment, 46
  planning, 46
  tapered polymer-coated wires, 47
  visibility, 46
  wire selection, 46–47
 indications and use
  CTA, 50–51
  IVUS, 51
 limitations, 44
 objectives, 43
 progress and safety, 48
 proximal cap, 45, 47


S. Rinfret (ed.), *Percutaneous Intervention for Coronary Chronic Total Occlusion: The Hybrid Approach*,
DOI 10.1007/978-3-319-21563-1

Antegrade wire escalation (AWE) (*cont.*)
  true lumen entry, 48–49
  wire selection
    newer generation wires, 48
    penetration force, 48
    polymer-coated wires, 47–48
    tactile feel, 48
    wire shaping, 48
Aortic dissection, 204
Aortocoronary dissection, 212
As Low As Reasonably Achievable (ALARA) principle, 188

**B**

Balloon-assisted microdissection (BAM), 83
Balloon-assisted sub-intimal entry (BASE), 67–71
Blind stick technique, 67, 69–71
Blunt proximal caps, 142

**C**

Cardiac catheterization laboratory volume, 15
Cardiac surgery program, 15
Catheter support
  anchoring support, 164–165
  backup support, 161
  guide catheter extensions, 163–164
  guide catheter shape, 162–163
  guide catheter size, 161–162
  newer support catheters, 165
  sheath length, 165–166
CenterCross support catheter, 165
Chronic total occlusion angioplasty program
  "buddy" system, 14
  infrastructure
    administrative support, 16
    cardiac catheterization laboratory volume, 15
    cardiac surgery program, 15
    non-medical staff, 15–16
  operator selection, 13–14
  practicalities, 16–18
  training, 14–15
Chronic total occlusion percutaneous coronary intervention (CTO-PCI). *See also* Chronic total occlusion angioplasty program
  acute cardiac complications
    aortic dissection, 204
    coronary perforation, 193, 195–200
    donor vessel injury, 200–203
    equipment loss/entrapment, 203
    periprocedural myocardial infarction, 204
    target vessel injury, 200, 203
  acute non-cardiac complications
    contrast induced nephropathy, 204
    radiation injury, 204–205
  benefits, 1–2
  completeness of revascularization, 2–3
  CTO segment, 33–34
  frequency of complications, 193–194
  guidelines, 6–7
  LV function, 4–5
  myocardial electrical stability, 5
  procedural success and complications, 5
  proposed algorithm, 7–8
  randomized control tria, 2
  surgical revascularization, 1
  survival, 3–4
  symptoms and quality of life, 2
  trapping balloon technique, 39–40
  wire manipulation techniques
    antegrade dissection reentry, 39
    controlled drilling, 35
    guidewire handling techniques, 34
    knuckled wire, 38
    penetration, 35–37
    sliding and drilling, 34–35
Collateral channels (CC)
  epicardial collaterals, 90, 92
  interventional *vs.* non-interventional epicardial collateral channels, 90, 93
  intramyocardial collaterals, 92, 93
  LAD CTO collateral patterns, 94
  LCx CTO collateral patterns, 94
  RCA CTO collateral patterns, 93–94
  Rentropp score, 90
  septal collateral, 89–90
  surfing technique, 89
  Werner classification, 90–91
Collateral vessel injury, 214–215
Common femoral artery (CFA) access, 167
Complication management equipment, 30
Confianza Pro 12 wire, 73–74
Contrast guided-STAR technique, 82
Contrast-induced acute kidney injury
  definitions, 179–180
  incidence, 180–181
  intra-procedural strategies
    coronary sinus contrast media extraction, 185
    follow up, 185
    forced diuresis, 184–185
    general measures, 183
    procedural techniques, 183–184
  pre-procedural strategies
    calculation of maximum allowable contrast dose, 182–183
    CTO road mapping, 183
    hemodialysis and hemofiltration, 183
    hydration, 182
    N-acetylcysteine, 183
    patient selection, 182
    sodium bicarbonate, 183
    statins, 183
  prognostic impact, 181–182
  risk factors, 180–181
Contrast induced nephropathy (CIN), 204
Coronary angiography, 87–88
Coronary artery bypass grafting (CABG), 2–3
Coronary perforation
  classification, 208
  collateral vessel perforation, 196
  coronary vessel locations, 195
  distal target vessel perforation, 196
  Ellis classification, 195
  epicardial coronary vessel perforation, 196–200
  hemodynamics, 200
  incidence, 207
  ping pong guide technique, 195
  potential consequences, 207
  predictors, 207–208
  prevention
    adjunctive medications, 208
    angiographic technique, 208
    gear perforation, 209

pre-procedure, 208
retrograde-specific considerations, 209
wire manipulation, 209
septal hematomas, 196
stent delivery balloon, 195
stiff and polymer-jacketed guidewires, 193
tamponade, 195
Corsair catheter, 21–22
CrossBoss catheter, 24, 28, 54–55, 73–74. *See also* Antegrade dissection/re-entry (ADR) approach
CTO operator
data, 223–224
education, 224
initial case selection, 225
learning, 226
mentoring, 224
outcomes tracking, 225
prevention, 225
program, 224
referral pattern, 225–226
CTO PCI equipment
checklist, 19–20
complication management equipment, 30
dissection/re-entry equipment, 24, 27–28
guide catheter extensions, 27, 29
guide catheters, 20
guidewires, 22–27
intravascular ultrasound, 28
microcatheters, 20–21
Corsair, 21–22
Finecross, 21–22
MultiCross, 21–22
Prodigy, 21–22
TurnPike, 22
Venture, 21–22
radiation protection equipment, 30
sheaths, 19
snares, 27
stents, 30
"uncrossable-undilatable" lesions, 28, 30

D
Device entrapment
bail-out strategies, 217–218
complication management, 221
embolized equipment, 221
incidence, 217
microcatheters, balloons and stents, 219–220
retrograde scenarios, 220
risk factors, 218–219
Rotablator burr, 220
trapped balloons, 220
trapped microcatheters, 220
trapped stents, 220
trapped wires, 219
wires, 219
Dissection/re-entry equipment, 24, 27–28
Distal anchor technique, 164
Donor vessel injury, 200–203, 212–214
Donor vessel ischemia, 213

E
Embolized equipment, 221
Epicardial CC crossing
angiographic projections, 99
FineCross, 100
Ping-pong catheter technique, 101–103
Sion wire, 101
Expanded hybrid approach
antegrade subintimal catheter
blind stick and swap technique, 150, 152–154
definition, 149
Knuckle-Boss technique, 150
wire redirect, 149
blunt proximal caps, 142
Corsair, not crossing collateral channel retrograde, 155–157
device-uncrossable antegrade/retrograde cap
definition, 148
suggested approaches, 148–149
enhanced hybrid CTO PCI algorithm, 143
hematoma compression
blind stick and swap technique, 145–146, 151
definition, 150
Knuckle-Boss technique, 150–154
STRAW technique, 150–151
key factors, 142
original hybrid algorithm, 142
proximal cap ambiguity, 143, 155–157
R-CART, 142
retrograde anatomic ambiguity, 158
reverse CART re-entry failure, 157
standard guidewire escalation techniques
bailout, 147–148
break the cap, 144, 148
definition, 143
end around, 143–148
stingray balloon antegrade
definition, 154
suggested approach, 154–155
wire externalization, 158

F
Finecross catheter, 21–22
Forced diuresis, 184–185
6 Fr guiding catheter, 172
8 Fr guiding catheter, 172

G
Graft crossing
flush ostial graft occlusion, 104–105
GuideLiner/GuideZilla, 105
Miracle 12 wire, 104
native artery CTO treatment, 95, 103
occluded graft, 96, 104
safe environment, 102
Venture catheter, 103
Grenadoplasty, 83
Guide catheter extensions, 27, 29
Guide catheters, 20, 107–109, 119–120, 123–124
Guide catheter size, 161–162
GuideLiner catheter, 163
Guidewires, 22–27
Guiding catheter
advancement and manipulation, 172–173
commercially available sheathless, 173, 177
selection, 170–172
without introducer sheath, 173–176

**H**
HeartRail coronary guiding catheter extension, 163–164
Hematoma compression
  blind stick and swap technique, 145–146, 151
  definition, 150
  Knuckle-Boss and blind stick and swap technique, 150–154
  STRAW technique, 150–151
Hemodialysis and hemofiltration, 183
High gram weight wires, 47
Hybrid algorithm and transradial approach, 173–176

**I**
Impenetrable cap, 67–68, 72
Implantable cardioverter-defibrillator (ICD), 5
In-stent chronic total occlusions (IS CTOs)
  angiographic appearance
    CrossBoss catheter, 135–136
    long in-stent occlusion, 135–136
    stent thrombosis, 135, 137–138
    tapered proximal cap, 134–135
  clinical impact, 133
  pathophysiology, 134
  prevalence, 134
  problem-solving strategies
    sub-stent subintimal strategy, 139–140
    sub-stent wiring, 139
  treatment algorithm
    Confianza Pro 12, 135–136
    CrossBoss catheter, 135–136
    knuckled wires, 139
    ostial location, 135
    Pilot 200, 135
    stent thrombosis, 137–139
    Tornus/Corsair microcatheters, 138
    Venture catheter, 138
In-stent occlusive restenosis, 134
In-stent restenosis (ISR), 134
Internal mammary artery, 126
Intra-myocardial non-septal collateral channel, 89, 92–93
Intra-occlusion microinjection of contrast
  alternative uses, 83–84
  contrast guided-STAR technique, 82
  STAR technique, 81–82
  storm cloud dissection, 82, 84
  tubular dissections, 82
Intravascular ultrasound (IVUS), 28, 49
Ipsilateral collaterals, 102–103, 126
Ischemic complications
  collateral vessel injury, 214–215
  donor vessel injury, 212–214
  overview, 211
  target CTO vessel injury, 211–212
IS CTOs. *See* In-stent chronic total occlusions (IS CTOs)

**K**
Knuckle-Boss technique, 73

**L**
LAD/LCX CTOs, 102–103, 114–117, 126
Lead aprons, 188
Left ventricular (LV) function, 4–5
Limited Antegrade Subintimal Tracking (LAST) technique, 54
LV ejection fraction (LVEF), 4–5

**M**
Medium weight highly torqueble wires, 47
Medium weight wires, 47
Microcatheters, 20–21
  Corsair, 21–22
  Finecross, 21–22
  MultiCross, 21–22
  Prodigy, 21–22
  TurnPike, 22
  Venture, 21–22
Mother-and-child catheter, 106
MultiCross catheter, 21–22, 165
Myocardial electrical stability, 5

**N**
N-acetylcysteine, 183

**O**
Occluded graft, 104, 105, 121
Over-the-wire (OTW) equipment, 46

**P**
Patient positioning for radial artery access, 169–170
Periprocedural myocardial infarction, 204
Pilot 200 wire, 74
Ping-pong catheter technique, 101–103
Ping pong guide technique, 195
Polymer-coated wires, 47–48
Post CABG CTOs, 125–130
Prodigy catheter, 21–22, 165
Progress 200 T wires, 74
Proximal cap
  ambiguity, 61, 143, 155–157
  anatomy, 44–45
  assessment, 45, 47
Proximal vessel anchor technique, 164

**R**
RA access. *See* Radial artery (RA) access
Radial artery (RA) access
  guiding catheter
    advancement and manipulation, 172–173
    commercially available sheathless, 173, 177
    selection, 170–172
    without introducer sheath, 173–176
  hybrid algorithm and transradial approach, 173–176
  patient positioning and gaining access, 169–170
  rationale, 167–168
  selection, 168–169
  sheath selection, 169–170
Radiation exposure complications, 185
  deterministic effects, 186–187
  intra-procedural strategies, 188
  operators, 187
  post-procedural strategies and follow up, 189
  pre-procedural strategies, 187–188
  radiation doses, 186
  stochastic effects, 186–187
Radiation injury, 204–205
Radiation protection equipment, 30
Radiation safety program, 188
Radiation-specific glasses, 188

RenalGuard system, 184–185
Residual Syntax score (rSS), 3
Retrograde approach
  coronary angiography, 87–88
  distal cap
    collateral channels, 89–94
    surgical grafts, 95–96
  procedure set up, 88–89
  step-by-step approach
    CTO crossing, 105–123
    epicardial CC crossing, 99–103
    graft crossing, 95, 96, 102–105
    internal mammary artery, 121–123, 126
    LAD/LCX CTOs, 102–103, 114–117, 126
    microcatheter, 99–101
    opening and stenting CTO, 123–125
    post CABG CTOs, 125–130
    retrograde wire connection, 107–108, 119–120, 123–124
    septal CC, 89–91, 96–99
Retrograde wire connection
  6–8 French 90 cm JR 4 guide, 123
  meticulous technique, 123
  microcatheter, 120
  retrograde dissection and re-entry, 107–108, 119–120
  RG3, 119
  RotaWire, 119
  snaring, 123–124
Reverse CART (R-CART), 106, 113
Rotablator burr, 220
Rotational atherectomy, 50

S
Scratch and go technique, 66–67
Seattle Angina Questionnaire (SAQ), 2
Septal CC crossing
  anatomic considerations, 96
  CC0, CC1 channels, 91, 98
  FineCross, 98
  invisible, 97
  left anterior oblique, 98
  septal surfing, 98–99
  stains, 98
  surfing technique, 89, 97
Sheath length, 165–166
Sheaths, 19
Shin leg covers, 188
Side branch anchor technique, 164
Side holed catheters, 163
Snares, 27
Sodium bicarbonate, 183
Standard guidewire escalation techniques
  bailout, 147–148
  break the cap, 144, 148
  definition, 143
  end around, 143–148
Statins, 183
Stents, 30
Stick and drive technique, 58, 60–61
Stick and swap technique, 58, 62–63
Stingray balloon, 24, 28. *See also* Antegrade dissection/re-entry (ADR) approach
  definition, 154
  suggested approach, 154–155
Storm cloud dissection, 82, 84
Subintimal tracking and re-entry (STAR) technique, 54, 81–82
Subintimal transcatheter withdrawal (STRAW) technique, 150–151
Subintimal wire passage, 53
Sub-stent subintimal strategy, 139–140
Sub-stent wiring, 139
Support catheters, 165
Surgical grafts, 95–96

T
Tapered polymer-coated wires, 47
Target vessel injury, 200, 203, 211–212
Thrombosis, 134
Thyroid shielding, 188
Tornus™ catheter, 28, 30, 50
Trapped balloons, 220
Trapped microcatheters, 220
Trapped stents, 220
Trapped wires, 219
Trapping balloon technique, 39–40, 162
True-to-true (TTT) antegrade approach
  aggressive antegrade dilation, 118
  Confianza Pro 12, 106, 109
  Fielder XT, 106
  kissing wires, 105
  MAC catheter, 118–119
  mother-and-child catheter, 106
  proximal LAD CTO, 112, 114–117
  rapid exchange balloon, 109
  retrograde dissection and re-entry, 106–112
  reverse CART, 106, 113
  tortuous and long CTO, 106, 113
Tubular dissections, 82
TurnPike catheter, 22
TwinPass catheter, 125

U
Uncrossable lesion, 72
"Uncrossable-undilatable" lesions, 28, 30

V
Venture catheter, 21–22

W
Wire manipulation, 209
  antegrade dissection reentry, 39
  controlled drilling, 35
  guidewire handling techniques, 34
  knuckled wire, 38
  penetration, 35–37
  sliding and drilling, 34–35

# Praktische Anleitung

zum

# Photometrieren

von

G. Schuchardt

**Mit 23 Abbildungen**

BERLIN
Verlag von M. Krayn
1909

# Vorwort.

Im „Journal für Gasbeleuchtung", Jahrgang 1908, Heft 18, veröffentlichte ich eine kleine Arbeit über Lichtmessung in der Gasbrennerfabrikation. Dieses zeitigte eine ganze Reihe von Anfragen über praktische Einrichtung eines Photometerzimmers, Arbeitsweise, Berechnung usw., die mir zeigten, daß bei der umfangreichen Literatur über Photometrie eine praktische Anleitung fehlt.

Mit vorliegendem Werkchen will ich daher, gestützt auf eine mehrjährige praktische Tätigkeit, dem Praktiker eine übersichtliche, leicht verständliche Anleitung zur Lichtmessung geben.

Möge diese Arbeit ihren Zweck nicht verfehlen und recht viele Freunde in der Praxis finden.

Der Verfasser.

# Inhalt.


| | Seite |
|---|---|
| Vorwort | 3 |
| Inhalt | 5 |
| Illustrationsverzeichnis | 6 |
| Einleitung | 7 |
| Das Photometerzimmer | 9 |
| Apparate und Meßinstrumente | 11 |
| Berechnung | 28 |
| Messungen der Lichtstärke: | |
| 1. Gasbrenner für niedrigen Druck | 34 |
| 2. „ „ hohen Druck | 36 |
| 3. Dochtlampen | 37 |
| 4. Elektrische Lampen | 39 |
| Flächen-Helligkeitsmessungen | 41 |
| Versuchsraum | 44 |
| Tabelle für Berechnungen | 46 |
| Bezugsregister | 50—56 |

# Illustrationsverzeichnis.


| | | Seite |
|---|---|---|
| Abbildg. | 1. Photometerzimmer | 10 |
| „ | 2. Spiegelapparat nach Prof. Drehschmidt | 11 |
| „ | 3. „ „ „ Martens | 13 |
| „ | 4. Gasmesser | 14 |
| „ | 5 und 6. Manometer | 16 |
| „ | 7. Hefnerlampe | 18 |
| „ | 8. Stromkreis | 20 |
| „ | 9. Photometerbank | 22 |
| „ | 10. Photometeraufsatz von Lummer & Brodhun | 23 |
| „ | 11. Würfel desselben | 24 |
| „ | 12. Photometeraufsatz v. Franz Schmidt & Haensch | 24 |
| „ | 13. Optisches Bild desselben | 25 |
| „ | 14. Webers Photometer | 26 |
| „ | 15. Würfel und optisches Bild | 27 |
| „ | 16. Darstellung für die räumliche Lichtverteilung | 29 |
| „ | 17. Lichtkurve | 32 |
| „ | 18. Rechenstab | 33 |
| „ | 19. Farbige Abbildung des Gesichtsfeldes im Photometeraufsatz v. Franz Schmidt & Haensch | 35 |
| „ | 20. Hermanns Betriebsphotometer | 38 |
| „ | 21. Rotierender Apparat von Brodhun | 40 |
| „ | 22. Webers Photometer | 42 |
| „ | 23. Versuchsraum | 44 |

# Einleitung.

Die zumeist sehr primitiven photometrischen Einrichtungen, mit denen man in der Praxis arbeitet, genügten wohl, solange man es noch mit verhältnismäßig schwachen Lichtquellen zu tun hatte, zu annähernden Messungen; der moderne Betrieb kommt mit denselben aber nicht mehr aus, seitdem unsere Lichtquellen eine Lichtstärke von 5000 und mehr Kerzen erreicht haben, seitdem man sich nicht mehr darauf beschränken kann, die Lichtstrahlen in horizontaler Richtung zu messen, sondern die räumliche Lichtstärke einer Lichtquelle zu bestimmen ist, die für die Beurteilung und zum Vergleich mit anderen Lichtquellen maßgebend ist.

Diesen Anforderungen muß zunächst in der Größe des Photometerzimmers Rechnung getragen werden.

# Das Photometerzimmer.

Für Gasanstalten[1]) ist die Größe des Photometerzimmers auf eine Länge von 4 m, eine Breite von 2,6 m als Mindestmaß angegeben, größer dürften die Photometerräume aber in den Lampenfabriken selten sein. Es leuchtet wohl ohne weiteres ein, daß ein solcher Raum für die Messung z. B. einer Preßgaslampe mit stündlichem Verbrauch von nahezu 2½cbm Gas unzulänglich ist. Die Verhältnisse, unter denen die Lampe hier brennt, hinsichtlich Temperatur und Luft, sind durchaus anomal und beeinflussen das Brennen einer Lampe ungünstig, ganz abgesehen davon, daß auch die Messung großer Lichtquellen in einem solch kleinen Raume zu ungenauen Resultaten führen muß.

Das moderne Photometerzimmer soll aber derartig geräumig sein, daß in demselben jede Messung exakt ausgeführt werden kann. Abbildung 1 stellt eine Teilansicht eines Photometerzimmers einer großen Lampenfabrik[2]) dar, das eine Länge von 9 m, eine Breite und eine Höhe von 4 m hat.

Trotzdem am Boden sowie an der Decke große Luftlöcher vorhanden, steigt die Temperatur des Raumes schnell. Als Mindestmaß muß daher eine Länge von 12 m und eine Breite von 6 m bei 4 m Höhe gefordert werden. Der Abzug der Abgase ist dabei noch durch Ventilatoren zu beschleunigen.

Um jeden Reflex auszuschließen, ist der Raum am besten grauschwarz zu streichen; helle Gegenstände verhängt man mit schwarzen Tüchern.

---

[1]) G. F. Schaar's Kalender für das Gas- und Wasserfach. Jahrgang 1909, zweiter Teil Seite 68.

[2]) Lampenfabrik von Ehrich & Graetz, Berlin-Treptow, Elsenstr. 92/93.

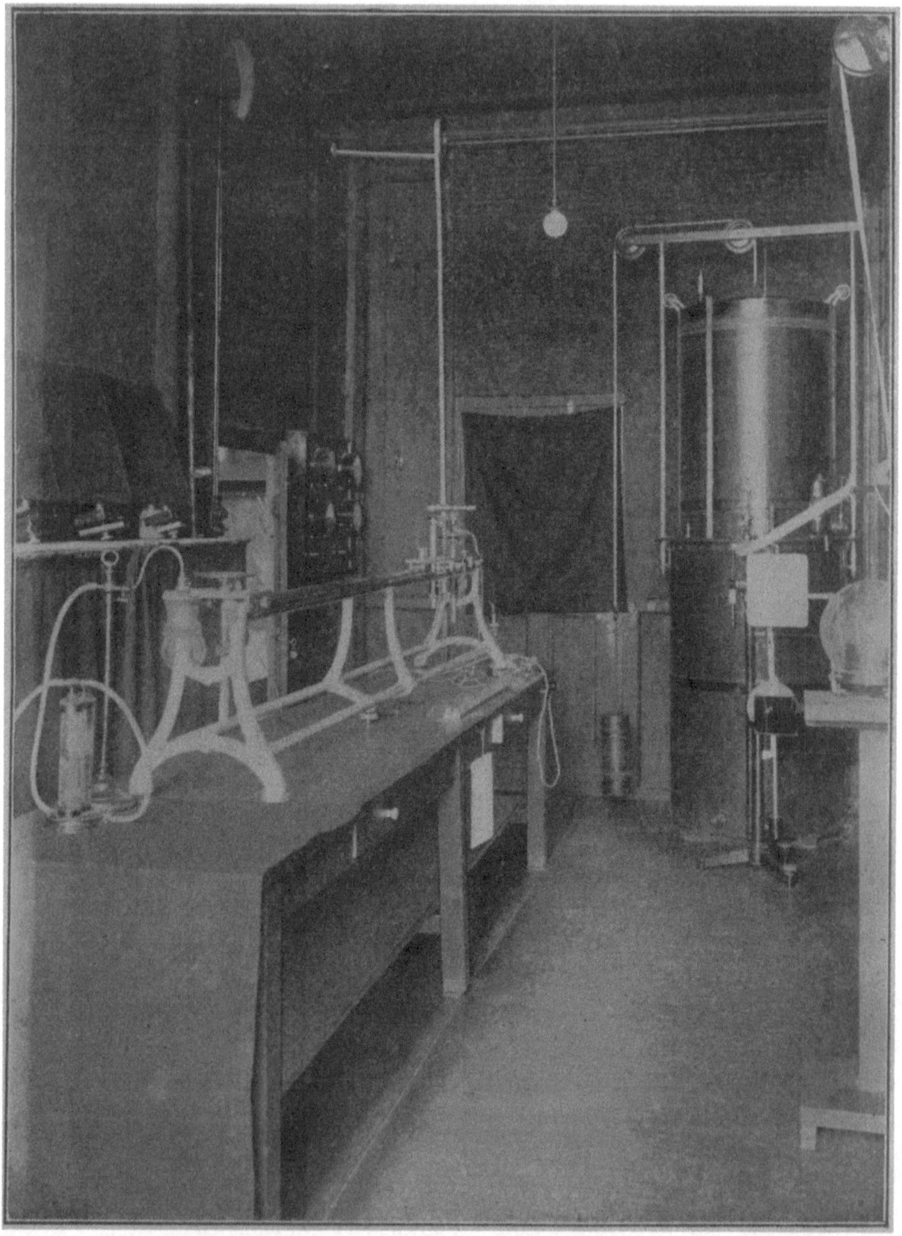

Abbildung 1.

links Photometerbank

rechts Cubicierapparat, (siehe Seite 16).

## Apparate und Meßinstrumente.

Den Photometertisch richtet man praktisch auf Schienen fahrbar ein, und zwar so, daß man auf allen Seiten bequem an dem Tische hantieren kann. In der Mitte der Schienen an beiden Enden des Zimmers finden

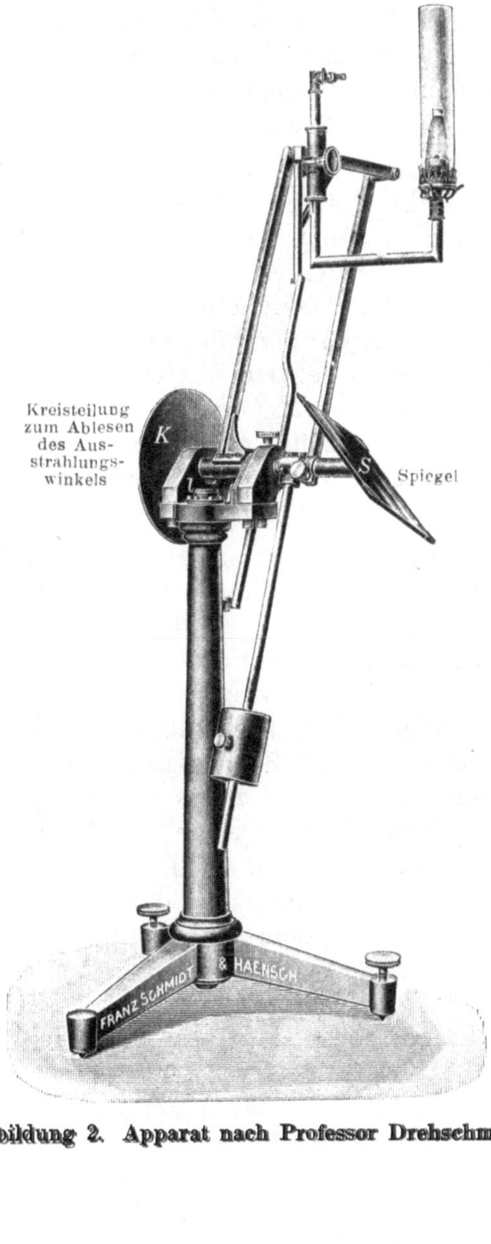


**Abbildung 2. Apparat nach Professor Drehschmidt.**

die Spiegelvorrichtungen ihre feste Aufstellung, so daß der Tisch in jeder Entfernung von denselben aufgestellt werden kann. Meist benutzt wird für Brenner der Spiegelapparat[1]) nach Prof. Drehschmidt, Tegel, für Lampen derjenige nach Prof. Martens. Die Spiegelvorrichtung für Brenner besteht nur aus einem Spiegel, der unter 45° gegen die Achse der Photometerbank geneigt ist. Die Einrichtung ist so getroffen, daß der Brenner um den Spiegel herumgedreht und der Ausstrahlungswinkel des Brenners auf dem Teilkreise hinter dem Spiegel abgelesen wird.

Der Apparat für Lampen besteht aus einer Anordnung von zwei Spiegeln, die um die Lampe gedreht werden. Die Lampe wird an einem Drahtseil hinter dem Apparat aufgehängt in Höhe der Achse des vorderen Spiegels. Das Licht fällt auf den seitlichen Spiegel und wird von diesem auf den unter 45 ° zur Photometerachse geneigten vorderen Spiegel reflektiert. Zwischen Lampe und Spiegelapparat stellt man einen schwarzgestrichenen Schutzschirm zweckmäßig aus Asbestpappe. Die Ablesung des Ausstrahlungswinkels ist wie bei dem kleinen Apparat.

Sind die Spiegel nicht im Gebrauch, so hält man dieselben sorgsam mit weichen schwarzen Tüchern verdeckt, vor den Messungen wischt man vorsichtig mit einem weichen Staubtuch über. Da die Entfernung des Brenners resp. der Lampe bei beiden Apparaten stets konstant ist, so hat man dieselbe nur einmal festzulegen. Es geschieht dies, indem man mittels Bandmaßes von der Brenner- resp. Lampenachse nach der resp. den Spiegelmitten mißt. Die Entfernung vom Spiegel zur Photometerbank ermittelt man von Fall zu Fall. Man stellt hierbei den Spiegel auf den Nullpunkt und mißt von der Mitte der Spiegelkante nach dem Nullpunkte der Skala der Photometerbank. Da die Spiegel einen Teil des Lichtes absorbieren, wird dieser Betrag durch die Messung derselben Lampe oder des Brenners einmal mit, das andere Mal ohne Spiegelapparat gemessen. Aus der

---

[1]) Journal für Gasbeleuchtung. Jahrgang 1905, No. 38, Seite 814.

Differenz ergibt sich der sogenannte Absorptionskoeffizient, den man bei der Berechnung einzusetzen hat. Dieser Absorptionskoeffizient muß von Zeit zu Zeit kontrolliert werden, da er sich im Laufe der Zeit ändert.

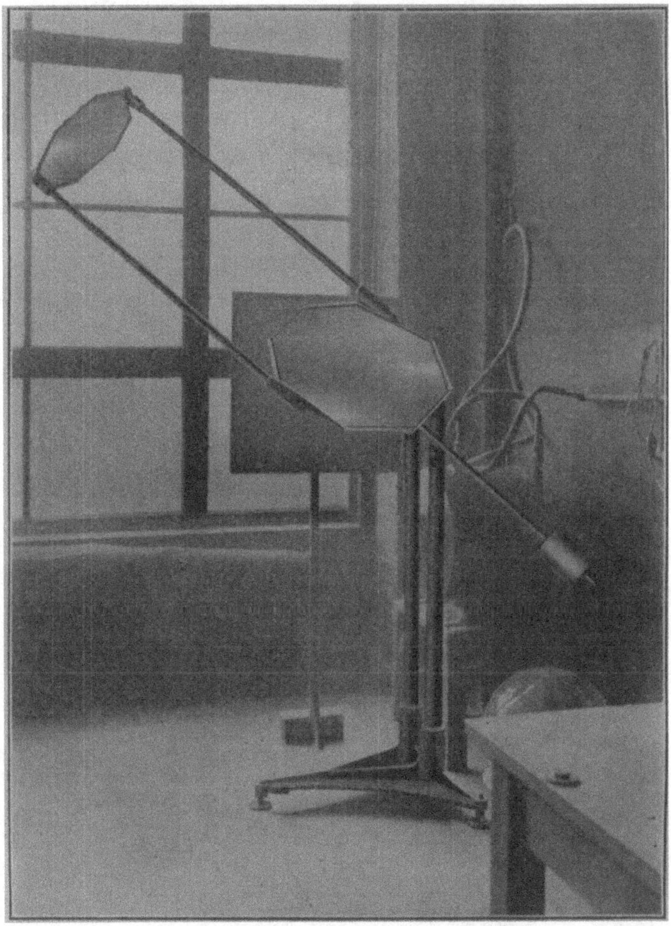

Abbildung 3. Spiegelapparat für Lampen von Professor Martens.

Neben oder hinter die Spiegelapparate placiert man die Gasmesser (Abbildung 4).

Die Gasmesser müssen wagerecht aufgestellt sein, was mit Hilfe der Justierschrauben und der Wasserwage genau zu erreichen ist. Besondere Aufmerksamkeit ist auch dem Auffüllen mit reinem Wasser zu widmen, das von Zeit zu Zeit zu geschehen hat. Das Auffüllen geschieht durch die hinter dem Zifferblatt angebrachte Füllschraube bei offenem Ein- und Ausgang, nachdem

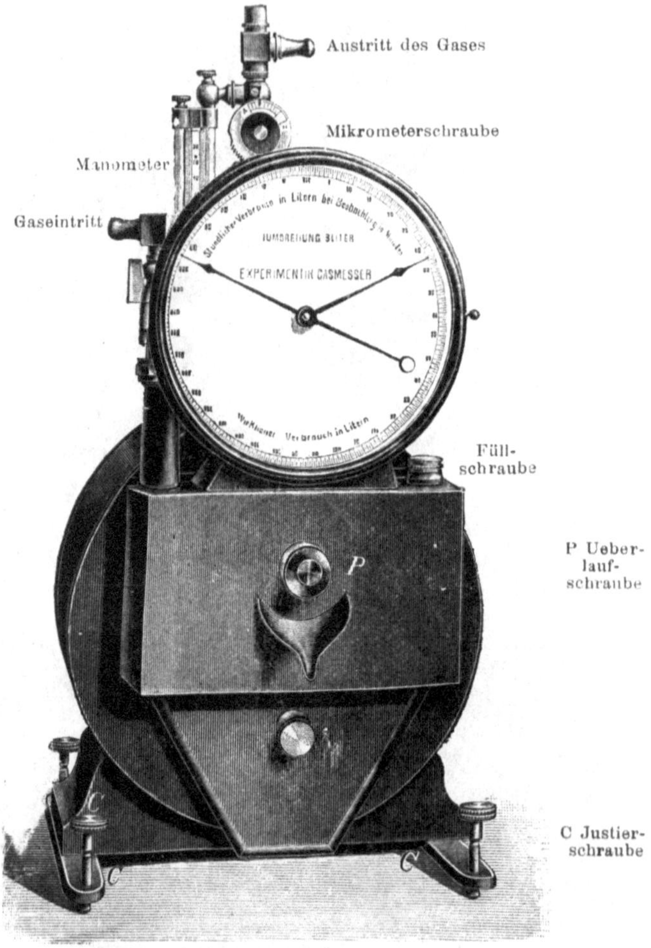


Abbildung 4.

man vorher die Schlauchverbindung mit der Gasleitung gelöst hat Das überschüssige Wasser läßt man aus der an der Vorderseite befindlichen Ueberlauföffnung abtropfen, ehe man die Schrauben wieder aufsetzt. Das Zifferblatt hat bei kleinen Experimentiergasmessern zwei Zeiger, der kürzere gibt den wirklichen Gasverbrauch an, der längere läuft 60mal schneller und gestattet so bei Beobachtung einer Minute, den stündlichen Verbrauch abzulesen.

Ist der längere Zeiger während einer Minute von 0 bis Teilstrich 100 gegangen, so ist der stündliche Gasverbrauch 100 l.

Der Gasmesser für Preßgas hat nur einen Zeiger. Hier liest man die Dauer eines ganzen Umganges des Zeigers ab. Hat man z. B. für eine Umdrehung des Zeigers, die gleich 100 l ist, 10 Minuten abgelesen, so ist der Stundenverbrauch 6mal so viel gleich 600 l Preßgas, d. h. einem Gas, das auf einen bestimmten Druck komprimiert ist. Gewöhnlich preßt man das Gas auf 100 mm Quecksilbersäule. Da das Quecksilber 13,6 mal schwerer ist als Wasser, so entspricht das einer Wassersäule von 1360 mm. Der Druck in den Gasleitungen nicht komprimierten Gases schwankt außerordentlich, meist in den Grenzen von 20-80 mm Wassersäule, als normalen Druck nimmt man für die Lichtmessungen 40 mm Wassersäule an. Auf diesen Druck reduziert man Preßgas.

Der Faktor zur Umrechnung von Preßgas von 1360 mm auf Gas von normalem Druck von 40 mm Wassersäule ist 1,13. Die oben gefundene Zahl 600 wäre demnach mit 1,13 zu multiplizieren, und würde der Verbrauch 678 l betragen. Diese Zahl ist dann der Berechnung der Oekonomie zugrunde zu legen. Es ist nötig, stets den Gasdruck, unter dem eine Lichtmessung ausgeführt ist, anzugeben.

Zur Ablesung des Druckes bedient man sich U-förmiger Manometer. Für niedrigen Druck wird das Manometer bis zum Nullpunkt mit Wasser gefüllt, bei Preßgas mit Quecksilber.

Die Oberfläche des Wassers, einer benetzenden Flüssigkeit, erscheint konkav durch die Adhäsion an den Rohrwandungen, des Quecksilbers dagegen, das das Glas nicht benetzt, konvex (Abbildung 5 und 6). Demgemäß ist abzulesen. Stände die Flüssigkeit auf Teilstrich 20 in beiden Schenkeln, so betrüge der Druck 40 mm Wasser- oder Quecksilbersäule.

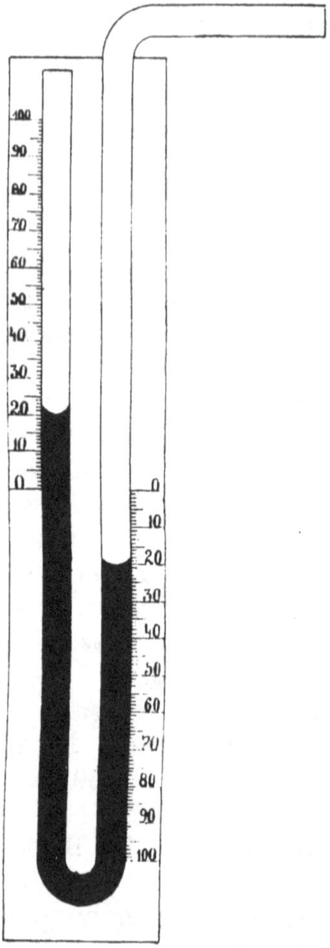


40 mm Wassersäule.

Abbildung 5.

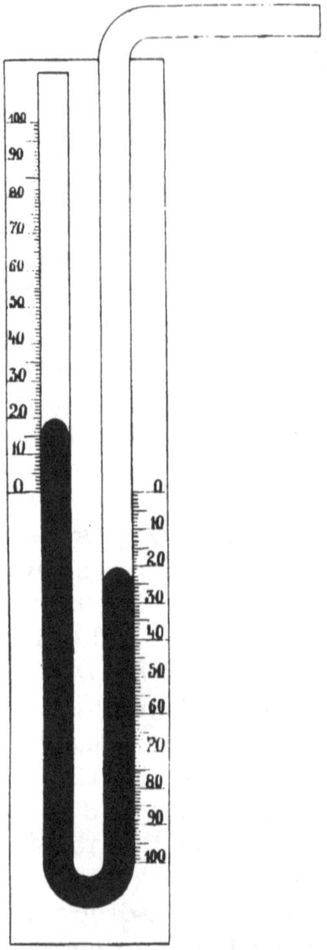


40 mm Quecksilbersäule.

Abbildung 6.

Da man oft in die Lage kommt, mit einem höheren Gasdruck, als in der Leitung vorhanden, arbeiten zu müssen, da ferner der Gasdruck namentlich zu Zeiten plötzlicher größerer Entnahme stark schwankt, bedient man sich des Kubizierapparates (s. Seite 10).

Derselbe besteht aus einem Wasserbehälter, in welchen eine Glocke eintaucht. Die Glocke ist mit einer Kette von bestimmtem Gewicht verbunden, die über eine

Rolle läuft und am Ende eine Auflage für die Gewichtsplatten hat.

Mittels der Plattengewichte läßt sich jeder Druck für Brenner oder Lampen, die bei niedrigem Druck, d. h. bis 100 mm Wassersäule, brennen, einstellen. Der Gewichtsverlust, der durch das Einsinken der Glocke in den Wasserbehälter entsteht, wird durch das Gewicht des hinzukommenden Teiles der Kette ausgeglichen, so daß der einmal eingestellte Druck immer konstant bleibt. Man wird daher zweckmäßig stets mit dem Kubizierapparat arbeiten.

Soll der Apparat gefüllt werden, so öffnet man den Hahn für die Gaszuleitung und legt alle Gewichtsplatten auf. Die Glocke wird durch das Gewicht hochgezogen und mit Gas gefüllt. Da in dem Apparat und in der Zuleitung, namentlich wenn der Apparat längere Zeit nicht benutzt ist, stets Luft vorhanden, was sich beim Brenner durch unruhiges Brennen bemerkbar machen würde, so entleert man den Behälter erst noch einmal. Man schließt die Zuleitung und öffnet den Auslaßhahn, nachdem man die Gewichtsplatten abgenommen. Das entweichende Gas läßt man aus einem Hahn der Ableitung abbrennen. Ist die Glocke völlig eingetaucht, so schließt man die Ableitung wieder, beschwert die Gewichtsauflage mit den Platten, öffnet die Gaszuleitung und füllt den Apparat wieder mit Gas. Die Glocke trägt eine Skala, die den Inhalt derselben angibt. Hierdurch ist man in den Stand gesetzt, den Gasverbrauch eines Brenners oder einer Lampe direkt ohne Gasmesser ablesen zu können. Hat der zu messende Brenner 10 Minuten gebrannt, so liest man unter Einstellung der Sekundenuhr den Stand der Glocke ab, nach Beendigung der Messung liest man wiederum unter Arretierung der Uhr ab.

Die Differenz zeigt den Gasverbrauch. Hätte der Zeiger der Skala auf Teilstrich 100 gestanden und stände bei Arretierung auf Teilstrich 150, so wären 50 l verbraucht. Man hat nur nötig, auf der Uhr die Zeit abzulesen, die z. B. 29 Minuten 20 Sekunden betragen, so würde der stündliche Gasverbrauch 102 l sein nach dem einfachen Ansatz:

in 29 Min. 20 Sek. = 1760 Sek. 50 l

in 1 Stunde = 3600 „ ?

$$\frac{50 \cdot 3600}{1760} = 102 \text{ l.}$$

Die Einheit für die Lichtmessung ist die Hefnerkerze, d. h. die horizontale Lichtstärke einer mit Amylacetat gespeisten Dochtlampe (s. Abbildung 7), deren Flammen-

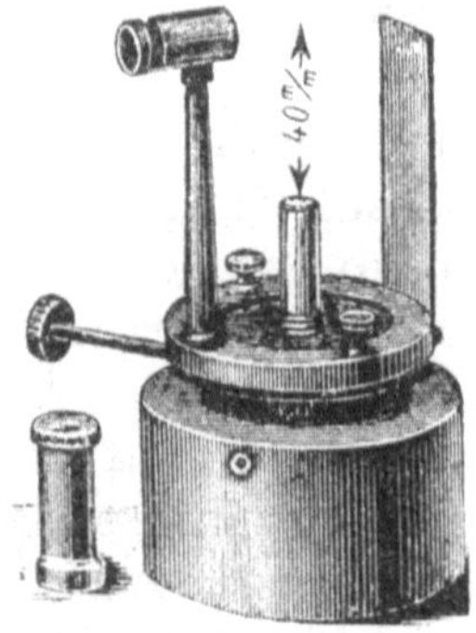


Abbildung 7.

höhe 40 mm beträgt. Zum Vergleich mit den anderweit üblichen Lichteinheiten diene die nachstehende Tabelle nach Angaben der internationalen Lichtmeßkommission.

**Vergleich der Lichteinheiten.**

(Tabelle der internationalen Lichtmeßkommission.)

| | HK | V. K. | E. K | 10 K. P | Carcel |
|---|---|---|---|---|---|
| Hefnerkerze . . . | 1 | 0,833 | 0,877 | 0,098 | 0,092 |
| Vereinskerze . . . | 1,20 | 1 | 1,05 | 0,109 | 0,111 |
| Englische Kerze . . | 1,14 | 0,95 | 1 | 0,104 | 0,105 |
| Harcourts 10-Kerzen-Pentanlampe . . | 11,00 | 9,16 | 9,6 | 1 | 1,0 |
| Carcellampe . . . | 10,80 | 9,0 | 9,5 | 0,98 | 1 |

Der Gebrauch der Lampe ist sehr einfach. Man füllt dieselbe mit Amylacetat, das zur Verhütung der Zersetzung in einer dunklen Flasche aufbewahrt wird, und läßt den Docht gut aufsaugen, sodann zündet man an und läßt bis zur Messung ca. 15 Minuten brennen; während dieser Zeit reguliert man die Flammenhöhe ein, indem das Auge in Höhe des Flammenmaßes über die Scheide in dem Röhrchen sieht, mit der die Spitze der Flamme abschneiden muß. Nach dem Gebrauch setzt man stets den Verschlußdeckel auf das Dochtrohr. Mit der Dochtlehre und dem optischen Flammenmaß kontrolliert man von Zeit zu Zeit die richtige Stellung des Dochtrohres zum Flammenmesser. An Stelle des letzteren schraubt man das Flammenmaß auf und setzt auf das Dochtrohr die Dochtlehre; zwischen dem oberen Rande des Dochtrohres und der Decke des inneren Hohlraumes der Lehre muß eine feine, weniger als 0,1 mm breite Lichtlinie sichtbar sein. Das Bild der Schneide der Lehre muß bei dem optischen Flammenmesser mit dem Strich auf der matten Scheibe zusammenfallen.

Zu den eigentlichen Messungen benutzt man jedoch nicht die Hefnerlampe, sondern elektrische Lampen von 3, 4, 5 oder mehr Kerzen[1]). Die Lampen mißt man mittels der Hefnerlampe und kontrolliert ihre Lichtstärke von Zeit zu Zeit. Hierzu benötigt man einen geeigneten Regulierwiderstand und ein Spiegelgalvanometer. Beide ordnet man am besten auf der Mitte des Photometertisches an, den Akkumulator für die elektrische Lampe unter dem Tische. Zur Aichung wird die Vergleichslampe gleichfalls erst einige Minuten gebrannt und dann die Spannung resp. Stromstärke, bei der die Lampe die verlangte Helligkeit hat, abgelesen. Hierbei ist zu beachten, daß die Lampe stets mit Unterspannung brennt. Auf solche Weise brennt die elektrische Lampe lange Zeit konstant mit derselben Spannung und Helligkeit.

Für die Messungen von elektrischen Lampen ist an der Wand eine Schalttafel anzubringen, die je ein Ampère- und Voltmeter für Gleichstrom- und Wechselstrom hat.

---

[1]) Kohlen- oder Metallfadenlampen. Metallfadenlampen wendet man vorzugsweise bei Glühlicht und Bogenlampen an, da die Farbenkontraste nicht so groß sind.

Ampère- und Voltmeter sind Apparate, die sich nur durch ihre Skala und höheren Widerstand unterscheiden, sonst gleich sind. Das Ampèremeter schaltet man in den Hauptstrom, das Voltmeter dagegen entsprechend seinem Zwecke, den Spannungsunterschied an zwei Stellen eines Stromkreises zu messen, in eine Stromverzweigung. Schematisch würde das so aussehen:

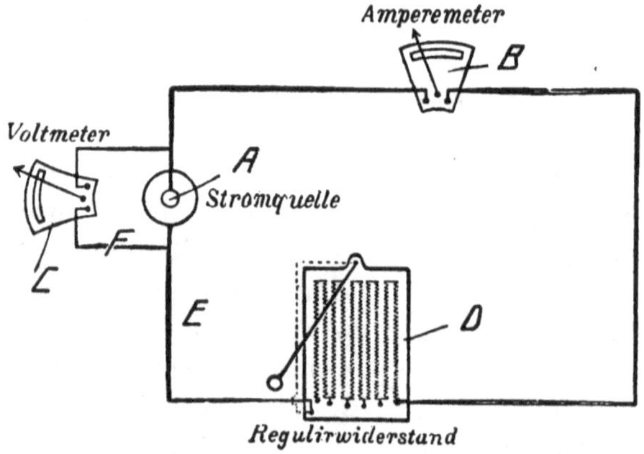


Abbildung 8.

A stelle die Stromquelle dar; E ist der Hauptstrom, der durch den Regulierwiderstand D beliebig ein- und ausgeschaltet werden kann und dessen Stärke auf dem Ampèremeter B abgelesen wird; F ist der Zweigstrom, in dem das Voltmeter C liegt. Die Konstruktion der Messer ist im Prinzip folgende: Ampère- wie Voltmeter enthalten eine Drahtrolle. Mit dieser Drahtrolle steht ein Winkelhebel in Verbindung, an dessen einem Ende der Zeiger des Instruments angebracht, an dessen anderem ein kurzes Eisenstäbchen über der Oeffnung der Drahtrolle hängt. Geht der Strom durch die Drahtrolle, so wird das Eisenstäbchen mehr oder weniger in die Oeffnung der Drahtrolle hineingezogen, wodurch der Zeiger betätigt wird. Zu genauerem Studium sei hier auf die trefflichen Bücher von Graetz[2]) hingewiesen.

---

[2]) Kurzer Abriß der Elektrizität von Prof. Dr. L. Graetz, Stuttgart, Verlag J. Engelhorn, und die Elektrizität und ihre Anwendungen von Prof. Dr. L. Graetz, Stuttgart, Verlag J. Engelhorn.

Der wichtigste Apparat ist die Photometerbank. Abbildung 9 zeigt eine große Photometerbank, wie sie von der Firma Franz Schmidt und Haensch, Berlin, gebaut wird.

I, II, III sind die verschiebbaren Wagen, die vermittels Rollen auf der Bank hin und her geschoben werden und durch Klemmvorrichtungen k festgestellt werden können. Auf dem Wagen I findet die zu messende Lampe ihre Aufstellung, der Wagen II trägt den eigentlichen Photometeraufsatz oder Photometerschirm, auf Wagen III wird die Hefnerlampe aufgestellt resp. die elektrische Vergleichslampe. Alle drei Wagen sind in der Höhe verstellbar durch die Triebvorrichtung t T, die Platten, die die Lampen tragen, sind auch um ihre Achse drehbar. Bei Messungen, bei denen die zu messende Lampe auf der Photometerbank steht, stellt man eine Reihe von schwarzen Schirmen B in der abgebildeten Weise auf zur Abblendung aller nicht horizontalen Lichtstrahlen.

Wagen II und III, Normallampe N und Photometerschirm L B sind fest miteinander verbunden.

Die Entfernung zwischen Photometerschirm und Normallampe ist also bekannt; es ist nur die Entfernung vom Photometerschirm bis zu der zu messenden Lampe zu ermitteln. Man gewöhne sich daran, in dieser Weise zu messen und nicht durch Verschieben des Photometerschirmes zwischen beiden Lichtquellen beide Entfernungen einzustellen. Anscheinend ist diese Einstellung leichter, da die Grenze, wo der Photometerschirm von der einen oder der anderen Lichtquelle stärker beleuchtet wird, auf einer kürzeren Strecke liegt, als wenn Vergleichslampe und Photometerschirm zusammen verschoben werden. Dafür muß aber in ersterem Falle zur Erlangung eines genauen Resultats die Einstellung sehr scharf erfolgen. Dies ist leicht verständlich, wenn man die Berechnung berücksichtigt.

Die Photometerbank ruht auf fünf Schrauben, mittels deren man dieselbe genau horizontal einstellt. Die gewöhnliche Länge der Bank beträgt 2,6 m. Zur Ablesung der Entfernungen ist auf dem einen Längsrohr

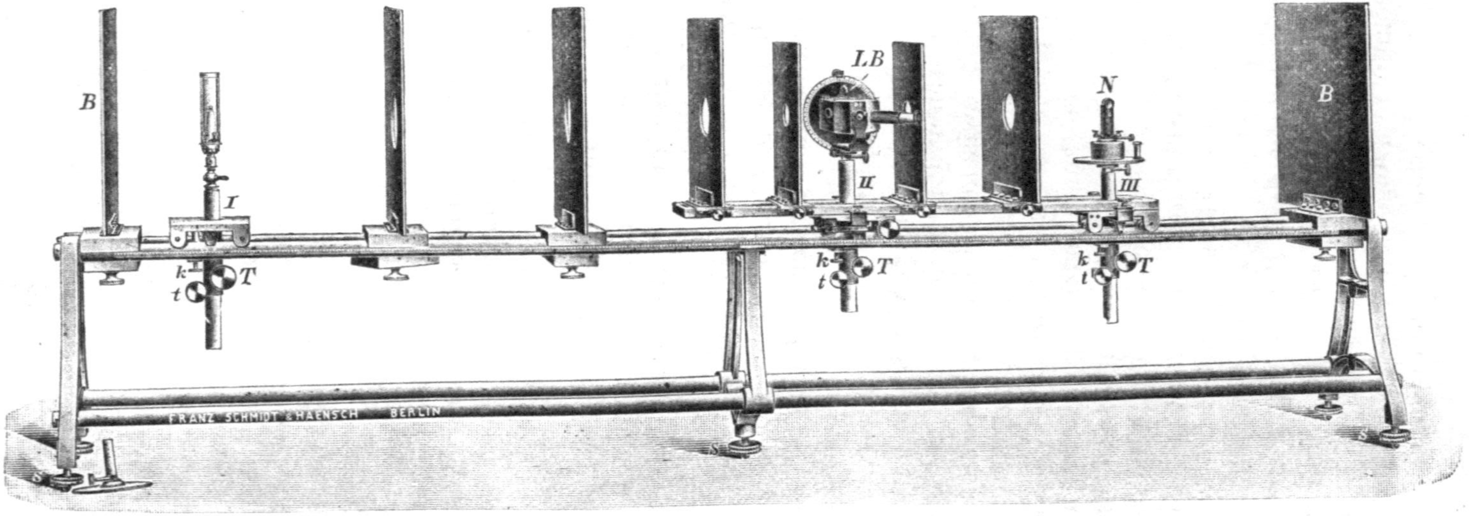


Abbildung 9.

eine Millimeterskala eingeritzt. Um den jeweiligen Stand der Wagen während der Messung ablesen zu können, läßt man sich unter jedem Wagen eine kleine elektrische Lampe anbringen, mittels derer man die Indizes der Wagen und die Skala beleuchten kann.

Der vielfach gebräuchliche Photometeraufsatz von Lummer und Brodhun sei schematisch dargestellt:

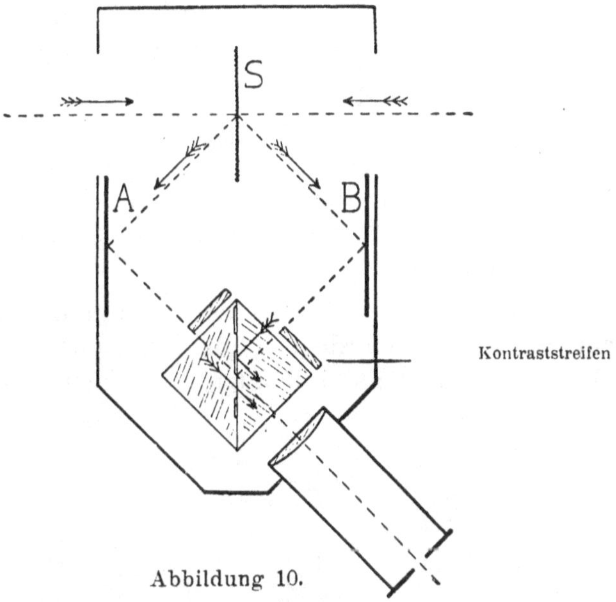


Abbildung 10.

Abbildung 10 zeigt den Schirm S, eine Gipsplatte, auf den die Lichtstrahlen der Normallampe und der zu messenden Lampe fallen. Bedingung ist, daß die Strahlen unter demselben Winkel auffallen; dieselben werden auf die rechts und links angebrachten Spiegel A und B und von hier aus auf den Lummer-Brodhun-Würfel reflektiert. Derselbe besteht aus zwei rechtwinkligen Prismen, die mit ihren Hypotenusenflächen aufeinander liegen. Die Fläche des linken Prismas ist an einigen Stellen geätzt. An diesen Stellen werden die von rechts kommenden Strahlen der einen Lichtquelle reflektiert, während sie die Strahlen der anderen Lichtquelle nicht durchlassen. Diese passieren die nicht geätzten Stellen. Man sieht also die nicht vertieften Stellen von der linken Seite des Schirmes beleuchtet, die vertieften von der rechten Seite. Abbildung 11 zeigt den Würfel und das optische

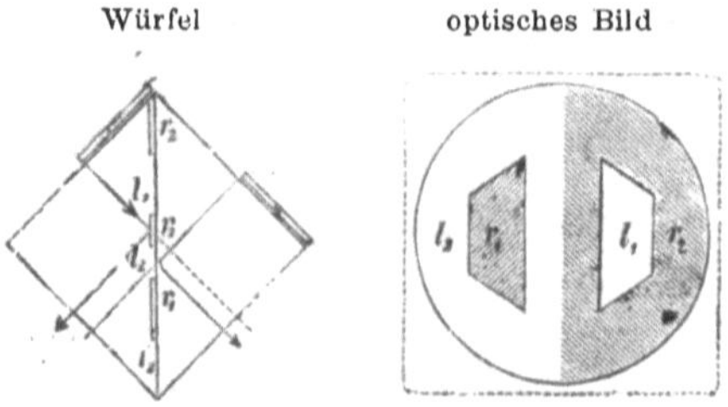


Abbildung 11.

Bild, das man mit demselben erhält. Die Pfeile geben die Richtung der Strahlen an, r und l die Strahlen derselben Lichtquelle.

Die exakte Einstellung des Lummer-Brodhun-Photometeraufsatzes erfordert schon ziemliche Uebung; weit leichter ist dieselbe mit dem Photometeraufsatze von

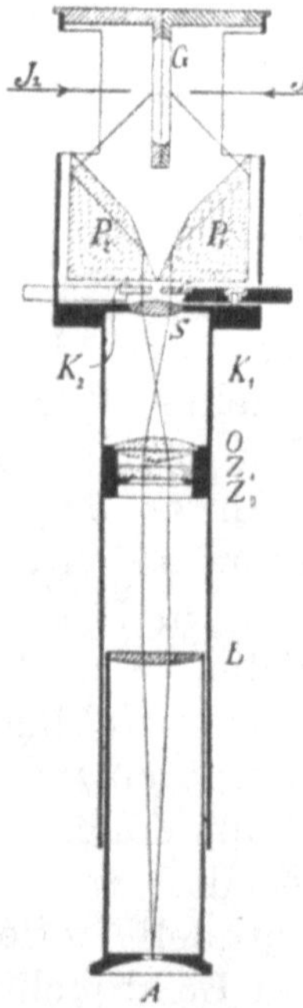


Abbildung 12.

Franz Schmidt und Haensch[3]). Derselbe eignet sich besonders für die Zwecke der Praxis (Abbildung 12).

Die Lichtstrahlen $J_1$ und $J_2$ treffen von rechts und links auf den Gipsschirm, werden auf die Prismen $P_1$ $P_2$ reflektiert und gelangen durch ein Linsensystem S O $Z_1$ $Z_2$ und die Lupe L zum Auge A. Die Farben der Felder können zur leichteren Einstellung durch kleine Vorschlaggläser $K_1$ $K_2$ kontrastiert werden. Das optische Bild zeigen die Figuren 1, 2, 3.

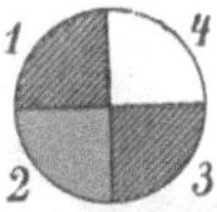


Fig. 1

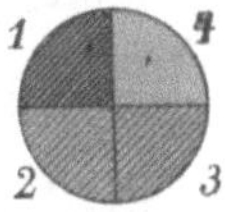


Fig. 2

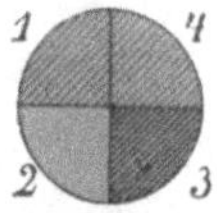


Fig. 3

Abbildung 13.

Fig. 1. Richtige Einstellung.
Fig. 2. Stellung des Photometers, bei der die Beleuchtung der zueinandergehörigen Felder 1 und 2 zu dunkel erscheint.
Fig. 3. Stellung des Photometers, bei der die Beleuchtung der zueinandergehörigen Felder 1 und 2 zu hell erscheint.

Sind sehr stark verschiedenfarbige Lichtquellen zu messen, so kann man sich eines Flimmerphotometeraufsatzes bedienen; ein geübtes Auge wird indes mit der Metallfadenlampe als Vergleichslampe meistens auskommen.

Das Weber-Photometer (Abbildung 14) benutzt man zu Flächenhelligkeitsmessungen. Als Vergleichslichtquelle dient hier eine Benzinlampe. Zu verwenden ist ein bestimmtes Benzin, das dem Instrument beigegeben ist. Reines Benzin z. B. gibt bis 50 % falsche Werte. Die Flammenhöhe beträgt 20 mm, die auf einer Skala im Innern des Lampengehäuses abgelesen werden. Nach einigen Minuten Brenndauer hat sich das Lampengehäuse erwärmt; man sieht durch das Fensterchen des Flammenmaßes q und stellt die Höhe der Flamme mittels der Triebschraube genau ein. Zu Messungen im Freien benutzt man jedoch die Benzinlampe wegen der unvermeidlichen Schwankungen nicht mehr, sondern wie auf der Photometerbank eine elektrische Vergleichslampe. Die Lampe ist dann in das Lampengehäuse eingebaut

---

3) Journal für Gas und Wasser (1900) 43.

und wird von einem Akkumulator gespeist. Die Stromstärke wird gleichsfalls auf einem Ampèremeter abgelesen und mittels eines kleinen Regulators eingestellt.

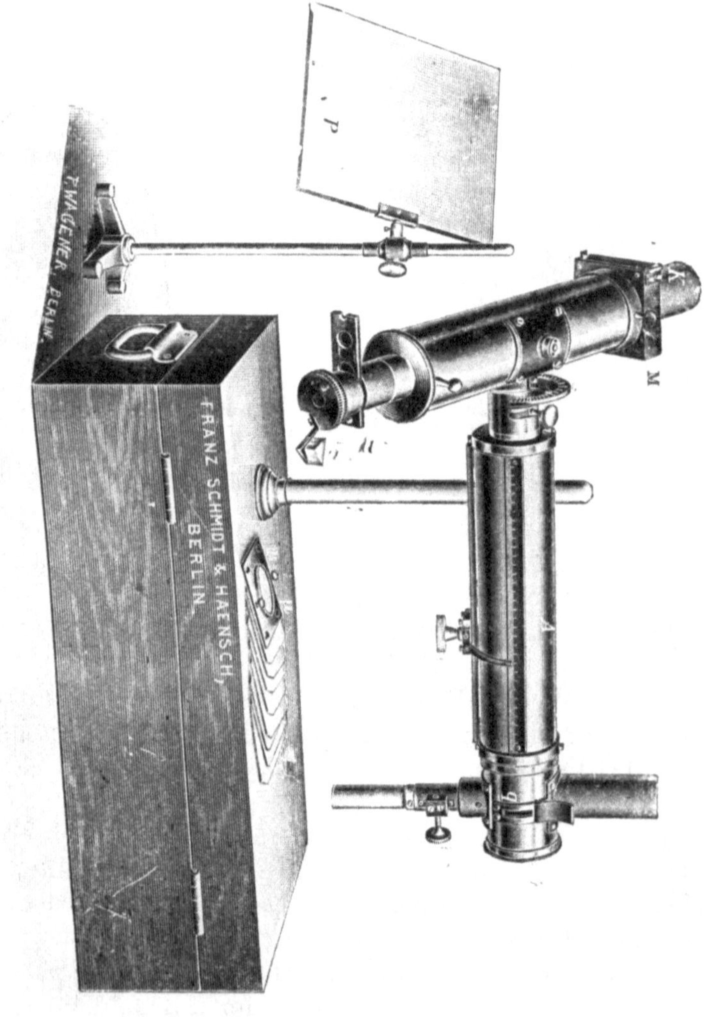


Abbildung 14. Weber'sches Photometer, fertig montiert zur Messung.

In dem um die Kreisteilung drehbaren Rohre ist ein Lummer-Brodhun-Würfel angeordnet, der das optische Bild (Abbildung 15) zeigt.

Das Licht von der Vergleichslampe wird durch Verschiebung einer Milchglasplatte geändert, das der zu messenden Lichtquelle durch auswechselbare Milchglasplatten, die in den Kasten M eingeschoben werden. Die dem Photometer beigegebenen Platten sind numeriert. 1 und 2 sind Rauchgläser, 3, 4, 5, 6, 7 Milchgläser, deren Konstanten für die Berechnung in der Gebrauchsanweisung angegeben sind. Man schiebt die Gläser so in den Kasten M ein, daß die Zahl dem Beobachter zugekehrt ist. Für Flächenhelligkeitsmessungen in vertikaler oder horizontaler Lage benutzt man den weißen Schirm P oder die Milchglasplatte, die man auf den Kasten M aufsetzen kann; für Messungen von Lichtstärken, zu denen man das Photometer eventuell auch benutzen kann, dient ein Tubus K, der an Stelle der Milchglasplatte auf den Kasten aufgeschoben wird. Die Schwächung des Lichtes erfolgt in beiden Fällen in gleicher Weise.

c Lichtstrahlen der einen
d Lichtstrahlen der anderen Lichtquelle

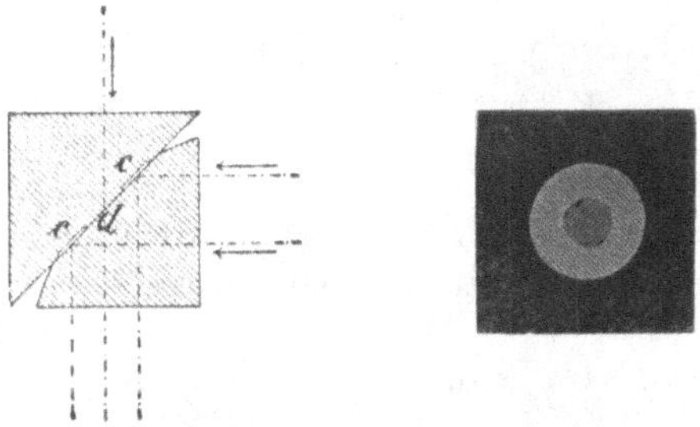


Abbildung 15.
Optisches Bild des Lummer-Brodhun-Würfels.
In vielen Fällen wird der Kontrastwürfel Abbildung 12 angewendet.

Zu erwähnen sei hier noch der Beleuchtungsmesser von Martens[4]), der sehr handlich, aber doch nicht in allen Fällen verwendbar, und die Straßenphotometer von Brodhun und Bechstein. Des hohen Preises wegen — das erstere kostet 1050 M., das Universalphotometer (Bechstein) 760 M. — dürfte man sich nur ausnahmsweise in der Praxis zur Anschaffung derselben verstehen, abgesehen natürlich von staatlichen oder städtischen Anstalten, die oft Messungen auf den Straßen vorzunehmen haben; meist wird man sich in diesem Falle des Weber-Photometers bedienen.

---

[4]) Journal für Gas und Wasser 1908.

## Berechnung.

Die Berechnung der durch die Messungen ermittelten Zahlen basiert auf dem Keplerschen Gesetz: Die Stärke der Erleuchtung oder die Lichtintensität nimmt mit wachsender Entfernung von der Lichtquelle ab, und zwar im umgekehrten Verhältnis des Quadrats der Entfernung. Ist die Helligkeit, mit welcher eine Fläche durch eine Lichtquelle in 1 m Entfernung beleuchtet wird, gleich 1 Kerze, so ist ihre Helligkeit in 2 m Entfernung gleich ¼ Kerze und umgekehrt in ½ m Entfernung gleich 4 Kerzen.

L und $L_1$ stellen die beiden Lichtquellen dar, die auf dem Photometer verglichen werden sollen, P ist der Photometerschirm.

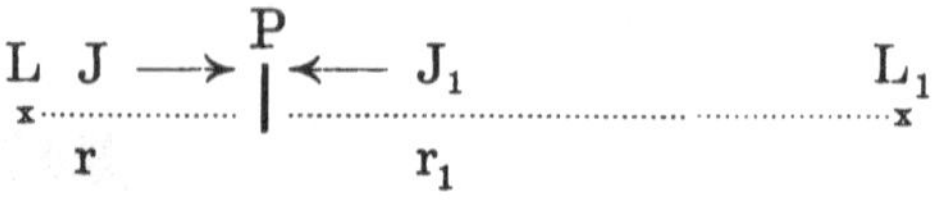


Sind r und $r_1$ die Entfernungen der beiden Lichtquellen von dem Photometerschirm, so ist die Beleuchtung von links $\frac{J}{r^2}$, von rechts $\frac{J_1}{r_1^2}$.

L stelle die Lichteinheit 1 dar und r sei = 50 mm, $r_1$ = 200 mm; wenn der Photometerschirm P von L wie $L_1$ gleich stark beleuchtet wird, dann ist

$$L_1 = \frac{r_1^2}{r^2} = \frac{200 \times 200}{50 \times 50} = 4 \times 4$$

= 16 Kerzen, da L = 1 Kerze ist; wäre L dagegen = 4 Kerzen, so wäre 16 noch mit 4 zu multiplizieren, also = 64 Kerzen.

Da man sich bislang meist mit der Messung in einer Richtung, der horizontalen, begnügte, kam man mit dieser sehr einfachen Berechnung aus; die Rechnung wird aber komplizierter, sobald eine Lichtquelle unter verschiedenen Ausstrahlungswinkeln gemessen wird und die mittlere räumliche Lichtstärke berechnet werden muß. Hauptsächlich kommt für die Praxis die mittlere räumliche Lichtstärke der unteren Hemisphäre in Frage.

Unter mittlerer räumlicher Lichtstärke versteht man die Lichtstärke, die eine Lichtquelle nach allen Richtungen des Raumes ausstrahlen müßte, wenn die ausgestrahlte Lichtmenge sich gleichmäßig auf den Raum verteilte.

Diesen Wert muß man ermitteln, um die Oekonomie einer Lampe berechnen zu können und ferner aber auch verschiedene Lichtquellen in ihrem Effekt miteinander vergleichen zu können.

In der Praxis ist die graphische Ermittlung der räumlichen Lichtstärke zu umständlich; es sei hier auf die Verfahren von Liebenthal und Rousseau verwiesen.[1]) Deshalb wählt man das kürzere rechnerische Verfahren, das mit Hilfe eines Rechenschiebers schneller auszuführen ist.

Die Ableitung der Berechnungsformel wird durch folgende Darstellung verständlich:

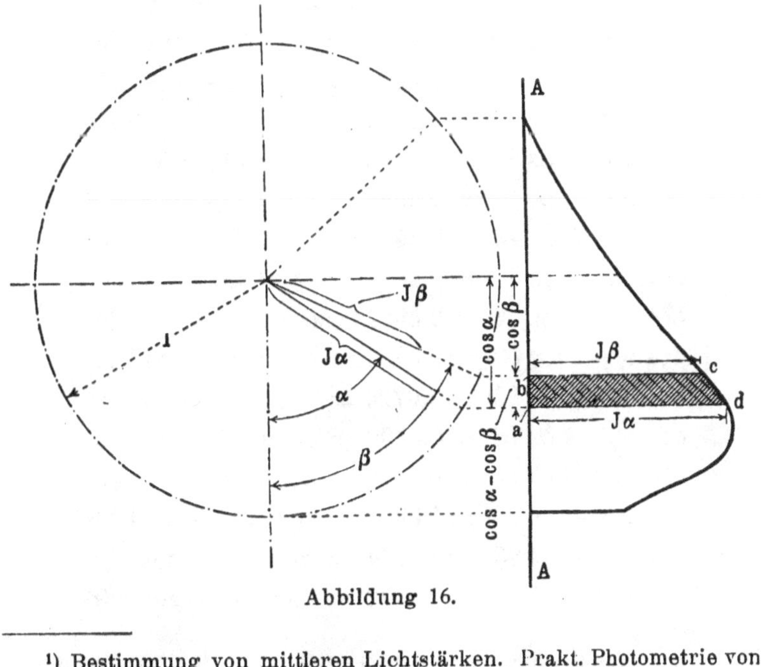


Abbildung 16.

[1]) Bestimmung von mittleren Lichtstärken. Prakt. Photometrie von Dr. E. Liebenthal, Braunschweig, Fr. Vieweg & Sohn. 1907.

$J\alpha$ und $J\beta$ sind die Lichtstärken unter den Winkeln $\alpha$ und $\beta$. Die Projektion des Bogenstückes $\beta-\alpha$ auf die Gerade AA ist gleich $\cos\alpha - \cos\beta$. Das Trapez abcd hat den Inhalt:

$$\frac{J\alpha + J\beta}{2}(\cos\alpha - \cos\beta).$$

Wenn die Lichtstärke von 5° zu 5° bestimmt ist, ergibt sich die mittlere Lichtstärke der unteren Hemisphäre aus der Formel:[2])

$$J_0 = {}^1/_2 [(J_0 + J_5)(\cos 0^0 - \cos 5^0) + (J_5 + J_{10})(\cos 5^0 - \cos 10^0) + \ldots\ldots + (J_{85} + J_{90})(\cos 85^0 - \cos 90^0)].\ _2)$$

Zur schnelleren Ausrechnung stellt man sich eine Tabelle der Kosinus-Differenzen zusammen:

| | | |
|---|---|---|
| cos 0°—cos 5° = | **0,0038** | = cos 180°—cos 175° |
| cos 5°—cos 10° = | **0,0114** | = cos 175°—cos 170° |
| cos 10°—cos 15° = | **0,0189** | = cos 170°—cos 165° |
| cos 15°—cos 20° = | **0,0262** | = cos 165°—cos 160° |
| cos 20°—cos 25° = | **0,0334** | = cos 160°—cos 155° |
| cos 25°—cos 30° = | **0,0403** | = cos 155°—cos 150° |
| cos 30°—cos 35° = | **0,0468** | = cos 150°—cos 145° |
| cos 35°—cos 40° = | **0,0532** | = cos 145°—cos 140° |
| cos 40°—cos 45° = | **0,0589** | = cos 140°—cos 135° |
| cos 45°—cos 50° = | **0,0643** | = cos 135°—cos 130° |
| cos 50°—cos 55° = | **0,0692** | = cos 130°—cos 125° |
| cos 55°—cos 60° = | **0,0736** | = cos 125°—cos 120° |
| cos 60°—cos 65° = | **0,0774** | = cos 120°—cos 115° |
| cos 65°—cos 70° = | **0,0806** | = cos 115°—cos 110° |
| cos 70°—cos 75° = | **0,0832** | = cos 110°—cos 105° |
| cos 75°—cos 80° = | **0,0852** | = cos 105°—cos 100° |
| cos 80°—cos 85° = | **0,0864** | = cos 100°—cos 95° |
| cos 85°—cos 90° = | **0,0872** | = cos 95°—cos 90° |

[2]) Voit, Wiener Ausstellungsbericht S. 140, Paul Högner, Lichtstrahlung und Beleuchtung, Braunschweig, Fr. Vieweg & Sohn, 1906.

Mit Hilfe dieser Formel berechnet sich die mittlere untere räumliche Lichtstärke einer Lampe wie folgt:

| Ausstrahlungswinkel Grad | Lichtstärken HK | Summe der Lichtstärken HK | Produkt aus Summe der Lichtstärken und Differenz der Winkel s. Seite 30 |
|---|---|---|---|
| 0 | 126 | 126 + 130 = 256 | 256 × 0,0038 = 0,97 |
| 5 | 130 | 130 + 131 = 261 | 261 × 0,0114 = 2,97 |
| 10 | 131 | 264 | 4,98 |
| 15 | 133 | 267 | 6,99 |
| 20 | 134 | 268 | 8,95 |
| 25 | 134 | 269 | 10,84 |
| 30 | 135 | 271 | 12,68 |
| 35 | 136 | 274 | 14,58 |
| 40 | 138 | 273 | 16,07 |
| 45 | 135 | 269 | 17,29 |
| 50 | 134 | 268 | 18,54 |
| 55 | 134 | 268 | 19,72 |
| 60 | 134 | 266 | 20,58 |
| 65 | 132 | 263 | 21,19 |
| 70 | 131 | 251 | 20,88 |
| 75 | 120 | 232 | 19,76 |
| 80 | 112 | 222 | 19,18 |
| 85 | 110 | 216 | 18,83 |
| 90 | 106 | | 255,00 |

$J_{\smile} = \frac{255}{2} = 127,5$ HK = der mittleren unteren räumlichen Lichtstärke.

Mit $J_{\smile}$ bezeichnet man die mittlere untere räumliche Lichtstärke
„ $J_{\bigcirc}$ „ „ „ „ sphärische Lichtstärke
„ $J_h$ „ „ „ horizontale Lichtstärke.

Ein übersichtliches Bild von obigem Zahlenmaterial erhält man durch die graphische Aufzeichnung (Abbildung 17). Gewöhnlich verwendet man zum Kurvenzeichnen Millimeterpapier. Auf der Zeichnung sind je 6,5 mm = 10 Kerzen gesetzt. Die Radien bezeichnen die Ausstrahlungswinkel, unter denen die Lampe gemessen worden ist. Man trägt die Zahlen der Lichtstärken durch Punkte auf den Radien auf und verbindet die Punkte durch eine Linie.

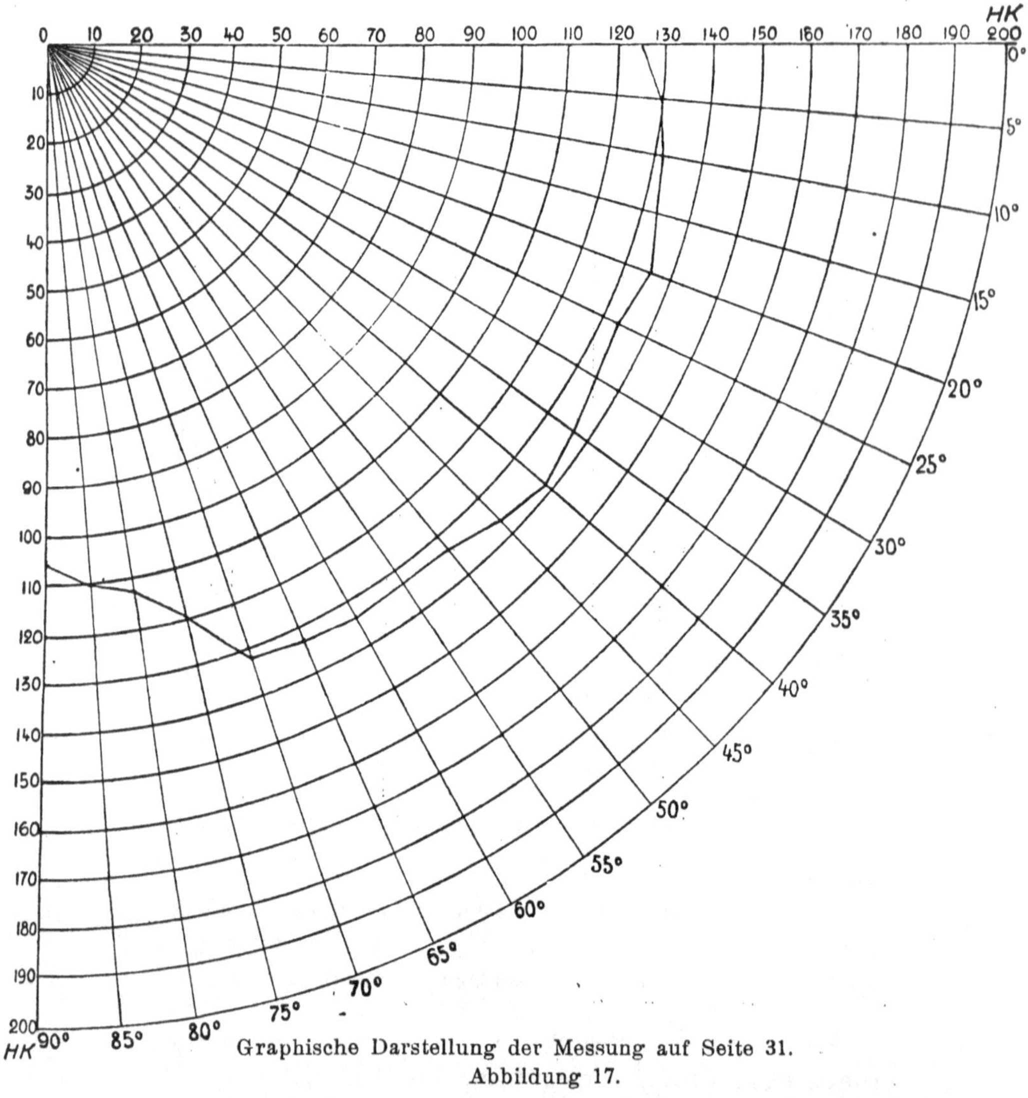


Graphische Darstellung der Messung auf Seite 31.
Abbildung 17.

Es sei weiter eine Methode zur Bestimmung der mittleren sphärischen Intensität einer Lichtquelle angeführt von Dipl.-Ing. Ernst W. Weinbeer, Berlin.[4])

---

[4]) Elektrotechn. Anzeiger No. 63. 1908.

Während die Bestimmung der mittleren sphärischen oder hemisphärischen Intensität einer Lichtquelle nach Rousseau die Anwendung eines Planimeters zum Auswerten eines Flächenstückes erforderte, gab Kenelly (El. World, Nr. 13, 1908) eine Konstruktion, das „Kenelly-Diagramm", an, die sich mit Lineal und Zirkel ausführen ließ und die mittlere hemisphärische Intensität als direkt abgreifbare Liniengröße ergab. Diese Konstruktion, die darauf beruhte, daß der von einer Lichtquelle innerhalb der von der Vertikalen aus gemessenen räumlichen Winkel $\varphi_1$ und $\varphi_2$ ausgestrahlte Lichtstrom $= 2\pi I (\cos \varphi_1 - \cos \varphi_2)$ ist, gab dem Verfasser dieses die Anregung zur Konstruktion eines Rechenschiebers zur Bestimmung der mittleren Intensität, der in seiner ursprünglichen Form in untengenannter Zeitschrift[5]) beschrieben wurde und nachstehend in seiner endgültigen Gestalt (Modell) abgebildet ist.

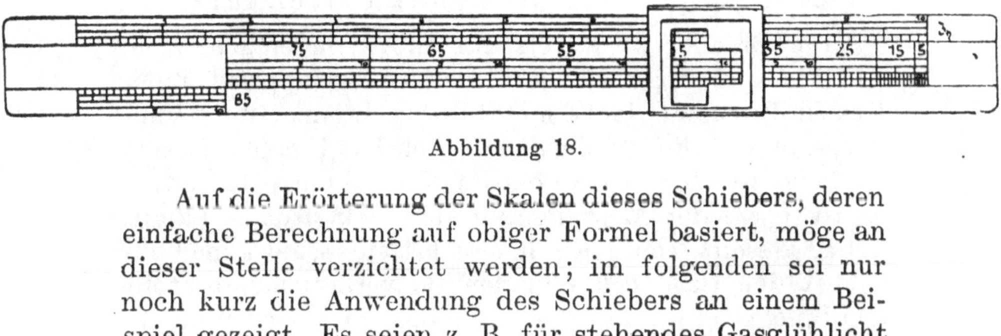


Abbildung 18.

Auf die Erörterung der Skalen dieses Schiebers, deren einfache Berechnung auf obiger Formel basiert, möge an dieser Stelle verzichtet werden; im folgenden sei nur noch kurz die Anwendung des Schiebers an einem Beispiel gezeigt. Es seien z. B. für stehendes Gasglühlicht die in nachstehender Tabelle gegebenen Intensitäten photometrisch bestimmt worden:

| Winkel gegen die Vertikale | Intensitäten | Winkel gegen die Vertikale | Intensitäten |
|---|---|---|---|
| Grad | HK | Grad | HK |
| 85 | 87 | 35 | 44 |
| 75 | 83 | 25 | 35 |
| 65 | 76 | 15 | 25 |
| 55 | 67 | 5 | 0 |
| 45 | 56 | | |

Man stellt nunmehr mit der Stirnkante des Mittelschiebers an der unteren, mit „85" bezeichneten Skala

[5]) The Illuminatig Engineer, London, Juli 1908.

die Intensität 87 ein, sodann mit dem Läufer an der Skala „75“ den Wert 83, auf die so erhaltene Läuferstellung die Stirnkante der Skala „65“, auf dieser Skala mit dem Läufer wieder den Wert 76, und so fort, bis man sämtliche Intensitäten „addiert“ hat, worauf man mittels des Läufers an der obersten Skala den Wert der mittleren hemisphärischen Intensität, im vorliegenden Falle etwa 65 HK, abliest. Die Ausführung sämtlicher Einstellungen bis zur Ablesung des Endresultats nimmt etwa 40 Sekunden in Anspruch, eine Zeit, die durch irgendwelche graphischen Konstruktionen wohl schwerlich erreicht werden könnte.

## Messungen.

Das Photometrieren des Gases ist so eingehend angegeben[1]), daß dies hier übergangen werden kann.

### Messung eines stehenden Brenners.

Der Brenner wird stets nur mit Zylinder gemessen. Abbildung 2 zeigt den auf dem Spiegelapparat montierten Brenner. Nachdem man den Brenner mit Glühkörper und Zylinder einige Minuten hat brennen lassen, während welcher Zeit auch die Normallampe brennt — es ist vor jeder Messung mit der elektrischen Lampe nötig, dieselbe warm werden zu lassen —, liest man zunächst den Gasdruck und den Gasverbrauch ab, stellt den Spiegel in die auf der Abbildung gegebene Stellung und geht mit dem Brenner von $5^0$ zu $5^0$ resp. $10^0$ zu $10^0$ nach unten.

Das Einstellen des Photometerschirmes — für die Praxis empfiehlt sich der Gebrauch des Photometeraufsatzes von Franz Schmidt und Haensch — geschieht in folgender Weise:

Der Photometerschirm stehe an einem Punkte, wo die eine Seite des Gesichtsfeldes dunkel erscheint, so suche man zunächst die beiden Punkte, wo in dem Gesichtsfelde ein deutlicher Farbenumschlag zu konstatieren ist.

---

[1]) Kalender für Gas- und Wasserfach.

Figur 2 zeigt den Punkt, wo der Schirm von links stärker beleuchtet wird wie von rechts.

Figur 3 zeigt den Punkt, wo der Schirm von rechts stärker beleuchtet wird.

Ist der Photometerschirm auf einen dieser Punkte eingestellt, so führt man den Schirm langsam in der entgegengesetzten Richtung, bis man auf den Punkt kommt, wo die gegenüberliegenden beiden Felder die gleiche Helligkeit zeigen (Figur 1, farbige Abbildung 19).

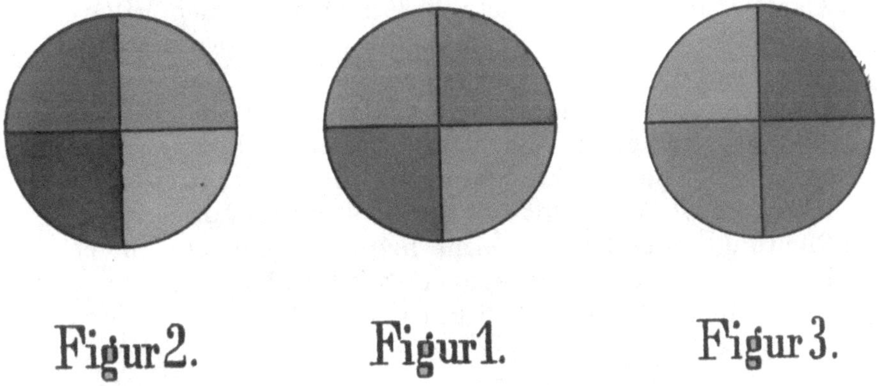


Abbildung 19.

Diesen Punkt liest man auf der Skala der Photometerbank ab. Der Anfänger wiederholt die Einstellung, indem er von dem anderen Umschlagspunkte ausgeht. Decken sich beide Einstellungen nicht, so lasse man sich nicht verleiten, durch rasches Hin- und Herschieben des Photometerschirmes den richtigen Punkt ermitteln zu wollen. Namentlich der Anfänger wird auf diesem Wege zu keinem exakten Resultat kommen.

Beim Invertbrenner erfordert die Einregulierung desselben einige Uebung.

Nachdem man den Brenner an dem Stativ angeschraubt hat, läßt man denselben einige Augenblicke ohne Glühstrumpf brennen zur Beobachtung des Flammenkegels. Währenddessen überzeugt man sich, daß der Brenner gasdicht angeschlossen ist. Hebt sich der grüne Kegel in der Flamme scharf ab, so ist man sicher, daß der Brenner funktioniert. Jetzt setzt man den Glühstrumpf auf, desgleichen Zylinder und Glocke und läßt den Brenner heiß werden.

Nach Verlauf von 10 Minuten reguliert man den Brenner auf beste Leuchtkraft ein, d. h. man gibt dem Brenner so viel Gas, daß der Glühstrumpf vollständig ausgefüllt ist, und liest den Gasverbrauch und Gasdruck ab.

Bei Invertbrennern ist es üblich, nur die untere Hemisphäre zu messen. Die Messung wird stets mit einer Klarglasglocke ausgeführt. Mißt man mit einer Milchglasglocke zum Beispiel, so ist die Lichtabsorption derselben zu bestimmen. Dieses geschieht in der Weise, daß man eine Messung mit einer Klarglasglocke und eine mit der Milchglasglocke unter denselben Bedingungen ausführt. Die Differenz ergibt die Absorption der letzteren. Man beginnt mit der Messung in horizontaler Richtung; der Brenner steht hier wie beim stehenden Brenner seitlich vom Spiegel und wird nach oben geführt, bis er senkrecht über dem Spiegel steht.

## Preßgaslampen.

Die Lampe wird an einem Drahtseil hinter dem Spiegel (Abbildung 3) aufgehängt, mit der Gasleitung verbunden und zentriert vermittels eines in die Horizontalachse des vorderen Spiegels einzuschraubenden Stabes. Die Spitze dieses Stabes muß bei richtiger Lampenhöhe Mitte Glühkörper zeigen. Ist die Lampe zentriert, so gibt man Gas und untersucht, ob dieselbe in allen Teilen gasdicht ist. Wie bei jedem Invertbrenner brennt man hierauf die Flammen ohne Glühkörper, um zu sehen, ob Düsen, Siebe, Luftregulierung in Ordnung. Der Kegel der Flamme ist bei Preßgas nicht grün, sondern blau. Die Glühkörper für Preßgasbrenner sind nicht kollodiniert, das Veraschen und Formen nimmt man an der Lampe vor. Hierbei ist auf folgendes zu achten: Der Körper wird am Tragering und Spitze gefaßt und vorsichtig etwas gedehnt und unmittelbar unter dem Ring etwas geweitet. Diese Manipulation ist aber nur mit trockenen und sauberen Fingern vorzunehmen, will man die höchste Leuchtkraft des Glühkörpers erzielen. Sind der oder die Glühkörper an dem Brenner aufgehängt, so öffnet man die Gaszuleitung und entzündet unter vollem Druck die Körper. Die besten Formen erzielt man, wenn es beim Anzünden gelungen, die Flamme in den Glühkörper an den Brennerkopf zu bringen; brennt das Gewebe erst von außen ab, so schlägt die Flamme nach dem Veraschen explosionsartig zum Brennerkopf zurück, wodurch Risse im Körper entstehen, die denselben zu Messungen ungeeignet machen. Zu dem Zwecke entzündet man den Körper unmittelbar unter dem Tragring; in den meisten Fällen schlägt die Flamme sofort zum Brennerkopf.

Dieses sofortige Hineinschlagen der Flamme in den Glühkörper unterstützt man aber noch dadurch, daß man direkt unterhalb des Tragringes einen Zündfaden durch das Gewebe zieht.

Haben sich die Körper gut zylindrisch geformt, so läßt man dieselben klar brennen, wie man überhaupt vor einer Brenndauer von 30 Minuten nicht mit den Messungen beginnt. Ist die Lampe heiß geworden, reguliert man die Luft ein, am besten in der Weise, daß ein Beobachter auf dem Photometer den besten Lichteffekt feststellt. Hierauf wird der Gasverbrauch bestimmt (wie Seite 15 angegeben) und die untere Hemisphäre wie beim Invertbrenner für niederen Druck gemessen (s. Beschreibung des großen Spiegelapparates).

Die Oekonomie einer Gaslampe berechnet sich aus dem Gasverbrauch und der Kerzenstärke.

Hat eine Lampe eine mittlere räumliche Lichtstärke von 2000 HK bei einem Gasverbrauch von 1000 l, so ist die Oekonomie $\frac{1000}{2000} = 0{,}5$, d. h. 0,5 l geben 1 HK (Hefnerkerze).

### Dochtlampen.

Zur exakten Messung einer Dochtlampe ist es nötig, einen neuen Docht einzuziehen und zur Erzielung einer ganz gleichmäßigen Oberfläche — hiervon ist bei

Petroleumlampen in erster Linie ein gutes Brennen abhängig — denselben in trockenem Zustande bis auf das Dochtrohr mit einem glühenden Eisen abzusengen, niemals abschneiden. Das Bassin wird hierauf gefüllt, der Brenner aufgesetzt und auf einer Präzisionswage gewogen. Hat sich der Docht voll Brennstoff gesaugt, wozu ein einstündiges Stehen erforderlich ist, zündet man die Lampe an und stellt die Sekundenuhr ein. Mit zunehmender Erwärmung bringt man die Flamme auf die größtmögliche Höhe und führt bei eingetretener Konstanz die photometrischen Messungen auf der Photometerbank aus, wobei man nur den Zylinder aufsetzt. In der Praxis begnügt man sich allgemein mit der Messung mittlerer horizontaler Lichtstärken. Zur Ermittlung derselben drehe ich den Teller des Photometerwagens, auf dem die Lampe steht, nach jeder Messung um 45° und nehme aus den gefundenen Zahlen das arithmetische Mittel. Beim Löschen der Lampe wird die Sekundenuhr arretiert. Nachdem die Lampe erkaltet ist, wird Bassin mit Brenner wiederum gewogen. Die Differenz der ersten und zweiten Wägung ergibt den Verbrauch der Brennflüssigkeit für die abgelesene Zeit und wird derselbe dann auf die Stunde berechnet, wie Seite 17 angegeben.

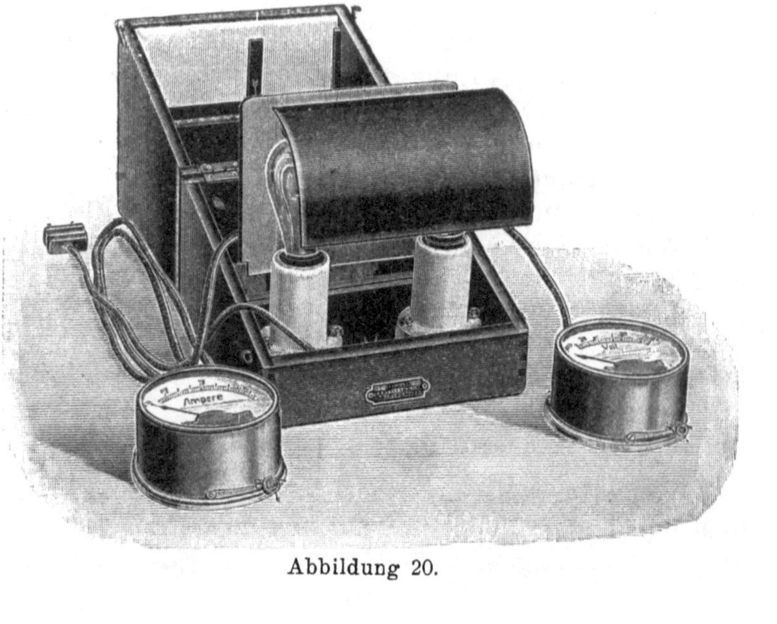


Abbildung 20.

## Elektrische Lampen.

Von allen Messungen ist die der elektrischen Lampe wohl die einfachste. Nirgends wird wohl aber auch so viel photometriert wie in einer Glühlampenfabrik, da hier jede Lampe gemessen wird, ehe dieselbe auf Lager wandert.

Dem Bedürfnis nach einem handlichen, einfachen und billigen Photometer, welches gestattet, elektrische Glühlampen mit einer für die Praxis ausreichenden Genauigkeit auf Leuchtkraft und Wattverbrauch zu prüfen, ist durch Herrmanns Betriebsphotometer (Abbild. 20) Rechnung getragen. Die Messung kann in jedem, auch unverdunkelten, Raume ohne irgendwelche photometrische Vorkenntnis ausgeführt werden. Die Lichtstärken der Lampen werden nach Einstellung des beweglichen schattenmachenden Körpers an einer Skala direkt abgelesen. Nähere Beschreibungen und Preislisten versendet die Firma: Land- und Seekabelwerke, Aktiengesellschaft, Abt. Apparatebau, Cöln-Nippes, welche die Herstellerin dieses Photometers ist.

Zu genaueren Messungen benutzt man je zwei quadratische ebene Silberspiegel von 13 cm Seitenlänge und 2—5 mm Dicke, die in einem Winkel von 120° zueinander stehen. Diese beiden Spiegel stellt man an den beiden Enden der Photometerbank auf und stellt Vergleichslampe wie zu messende Lampe in gleicher Entfernung davor auf, und zwar beträgt die Entfernung der Lampenachse bis zur Scheitelachse des Spiegels 9 cm.

Statt der Winkelspiegel benutzt man aber bei den Verschiedenheiten der Lichtstärke in einer Glühlampe besser den rotierenden Apparat von Brodhun[2]) (Abbildung 21).

Die zu messende Lampe steht fest; ihre Achse ist horizontal und liegt in der Verlängerung der Bankachse. Die beiden Spiegel sind gegen die Lampenachse um 45°

[2]) Liebenthal prakt. Photometrie, S. 333.

geneigt und werden um die letztere mittels des Elektromotors in so schnelle Rotation (etwa 4mal in der Sekunde) versetzt, daß im Photometer ein kontinuierlicher Eindruck entsteht. Durch den mit zwei Oeffnungen versehenen mitrotierenden Schirm werden die direkten Strahlen abgeblendet.

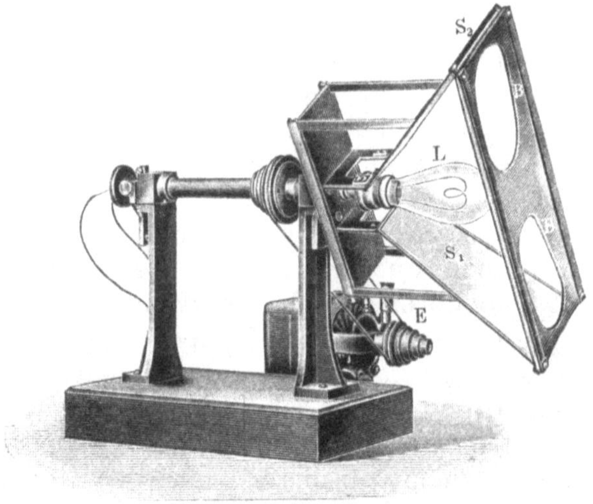


Abbildung 21.

E Motor, L Lampe, $S_1$, $S_2$ Spiegel, B rotierender Schirm.

Man mißt hier die Summe der mittleren Lichtstärken der rotierenden Spiegelbilder.

Die Oekonomie der Glühlampen berechnet man auf die mittlere horizontale Lichtstärke, die der Bogenlampen auf die mittlere räumliche.

Wie bei Gaslampen Gasdruck und Gasverbrauch anzugeben ist, gibt man bei elektrischen Lampen Stromstärke und Stromspannung an:

$$\frac{\text{Stromstärke} \times \text{Stromspannung}}{\text{Lichtstärke}} = \text{Oekonomie der Lampe.}$$

Z. B. eine Lampe hätte eine mittlere horizontale Lichtstärke von 44 Hefnerkerzen bei einer Stromstärke von 0,4 Ampère und einer Spannung von 220 Volt, so wäre der Verbrauch 0,4 $\times$ 220 = 88 Watt und die Oekonomie der Lampe $\frac{0{,}4 \times 220}{44} = 2{,}0$, d. h. 2 Watt pro Hefnerkerze.

## Flächenhelligkeitsmessungen.

Die Flächenhelligkeit, die man mit einer Lichtquelle erhält, deren Lichtstärke gemessen, kann berechnet werden nach folgender Formel:

$$\text{Flächenhelligkeit E. im Punkte M} = \frac{J \times \sin\alpha}{h^2 + x^2}$$

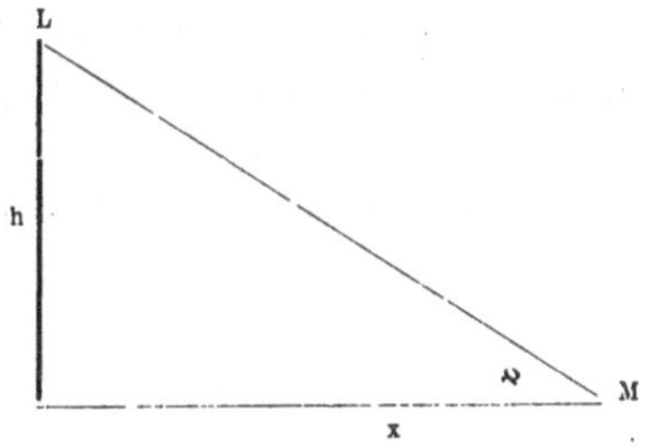


Wenn L bezeichnet die Lichtquelle, deren Lichtintensität J ist,

h die Aufhängehöhe,

x die Entfernung vom Fußpunkt der Lichtquelle,

α der Winkel, unter dem die Lichtstrahlen auf Punkt M auftreffen.

Der berechnete Wert wird aber in der Praxis niemals genau zutreffen, da Reflexe, Schattenwirkungen bei der wirklichen Flächenhelligkeit mitsprechen, die in der Rechnung nicht berücksichtigt sind. Genaue Zahlen kann man daher nur durch einwandfreie Flächenhelligkeitsmessungen bekommen.

Die Frage, ob die horizontale oder vertikale Beleuchtung für die Beurteilung der Güte einer Beleuchtung maßgeblich ist, soll hier nicht erörtert werden, bei den Messungen müssen beide in gleicher Weise berücksichtigt werden. Die Messungen nimmt man mit dem Seite 25 beschriebenen Weberphotometer oder mit dem Straßenphotometer von Bechstein[1]) vor.

Die Einheit „Lux“, welche man der Flächenhelligkeit zugrunde legt, ist die Meterkerze, d. h. die Helligkeit, die durch eine Hefnerkerze in einer Entfernung von 1 m auf einer zur Strahlungsrichtung senkrechten Fläche hervorgerufen wird.

[1]) Zeitschrift für Instrumentenkunde. Juni 1907.

Zu Messungen im Freien wird man sich der Einfachheit halber der Milchglasplatte bedienen.

Bei Messung der horizontalen Flächenhelligkeit hat das Photometer die skizzierte Stellung (Abbildung 22); soll die vertikale gemessen werden, so dreht man das Rohr mit dem Lummer-Brodhun-Würfel um 90°. Man beginnt mit der Messung unter der zu messenden Lichtquelle und macht dann in geeigneten Abständen horizontale und vertikale Messungen. Bei Messungen der Straßenbeleuchtung wählt man zweckmäßig die Mitte der Straße und mißt in Abständen von 1 m.

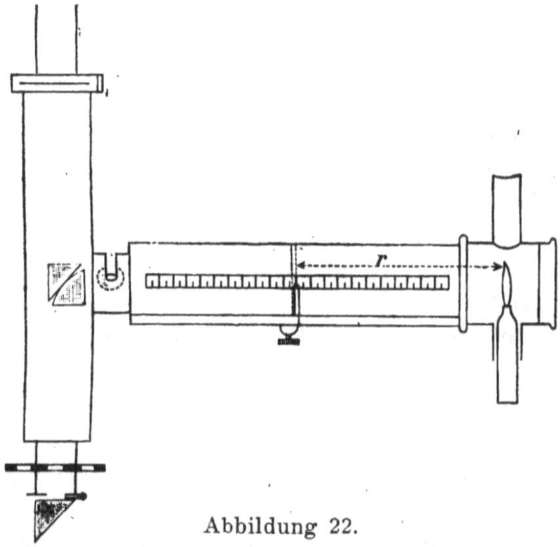


Abbildung 22.

Die Berechnung der Beleuchtungsstärke geschieht nach der Formel:

$$E = \frac{C^1 \; 10\,000 \text{ Meterkerzen.}}{r^2}$$

Die Werte für $C^1$ (Konstante der Milchglasscheibe sowie die der anderen Schwächungsplatten) sind für jeden Apparat angegeben. Der Faktor $10\,000 = 100 \times 100$ kommt daher, daß für die Flächenhelligkeit die Längeneinheit = 1 m ist, während die Entfernung der Vergleichslichtquelle in Zentimetern gemessen wird.

Reicht die Milchglasplatte zur Einstellung auf

gleiche Helligkeit nicht aus, so schiebt man weitere Platten zur Schwächung ein.

Ist der Farbenunterschied der Vergleichslichtquelle und der zu messenden Lichtquelle sehr groß, dann schaltet man vor das Okular abwechselnd ein rotes und ein grünes Glas vor. Es sei R das im roten, G das im grünen Lichte erhaltene Resultat, so bildet man den Quotienten $\frac{G}{R}$ und nimmt aus nachstehender Tabelle den Faktor, den man in die Berechnungsformel $E = k \times R$ einsetzt.

**Tabelle nach L. Weber zur Photometrie gefärbten Lichtes.**

| $\frac{G}{R}$ | k | $\frac{G}{R}$ | k | $\frac{G}{R}$ | k | $\frac{G}{R}$ | k | $\frac{G}{R}$ | k | $\frac{G}{R}$ | k |
|---|---|---|---|---|---|---|---|---|---|---|---|
| **0,0** | | **1,0** | **1,00** | **2,0** | **1,60** | **3,0** | **2,02** | **4,0** | **2,33** | **5,0** | **2,60** |
| 0,1 | | 1,1 | 08 | 2,1 | 65 | 3,1 | 05 | 4,1 | 36 | 5,1 | 62 |
| 0,2 | | 1,2 | 15 | 2,2 | 70 | 3,2 | 08 | 4,2 | 39 | 5,2 | 64 |
| 0,3 | 0,50 | 1,3 | 22 | 2,3 | 75 | 3,3 | 11 | 4,3 | 42 | 5,3 | 67 |
| 0,4 | 56 | 1,4 | 28 | 2,4 | 80 | 3,4 | 15 | 4,4 | 44 | 5,4 | 69 |
| **0,5** | **0,64** | **1,5** | **1,34** | **2,5** | **1,84** | **3,5** | **2,18** | **4,5** | **2,47** | **5,5** | **2,71** |
| 0,6 | 72 | 1,6 | 40 | 2,6 | 88 | 3,6 | 20 | 4,6 | 49 | 5,6 | |
| 0,7 | 80 | 1,7 | 46 | 2,7 | 92 | 3,7 | 24 | 4,7 | 52 | 5,7 | |
| 0,8 | 87 | 1,8 | 50 | 2,8 | 96 | 3,8 | 27 | 4,8 | 55 | 5,8 | |
| 0,9 | 94 | 1,9 | 55 | 2,9 | 99 | 3,9 | 30 | 4,9 | 57 | 5,9 | |

Beispielsweise hätte man abgelesen bei der ersten Einstellung mit rotem Glas r = 12 cm. Die Konstante für die Milchglasplatte sei = 0,5, so wäre

$$R = \frac{0{,}5\ 100 \times 100}{12 \times 12} = 34{,}70.$$

Die Einstellung mit grünem Glas

$$G = \frac{0{,}5\ 100 \times 100}{11 \times 11} = 41{,}32.$$

$\frac{G}{R} = 1{,}19$ k aus der Tabelle 1,2 = 1,15.

Ist die Farbe der zu messenden Lichtquelle und der Vergleichslampe gleich, so ist Faktor k = 1. Die Ablesung kann dann mit jedem Glase gemacht werden.

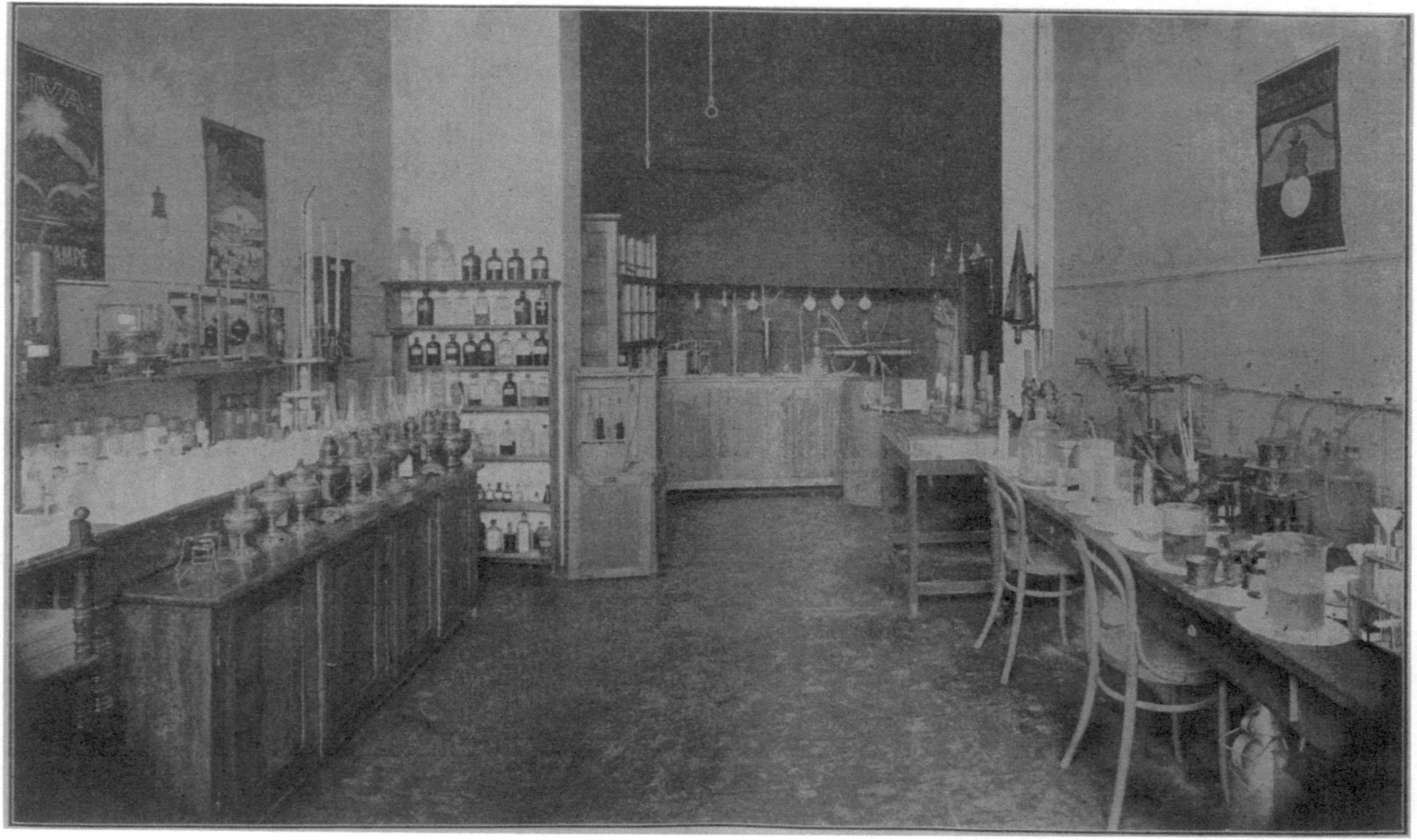

Abbildung 23.

## Versuchsraum.

An das oder die Photometerzimmer anschließend — ein Großbetrieb dürfte mit einem Zimmer schwerlich auskommen, ganz abgesehen von den kleinen Photometerkammern, deren man bei der Fabrikation von elektrischen Glühlampen einer ganzen Anzahl bedarf —, richtet man zweckmäßig einen Raum ein, in dem man die Vorbereitungen für die photometrischen Messungen ausführen kann. Abbildung 23 zeigt einen solchen Raum. In dem schwarz gestrichenen Teil sind Rampen für Gassowohl wie für elektrische Lampen vorgesehen.

Hier werden vor allem Dauerversuche vorgenommen, die durch photometrische Messungen kontrolliert werden müssen.

Für Lampen für flüssige Brennstoffe ist der viereckige Tisch rechts vor der Rampe eingerichtet. Auf einem Holzgestell ist ein Blechkasten, der mit Sand gefüllt ist, aufgesetzt, dessen Deckel durchlocht ist. Bei Explosionen nimmt der Sand die Flüssigkeit auf und die Flamme kann leicht erstickt werden.

Der vordere Teil des Raumes ist hell gestrichen, die Mitte ist frei, so daß hier Flächenhelligkeitsmessungen mit kleinen Lichtquellen ausgeführt werden können.

## Tabellen zum praktischen Gebrauch.

Nr. 1 für Messungen, die auf der Bank ausgeführt werden. Die zu messende Lampe steht auf Teilstrich 20, die Vergleichslichtquelle auf Teilstrich 250. x gibt die Stellung des Photometerschirmes an. Die Vergleichslichtquelle hat eine Stärke von 4 Hefnerkerzen.

Nr. 2 für Messungen, bei denen Vergleichslampe und Photometerschirm fest verbunden sind. Die Vergleichslichtquelle kann 1, 2, 3, 4, 5, 10 Kerzen betragen.

Nr. 3 für Messungen großer Lichtquellen. Die Vergleichslichtquelle hat eine Stärke von 4 Hefnerkerzen.

Bei Tabelle 2 und 3 sind die Kerzenstärken auf ganze Zahlen abgerundet.

## Photometrische Tabelle 1.

### Einstellung auf der Photometerbank.

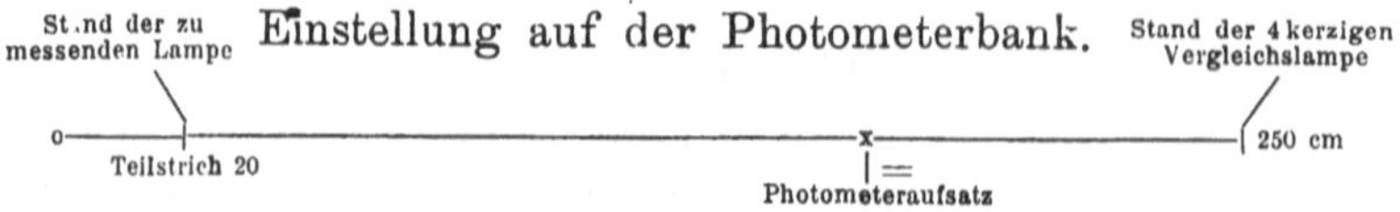


| | HK | | HK | | HK | | HK | | HK |
|---|---|---|---|---|---|---|---|---|---|
| x = 160 | 9,6 | x = 187 | 28,1 | x = 200,5 | 53,1 | x=209,5 | 87,5 | x=212,2 | 103,4 |
| 161 | 10,0 | 188 | 29,3 | 200,6 | 53,4 | 209,6 | 88,1 | 212,3 | 104,0 |
| 162 | 10,4 | 189 | 30,7 | 200,7 | 53,7 | 209,7 | 88,6 | 212,4 | 104,8 |
| 163 | 10,8 | 190 | 32,1 | 200,8 | 54,0 | 209,8 | 89,1 | 212,5 | 105,4 |
| 164 | 11,2 | 191 | 33,6 | 200,9 | 54,2 | 209,9 | 89,7 | 212,6 | 106,1 |
| 165 | 11,6 | 192 | 35,2 | 201,0 | 54,5 | 210,0 | 90,2 | 212,7 | 106,8 |
| 166 | 12,0 | 193 | 36,8 | 201,1 | 54,8 | 210,1 | 90,8 | 212,8 | 107,5 |
| 167 | 12,5 | 194 | 38,6 | 201,2 | 55,1 | 210,2 | 91,3 | 212,9 | 108,1 |
| 168 | 13,0 | 195 | 40,5 | 201,3 | 55,4 | 210,3 | 91,9 | 213,0 | 108,8 |
| 169 | 13,5 | 196 | 42,4 | 201,4 | 55,7 | 210,4 | 92,4 | 213,1 | 109,5 |
| 170 | 14,0 | 197 | 44,6 | 201,5 | 56,0 | 210 5 | 93,0 | 213,2 | 110,2 |
| 171 | 14,6 | 198 | 46,8 | 201,6 | 56,3 | 210,6 | 93,6 | 213,3 | 111,0 |
| 172 | 15,1 | 199 | 49,2 | 201,7 | 56,6 | 210,7 | 94,1 | 213,4 | 111,7 |
| 173 | 15,8 | 199,1 | 49,5 | 201,8 | 56,9 | 210,8 | 94,7 | 213,5 | 112,4 |
| 174 | 16,4 | 199,2 | 49,7 | 201,9 | 57,2 | 210,9 | 95,3 | 213,6 | 113,1 |
| 175 | 17,0 | 199,3 | 50,0 | 202,0 | 57,5 | 211,0 | 95,9 | 213,7 | 113,9 |
| 176 | 17,7 | 199,4 | 50,2 | 203,0 | 60,6 | 211,1 | 96,5 | 213,8 | 114,7 |
| 177 | 18,5 | 199,5 | 50,5 | 204,0 | 64,0 | 211,2 | 97,1 | 213,9 | 115,4 |
| 178 | 19,2 | 199,6 | 50,8 | 205,0 | 67,6 | 211,3 | 97,7 | 214,0 | 116,0 |
| 179 | 20,0 | 199,7 | 51,0 | 206,0 | 71,4 | 211,4 | 98,3 | 215,0 | 124,0 |
| 180 | 20,9 | 199,8 | 51,3 | 207,0 | 75,6 | 211,5 | 98,9 | 216,0 | 132,9 |
| 181 | 21,7 | 199,9 | 51,5 | 208,0 | 80,1 | 211,6 | 99,5 | 217,0 | 142,5 |
| 182 | 22,7 | 200,0 | 51,8 | 209,0 | 85,0 | 211,7 | 100,2 | 218,0 | 153,0 |
| 183 | 23,6 | 200,1 | 52,1 | 209,1 | 85,5 | 211,8 | 100,9 | 219,0 | 164,0 |
| 184 | 24,7 | 200,2 | 52,3 | 209,2 | 86,0 | 211,9 | 101,4 | 220,0 | 177,7 |
| 185 | 25,7 | 200,3 | 52,6 | 209,3 | 86,5 | 212,0 | 102,0 | | |
| 186 | 26,9 | 200,4 | 52,9 | 209,4 | 87,0 | 212,1 | 102,7 | | |

## Tabelle 2.

| Entfernung der zu messenden Lampe vom Photometerschirm | | Entfernung der Vergleichslampe vom Photometerschirm 40 cm | | | | | |
|---|---|---|---|---|---|---|---|
| | | 1 HK | 2 HK | 3 HK | 4 HK | 5 HK | 10 HK |
| cm | | | | | | | |
| 200 | HK = | 25,0 | 50,0 | 75,0 | 100,0 | 125,0 | 250,0 |
| 205 | | 26,0 | 52,0 | 79,0 | 105,0 | 131,0 | 262,0 |
| 210 | | 28,0 | 55,0 | 83,0 | 110,0 | 138,0 | 275,0 |
| 215 | | 29,0 | 58,0 | 86,0 | 115,0 | 144,0 | 288,0 |

| Entfernung der zu messenden Lampe vom Photometerschirm | | Entfernung der Vergleichslampe vom Photometerschirm 40 cm | | | | | |
|---|---|---|---|---|---|---|---|
| | | 1 HK | 2 HK | 3 HK | 4 HK | 5 HK | 10 HK |
| cm | | | | | | | |
| 220 | HK = | 30,0 | 60,0 | 91,0 | 121,0 | 151,0 | 302,0 |
| 225 | | 32,0 | 63,0 | 95,0 | 126,0 | 158,0 | 316,0 |
| 230 | | 33,0 | 66,0 | 99,0 | 132,0 | 165,0 | 330,0 |
| 235 | | 35,0 | 69,0 | 104,0 | 138,0 | 173,0 | 345,0 |
| 240 | | 36,0 | 72,0 | 108,0 | 144,0 | 180,0 | 360,0 |
| 245 | | 38,0 | 75,0 | 113,0 | 150,0 | 188,0 | 375,0 |
| 250 | | 39,0 | 78,0 | 117,0 | 156,0 | 195,0 | 390,0 |
| 255 | | 41,0 | 81,0 | 122,0 | 162,0 | 203,0 | 406,0 |
| 260 | | 42,0 | 84,0 | 127,0 | 169,0 | 211,0 | 422,0 |
| 265 | | 44,0 | 88,0 | 132,0 | 176,0 | 220,0 | 439,0 |
| 270 | | 46,0 | 91,0 | 137,0 | 182,0 | 228,0 | 455,0 |
| 275 | | 47,0 | 94,0 | 142,0 | 189,0 | 236,0 | 472,0 |
| 280 | | 49,0 | 98,0 | 147,0 | 196,0 | 245,0 | 490,0 |
| 285 | | 51,0 | 101,0 | 152,0 | 203,0 | 254,0 | 507,0 |
| 290 | | 53,0 | 105,0 | 158,0 | 210,0 | 263,0 | 525,0 |
| 295 | | 54,0 | 109,0 | 163,0 | 217,0 | 272,0 | 543,0 |
| 300 | | 56,0 | 112,0 | 169,0 | 225,0 | 281,0 | 562,0 |
| 305 | | 58,0 | 116,0 | 174,0 | 232,0 | 291,0 | 581,0 |
| 310 | | 60,0 | 120,0 | 180,0 | 240,0 | 300,0 | 600,0 |
| 315 | | 62,0 | 124,0 | 186,0 | 248,0 | 310,0 | 620,0 |
| 320 | | 64,0 | 128,0 | 192,0 | 256,0 | 320,0 | 640,0 |
| 325 | | 66,0 | 132,0 | 198,0 | 264,0 | 330,0 | 660,0 |
| 330 | | 68,0 | 136,0 | 204,0 | 272,0 | 340,0 | 680,0 |
| 335 | | 70,0 | 140,0 | 210,0 | 280,0 | 351,0 | 701,0 |
| 340 | | 72,0 | 144,0 | 217,0 | 289,0 | 361,0 | 722,0 |
| 345 | | 74,0 | 149,0 | 223,0 | 298,0 | 372,0 | 744,0 |
| 350 | | 77,0 | 153,0 | 230,0 | 306,0 | 383,0 | 765,0 |
| 355 | | 79,0 | 157,0 | 236,0 | 315,0 | 394,0 | 787,0 |
| 360 | | 81,0 | 162,0 | 243,0 | 324,0 | 405,0 | 809,0 |
| 365 | | 83,0 | 166,0 | 250,0 | 333,0 | 416,0 | 832,0 |
| 370 | | 86,0 | 171,0 | 257,0 | 342,0 | 428,0 | 855,0 |
| 375 | | 88,0 | 176.0 | 263,0 | 351,0 | 439,0 | 878,0 |
| 380 | | 90,0 | 180,0 | 271,0 | 361,0 | 451,0 | 902,0 |
| 385 | | 93,0 | 185,0 | 278,0 | 370,0 | 463,0 | 926,0 |
| 390 | | 95,0 | 190,0 | 285,0 | 380,0 | 475,0 | 950,0 |

| Entfernung der zu messenden Lampe vom Photometerschirm | Entfernung der Vergleichslampe vom Photometerschirm 40 cm | | | | | |
|---|---|---|---|---|---|---|
| | 1 HK | 2 HK | 3 HK | 4 HK | 5 HK | 10 HK |
| cm | | | | | | |
| 395 HK = | 98,0 | 195,0 | 293,0 | 390,0 | 488,0 | 975,0 |
| 400 | 100,0 | 200,0 | 300,0 | 400,0 | 500,0 | 1000,0 |
| 405 | 103,0 | 205,0 | 308,0 | 410,0 | 513,0 | 1025,0 |
| 410 | 105,0 | 211,0 | 316,0 | 421,0 | 527,0 | 1053,0 |
| 415 | 108,0 | 215,0 | 323,0 | 430,0 | 538,0 | 1076,0 |
| 420 | 110,0 | 220,0 | 331,0 | 441,0 | 551,0 | 1102,0 |
| 425 | 113,0 | 226,0 | 339,0 | 452,0 | 565,0 | 1129,0 |
| 430 | 116,0 | 231,0 | 347,0 | 462,0 | 578,0 | 1155,0 |
| 435 | 118,0 | 236,0 | 355,0 | 473,0 | 591,0 | 1182,0 |
| 440 | 121,0 | 242,0 | 363,0 | 484,0 | 605,0 | 1210,0 |
| 445 | 124,0 | 247,0 | 371,0 | 494,0 | 618,0 | 1236,0 |
| 450 | 127,0 | 253,0 | 380,0 | 506,0 | 633,0 | 1265,0 |
| 455 | 129,0 | 259,0 | 388,0 | 518,0 | 647,0 | 1294,0 |
| 460 | 132,0 | 264,0 | 396,0 | 528,0 | 661,0 | 1321,0 |
| 465 | 135,0 | 270,0 | 405,0 | 541,0 | 676,0 | 1352,0 |
| 470 | 138,0 | 276,0 | 414,0 | 552,0 | 690,0 | 1380,0 |
| 475 | 141,0 | 282,0 | 423,0 | 564,0 | 705,0 | 1410,0 |
| 480 | 144,0 | 288,0 | 432,0 | 576,0 | 720,0 | 1440,0 |
| 485 | 147,0 | 294,0 | 441,0 | 588,0 | 735,0 | 1470,0 |
| 490 | 150,0 | 300,0 | 450,0 | 600,0 | 750,0 | 1500,0 |
| 495 | 153,0 | 306,0 | 449,0 | 612,0 | 765,0 | 1530,0 |
| 500 | 156,0 | 312,0 | 468,0 | 624,0 | 780,0 | 1560,0 |

## Tabelle 3.

| Entfernung der zu messenden Lampe vom Photometerschirm | Entfernung der 4 HK Vergleichslampe vom Photometerschirm **35 cm** | Entfernung der zu messenden Lampe vom Photometerschirm | Entfernung der 4 HK Vergleichslampe vom Photometerschirm **35 cm** |
|---|---|---|---|
| cm | | cm | |
| 500 HK = | 816 | 530 HK = | 917 |
| 510 | 849 | 540 | 952 |
| 520 | 883 | 550 | 988 |

| Entfernung der zu messenden Lampe vom Photometerschirm | Entfernung der 4 HK Vergleichslampe vom Photometerschirm **35 cm** | Entfernung der zu messenden Lampe vom Photometerschirm | Entfernung der 4 HK Vergleichslampe vom Photometerschirm **35 cm** |
|---|---|---|---|
| cm | | cm | |
| 560 HK = | 1024 | 890 HK = | 2586 |
| 570 | 1060 | 900 | 2645 |
| 580 | 1100 | 910 | 2700 |
| 590 | 1136 | 920 | 2764 |
| 600 | 1175 | 930 | 2824 |
| 610 | 1215 | 940 | 2885 |
| 620 | 1255 | 950 | 2947 |
| 630 | 1296 | 960 | 3009 |
| 640 | 1337 | 970 | 3072 |
| 650 | 1379 | 980 | 3136 |
| 660 | 1422 | 990 | 3200 |
| 670 | 1465 | 1000 | 3265 |
| 680 | 1510 | 1005 | 3298 |
| 690 | 1555 | 1010 | 3331 |
| 700 | 1600 | 1015 | 3372 |
| 710 | 1646 | 1020 | 3397 |
| 720 | 1693 | 1025 | 3430 |
| 730 | 1740 | 1030 | 3464 |
| 740 | 1788 | 1035 | 3498 |
| 750 | 1837 | 1040 | 3531 |
| 760 | 1886 | 1045 | 3560 |
| 770 | 1936 | 1050 | 3600 |
| 780 | 1986 | 1055 | 3634 |
| 790 | 2038 | 1060 | 3660 |
| 800 | 2090 | 1065 | 3704 |
| 810 | 2142 | 1070 | 3738 |
| 820 | 2196 | 1075 | 3773 |
| 830 | 2250 | 1080 | 3808 |
| 840 | 2304 | 1085 | 3844 |
| 850 | 2359 | 1090 | 3879 |
| 860 | 2415 | 1095 | 3915 |
| 870 | 2470 | 1100 | 3951 |
| 880 | 2528 | | |

Paß & Garleb G. m. b. H., Berlin W. 57.